Principles and Practice
of
ENDODONTICS

Principles and Practice
of
ENDODONTICS

THIRD EDITION

RICHARD E. WALTON, DMD, MS

Professor
Department of Endodontics
The University of Iowa
College of Dentistry
Iowa City, Iowa

MAHMOUD TORABINEJAD, DMD, MSD, PhD

Professor and Program Director
Department of Endodontics
School of Dentistry
Loma Linda University
Loma Linda, California

W.B. SAUNDERS COMPANY
A Harcourt Health Sciences Company
Philadelphia   London   New York   St. Louis   Sydney   Toronto

W.B. SAUNDERS COMPANY
A Harcourt Health Sciences Company

The Curtis Center
Independence Square West
Philadelphia, Pennsylvania 19106-3399

Library of Congress Cataloging-in-Publication Data

Walton, Richard E., 1939-
  Principles and practice of endodontics / Richard E. Walton, Mahmoud Torabinejad.--
3rd ed.
    p. ; cm.
  Includes bibliographical references and index.
  ISBN 0-7216-9160-9
    1. Endodontics. I. Torabinejad, Mahmoud. II. Title.
  [DNLM: 1. Root Canal Therapy. 2. Endodontics. WU 230 W241p 2002]
  RK351 .W35 2002
  617.6'342--dc21   2001042814

Editor-in-Chief: John Schrefer
Editor: Penny Rudolph
Developmental Editor: Jaime Pendill
Project Manager: Patricia Tannian
Production Editor: John Casey
Book Designer: Reneé Duenow

PRINCIPLES AND PRACTICE OF ENDODONTICS   ISBN: 0–7216–9160-9

Last digit is the print number: 9   8   7   6   5   4   3   2   1

Contributors

Frances M. Andreasen, DDS
Associate Professor of Dental Traumatology
Pediatric Dentistry and Oral and Maxillofacial Surgery
Dental School, Health Sciences Faculty
Copenhagen University
Copenhagen, Denmark

Jens O. Andreasen, DDS, Odont. Dr.
Associate Director
Department of Oral and Maxillofacial Surgery
University Hospital
Copenhagen, Denmark

Leif K. Bakland, DDS
Professor and Chair, Department of Endodontics
Dean for Advanced Education
School of Dentistry, Loma Linda University
Loma Linda, California

J. Craig Baumgartner, DDS, MS, PhD
Professor and Chairman, Department of
    Endodontology
Director, Advanced Education Program—Endodontics
Oregon Health Sciences University
Portland, Oregon

Stephen Cohen, MA, DDS
Adjunct Professor, Department of Endodontics
University of the Pacific
School of Dentistry
San Francisco, California

Shimon Friedman, DMD
Professor, Department of Endodontics
Faculty of Dentistry
University of Toronto
Toronto, Ontario, Canada

Gerald N. Glickman, DDS, MS, MBA
Professor and Chairman, Department of Endodontics
Director, Graduate Program in Endodontics
University of Washington School of Dentistry
Seattle, Washington

Kenneth M. Hargreaves, DDS, PhD
Professor and Chair, Department of Endodontics
Professor, Department of Pharmacology
University of Texas Health Science Center at San
    Antonio
San Antonio, Texas

Gerald W. Harrington, DDS, MSD
Professor Emeritus, Department of Endodontics
University of Washington
Seattle, Washington

Graham Rex Holland, BDS, PhD
Professor, Department of Cariology
Restorative Sciences and Endodontics
School of Dentistry, University of Michigan
Ann Arbor, Michigan

Jeffrey W. Hutter, DMD, MEd
Chair, Department of Endodontics
Director, Postdoctoral Program in Endodontics
Goldman School of Dental Medicine
Boston University
Boston, Massachusetts

William T. Johnson, DDS, MS
Professor, Department of Family Dentistry
The University of Iowa College of Dentistry
Iowa City, Iowa

Keith V. Krell, DDS, MS, MA
Clinical Associate Professor, Department of
    Endodontics
The University of Iowa College of Dentistry
Iowa City, Iowa

Ronald R. Lemon, DMD
Professor and Chairperson, Department of
    Endodontics
School of Dentistry, Louisiana State University
New Orleans, Louisiana

Neville J. McDonald, BDS, MS
Clinical Professor and Division Head, Endodontics
Department of Cariology, Restorative Sciences and
    Endodontics
School of Dentistry, University of Michigan
Ann Arbor, Michigan

Harold H. Messer, BDSc, MDSc, PhD
Professor of Restorative Dentistry
School of Dental Medicine
University of Melbourne
Melbourne, Victoria, Australia

Thomas R. Pitt Ford, BDS, PhD
Professor of Endodontology
GKT Dental Institute
King's College
London, England

Alfred W. Reader, DDS, MS
Professor and Program Director, Department of
    Graduate Endodontics
Ohio State University
Columbus, Ohio

Eric M. Rivera, DDS, MS
Associate Professor and Graduate Program Director
    and Head
Department of Endodontics
The University of Iowa College of Dentistry
Iowa City, Iowa

Ilan Rotstein, CD
Associate Professor
Chair of Surgical, Therapeutic, and Bioengineering
    Sciences
University of Southern California School of Dentistry
Los Angeles, California

Gerald L. Scott, DDS
Clinical Assistant Professor, Department of Endodontics
Director, Emergency Clinic
The University of Iowa College of Dentistry
Iowa City, Iowa

Shahrokh Shabahang, DMD
Assistant Professor, Department of Endodontics
School of Dentistry, Loma Linda University
Loma Linda, California

Asgeir Sigurdsson, DDS, MS
Associate Professor and Graduate Program Director,
    Department of Endodontics
University of North Carolina School of Dentistry
Chapel Hill, North Carolina

Denis E. Simon III, DDS, MS
Associate Professor of Clinical Endodontics
Louisiana State University Health Science Center
School of Dentistry
New Orleans, Louisiana

David R. Steiner, DDS, MSD
Affiliate Professor, Graduate Endodontic Program
University of Washington School of Dentistry
Seattle, Washington

Calvin D. Torneck, DDS, MS, FRCD(C)
Professor, Department of Endodontics
Faculty of Dentistry
University of Toronto
Toronto, Ontario, Canada

Henry O. Trowbridge, DDS, PhD
Professor Emeritus, Department of Pathology
University of Pennsylvania
Philadelphia, Pennsylvania

Frank J. Vertucci, DMD
Professor and Chairman, Department of Endodontics
College of Dentistry, University of Florida
Gainesville, Florida

James A. Wallace, DDS, MDS, MSD, MS
Director, Department of Endodontics
University of Pittsburgh School of Dental Medicine
Pittsburgh, Pennsylvania

Lisa R. Wilcox, DDS, MS
Adjunct Associate Professor, Department of Endodontics
The University of Iowa College of Dentistry
Iowa City, Iowa

Peter R. Wilson, MDS, MS, PhD
Associate Professor
University of Melbourne School of Dental Science
Melbourne, Victoria, Australia

Preface

Endodontics deals with the diagnosis and treatment of pulpal and periradicular diseases. It is a discipline that includes different procedures and as such is based on two inseparable bodies—art and science. Many advances have been made in both the scientific and technologic aspects of endodontics since the publication of the second edition of this book 6 years ago. Despite these changes, the basic principles and practice of root canal therapy—eradication of root canal irritants, obturation of the root canal system, and preservation of the natural dentition—remain unchanged.

This edition contains important and significant new endodontics information that has been collected within the last 6 years. The new and updated information in this completely revised edition is essential for those who elect general practice and intend to treat uncomplicated cases. Although many changes have been made in content, the overall emphasis and organization of this edition are the same as the first two editions and are designed for dental students and general practitioners. We combined the chapters on diagnosis and treatment planning and added two new chapters on endodontic therapeutics and geriatric endodontics to reflect changes in practice. To familiarize our readers with the biology of pulp and periradicular tissues, which is an essential part of endodontic practice, we have included a few chapters that cover embryology, anatomy, histology, physiology, pharmacology, pathology, and microbiology.

The chapters remain relatively concise and contain updated information and references. Several color figures have been added to provide better visualization for the reader. To integrate the principles of biology and the practice of endodontics, we invited well-recognized contributing authors who have direct association with predoctoral endodontic education. The contributors were asked to be precise and up to date and to provide information that could be presented in a 1-hour lecture or seminar. The intent of our textbook is to teach predoctoral students and general practitioners how to diagnose and treat uncomplicated endodontic cases. This text is designed to be neither a cookbook nor a preclinical laboratory technique manual.

We thank the contributing authors for their dedication to teaching and for improving the lives of patients by preserving their natural dentition. We also express appreciation of the staff at Harcourt, whose collaboration and hard work helped us to complete this edition. In addition, we recognize the many colleagues and students who gave us helpful suggestions and contributed material to improve the quality of this text, which has become one of the most popular in our field. Please keep these suggestions coming. We appreciate the suggestions; they will be incorporated in our future editions.

RICHARD E. WALTON
MAHMOUD TORABINEJAD

Contents

1 / Scope of Undergraduate Teaching in Endodontic Education, *1*
Richard E. Walton and Mahmoud Torabinejad

2 / Biology of the Dental Pulp and Periradicular Tissues, *3*
Calvin D. Torneck and Mahmoud Torabinejad

3 / Pulp and Periradicular Pathosis, *27*
Mahmoud Torabinejad

4 / Diagnosis and Treatment Planning, *49*
Richard E. Walton and Mahmoud Torabinejad

5 / When and How To Refer, *71*
Mahmoud Torabinejad and Denis E. Simon III

6 / Patient Education, *87*
Stephen Cohen and Mahmoud Torabinejad

7 / Local Anesthesia, *99*
Richard E. Walton and Alfred W. Reader

8 / Isolation, *118*
Gerald L. Scott

9 / Endodontic Radiography, *130*
Richard E. Walton

10 / Endodontic Instruments, *151*
Keith V. Krell

11 / Internal Anatomy, *166*
Richard E. Walton and Frank J. Vertucci

12 / Access Preparation and Length Determination, *182*
Richard E. Walton

13 / Cleaning and Shaping, *206*
Richard E. Walton and Eric M. Rivera

14 / **Obturation,** *239*
Richard E. Walton and William T. Johnson

15 / **Preparation for Restoration and Temporization,** *268*
Harold H. Messer and Peter R. Wilson

16 / **Endodontic Microbiology,** *282*
J. Craig Baumgartner

17 / **Endodontic Emergencies,** *295*
Richard E. Walton and Jeffrey W. Hutter

18 / **Procedural Accidents,** *310*
Mahmoud Torabinejad and Ronald R. Lemon

19 / **Evaluation of Success and Failure,** *331*
Asgeir Sigurdsson

20 / **Orthograde Retreatment,** *345*
Shimon Friedman

21 / **Preventive Endodontics: Protecting the Pulp,** *369*
Henry O. Trowbridge

22 / **Management of Incompletely Formed Roots,** *388*
Thomas R. Pitt Ford and Shahrokh Shabahang

23 / **Bleaching Discolored Teeth: Internal and External,** *405*
Ilan Rotstein and Richard E. Walton

24 / **Endodontic Surgery,** *424*
Neville J. McDonald and Mahmoud Torabinejad

25 / **Management of Traumatized Teeth,** *445*
Leif K. Bakland, Frances M. Andreasen, and Jens O. Andreasen

26 / **Periodontal-Endodontic Considerations,** *466*
Gerald W. Harrington and David R. Steiner

27 / **Endodontic Adjuncts,** *485*
Gerald N. Glickman and James A. Wallace

28 / **Longitudinal Tooth Fractures,** *499*
Richard E. Walton

29 / **Differential Diagnosis of Orofacial Pain,** *520*
Graham Rex Holland

30 / **Endodontic Therapeutics,** *533*
Kenneth M. Hargreaves and J. Craig Baumgartner

31 / **Geriatric Endodontics,** *545*
Richard E. Walton

Appendix: Pulpal Anatomy and Access Preparations, *561*
Lisa R. Wilcox

Principles and Practice
of
ENDODONTICS

Scope of Undergraduate Teaching in Endodontic Education

T he accepted definition of endodontics is "That branch of dentistry concerned with the morphology, physiology, and pathology of the human dental pulp and periradicular tissues. Its study and practice encompass the basic and clinical sciences including biology of the normal pulp, the etiology, diagnoses, prevention, and treatment of diseases and injuries of the pulp and associated periradicular tissues."[1]

In addition to these knowledge areas, the graduating dentist must be able to critically evaluate his or her level of competency as a diagnostician and clinician. Based on this evaluation, the graduate must recognize the effect of his or her own limitations in managing patients with conditions for which he or she possesses less than a competency level of skill; those patients are referred to the appropriate specialist for consultation and/or treatment.

The purpose of this textbook is to supply the undergraduate dental student with basic knowledge in endodontics. This information is necessary to successfully complete an endodontic curriculum in preparation for graduation. The knowledge and skills are needed by the general practitioner to prevent, diagnose, and treat pulpal and/or periradicular pathoses and to recognize other related disorders.

Principles and Practice of Endodontics is based on the *Curriculum Guidelines for Endodontics* for predoctoral students. These guidelines were developed by The American Association of Dental Schools Section on Endodontics, in response to a request from the American Dental Association's Council on Dental Education.[2,3]

The *Guidelines* represent a matrix for developing an undergraduate endodontic curriculum. They specify that endodontic teaching has a basis in, and interrelates with, biomedical sciences. In addition, clinical treatment must integrate closely with other disciplines. This matrix would be universal. A recent survey of dental schools in North America and Europe showed consensus of undergraduate teaching in endodontics.[4]

Undergraduate Curriculum

As a prerequisite to or in conjunction with endodontic training, the student should have knowledge of (1) oral anatomy and histology; (2) infection, inflammation, healing, and repair; (3) microbiology and immunology; (4) pain; (5) radiology; (6) caries and other pulpal irritants; (7) therapeutic agents; (8) systemic diseases; (9) medical emergencies; and (10) management of medically compromised patients.

Upon completion of predoctoral instruction, the graduating dentist must be able to manage uncomplicated endodontic procedures as a general practitioner. In preparation for this, the core curriculum for undergraduates must include (1) diagnosis and treatment planning, (2) management of the vital pulp, (3) uncomplicated root canal treatment, (4) management of procedural errors, (5) determination of success or failure, (6) primary management of trauma, (7) internal bleaching of discolored teeth, (8) management of emergencies, and (9) management of uncomplicated retreatments.

The graduating dentist should also be familiar with other endodontic procedures, recognizing their role in the treatment of patients. Most of these should be referred to the endodontist for management. These include (1) challenging diagnoses, (2) complicated root canal treatment,

(3) complicated emergency management, (4) difficult retreatment, (5) long-term management of trauma, (6) endodontic-periodontic interrelationships, (7) endodontic-orthodontic problems, (8) open apex management, (9) complicated cracked tooth, (10) endodontic surgery, and (11) intentional replantation.

The graduate must be able to perform self-evaluation. This is a critical evaluation of his or her level of competency diagnostically and technically. The end result is independent thinking and action; the ultimate benefit is providing quality care to the patient.

REFERENCES

1. American Association of Endodontists: Appropriateness of Care and Quality Assurance Guidelines, ed 3, Chicago, The Association, 1998, p.3.
2. American Association of Dental Schools, Section on Endodontics: Curriculum Guidelines for Endodontics, *J Dent Educ* 50:190, 1986.
3. Curriculum Guidelines for Endodontics, *J Dent Educ* 57:251, 1993.
4. Qualtrough A, Whitworth J, Dummer P: Preclinical endodontology: an international comparison, *Int Endodon J* 32:406, 1999.

Calvin D. Torneck and Mahmoud Torabinejad

2

Biology of the Dental Pulp and Periradicular Tissues

LEARNING OBJECTIVES

After reading this chapter, the student should be able to:

1 / Describe the development of pulp from its embryologic stage to its fully developed state.

2 / Describe the process of root development and maturation of the apical foramen.

3 / Recognize the anatomic regions of pulp.

4 / List cell types in pulp and state their function.

5 / Describe the fibrous and nonfibrous components of the extracellular matrix of pulp.

6 / Describe the blood vessels and lymphatics of pulp.

7 / List the neural components of pulp and describe their distribution and function.

8 / Discuss theories of dentin sensitivity.

9 / Describe pathways of efferent nerves from pulp to the central nervous system.

10 / Describe changes in pulp morphology that occur with age.

11 / Describe the structure and function of periradicular tissues.

OUTLINE

Embryology of the Dental Pulp
  Early Development of Pulp
  Root Formation
  Formation of Lateral Canals and Apical
    Foramen
  Formation of Periodontium

Anatomic Regions and Their Clinical
  Importance

Pulp Function
  Induction
  Formation
  Nutrition
  Defense
  Sensation

Histology

Cells of the Dental Pulp
  Odontoblasts
  Preodontoblasts
  Fibroblasts
  Undifferentiated (Reserve) Cells
  Cells of the Immune System

Extracellular Components
  Fibers
  Ground Substance
  Calcifications

Blood Vessels
  Afferent Blood Vessels (Arterioles)
  Efferent Blood Vessels (Venules)
  Vascular Physiology
  Lymphatics

Innervation
  Neuroanatomy
  Developmental Aspects of Pulp Innervation
  Theories of Dentin Hypersensitivity

Age Changes in the Dental Pulp
  Morphologic Changes
  Physiologic Changes

Periradicular Tissues
  Cementum
  Cementoenamel Junction
  Periodontal Ligament
  Alveolar Bone

Dental pulp is the soft tissue located in the center of the tooth. It forms, supports, and is an integral part of the dentin that surrounds it. The *primary function* of the pulp is formative; it gives rise to odontoblasts that not only form dentin but interact with dental epithelium, early in tooth development, to initiate the formation of enamel. Subsequent to tooth formation, pulp provides several *secondary functions* related to tooth sensitivity, hydration, and defense. Injury to pulp may cause discomfort and disease. Consequently the health of the pulp is important to the successful completion of restorative and prosthetic dental procedures. In restorative dentistry, for example, the size and shape of the pulp must be considered to determine cavity depth. The size and shape of the pulp, in turn, may be influenced by the stage of tooth development (related to patient age). The stage of tooth development may also influence the type of the pulp treatment rendered when a pulp injury occurs. Procedures routinely undertaken on a fully developed tooth are not always practical for a tooth that is only partially developed. In such cases special procedures not often used for the mature tooth are applied. Because the symptoms as well as the radiographic and clinical signs of pulp disease are not always readily differentiated from the signs and symptoms of other dental and nondental diseases, a knowledge of the biology of the pulp also is essential for the development of a rational treatment plan. For example, the appearance of periodontal lesions of endodontic origin can be similar to that of lesions induced by primary disease of periodontium and lesions of nondental origin. An inability to recognize this similarity may lead to misdiagnosis and incorrect treatment. Comprehensive descriptions of pulp embryology, histology, and physiology are available in several dental texts. This chapter presents an overview of the biology of the pulp and the periodontium: development, anatomy, and function that affect pulp disease as well as periradicular disease and its related symptoms.

Embryology of the Dental Pulp

EARLY DEVELOPMENT OF PULP

Pulp originates from ectomesenchymal cells (derived from the neural crest) of the dental papilla. Dental pulp is identified when these cells mature and dentin has formed. Differentiation of odontoblasts from undifferentiated ectomesenchymal cells is accomplished through an interaction of cells and signaling molecules mediated through the basal lamina and the extracellular matrix.[1]

The expression of various growth factors from the cells of the inner enamel membrane initiates the differentiation process.[2] Several cell replications are required before an odontoblast appears. In tooth development, only the cells next to basal lamina replicate fully into odontoblasts. Not fully replicated daughter cells derived from odontoblasts remain in the subodontoblastic region as *preodontoblasts.* Under specific circumstances dictated by the environment, these cells can replicate and form odontoblasts when required.[3]

Formation of dentin by odontoblasts heralds the conversion of dental papilla to dental pulp. This formation begins with formation of extensive junctional complexes and gap junctions between odontoblasts and the deposition of unmineralized matrix at the cusp tip (Figure 2-1). Deposition progresses in a cervical (apical) direction in a rhythmic, regular pattern and averages about 4.5 μm/day.[4] Crown shape is predetermined by the proliferative pattern of the cells of the inner enamel epithelium. The first dentin formed is called mantle dentin. The deposition and size of the collagen fibers in mantle dentin are different from those for fibers of the circumpulpal dentin, which forms after the odontoblast layer is organized and which represents most of the dentin that is formed. Mineralization occurs shortly after matrix has formed. Normally, 10 to 47μm of the dentin matrix immediately adjacent to the odontoblast layer remains unmineralized and is referred to as *predentin.* Its absence may predispose the dentin to internal resorption by odontoclasts.

As crown formation occurs, vascular and sensory neural elements begin migrating into the pulp in a coronal direction. The ingrowth of unmyelinated sensory nerves (c fibers) occurs at about the same time as that of the myelinated sensory nerves (Aδ fibers). Eventually the myelinated nerves lose their myelin sheath and terminate in the subodontoblastic region as an unmyelinated plexus *(plexus of Raschkow).* This usually occurs after the tooth has erupted, and root formation has been completed.[5] Formation and mineralization of enamel begins at the cusp tip shortly after the dentin has formed, a further expression of epithelial-ectomesenchymal interactions in tooth formation.

ROOT FORMATION

The cells of the inner and outer enamel unite at a point known as the cervical loop. This delineates the end of the anatomical crown and the site where root formation begins. It is initiated by the apical proliferation of the two epithelial structures, which combine at the cervical loop to form a double layer of cells known as Hertwig's epithelial root sheath. The function of the sheath is similar to that of the inner enamel epithelium during crown formation. It provides the stimulus for the differentiation of odontoblasts, which form the dentin and the template to which the dentin is formed (Figure 2-2). Cell proliferation in the root sheath is genetically determined; its pattern regulates whether the root will be wide or narrow, straight or curved, long or short, or single or multiple. Multiple roots result when opposing parts of the root sheath proliferate horizontally as well as vertically. As horizontal segments join and continue to proliferate apically, an additional root or multiple roots are formed. The pattern of proliferation also determines whether the roots are separate or joined as can be noted in mandibular molars and maxillary premolars. Patterns of root sheath proliferation and progressive differentiation and maturation of odontoblasts are readily discernible when the developing root end is viewed microscopically (Figure 2-3).

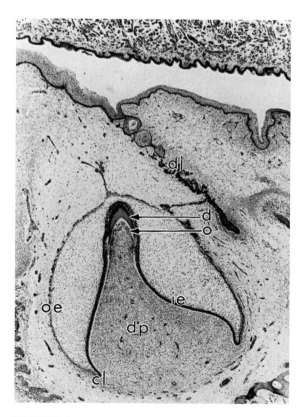

FIGURE 2-1
Late bell stage of tooth formation with early dentin formation. *dl,* Dental lamina; *d,* newly formed dentin; *o,* odontoblasts, *oe,* outer enamel epithelium; *ie,* inner enamel epithelium; *cl,* cervical loop; *dp,* dental papilla.

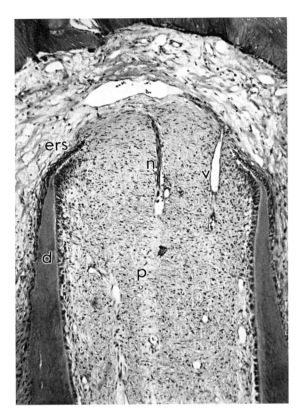

FIGURE 2-2
Apical region of developing incisor. *ers,* Epithelium root sheath; *p,* pulp; *d,* dentin; *n,* nerve; *v,* venule.

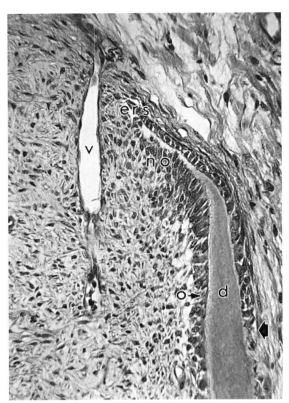

FIGURE 2-3
Higher-power photomicrograph of Hertwig's epithelial root sheath *(ers)* shown in Figure 2-2. New odontoblasts *(no)* are differentiating along the pulpal side of the root sheath and eventually forming dentin *(d).* Functioning odontoblasts *(o)* continue to form dentin after the root sheath begins to break up *(large arrowhead).* A venule *(v)* exits the pulp near the root sheath.

After the first dentin *(mantle dentin)* has formed, the underlying basement membrane breaks up, and the innermost root sheath cells secrete a hyaline-like material, presumed to be enameloid, over the newly formed dentin. After its mineralization this becomes the *hyaline layer of Hopewell-Smith.* This helps bind the soon-to-be-formed cementum to dentin.[6] Fragmentation of Hertwig's epithelial root sheath occurs shortly afterwards. This allows cells of the surrounding follicle to migrate and contact the newly formed dentin surface, where they differentiate into cementoblasts and initiate acellular cementum formation. This cementum ultimately serves as an anchor for the developing principal periodontal fibers (Figure 2-4). In many teeth, cell remnants of the root sheath persist in the periodontium in close proximity to the root after root development has been completed. These are the *epithelial cell rests of Malassez.* Normally functionless, in the presence of inflammation they can proliferate and may under certain conditions give rise to a radicular cyst.[7]

FORMATION OF LATERAL CANALS AND APICAL FORAMEN
Lateral Canals

Lateral canals (or, synonymously, accessory canals) are channels of communication between pulp and periodontal ligament. They form when a localized area of root sheath is fragmented before dentin formation. The result is direct communication between pulp and lateral periodontal ligament via a channel through the dentin. Lateral canals also can form when blood vessels, which normally pass between dental papilla and investing dental follicle, become entrapped in the proliferating epithelial root sheath. Lateral canals may be large or small or multiple or singular; they may occur anywhere along the root but predominate in the apical third. In molars they may extend from the pulp chamber to furcation. *Lateral canals*

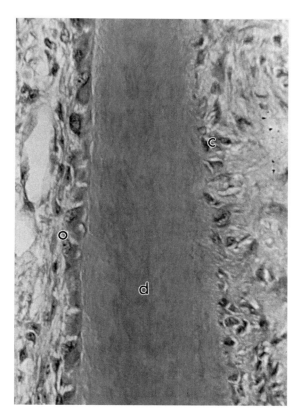

FIGURE 2-4
Higher-power photomicrograph of developing root shows cementoblasts *(c)* differentiating and producing cementum on dentin *(d)* subsequent to breakup of the epithelium root sheath. Odontoblasts *(o)* are forming dentin on the pulpal side of the dentin.

are clinically significant; like the apical foramen they represent pathways along which disease in pulp may extend to periradicular tissues and occasionally allow disease in periodontium to extend to pulp.

Apical Foramen

As the epithelial root sheath proliferates, it encloses more dental papilla until only a basal (apical) opening remains. This opening is the principal entrance and exit for pulpal vessels and nerves. During root formation the apical foramen is usually located at the end of the anatomic root. However, by the time tooth development has been completed, the apical foramen is smaller and more eccentric. This eccentricity becomes more pronounced when apical cementum is formed and changes again with the continued deposition of cementum associated with coronal wear and tooth drifting.

There may be one foramen or multiple foramina at the apex. Multiple foramina occur more often in multirooted teeth. When more than one foramen is present, the largest one is referred to as the apical foramen and the smaller ones as accessory canals (in combination, the *apical delta*). The diameter of the apical foramen in a mature tooth usually ranges between 0.3 and 0.6 mm. The largest diameters are found on the distal canal of mandibular molars and the palatal root of maxillary molars.[8] Foramen size is unpredictable, however, and cannot be accurately determined clinically.

FORMATION OF PERIODONTIUM

Tissues of the periodontium, which include the cementum, periodontal fibers, and the alveolar bone, arise from ectomesenchyme-derived fibrocellular tissue that surrounds the developing tooth *(dental follicle)*. After the mantle dentin has formed, enamel-like proteins are secreted into the space between the basement membrane and the newly formed collagen by the root sheath cells.[9] This area is not mineralized with the mantel dentin but does mineralize later and to a greater degree to form the *hyalin layer of Hopewell-Smith*. After mineralization has occurred, the root sheath undergoes fragmentation. This fragmentation allows cells from the follicle to proliferate through the root sheath, differentiate into cementoblasts, and produce cementum over the hyalin layer. Bundles of collagen, produced by fibroblasts in the central region of the follicle *(Sharpey's fibers)*, are embedded in the forming cementum and serve as an anchor for the soon-to-be-formed principal periodontal fibers.

Concomitantly, cells in the outermost area of the follicle differentiate into osteoblasts to form the bundle bone that also will serve as an anchor for the periodontal fibers. Later periodontal fibroblasts produce collagen that links the anchored fragments together to form the arrangement of principle periodontal fibers that suspend the tooth in its socket. Areas of the periodontium between the principal fibers remain as loose fibrous connective tissue through which nerves and vessels that supply the periodontium pass. Undifferentiated (or partly differentiated) cells are plentiful in the periodontium and possess the ability to form new cementoblasts, osteoblasts, or fibroblasts, in response to specific stimuli. Cementum formed after the formation of the principle periodontal fibers is of the cellular type and plays a lesser role in tooth support.

The blood supply to the periodontium is derived from the surrounding bone, gingiva, and pulpal vessels. It is extensive and supports the

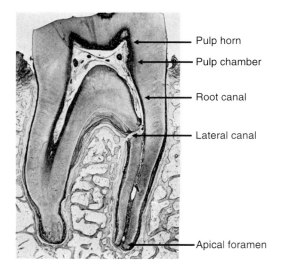

FIGURE 2-5
Anatomic regions of the root canal system highlighting the pulp horn(s), pulp chamber, root canal, lateral canal, and apical foramen. The pulp, which is present in the root canal system, communicates with the periodontal ligament primarily through the apical foramen and the lateral canal(s). (Courtesy Orban Collection.)

high level of cellular activity in the area. The pattern of innervation is similar to that of the vasculature. The neural supply consists of small unmyelinated sensory and autonomic nerves and larger myelinated sensory nerves. Some of the latter terminate as unmyelinated neural structures, which are thought to be nociceptors and mechanoreceptors. No proprioceptive properties have been attributed to these nerves.[10]

Anatomic Regions and Their Clinical Importance

The tooth has two principal anatomic divisions, root and crown, that join at the cervix *(cervical region)*. Pulp space is similarly divided into coronal and radicular regions. In general, the shape and the size of the tooth surface determine the shape and the size of the pulp space. Coronal pulp is subdivided into pulp horn and pulp chamber (Figure 2-5). Pulp horns extend from the chamber into the cuspal region. In some teeth, they are extensive and may be inadvertently exposed during routine cavity preparation.

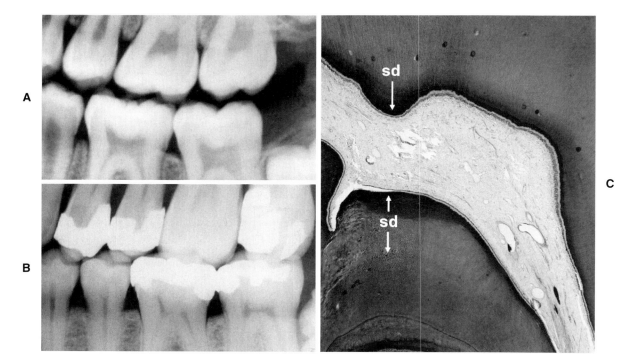

FIGURE 2-6
A and **B**, Radiographic changes noted in the shape of the pulp chamber over time. The posterior bitewing radiographs were taken 15 years apart. The shapes of the root canal systems have been altered as a result of secondary dentinogenesis and in instances where deep restorations are present, by the deposition of tertiary dentin. **C**, Human mandibular molar showing deposition of secondary dentin *(sd)* on the roof and floor of the pulp chamber; this tends to "flatten" the chamber.

As will be discussed later in this chapter under "Age Changes in the Dental Pulp," the pulp space becomes asymmetrically smaller over time, due to the continued, albeit slower, production of dentin. Principally there is a pronounced decrease in the height of the pulp horn and a reduction in the overall size of the pulp chamber. In molars the apical-occlusal dimension is reduced more than the mesial-distal dimension. Excessive reduction of the size of the pulp space is clinically significant and can lead to difficulties in locating, cleaning, and shaping the root canal system (Figure 2-6, *A to C*).

Anatomy of the root canal can vary not only between tooth types but also within tooth types. Although at least one canal must be present in each root, some roots have multiple canals, some comparable in size and others different. *Understanding and appreciating all aspects of root canal anatomy are essential prerequisites to root canal treatment.*

Variation in the size and location of the apical foramen influences the degree to which blood flow to the pulp may be compromised after a traumatic event. *In this situation, young, partially developed teeth have a better prognosis for pulp survival than teeth with mature roots* (Figure 2-7).

Posteruptive deposition of cementum in the region of the apical foramen creates a disparity between the radiographic apex and the apical foramen. It also creates a funnel-shaped opening to the foramen that is often larger in diameter than the intraradicular portion of the foramen. The narrowest portion of the canal has been referred to as the "*constriction*." However, a constriction is not clinically evident in all teeth.[11] Cementum contacts dentin inside the canal coronal to the cementum surface. That point is the *cementodentinal junction (CDJ)*. The CDJ level varies not only from tooth to tooth but also within a single root canal. One study estimated the junction to be located 0.5 to 0.75 mm coronal to the apical opening.[8] Theoretically, that is the point where the pulp terminates and the periodontal ligament begins. However, histologically and clinically it is not always possible to locate that point. Cleaning, shaping, and obturation of the root canal should terminate short of the apical foramen and remain confined to the canal to avoid unnecessary injury to the periapical tissues. *The determination of root length and the establishment of a working length are essential prerequisites to root canal preparation, for that reason. The radiograph and electronic apex locators are helpful in establishing the root length.*

Pulp Function

The pulp performs five functions, some formative and others supportive.

INDUCTION

Pulp participates in the initiation and development of dentin, which, when formed, leads to the formation of enamel. These events are interdependent in that enamel epithelium induces the differentiation of odontoblasts, and odontoblasts and dentin induce the formation of

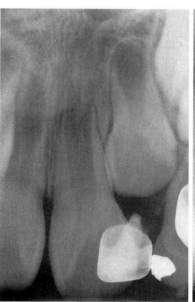

A

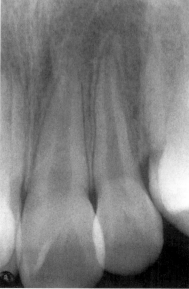

B

FIGURE 2-7
Changes in the anatomy of the tooth root and pulp space. **A,** A small crown-root ratio, thin dentin walls, and divergent shape in the apical third of the canal are seen. **B,** Four years later, a longer root, greater crown-root ratio, smaller pulp space, and thicker dentin walls with a convergent shape are seen.

enamel. Such epithelial-mesenchymal interactions are the essence of tooth formation.

FORMATION

Odontoblasts form dentin. These highly specialized cells participate in dentin formation in three ways: (1) by synthesizing and secreting inorganic matrix; (2) by initially transporting inorganic components to newly formed matrix; and (3) by creating an environment that permits mineralization of matrix. During early tooth development, primary dentinogenesis is generally a rapid process. After tooth maturation, dentin formation continues at a much slower rate and in a less symmetrical pattern *(secondary dentinogenesis)*. Odontoblasts can also form a dentin in response to injury, which may occur in association with caries, trauma, or restorative procedures. Generally this dentin is less organized than primary and secondary dentin and mostly localized to the site of injury. This dentin is referred to as *tertiary dentin*. Morphologically tertiary dentin has a variety of appearances. It is also referred to as reactive, reparative, irritation, or irregular dentin (Figure 2-8).

NUTRITION

Pulp supplies nutrients that are essential for dentin formation (for example, peritubular dentin) and hydration via dentinal tubules.

DEFENSE

As mentioned previously, odontoblasts form dentin in response to injury, particularly when the original dentin thickness has been reduced due to caries, attrition, trauma, or restorative procedures. Dentin can also be formed at sites where its continuity has been lost, such as a site of pulp exposure. This occurs through the induction, differentiation, and migration of new odontoblasts or odontoblast-like cells to the exposure site.[12,13] However, the structure of dentin produced in response to injury such as this may not resemble that of dentin produced physiologically and hence may not afford the same degree of protection to the underlying pulp tissue (Figure 2-9).

Pulp also has the ability to process and identify foreign substances and to elicit an immune response to their presence. This is typical of the response of the pulp to dentinal caries.

SENSATION

Pulp transmits neural sensations mediated through enamel or dentin to the higher nerve centers. These stimuli are usually expressed clinically as pain, although physiologic and psychophysiologic studies indicate that pulp can transmit sensations of temperature and touch.[14,15] Pulp also transmits sensations of deep pain, which may be initiated by disease, principally in-

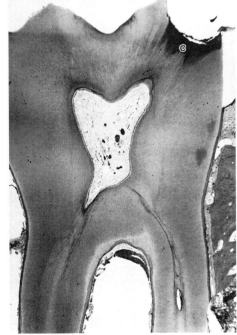

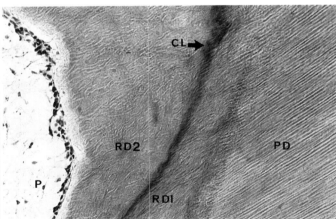

FIGURE 2-8

A, Reactive dentin formation under caries *(c).* Pulp displays chronic inflammation and tertiary dentinogenesis on the inner walls of the pulp space in the region of the dentinal tubules associated with the base of the carious lesion. **B,** Higher-power photomicrograph of tertiary dentin shown in **A.** *PD,* primary dentin; *RD1,* first period of tertiary dentin formation; *CL,* calciotraumatic line; *RD2,* second period of tertiary dentin formation. Note the progressive irregularities in tubule formation and changes in the morphology of the odontoblasts *(P)* in that region.

flammatory disease. Pulp sensation mediated through dentin and enamel is usually fast, sharp, and severe and is transmitted by Aδ fibers *(myelinated fibers)*. Sensation initiated within the pulp core and transmitted by the smaller c fibers is slower, duller, and more diffuse.

Histology

Dentin and pulp are really a tissue complex; therefore a discussion of pulp (particularly odontoblasts) should include a discussion of dentin formation and maturation. It should also be remembered that their histologic appearance varies chronologically and in accordance with their exposure to external stimuli.

Under light microscopy, a young, fully developed permanent tooth shows certain recognizable aspects of pulp architecture. In its outer (peripheral) regions subjacent to predentin there is the odontoblast layer. Internal to this layer is a relatively cell-free area (the zone of Weil). Internal to the cell-free zone is a higher concentration of cells (cell-rich zone). In the center is an area containing mostly pulp cells and major branches of nerves and blood vessels referred to as the pulp core (Figure 2-10).

Cells of the Dental Pulp

ODONTOBLASTS

Odontoblasts are the most distinctive cells of pulp. They form a single layer at its periphery and they synthesize the matrix, which is mineralized and becomes dentin. In the coronal part of the pulp space the odontoblasts are numerous and relatively large and columnar in shape. They number between 45,000 and 65,000/mm² in that area. In the cervical portion and midportion of the root their numbers are fewer and they are flattened (squamous) in appearance. Significantly, the morphology of the cell generally reflects its functional activity, with larger cells having a capacity to synthesize more matrix.[16] Odontoblasts are end cells and as such do not undergo further cell division (see "Preodontoblasts"). During their life span, which could equal the period of pulp vitality, they go through functional, transitional, and resting phases, all marked by differences in cell size and organelle expression.

The odontoblast consists of two major structural and functional components, the cell body and the cell process. The *cell body* lies subjacent to the unmineralized dentin matrix *(predentin)*. The *cell process* extends outwardly through a tubule in the predentin and dentin. The distance to which

it extends has been debated among anatomists for years. Some studies have shown that the process extends only part way through the dentin, while others have shown that it extends through the full thickness of the dentin and terminates at or close to the dentinoenamel junction (DEJ) or CDJ.[17,18] The extent to which the cell process has been found appears to be influenced by the method of investigation. Today the issue remains unresolved; it is likely that there is variation in its extent.

The cell body is the synthesizing portion of the cell and contains a basally located nucleus and an organelle structure in the cytoplasm that is typical of a secreting cell. During active dentinogenesis, endoplasmic reticulum and the Golgi apparatus are prominent with numerous mitochondria and vesicles (Figure 2-11). Cell bodies are joined by a variety of complex junctions consisting of gap junctions, tight junctions, and desmosomes whose locations are variable and determined by function.

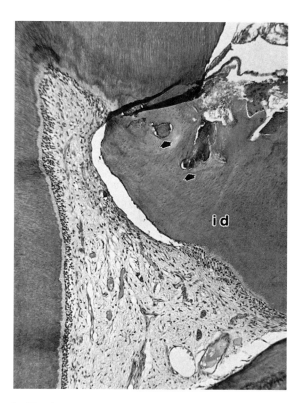

FIGURE 2-9
Photomicrograph of a mandibular permanent molar that was mechanically exposed earlier and capped with a paste of calcium hydroxide and saline. Tertiary (reparative) irregular dentin *(id)* at the site of exposure displays irregularities *(arrowheads)* that can be traced from surface to pulp. The clear area at the pulp surface below the irregular dentin is an artifact.

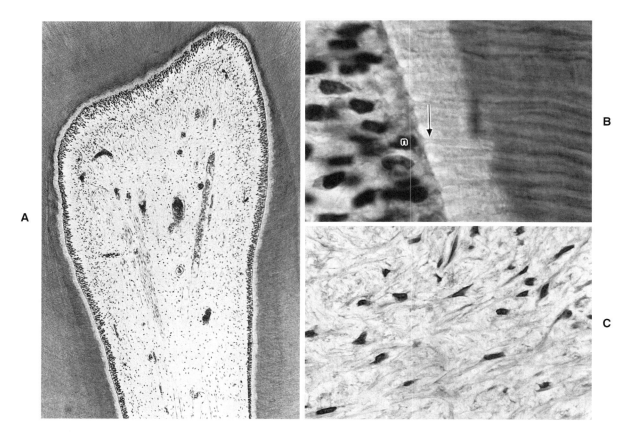

FIGURE 2-10
A, Mandibular premolar showing major features of dentin-pulp anatomy. From the periphery inward there is the mineralized dentin, predentin, odontoblasts, and cell-free and cell-poor zones of the pulp. The central pulp or pulp core is cellular and contains the major nerves and blood vessels of the pulp. **B,** Odontoblast-predentin interface at higher power. Odontoblast cell nuclei *(n)* are aligned along the predentin. The *arrow* indicates an odontoblast process in a tubule in predentin. **C,** High-power photomicrograph of fibroblasts in the pulp core. At this magnification only the nuclei are apparent interspersed between collagen fibers of the extracellular matrix.

The junctions isolate the site where dentin is formed and regulate the flow of substances into and out of the area.[19] Secretory products of the odontoblasts are released through the cell membrane at the peripheral end of the cell body and the basal end of the cell process.[20] Initially this includes organic components of the dentin matrix and mineralization crystals but subsequent to the initial mineralization of the dentin only matrix components are secreted. Odontoblasts are most active during primary dentinogenesis and during reparative dentin formation. Activity is substantially reduced during ongoing secondary dentinogenesis.

PREODONTOBLASTS

New odontoblasts can arise after an injury that results in a loss of existing odontoblasts. The prob-

ability is that preodontoblasts (cells that have partly differentiated along the odontoblast line) do exist and reside in the cell-rich zone. These precursor cells migrate to, and continue their differentiation at, the site of injury. To date, the specific circumstances leading to this type of replacement are unknown, although certain growth factors such as bone morphogenic protein (BMP) and transforming growth factor β in combination with other tissue components appear to initiate the change.[21]

FIBROBLASTS

Fibroblasts are the most common cell type and are seen in greatest numbers in the coronal pulp. They produce and maintain the collagen and ground substance of the pulp and alter the structure of the pulp in disease.[22] Like odontoblasts,

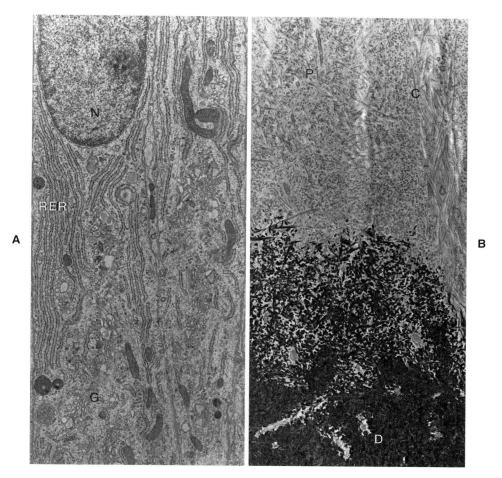

FIGURE 2-11
A, Odontoblast cell body. The nucleus *(N)* is proximal, and the numerous organelles such as rough endoplasmic reticulum *(RER)* and Golgi apparatus *(G),* which are responsible for synthesis of matrix components, occupy the central-distal regions. **B,** Predentin *(P)* shows the orientation of collagen *(C)* to the odontoblastic process, which is the secretory organ that extends through the predentin into the dentin *(D).* (Courtesy Dr. P. Glick and Dr. D. Rowe.)

the prominence of their cytoplasmic organelles changes according to their activity. The more active the cell, the more prominent the organelles and other components necessary for synthesis and secretion. Unlike odontoblasts, however, these cells do undergo apoptotic cell death and are replaced when necessary by the maturation of less differentiated cells.

UNDIFFERENTIATED (RESERVE) CELLS

These cells represent the cell pool from which connective tissue cells of the pulp are derived. These precursor cells are found in the cell-rich zone and in the pulp core in close association with blood vessels. They appear to be the first cells to divide after injury.[23] They are

reduced in number and this in concert with an increase in pulp calcification and blood flow reduces the regenerative capabilities of the pulp.

CELLS OF THE IMMUNE SYSTEM

Macrophages, T lymphocytes, and dendritic cells are also normal cellular inhabitants of the pulp.[24] Dendritic cells and their processes are found throughout the odontoblast layer and have a close association with vascular and neural elements. These cells are part of the surveillance and initial response system of the pulp. They capture and present antigens to the resident T cells and macrophages. Collectively this group of cells makes up approximately 8% of the cell population of the pulp.

Extracellular Components

FIBERS

Type I collagen is the predominant collagen in dentin whereas both type I and type III collagen are found within pulp in a ratio of approximately 55:45.[25] Type I collagen is synthesized exclusively by odontoblasts and incorporated into dentin matrix, whereas fibroblasts produce both the type I and type III collagen incorporated into pulp. Small amounts of type V collagen have also been found in pulp.[26] Fine reticular fibers are also found, but elastic and oxytalan fibers are not normally present.

The proportion of collagen types is constant in the pulp, but with age there is an increase in the overall collagen content and an increase in the organization of collagen fibers into collagen bundles. Normally, the apical portion of pulp contains more collagen than coronal pulp, facilitating pulpectomy with a barbed broach or endodontic file during endodontic treatment.

GROUND SUBSTANCE

Pulp ground substance is similar to that of other loose connective tissue. It is composed principally of glycosaminoglycans, glycoproteins, and water in the form of a sol-gel that supports the cells and acts as a medium for transport of nutrients and metabolites. Alterations in composition of ground substance caused by age or disease may interfere with normal cell activity and lead to irregularities in cell function and mineral deposition.

CALCIFICATIONS

Pulp stones or denticles were once classified as true or false depending on the presence or absence of a tubular structure. However, this classification has been challenged, and a new nomenclature based on the genesis of the calcification has been suggested.[27] Pulp stones have also been classified according to location. Three types of pulp stones have been described: *free stones,* which are surrounded by pulp tissue; *attached stones,* which are continuous with the dentin; and *embedded stones,* which are surrounded entirely by dentin, mostly of the tertiary type.

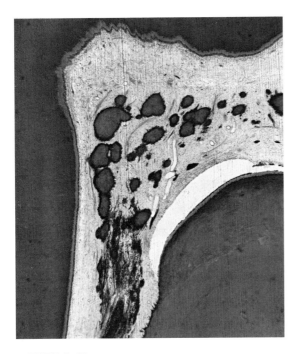

FIGURE 2-12
Pulp stones in the coronal pulp and linear, or diffuse, calcifications in the radicular portion. (Courtesy Dr. S. Bernick.)

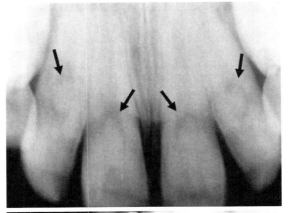

A

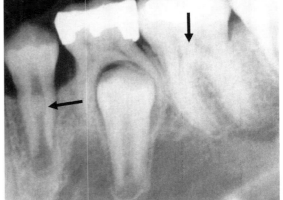

B

FIGURE 2-13
Multiple pulp stones *(arrows)* in the pulp chamber and root canals of the anterior (**A**) and posterior (**B**) teeth of a young patient.

Pulp stones may be seen in young and old patients and may occur in one or several teeth. They occur in normal pulp as well as in chronically inflamed pulp. Contrary to popular opinion, they are not responsible for painful symptoms, regardless of size.

Calcifications may also occur in the form of diffuse or linear deposits (Figure 2-12). These are associated with neurovascular bundles in the pulp core. This type of calcification is seen most often in the aged or chronically inflamed pulp. Depending on shape, size, and location, pulp calcifications may or may not be detected on a dental radiograph (Figure 2-13). *Large pulp stones are clinically significant in that they may block access to canals or the root apex during root canal treatment.*

Blood Vessels

Mature pulp has an extensive and unique vascular pattern that reflects its unique environment. The vessel network has been examined using a variety of techniques including India ink perfusion, transmission electron microscopy, scanning electron microscopy, and microradiography.[28–31]

AFFERENT BLOOD VESSELS (ARTERIOLES)

One and sometimes two afferent vessels enter the canal via each apical foramen. These vessels are of arteriolar diameter and are branches of the inferior alveolar artery, the superior posterior alveolar artery, or the infraorbital artery, which branch from the internal maxillary artery.

After the arteriole passes into the canal, there is a decrease in its smooth muscle coating and a corresponding increase in the size of the vessel lumen. This reduces the rate of blood flow. As the arterioles course toward the coronal pulp, they give off smaller branches (metarterioles and precapillaries) throughout the pulp (Figure 2-14). The most extensive branching occurs in the subodontoblastic layer of the coronal pulp where the vessels terminate in a capillary bed (Figure 2-15). The loops of some of these capillaries extend between odontoblasts and continue as venules. In addition, there is an extensive shunting system composed of arteriovenous and venovenous anastomoses; these shunts become active after pulp injury and repair.[32] All afferent vessels (except capillaries) and arteriovenous shunts have neuromuscular mechanisms to control regional blood flow. The endothelial cells also respond to a variety of endogenous and exogenous substances.

EFFERENT BLOOD VESSELS (VENULES)

Venules constitute the efferent (exit) side of the pulpal circulation and are slightly larger than the corresponding arterioles. Venules enlarge as they merge and advance toward the apical foramen. After exiting from the foramen, venules coalesce and drain posteriorly into the maxillary vein through the pterygoid plexus or anteriorly into the facial vein.

Efferent vessels are thin-walled and show only scanty smooth muscle. Because they are not innervated they are largely passive and nonconstrictive (Figure 2-16).

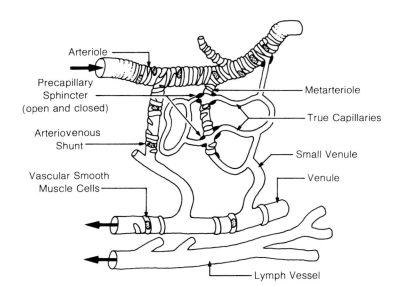

Arteriole

Precapillary Sphincter (open and closed)

Arteriovenous Shunt

Vascular Smooth Muscle Cells

Metarteriole

True Capillaries

Small Venule

Venule

Lymph Vessel

FIGURE 2-14
Schematic of the pulpal vasculature. Smooth muscle cells that surround vessels and precapillary sphincters selectively control blood flow. Arteriovenous shunts bypass capillary beds.

FIGURE 2-15
The dense capillary bed in the sub-odontoblastic region is shown by resin cast preparation and scanning electron microscopy. (Courtesy Dr. C. Kockapan.)

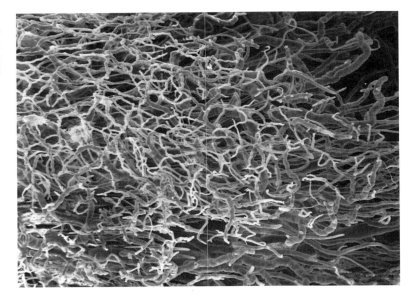

VASCULAR PHYSIOLOGY
Normal

The dental pulp is a highly vascularized tissue. Capillary blood flow in the coronal region is almost twice that of the radicular region. Blood supply is regulated by local factors as well as by sensory and sympathetic nerves. Smooth muscles on vessels have both α- and β-adrenergic receptors; therefore they respond by constricting when sympathetic nerves are stimulated or when vasoconstrictors are injected intravascularly.[33,34]

The presence of cholinergic pulp nerves has not been confirmed although the presence of vasoactive intestinal peptide, a neurokinin identified with cholinergic nerve activity, has been. Normally the blood flow through the peripheral capillary bed of a mature tooth is well below maximum capacity. Thus the full extent of the subodontoblastic capillary bed is not apparent when pulp is viewed by standard light microscopy. Capillaries become more apparent when the vasculature is experimentally perfused or when a hyperemia occurs.

Pulp tissue pressure has been measured at 6 mm Hg compared with a capillary pressure of 35 mm Hg and a venular pressure of 19 mm Hg. However, the lack of a reliable and consistent method of recording pulp tissue pressure makes the accuracy of these measurements questionable.[35]

Pathologic

As with similar types of connective tissue, pulpal injury appears to evoke a biphasic vascular response. This consists of an initial vasoconstriction followed by vasodilation and increased vascular permeability. This latter phase appears to be mediated by neuropeptides released from afferent pain fibers. Localized edema associated with leakage from the primary venules then occurs and raises the local tissue pressure. This, in turn, initiates a regional reduction in blood flow and lymph drainage that leads to an increase in tissue carbon dioxide and acidity.[36] To compensate, the vascular flow to the injured area is reduced by a redirection of blood into arteriovenous shunts and the efferent pulp vessels. This allows for slow resolution of tissue edema and restoration of a normal flow.[32] If the injury is severe enough, compensation cannot occur and local ischemia and a progressive extension of tissue destruction may result.

Recent studies have shown a reciprocal relationship between the vascular flow and nociceptive nerve activity.[37] An increased rate of flow may occur during certain stages of inflammation and contribute to a decrease in the pain threshold of the larger pulp nerves (Aδ fibers) and result in an increased response to thermal stimuli (hot and cold). Conversely, the restriction of blood flow can suppress the activity of the larger (Aδ) nerves and again change the nature of the pain experience.

Painful stimuli cause a release of substance P and calcitonin gene-related peptide from the nociceptive c fibers in the pulp core.[38] These peptides have vasoactive properties that can cause increased vascular permeability and edema. Because some teeth share afferent nerve fibers, a painful experience in one tooth can lead also to vascular changes in another. This pattern of inflammation is re-

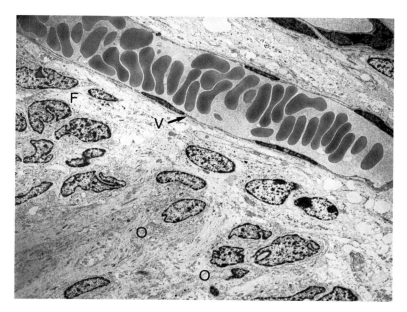

FIGURE 2-16
A small, thin-walled venule *(V)* filled with erythrocytes lies within the cell-free zone. The peripheral pulp is below, with odontoblasts *(O)* and fibroblasts *(F)*. (Courtesy Dr. T. Cipriano.)

ferred to as *neurogenic inflammation* and highlights the interdependence of normal tooth physiology.

LYMPHATICS

The presence of an active lymphatic system in the dental pulp was once a subject of debate. However, investigations performed at different times and with different techniques have confirmed its existence.[39-41] Lymphatic vessels arise as small, blind, thin-walled vessels in the coronal region. They pass through its middle and apical regions to exit as one or two larger vessels through the apical foramen (Figure 2-17). The lymphatic vessel walls are composed of an endothelium rich in organelles and granules. There are discontinuities in the walls of the vessels similar to those found in capillaries. However, unlike the blood vessels, there are also discontinuities in the subjacent basement membrane. These openings in the basement membrane and vessel walls permit passage of interstitial tissue fluid and, when necessary, lymphocytes into the negative-pressure lymph vessel.

The presence of lymphocytes and the absence of red blood cells in the lumen are characteristic findings (Figure 2-18). Lymphatics assist in the removal of inflammatory exudates and transudates as well as irritants such as cellular debris. After exiting from the pulp, some vessels join vessels from the periodontal ligament; all drain into regional lymph glands (submental, submandibular, or cervical) before emptying into the subclavian and internal jugular veins. *An understanding of lymphatic drainage assists in diagnosis of infection of endodontic origin.*

Innervation

The second and third divisions (V^2 and V^3) of the trigeminal nerve provide the principal sensory innervation to the pulp of maxillary and mandibular teeth, respectively. Mandibular premolars also can receive sensory branches from the mylohyoid nerve of V^3, which is principally a motor nerve. Branches from this nerve reach the teeth via small foramina on the lingual aspect of the mandible. Mandibular molars occasionally receive sensory innervation from the second and third cervical spinal nerves (C_2 and C_3).[42] This can create difficulties in anesthetizing these teeth with an inferior dental block injection only.

Cell bodies of trigeminal nerves are located in the trigeminal ganglion. Dendrites from these nerves synapse with neurons in the trigeminal nucleus at the base of the brain and upper spinal chord and then pass on to the higher centers.

Pulp also receives sympathetic (motor) innervation from T_1 and to some extent C_8 and T_2 via the superior cervical ganglion. These nerves enter the pulp space alongside the main pulp blood vessels. Other branches from the superior cervical ganglion supply the periodontium, oral mucosa, and skin.[43] Activation of these nerves causes vasoconstriction and reduction of pulpal blood flow. Without activation there is a passive vasodilation.

NEUROANATOMY
Pulpal and Dentinal Nerves

Sensory nerves supplying the dental pulp are mixed nerves containing both myelinated and

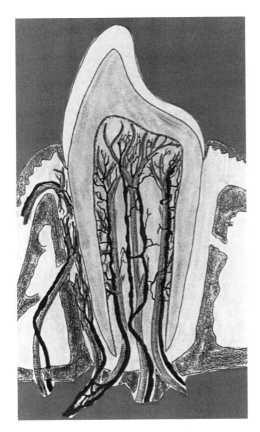

FIGURE 2-17
Lymph drainage *(black vessels)* is depicted in immature dental pulp. Note the confluence with periodontal lymphatics. (Courtesy Dr. A. Goerig.)

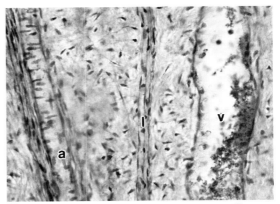

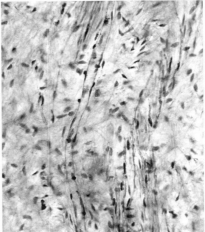

FIGURE 2-18
Lymphatic vessel in pulp *(l)* associated with an arteriole *(a)* and a venule *(v)*. (Courtesy Dr. S. Bernick.)

unmyelinated axons (Figure 2-19). Myelinated axons are classified according to diameter and conduction velocity. Among these the Aδ axons (diameter 1 to 6 μm), which are slow-conducting myelinated nerves, are the most numerous. A small percentage of the myelinated axons (1% to 5%) are faster-conducting Aβ axons (diameter 6 to 12 μm). The Aβ group can be touch or pressure sensitive. Myelinated sensory nerves give off an increasing number of branches as they ascend coronally. Ultimately they lose their myelin sheath and terminate as small unmyelinated branches either below the odontoblasts, around the odontoblasts, or alongside the odontoblast process in the dentinal tubule (Figure 2-20). There they form a syncytium of nerves called the subodontoblastic plexus of Raschkow (Figure 2-21). Stimulation of these fibers results in a fast, sharp pain that is relatively well localized. This plexus is best visualized histologically by the use of special staining methods.[44] The nerves that enter the dentinal tubules do not synapse with the process but remain in close proximity with it

for only part of its length. Approximately 27% of the tubules in the area of the pulp horn a of a young, mature tooth contain an intratubular nerve. These nerves occur less often in the middle (11%) and cervical portions (8%) of the crown and not at all in the root. Their incidence is higher in predentin than in mineralized dentin.[45]

Nonmyelinated nociceptive axons, or c fibers (diameter <1 μm), are the most numerous and are found chiefly in the pulp core. Their conduction velocity is slower than the Aδ fibers, and stimulation of these fibers produces pain that is slower in onset and dull and diffuse in nature.

DEVELOPMENTAL ASPECTS OF PULP INNERVATION

The types and relative number of nerves depend on the state of tooth maturity.[5,46] Myelinated nerves enter the pulp about the same time as un-

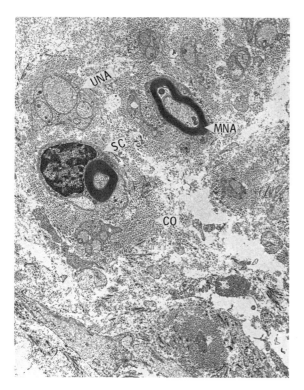

FIGURE 2-19
Pulp nerves in region of the pulp core. A group of unmyelinated *(UNA)* and myelinated *(MNA)* nerve axons are shown in cross section. A Schwann cell *(SC)* associated with one of the myelinated axons is evident. Nerves are surrounded by collagen fibers *(CO)*.

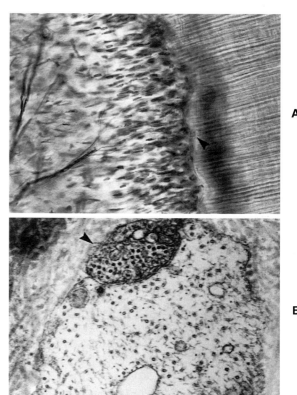

FIGURE 2-20
A, Silver-stained section of pulp in a young human molar demonstrates arborization of nerves in the subodontoblastic region and a nerve *(arrow)* passing between odontoblasts into the predentin area. (Courtesy Dr. S. Bernick.) **B,** Transmission electron micrograph demonstrates an unmyelinated nerve axon *(arrow)* alongside the odontoblast process in the dentin tubule at the level of the predentin. (Courtesy Dr. G. R. Holland.)

myelinated nerves but, in most instances, do not form the subodontoblastic plexus until some time after tooth eruption has occurred. Because normal responses to various pulp-testing modalities depend on a fully developed and functional subodontoblastic plexus of nerves, significant variations in responses of partially developed teeth to such testing modalities can occur. *This undermines the value of stimulatory tests for determining pulp status in young patients particularly after trauma.*[47]

Intratubular nerves as well as the overall number of pulpal nerves diminish with chronologic (55+ years) and physiologic tooth aging. *The significance of this reduction in terms of pulp response to testing is undetermined.*

Pathways of Transmission from Pulp to Central Nervous System

Mechanical, thermal, and chemical stimuli initiate an impulse that travels along the pulpal axons in the maxillary (V^2) or mandibular (V^3) branches of the trigeminal nerve to the trigeminal (Gasserian) ganglion, which contains the cell body of the neuron. Dendrites from the ganglion then pass centrally and synapse with second-level neurons in the trigeminal nuclear complex located at the base of the medulla and the upper end of the spinal cord. Most of the painful stimuli that originate in the dental pulp are conducted along axons that synapse with neurons in the spinal portion of the complex most notably, the subnucleus caudalis. Other stimuli travel along axons that synapse with neurons that are located in other spinal nuclei (oralis and interoralis) and in the main sensory nucleus located in the base of the brain.

Some neurons in the trigeminal nuclear complex receive only nociceptive impulses; these are know as nociceptive specific neurons; others, known as wide dynamic range neurons, receive both nociceptive and tactile input. Several peripheral axons may converge on a single secondary

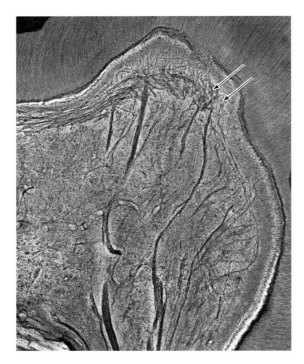

FIGURE 2-21
Silver-stained section of pulp in a young human molar. Large nerve bundles can be identified in the pulp core. These branch and form the subodontoblastic plexus (plexus of Raschkow), identified by *arrows* in the cell-free zone. (Courtesy Dr. S. Bernick.)

neuron, bringing input from several peripheral areas to one second-level site.[48] Information into and out of that neuron is determined by the interaction of stimuli conducted along larger and smaller fibers and the modulating effect of descending input from higher centers of the brain. This can markedly influence the pain experience in terms of intensity and localization.[49] Information recorded at the second-level site then travels to reflex centers and to the opposite side of the brain where it is carried via the trigeminothalamic tract to the thalamus and the cortex. *Pain can be modified by psychologic as well as neurologic factors; the complexity of all the combinations possible makes the experience distinctive to each individual.*

THEORIES OF DENTIN HYPERSENSITIVITY

Pain elicited by scraping or cutting of dentin or by application of cold or hypertonic solutions gives the impression that there may be a nerve pathway from the central nervous system to the DEJ. However, no direct pathway has been identified; application of pain-producing substances such as histamine, acetylcholine, or potassium chloride to the dentin surface fails to produce pain. Furthermore, when pain exists, application of local anesthetic to dentin gives no relief.

Because of variations in the response of dentin to normal sensory stimuli, the mechanism responsible for its sensitivity is unknown. Several theories have been proposed. Each theory has shortcomings, which supports the premise that more than one mechanism may be responsible. The three mechanisms that have been considered are (1) *direct innervation of dentin*, (2) *odontoblasts as receptors*, and (3) *hydrodynamic theory* (Figure 2-22).

Direct Innervation

Nerves are present in dentin. However, these nerves are present only in the predentin and the inner third of the mineralized dentin. They are not present in the outer third, at the DEJ or the DCJ, which appear to be highly sensitive areas. Furthermore, unlike other innervated sites, when pain-producing and pain-relieving substances are applied to dentin they fail to elicit an action potential (nerve response). The consensus, therefore, is that although nerves of trigeminal origin are found in dentin, direct stimulation of these nerves is unlikely to be the principal mechanism involved in dentin sensitivity.

Odontoblasts as Receptors

This theory was initially considered when it was discovered that odontoblasts were of neural crest origin and that staining of odontoblasts for acetylcholine was positive. However, later research showed that the odontoblast process extended only part way through dentin and that the membrane potential of the odontoblast was too low to permit transduction. The theory, however, did regain some credibility when it was discovered that in some teeth the process did extend through the full thickness of dentin and that gap junctions (which permit electronic coupling) did exist between odontoblasts and possibly between odontoblasts and nerves.[50] Currently, there is little support for the transduction theory.

Hydrodynamic Theory

The hydrodynamic theory, as originally proposed by Brännström and Aström,[51] satisfies most of the experimental and morphologic data associated with dentin sensitivity. The theory postulates that rapid movement of fluid in the dentinal tubules (inward or outward) results in distortion of nerve endings in the subodontoblastic nerve

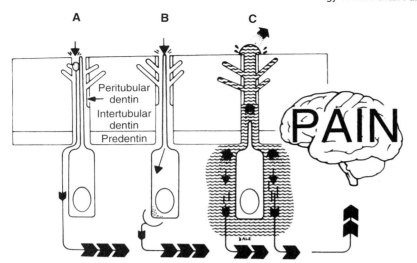

FIGURE 2-22
Schematic drawing of theoretic mechanisms of dentin sensitivity. *A,* Classic theory (direct stimulation of nerve fibers in the dentin). *B,* Odontoblasts as a mediator between the stimuli and the nerve fibers. *C,* Fluid movement as proposed in hydrodynamic theory. (Modified from Torneck CD: Dentin-pulp complex. In Ten Cate AR, editor, *Oral histology,* ed 4, St Louis, 1994, Mosby.)

plexus (plexus of Raschkow) that generates an neural impulse and a sensation of pain. When dentin is cut, or when hypertonic solutions are placed on a cut dentin surface, fluid moves outward and pain is initiated. Procedures that block tubules (such as applying resin to the dentin surface or the buildup of crystals within the tubule lumen appear to interrupt fluid flow and reduce sensitivity.[52]

In intact teeth the application of hot and cold to the tooth surface produces different contraction rates in dentin and dentinal fluid; this results in fluid movement and initiation of pain. This response is exaggerated when dentin is exposed.

The hydrodynamic theory has been accepted but not without obvious criticism. It requires the presence of a subodontoblastic nerve plexus, yet dentin hypersensitivity occurs in teeth with a severely damaged pulp. The "fluid" in the tubules of intact dentin may be a relatively dense hydrogel with little hydraulic conductivity rather than simple tissue fluid as first proposed by Brannström. Finally sensitivity produced by application of hot and cold can be explained by the presence of pulp thermoreceptors and by the hydrodynamic theory.

Age Changes in the Dental Pulp

Pulp, like other connective tissues, undergoes changes with time. Some of these changes are natural (chronologic), whereas others may be a result of injury (pathophysiologic) such as caries, periodontal disease, trauma, or restorative dental procedures. Regardless of the cause, changes in pulp appearance (morphologic changes) and in pulp function (physiologic changes) do occur.

MORPHOLOGIC CHANGES

The most obvious morphologic change seen in chronologic aging of the pulp is a progressive reduction in the volume of cellular elements in the pulp space. This occurs as a result of continued deposition of dentin (secondary and tertiary dentinogenesis) and pulp stone formation. Secondary dentin formation is asymmetrical. In the pulp chamber of molars, for example, there is greater deposition on the roof and floor than on the proximal, facial, and lingual (palatal walls). Root canals also become smaller and threadlike in size. Pulp stone formation reduces the space further and restricts access to the apical foramen. Contrary to popular belief, no correlation has been established between pulp stones and dental pain. Pulp volume may also be disproportionately reduced by the deposition of irregular (reparative) dentin in response to odontoblast injury. While the radiographic image of teeth affected by injury may show absence of a pulp space, histologic examination of these teeth often reveals one to be present.[53]

Aging also results in a reduction in number of pulp cells. Between the ages of 20 and 70, cell density decreases by approximately 50%. This reduction affects all cells, from the highly differentiated odontoblast to the undifferentiated reserve cell. In addition, reduced formative activity leads to a reduction in the size and synthesizing capacity of odontoblasts.

The number of nerves and blood vessels is also decreased. Furthermore blood vessels often display arteriosclerotic changes, and an increased incidence of calcification in the collagen bundles that surround the larger vessels and nerves. *The decrease in sensory innervation may be partially responsible for a deceased responsiveness to pulp testing in older patients.*

PHYSIOLOGIC CHANGES

Aging of the pulp-dentin complex results in a decrease in dentin permeability through a progressive reduction in tubule diameter (dentin sclerosis) and through a decrease in tubule patency (dead tract formation). This provides a more protected environment for the pulp and may diminish the injurious effect of conditions such as caries, attrition, and periodontal disease.

Periradicular Tissues

The periodontium, the tissues surrounding and investing the root of the tooth consists of the cementum, periodontal ligament, and alveolar bone (Figure 2-23). These tissues originate from the dental follicle that surrounds the enamel organ; their formation is initiated when root development begins. After the tooth has erupted, the cervical portion of the tooth is in contact with the epithelium of the gingiva, which in combination with reduced dental epithelium on the enamel forms the *dentogingival junction*. When intact, this junction protects the underlying periodontium from potential irritants in the oral cavity.

The pulp and the periodontium form a continuum at sites along the root where blood vessels enter and exit the pulp such as the apical foramen and lateral and accessory canals (Figure 2-24). At times it is difficult to determine where the pulp ends and the periodontium begins.

CEMENTUM

Cementum is a bone-like tissue that covers the root and provides attachment for the principal periodontal fibers. Several types of cementum have been identified.

1. *Primary acellular intrinsic fiber cementum.* This is the first cementum formed, and it is present before principle periodontal fibers are fully formed. It extends from the cervical margin to the cervical third of the tooth in some teeth and around the entire root in others (incisors and cuspids). It is more mineralized on the surface than near the dentin and it contains collagen produced initially by cementoblasts and later by the fibroblasts.

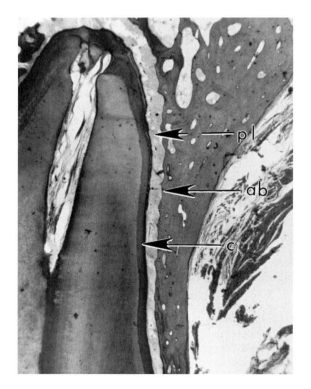

FIGURE 2-23
Maxillary root surrounded by periodontal ligament *(pl)* and alveolar bone proper *(ab)*. Periodontal fibers are inserted into cementum *(c)* on the tooth and into alveolar bone.

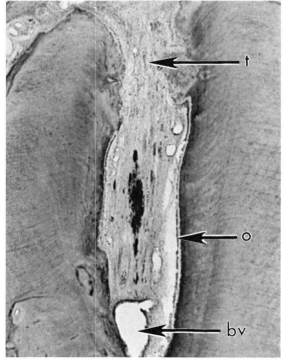

FIGURE 2-24
Apical region of maxillary incisor showing apical foramen. *t,* Transitional tissue between periodontal ligament and pulp; *o,* odontoblasts; *bv,* blood vessel.

2. *Primary acellular extrinsic fiber cementum.* This is cementum that continues to be formed about the primary periodontal fibers after they have been incorporated into primary acellular intrinsic fiber cementum.

3. *Secondary cellular intrinsic fiber cementum.* This cementum is bone-like in appearance and only plays a minor role in fiber attachment. It occurs most often in the apical part of the root of premolars and molars.

4. *Secondary cellular mixed fiber cementum.* This is an adaptive type of cellular cementum that incorporates periodontal fibers as they continue to develop. It is variable in its distribution and extent and can be recognized by the inclusion of cementocytes, its laminated appearance, and the presence of cementoid on its surface.

5. *Acellular afibrillar cementum.* This is the cementum seen on enamel, which plays no role in fiber attachment.

Although sometimes cellular, cementum is not vascularized and appears to resist resorption more than bone. Cementum formation is a continuing process and is influenced by changes in tooth position and function.

As mentioned earlier in this chapter the junction between the cementum and the dentin *(cementodentinal junction)* is ill defined and not uniform throughout its circumference. Despite this the CDJ is often cited as the point at which root canal procedures should terminate especially when the status of the periodontium is normal. *Although many practitioners debate the probabilities and practicalities of achieving this goal, most agree that it is essential to measure canal length accurately and to restrict all procedures to the determined canal length.*

Despite the relative resistance of cementum, inflammatory lesions in the periodontal ligament and surrounding bone can cause cementum resorption. If inflammation is eliminated, however, resorption sites generally undergo repair and the integrity of the periodontium is restored. Mechanical pressure such as orthodontic movement can cause cementum resorption. This is a noninflammatory type of resorption and also can undergo repair after pressures have returned to physiologic levels. Occasionally cementum undergoes resorption without an identifiable cause. This is referred to as idiopathic resorption. This resorption can be self-limiting or it may progress and lead to loss of dentin.

CEMENTOENAMEL JUNCTION

It was once thought that the junction between enamel and cementum occurred in one of three patterns at the cervical part of the tooth: (1) butt junction, (2) gap between the two, and (3) overlap of cementum on enamel. Recent studies however, have shown that all three appear to occur at different sites along the CEJ when the circumference of the junction is examined.[53] *It is possible that a significant discrepancy between cementum and enamel at the CEJ can lead to an increased risk of dentin sensitivity.*

PERIODONTAL LIGAMENT

Periodontal ligament (PDL), like dental pulp, is a specialized connective tissue. Its function relates in part to the presence of specially arranged bundles of collagen fibers that support the tooth in the socket and absorb the forces of occlusion from being transmitted to the surrounding bone. The PDL space is small, varying from an average of 0.21 mm in young teeth to 0.15 mm in older teeth.[48] Its uniformity (as visualized in a radiograph) is one of the criteria used to determine its health.

Lining the periodontal space are cementoblasts and osteoblasts. Interwoven between the principal periodontal fibers is a loose connective tissue that contains fibroblasts, reserve cells, macrophages, osteoclasts, blood vessels, nerves, and lymphatics. Epithelial cell rests of Malassez are also present (Figure 2-25). As already noted, these cells are of no known significance in the healthy periodontium but can, during inflammatory states, proliferate and give rise to cyst formation.

The vasculature of the periodontium is extensive and complex. Arterioles that supply the PDL arise from the superior and inferior alveolar branches of the maxillary artery in the cancellous bone. These arterioles pass through small openings in the alveolar bone of the socket, at times accompanied by nerves, and extend upward and downward throughout the periodontal space. They are more prevalent in posterior than anterior teeth. Other vessels arise from the gingiva or from dental vessels that supply the pulp; these latter vessels branch and extend upward into the periodontal space before the pulpal vessels pass through the apical foramen. The degree of collateral blood supply to the PDL and the depth of its cell resources impart an excellent potential for its repair subsequent to injury, a potential that is retained for life in the absence of systemic or prolonged local disease.

The periodontium receives autonomic and sensory innervation. Autonomic nerves are sympathetic nerves that arise from the superior cervical ganglion and terminate in the smooth muscle of the periodontal arterioles. Activation of the sympathetic fibers induces constriction of the vessels. As in the pulp, there is no convincing evidence that a parasympathetic nerve supply exists.

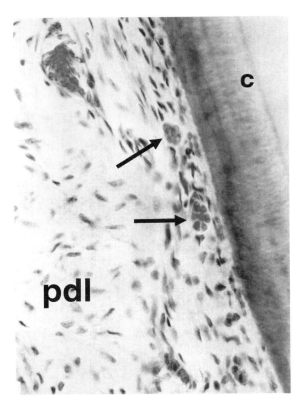

FIGURE 2-25
Epithelial cell rests of Malassez *(arrows)*, in the periodontal space at the level of mid root. *pdl*, Periodontal ligament, *c*, cementum.

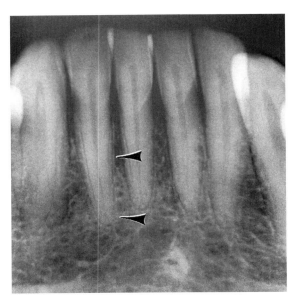

FIGURE 2-26
Mandibular anterior teeth with normal, uniform periodontal ligament space and identifiable lamina dura *(arrows)*. This usually, but not always, indicates the absence of periradicular inflammation.

Sensory nerves that supply the periodontium arise from the second and third divisions (V^2 and V^3) of the trigeminal nerve. They are principally mixed nerves of large and small diameter. Large fibers are $A\beta$ fibers, whereas small fibers are $A\delta$ fibers and unmyelinated C fibers. Small fibers terminate as free endings and mediate pain sensation. Large fibers are mechanoreceptors and terminate in special endings throughout the ligament but are in greatest concentration in the apical third of the periodontal space.[54] These are highly sensitive and record pressures in the ligament associated with micro and macro tooth movements.[55] The ability of patients to identify inflammation in the periodontium is a learned experience not a physiologic one.

ALVEOLAR BONE

The bone of the jaws is referred to as the *alveolar process*. Bone that lines the socket and into which the principle periodontal fibers are anchored is referred to as *alveolar bone proper* (bundle bone, cribriform plate). Alveolar bone is perforated to accommodate vessels, nerves, and investing connective tissues that pass from the cancellous portion of the alveolar process to the periodontal space. Despite these perforations alveolar bone proper is denser than the surrounding cancellous bone and has a distinct opaque appearance when imaged in a dental radiograph. On the radiograph, alveolar bone proper is referred to as lamina dura (Figure 2-26). Its presence is equated with periodontal health and its absence (attenuation) with disease. However, radiographic changes associated with periradicular inflammatory disease usually follow, rather than accompany the disease. The lesion is usually present before it is visible radiographically. Significant bone loss is necessary before a radiographic image is seen.

Alveolar bone proper is principally lamellar bone that continually adapts to the stress of tooth movements. Because pressures are not constant, bone is constantly remodeling (bone resorption and apposition). *Current concepts of host response to periodontal infections identify an alteration in this bone remodeling as the principal cause of the associated bone loss.*[56]

REFERENCES

1. Ruch JV: Odontoblast differentiation and the formation of the odontoblast layer, *J Dent Res* 64:489, 1985.
2. Begue-Kirn C, Smith AJ, Loriot M, et al: Comparison analysis of TGFβ1, BMPs, IGF1, msxs, osteonectin,

and bone sialoprotein gene expression during normal and in vitro-induced odontoblast differentiation, *Int J Dev Biol* 38:405, 1994.

3. Ruch JV: Patterned distribution of differentiating dental cells: Facts and hypotheses, *J Biol Buccale* 18:91, 1990.

4. Kawasaki K, Tanaka S, Ishikawa T: On the daily incremental lines in human dentine, *Arch Oral Biol* 24:939, 1980.

5. Johnsen DC, Harshburger J, Rymer HD: Quantitative assessment of neural development in human premolars, *Anat Rec* 205:421, 1983.

6. Lindskog S: Formation of intermediate cementum. II. A scanning electron microscopic study of the epithelial root sheath of Hertwig in the monkey, *J Craniofac Genet Dev Biol* 2:161, 1982.

7. Ten Cate AR: The epithelial cell rests of Malassez and genesis of the dental cyst, *Oral Surg Oral Med Oral Pathol* 34:956, 1972.

8. Kuttler Y: Microscopic investigation of root apices, *J Am Dent Assoc* 50:544, 1955.

9. Hammarström L: Enamel matrix, cementum development and regeneration, *J Clin Periodontol* 24:658, 1997.

10. Lambritchs I, Creemers J, van Steenberghe D: Morphology of neural endings in the periodontal ligament. An electron microscopic study, *J Periodontol Res* 27:191, 1992.

11. Min-Kai Wu, Wesselink PR, Walton RE: Apical terminus location of root canal treatment procedures, *Oral Surg Oral Med Oral Pathol Oral Radiol Endod* 89:99, 2000.

12. Schroeder U, Sundstrom B: Transmission election microscopy of tissue changes following experimental pulpotomy of intact human teeth and capping with calcium hydroxide, *Odontol Rev* 25:1, 1974.

13. Rutherford RB, Wahle J, Tucker M, et al: Induction of reparative dentine formation in monkeys by recombinant human osteogenic protein. *Arch Oral Biol* 38:571, 1993.

14. Narhi MVO: The characteristics of interdental sensory units and their responses to stimulation, *J Dent Res* 64:564, 1985.

15. Kollman W, Mijatovic E: Age dependent changes in thermoperception in human anterior teeth, *Arch Oral Biol* 30:711, 1985.

16. Couve E: Ultrastructural changes during the life cycle of human odontoblasts, *Arch Oral Biol* 31:643, 1986.

17. Brannström M, Garberoglio R: The dentinal tubules and the odontoblast process, a scanning electron microscopic study, *Acta Odontol Scand* 30:291, 1972.

18. Sigal MJ, Aubin JE, Ten Cate AR: A combined scanning electron microscopy and immunofluorescence study demonstrating that the odontoblast process extends to the dentinoenamel junction in human teeth, *Anat Rec* 210:453, 1984.

19. Turner DF, Marfurt CF, Sattelburg C: Demonstration of physiological barrier between pulpal odontoblasts and its perturbation following routine restorative procedures, *J Dent Res* 68:1262, 1989.

20. Koling A: Freeze fracture electron microscopy of simultaneous odontoblast exocytosis and endocytosis in human permanent teeth, *Arch Oral Biol* 32:153, 1987.

21. Tziafas D, Alvanou A, Panagiotakopoulos N, et al: Induction of odontoblast-like cell differentiation in dog dental pulps after in vivo implantation of dentin matrix components, *Arch Oral Biol* 40:883, 1995.

22. Torneck CD: Intracellular destruction of collagen in the human dental pulp, *Arch Oral Biol* 23:745, 1978.

23. Torneck CD, Wagner D: The effect of calcium hydroxide cavity liner on early cell division in the pulp subsequent to cavity preparation and restoration, *J Endod* 6:719, 1980.

24. Jontell M, Bergenholtz G: Accessory cells in the immune defense of the dental pulp, *Proc Finn Dent Soc* 88:345, 1992.

25. Linde A: Dentin matrix proteins: composition and possible functions in calcification, *Anat Rec* 224:154, 1989.

26. Tsuzaki M, Yamauchi M, Mechanic GL: Bovine dental pulp collagens: characterization of types III and V collagen, *Arch Oral Biol* 35:195, 1990.

27. Moss-Salentijn L, Hendricks-Klyvert M: Calcified structures in the human dental pulps, *J Endod* 14:184, 1988.

28. Kramer IRH: The vascular architecture of the human dental pulp, *Arch Oral Biol* 2:177, 1960.

29. Harris R, Griffin CJ: The ultrastructure of small blood vessels of the normal dental pulp, *Aust Dent J* 16:220, 1971.

30. Takahashi K, Kishi Y, Kim S: A scanning electron microscope study of the blood vessels of dog pulp using corrosion resin casts, *J Endod* 8:132, 1982.

31. Saunders RL, de CH: X ray microscopy of the periodontal and dental pulp vessels in the monkey and in man, *Oral Surg Oral Med Oral Pathol* 22:503, 1966.

32. Kim S: Microcirculation of the dental pulp in health and disease, *J Endod* 11:465, 1985.

33. Gazelius B, Olgart L, Edwall B, Edwall L: Non-invasive recording of blood flow in human dental pulp, *Endod Dent Traumatol* 2:219, 1986.

34. Tonder K, Naess G: Nervous control of blood flow in the dental pulp in dogs, *Acta Physiol Scand* 104:13, 1978.

35. Tonder KJH, Kvinsland I: Micropuncture measurements of interstitial fluid pressure in normal and inflamed dental pulp in cats, *J Endod* 9:105, 1983.

36. Heyeraas KJ, Kvinsland I: Tissue pressure and blood flow in pulp inflammation, *Proc Finn Dent Soc* 88(suppl):393, 1992.

37. Olgart L, Gazelius B: Effects of adrenalin and felypressin (octapressin) on blood flow and sensory nerve activity in the tooth, *Acta Odontol Scand* 35:69, 1977.

38. Grutzner E, Garry M, Hargreaves KM. Effect of injury on levels of immunoreactive substance P and CGRP, *J Endod* 18:553, 1992.

39. Walton R, Langeland K: Migration of materials in dental pulp of monkeys, *J Endod* 4:167, 1978.

40. Bernick S: Morphological changes in lymphatic vessels in pulpal inflammation, *J Dent Res* 56:841, 1977.

41. Marchetti C, Poggi P, Calligaro A, Casasco A: Lymphatic vessels in the healthy human dental pulp, *Acta Anat (Basel)* 140:329, 1991.

42. Bolding SL, Hutchins B: Histological evidence for a cervical plexus contribution to the cat mandibular dentition, *Arch Oral Biol* 38:619, 1993.

43. Mumford JM: *Orofacial pain: etiology, diagnosis and treatment*, ed 3, New York, 1982, Churchill-Livingstone.

44. Bernick S: Innervation of the human tooth, *Anat Rec* 101:81, 1948.

45. Lilja T: Innervation of different parts of predentin and dentin in young human premolars, *Acta Odont Scand* 37:339, 1979.

46. Peckham K, Torabinejad M, Peckham N: Presence of nerve fibers in the coronal odontoblast layer of teeth at various stages of root development, *Int Endod J* 24:303, 1991.

47. Klein H: Pulp responses to an electric pulp stimulator in the developing permanent anterior dentition, *J Dent Child* 45:23, 1978.

48. Dostrovsky JO: An electrophysiological study of canine, premolar and molar tooth pulp afferents and their convergence on medullary trigeminal neurons, *Pain* 19:1, 1984.

49. Sessle BJ, Hu JW, Amano N, Zhong G: Convergence of cutaneous, tooth pulp visceral, neck and muscle afferents into nociceptive and non-nociceptive neurons in trigeminal subnucleus caudalis (medullary dorsal horn) and its implications for referred pain, *Pain* 27:219, 1987.

50. Koling A, Rask-Andersen H: Membrane junctions in the subodontoblastic region, *Acta Odontol Scand* 41:99, 1983.

51. Brannström M, Astrom A: The hydrodynamics of the dentine: its possible relationship to dentinal pain, *Int Dent J* 22:219, 1972.

52. Pashley D: Dentin permeability and dentin sensitivity, *Proc Finn Dent Soc* 88:31, 1992.

53. Freeman E: Periodontium. In Ten Cate AR, editor: *Oral histology, development, structure, and function*, ed 4, St Louis, 1994, Mosby.

54. Cash RM, Linden RW: The distribution of mechanoreceptors in the periodontal ligament of the mandibular canine tooth of the cat, *J Physiol (Lond)* 330:439, 1982.

55. Cash RM, Linden RW: Effects of sympathetic nerve stimulation on intra-oral mechanoreceptor activity in the cat, *J Physiol (Lond)* 330:451, 1982.

56. Okada H, Murakami S, Cytokine expression in periodontal health and disease, *Crit Rev Oral Biol Med* 9:498, 1998.

Pulp and Periradicular Pathosis

LEARNING OBJECTIVES

After reading this chapter, the student should be able to:

1 / Identify etiologic factors causing pulp inflammation.

2 / Explain the mechanism of spread of inflammation in the pulp.

3 / Explain why pulp has difficulty in recovering from severe injury.

4 / List specific and nonspecific mediators of pulpal inflammation.

5 / Classify pulpal diseases and their clinical and histologic features.

6 / Describe the mechanisms and explain the consequences of the spread of pulpal inflammation into periradicular tissues and the subsequent inflammatory and immunologic responses.

7 / Classify periradicular lesions of pulpal origin.

8 / Identify and distinguish between histologic features and clinical signs and symptoms of acute apical periodontitis, chronic apical periodontitis, acute and chronic apical abscesses (suppurative apical periodontitis), and condensing osteitis.

9 / Describe the steps involved in repair of periradicular pathosis after successful root canal treatment.

10 / Identify and describe, in general, nonendodontic pathologic lesions that may simulate endodontic periradicular pathosis.

OUTLINE

Irritants
  Microbial Irritants
  Mechanical Irritants
  Chemical Irritants

Pulpal Pathosis
  Inflammatory Process
  Immunologic Response
  Lesion Progression

Classification of Pulpal Diseases
  Reversible Pulpitis
  Irreversible Pulpitis
  Hard Tissue Changes Caused by Pulpal
    Inflammation
  Pulpal Necrosis

Periradicular Pathosis
  Nonspecific Mediators of Periradicular
    Lesions
  Specific Mediators of Periradicular Lesions

Classification of Periradicular Lesions
  Acute Apical Periodontitis
  Chronic Apical Periodontitis
  Condensing Osteitis
  Acute Apical Abscess
  Chronic Apical Abscess (Suppurative Apical
    Periodontitis)

**Healing of Periradicular Lesions Following
  Root Canal Treatment**
  Extent of Healing
  Process of Healing

Nonendodontic Periradicular Pathosis
  Differential Diagnosis
  Normal and Pathologic Entities

Irritants

Irritation of pulpal or periradicular tissues results in inflammation. The major irritants of these tissues can be divided into living and nonliving irritants. The living irritants are various microorganisms and viruses. The nonliving irritants include mechanical, thermal, and chemical irritants.

MICROBIAL IRRITANTS

Microorganisms present in the dental caries are the main sources of irritation of the dental pulp and periradicular tissues. Carious dentin and enamel contain numerous species of bacteria such as *Streptococcus mutans*, lactobacilli, and *Actinomyces*.[1] The population of microorganisms decreases to few or none in the deepest layers of carious dentin.[2] However, direct pulp exposure to microorganisms is not a prerequisite for pulpal response and inflammation. Microorganisms in caries produce toxins that penetrate to the pulp through tubules. Studies have shown that even small lesions in enamel are capable of attracting inflammatory cells in the pulp.[3,4] As a result of the presence of microorganisms and their by-products in dentin, pulp is infiltrated locally (at the base of tubules involved in caries) primarily by chronic inflammatory cells such as macrophages, lymphocytes, and plasma cells. As the decay progresses toward the pulp, the intensity and character of the infiltrate change.

When actual exposure occurs, the pulp tissue is infiltrated locally by polymorphonuclear (PMN) leukocytes to form an area of liquefaction necrosis at the site of exposure (Figure 3-1).[5] After pulp exposure, bacteria colonize and persist at the site

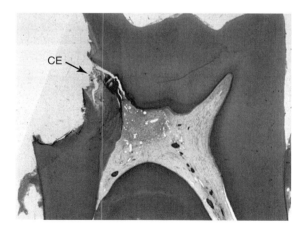

FIGURE 3-1
A localized inflammatory reaction containing mainly polymorphonuclear leukocytes *(arrow)* at the site of a carious pulpal exposure *(CE)*. The remainder of the coronal pulp is almost free of inflammatory cells. (Courtesy Dr. JH Simon.)

of necrosis. Pulpal tissue may stay inflamed for a long period of time and may undergo necrosis eventually or become necrotic quickly. This depends on several factors: (1) the virulence of bacteria, (2) the ability to release inflammatory fluids to avoid a marked increase in intrapulpal pressure, (3) host resistance, (4) amount of circulation, and (5) most important, lymph drainage. Yamasaki et al.[6] created pulpal exposure in rats and showed that necrosis extended gradually from the upper portion of pulp to the apex. A periapical lesion ensued after pulpal inflammation and necrosis. The lesions extended first horizontally and then vertically before their expansion ceased.

As a consequence of exposure to the oral cavity and to caries, pulp harbors bacteria and their byproducts. Pulp usually cannot eliminate these damaging irritants. At best, defenses temporarily halt or slow the spread of infection and tissue destruction. Sooner or later the damage will become extensive and will spread throughout the pulp. Then, bacteria or their by-products and other irritants from necrotic pulp will diffuse from the canal periapically, resulting in development of severe inflammatory lesions (Figure 3-2).

Bacteria play an important role in the pathogenesis of pulp and periradicular pathoses. A number of investigations have established that pulpal and/or periradicular pathosis does not develop without the presence of bacterial contamination.[7-10] Kakehashi et al.[7] created pulpal exposures in conventional and gnotobiotic (germ-free) rats. This procedure in the germ-free rats caused only minimal inflammation throughout the 72-day investigation. Pulpal tissue in these animals was not completely devitalized but rather showed calcific bridge formation by day 14, with normal tissue apical to the dentin bridge (Figure 3-3, A). In contrast, autoinfection, pulpal necrosis, and abscess formation

occurred by the eighth day in conventional rats (Figure 3-3, B).

Other investigators have examined the importance of bacteria in the development of periradicular lesions by sealing noninfected and infected

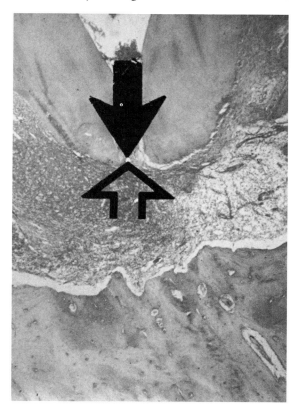

FIGURE 3-2
Egress of irritants *(closed arrow)* from the root canal into the periapical tissue causes inflammation *(open arrow)* and replacement of normal periradicular structures with a granulomatous tissue.

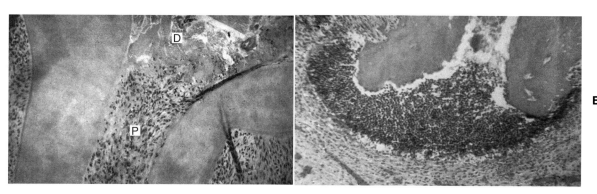

FIGURE 3-3
A, No inflammation is seen in an exposed pulp (P) of a germ-free rat. Food particles and other debris (D) are packed into the chamber. **B,** Periradicular lesion is apparent in a conventional rat after pulp exposure. (Courtesy Dr. H. Stanley.)

pulps in canals of monkeys.[8] After 6 to 7 months, clinical, radiographic, and histologic examination of teeth sealed with noninfected pulps showed an absence of pathosis in periradicular tissues, whereas teeth sealed with necrotic pulps containing certain bacteria showed periapical inflammation. The bacteriological investigations by Bergenholtz[9] and Sundqvist[10] examining the flora of human necrotic pulps support the findings of Kakehashi et al.[7] as well as those of Moller and Fabricius.[8] These studies examined previously traumatized teeth with necrotic pulps with and without periradicular pathosis. Canals in teeth without apical lesions were aseptic, whereas those with periapical pathosis had positive bacterial cultures.

Examination of the amount of microbial inoculum had demonstrated that higher levels of contamination led to greater inflammatory responses.[11] In contrast, lower levels of contamination led to milder responses and a tendency for healing and repair of pulpal and/or periapical tissues. A further relationship between the presence of bacteria and inflammatory reactions became apparent when bacteria were placed in cavities prepared in the dentin.[12] This experiment showed that bacterial compounds can permeate through the dentin and cause pulpal inflammation without direct pulpal exposure.

MECHANICAL IRRITANTS

In addition to bacterial irritation, pulp or periradicular tissues can also be irritated mechanically. Deep cavity preparations, removal of tooth structure without proper cooling, impact trauma, occlusal trauma, deep periodontal curettage, and orthodontic movement of teeth are the main thermal and physical irritants of the pulp tissue. If proper precautions are not taken, cavity or crown preparations damage subjacent odontoblasts (Figure 3-4). The number of tubules per unit surface area and their diameter increase closer to the pulp. As a result, dentinal permeability is greater closer to pulp than near the dentinoenamel junction or cementodentinal junction.[13,14] Therefore the potential for pulp irritation increases as more dentin is removed (i.e., as cavity preparation deepens). Pulp damage is roughly proportional to the amount of tooth structure removed as well as to the depth of removal.[15] Also, operative procedures without water coolant cause more irritation than those performed under water spray.[16] Reactions and vascular changes occurring in experimentally induced acute and chronic pulpitis demonstrated increased permeability and dilation of blood vessels in the early stages of pulpitis.[17]

Impact injury with or without crown or root fractures may cause pulpal damage (see Chapter 25). The severity of trauma and degree of apical closure are important factors in recovery of the pulp. Teeth undergoing mild to moderate trauma and those with immature apexes have a better chance of pulpal survival than those suffering severe injury or those with closed apexes.

Application of forces beyond the physiologic tolerance of the periodontal ligament during orthodontics results in disturbance of the blood and nerve supply of pulp tissue.[18,19] The resulting changes include atrophy of cells and alteration of nerve axons. In addition, orthodontic movement may initiate resorption of the apex, usually without a change in vitality. Deep scaling and curettage may injure apical vessels and nerves, resulting in pulpal damage (see Chapter 26).

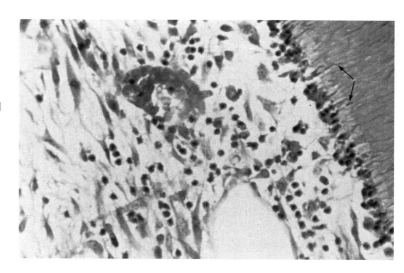

FIGURE 3-4
Crown preparation through enamel and into 1 mm of dentin resulted in aspiration of odontoblasts *(arrows)* into the tubules and infiltration of the pulp by PMN leukocytes and lymphocytes. The specimen was taken 48 hours after crown preparation.

The periradicular tissue can be mechanically irritated and inflamed by impact trauma, hyperocclusion, endodontic procedures and accidents, pulp extirpation, overinstrumentation, perforation of the root, and overextension of the filling materials. Mechanical irritation by instruments may occur during canal preparation. Inaccurate determination of canal length is usually the cause of overinstrumentation and inflammation. In addition, lack of an apical stop after cleaning and shaping can cause overextension of filling materials into the periapex, resulting in physical and chemical damage (Figure 3-5).

CHEMICAL IRRITANTS

Chemical irritants of the pulp include various dentin cleansing, sterilizing, and desensitizing substances as well as some of the substances present in temporary and permanent filling materials and cavity liners. Antibacterial agents such as silver nitrate, phenol with and without camphor, and eugenol were used in an attempt to "sterilize" the dentin after cavity preparations. However, their effectiveness as dentin sterilizers is questionable, and their cytotoxicity can cause inflammatory changes in underlying dental pulp.[20] Other irritating agents include cavity cleansers such as alcohol, chloroform, hydrogen peroxide, and various acids, chemicals present in desensitizers, cavity liners and bases, as well as temporary and permanent filling materials.

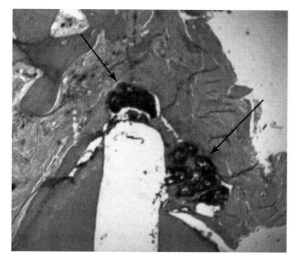

FIGURE 3-5
Improper instrumentation and extrusion of filling materials into the periapical tissues cause periradicular inflammation (*arrows*).

Antibacterial irrigants used during cleaning and shaping of root canals, intracanal medications, and some compounds present in obturating materials are examples of potential chemical irritants of periradicular tissues. Most irrigants and medicaments are toxic and are not biocompatible.[21,22]

Pulpal Pathosis

Apart from anatomic configuration and diversity of inflicted irritants, pulp reacts to these irritants as do other connective tissues. Pulpal injury results in cell death and inflammation. The degree of inflammation is proportional to the intensity and severity of tissue damage. Slight injuries, such as incipient caries or shallow cavity preparations, cause little or no inflammation in the pulp. In contrast, deep caries, extensive operative procedures, or persistent irritation usually produce more severe inflammatory changes. Depending on the severity and duration of the insult and the host response, the pulpal response ranges from transient inflammation (reversible pulpitis) to irreversible pulpitis and then to total necrosis. These changes often occur without pain and without the knowledge of patient or dentist.

INFLAMMATORY PROCESS

Irritation of the dental pulp results in activation of a variety of biologic systems such as nonspecific inflammatory reactions mediated by histamine, bradykinin, and arachidonic acid metabolites.[23] Also released are PMN lysosomal granule products (elastase, cathepsin G, and lactoferrin),[24] protease inhibitors such as antitrypsin,[25] and neuropeptides such as calcitonin gene-related peptide (CGRP) and substance P (SP).[26]

Unlike connective tissues in other parts of the body, normal and healthy dental pulps lack mast cells. However, these cells are found in inflamed pulp (Figure 3-6).[27] Mast cells contain histamine, leukotrienes, and platelet-activating factors. Physical injury to mast cells or bridging of two IgE molecules by an antigen on their cell surfaces results in the release of histamine and other bioactive substances present in mast cell granules. The presence of histamine in the blood vessel walls and a marked increase in histamine levels indicate the importance of histamine in pulpal inflammation.[28]

Kinins, which produce many signs and symptoms of acute inflammation, are produced when plasma or tissue kallikreins contact kininogens. Bradykinin, SP, and neurokinin A have been identified in dental pulp tissue using high-performance

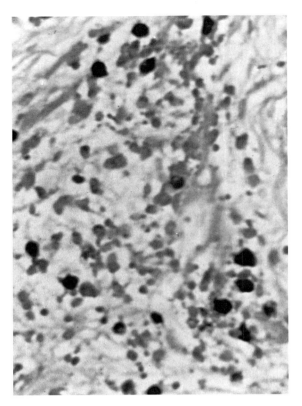

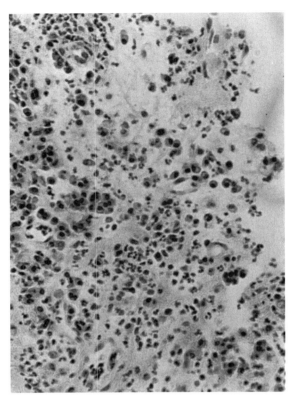

FIGURE 3-6
Mast cells are readily visible as dark-stained cells in this inflamed human dental pulp.

FIGURE 3-7
Numerous plasma cells stain positively for IgG in inflamed human dental pulp, indicating immunologic activity.

liquid chromatography.[29] A recent in vitro study showed that bradykinin evokes immunoreactive CGRP released from bovine dental pulp, which is also positively enhanced by prostaglandin E_2.[30] As a result of cellular damage, phospholipase A_2 causes release of arachidonic acid from cell membranes. Metabolism of arachidonic acid results in formation of various prostaglandins, thromboxanes, and leukotrienes. Various arachidonic acid metabolites have been found in experimentally induced pulpitis.[31] The presence of these metabolites in inflamed pulps[32,33] indicates that arachidonic acid metabolites participate in inflammatory reactions of the dental pulp.

The dental pulp is densely innervated with sensory fibers containing immunomodulatory neuropeptides such as SP and CGRP. Denervation of the rat molar pulp, caused by axotomy of the inferior alveolar nerve, resulted in enhanced pulp tissue damage and a decrease in infiltration of immunocompetent cells.[34] These findings indicate that pulpal nerves are protective in nature and that they may be involved in the recruitment of inflammatory/immunocompetent cells to the injured pulp.[34]

Mild to moderate pulpal injuries result in sprouting of sensory nerves with an increase in immunoreactive (i) CGRP.[26,35] However, severe injuries have the opposite effect, resulting in either reduction or elimination of iCGRP and SP.[35] These investigations indicate that pulpal neuropeptides undergo dynamic changes after injury. A number of recent studies have shown that stimulation of the dental pulp by caries results in the formation of various interleukins and recruitment of inflammatory cells to the site of injury.[36-40]

IMMUNOLOGIC RESPONSE

In addition to nonspecific inflammatory reactions, immune responses also may initiate and perpetuate pulpal diseases.[23] Potential antigens include bacteria and their by-products within dental caries, which directly (or via tubules) can initiate different types of reactions. Studies have shown that normal and uninflamed dental pulps contain immunocompetent cells such as T and B (fewer) lymphocytes, macrophages, and a substantial number of class II molecules expressing dendritic cells similar morphologically to macrophages.[34] Elevated levels of various immunoglobulins in inflamed pulps (Figure 3-7) show that these factors participate in defense mechanisms involved in protection of this

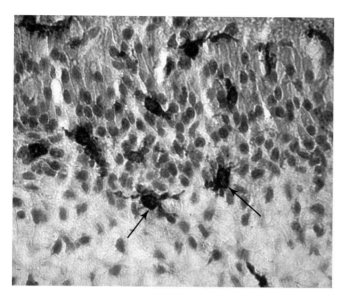

FIGURE 3-8
Many dendritic cells *(arrows)* are present in an inflamed dental pulp. (Courtesy Dr. M. Jontell.)

tissue.[41] Arthus-type reactions have been shown to occur in the dental pulp.[42] In addition, the presence of immunocompetent cells such as T lymphocytes, macrophages, and class II molecules expressing cells appearing as dendritic cells (Figure 3-8) in inflamed pulps indicates that delayed hypersensitivity reactions can also occur in this tissue.[34] Despite their protective mechanisms, immune reactions in the pulp can result in the formation of small necrotic foci and eventually total pulpal necrosis.

LESION PROGRESSION

Mild pulpal injuries may not result in significant changes. However, moderate to severe insults result in localized inflammation[43] and release of a high concentration of inflammatory mediators. An increase in protease inhibitors in moderately to severely inflamed pulp indicates the presence of natural modifiers.[25] As a consequence of release of a large quantity of inflammatory mediators, increased vascular permeability, vascular stasis, and migration of leukocytes to the site of injury occur. Available information shows that the sensory neuropeptide CGRP is responsible for the increase of blood flow during pulpal inflammation.[44]

Elevated capillary pressure and increased capillary permeability move fluid from blood vessels into the surrounding tissue. If removal of fluid by venules and lymphatics does not match filtration of fluid from capillaries, an exudate forms. The pulp is encased in rigid walls and forms a low-compliance system; therefore a small increase in tissue pressure causes passive compression and even complete collapse of the venules at the site of pulpal injury.[45] Pressure increases occur in small "compartmentalized" regions and progress slowly (Figure 3-9). Thus

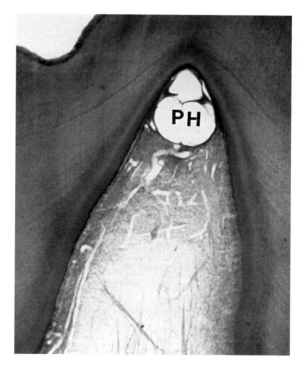

FIGURE 3-9
Irritation of pulp resulting from cavity preparation has resulted in destruction of tissue in pulp horn *(PH)*; note the band of inflammatory lines next to pulp necrosis. There is normal pulp subjacent to the inflammatory zone. (Courtesy Dr. N. Perrini).

pulp does not die by extensive increases in pressure with subsequent strangulation.[45,46]

Pain is often caused by different factors. Release of mediators of inflammation causes pain *directly* by lowering the sensory nerve threshold. These substances also cause pain *indirectly* by increasing both vasodilation in arterioles and vascular permeability in venules, resulting in edema and elevation of tissue pressure. This pressure acts directly on sensory nerve receptors.

Increased tissue pressure, the inability of pulp to expand, and the lack of collateral circulation may result in pulpal necrosis and the development of a subsequent periradicular pathosis.

Classification of Pulpal Diseases

Because there is little or no correlation between the histologic findings of pulpal pathosis and symptoms,[47,48] the diagnosis and classification of pulpal diseases are based on clinical signs and symptoms rather than on histopathologic findings. Pulpal conditions can be classified as reversible and irreversible pulpitis, hyperplastic pulpitis, and necrosis. Hard tissue responses include calcifications and resorption.

REVERSIBLE PULPITIS

By definition, reversible pulpitis is inflammation of the pulp that is not severe. If the cause is eliminated, inflammation will resolve and the pulp will return to normal. Mild or short-acting stimuli such as incipient caries, cervical erosion, or occlusal attrition, most operative procedures, deep periodontal curettage, and enamel fractures resulting in exposure of dentinal tubules can cause reversible pulpitis.

Symptoms

Reversible pulpitis is usually asymptomatic. However, when present, symptoms usually form a particular pattern. Application of stimuli such as cold or hot liquids or even air, may produce sharp transient pain. Removal of these stimuli, which do not normally produce pain or discomfort, results in immediate relief. Cold and hot stimuli produce different pain responses in normal pulp.[49] When heat is applied to teeth with uninflamed pulp, there is a delayed initial response; the intensity of pain increases as the temperature rises. In contrast, pain in response to cold in normal pulp is immediate; the intensity tends to decrease if the cold stimulus is maintained. Based on these observations, responses of both healthy and diseased pulps apparently result largely from changes in intrapulpal pressures.[49]

Treatment

Removal of irritants and sealing as well as insulating the exposed dentin or vital pulp usually result in diminished symptoms (if present) and reversal of the inflammatory process in the pulp tissue (Figure 3-10). However, if irritation of pulp continues or increases in intensity for reasons stated earlier, moderate to severe inflammation develops with irreversible pulpitis and eventually pulpal necrosis.

IRREVERSIBLE PULPITIS

Irreversible pulpitis is often a sequel to and a progression from reversible pulpitis. Severe pulpal damage from extensive dentin removal during operative procedures or impairment of pulpal blood flow caused by trauma or orthodontic movement of teeth may also cause irreversible pulpitis. Irreversible pulpitis is a severe inflammation that will not resolve even if the cause is removed. The pulp slowly or rapidly progresses to necrosis.

Symptoms

Irreversible pulpitis is usually asymptomatic, or the patient reports only mild symptoms. However, irreversible pulpitis may also be associated with intermittent or continuous episodes of spontaneous pain (with no external stimuli). Pain of irreversible pulpitis may be sharp, dull, localized, or diffuse and may last only for minutes or for hours. Localization of pulpal pain is more difficult than localization of periradicular pain and becomes more difficult as the pain intensifies. Application of external stimuli such as cold or heat may result in prolonged pain.

Accordingly, in the presence of severe pain, pulpal responses differ from those of uninflamed teeth or teeth with reversible pulpitis.[49] For example, application of heat to teeth with irreversible pulpitis may produce an immediate response; also, sometimes with the application of cold, the response does not disappear and is prolonged. Occasionally, application of cold in patients with painful irreversible pulpitis causes vasoconstriction, a drop in pulpal pressure, and subsequent pain relief. Although it has been claimed that teeth with irreversible pulpitis have lower thresholds to electrical stimulation, Mumford[50] found similar pain perception thresholds in inflamed and uninflamed pulp.

Tests and Treatment

If inflammation is confined and has not extended periapically, teeth respond within normal limits to palpation and percussion. Extension of inflammation to the periodontal ligament causes percussion sensitivity and better localization of pain. Root canal treatment or extraction is indicated for teeth with signs and symptoms of irreversible pulpitis.

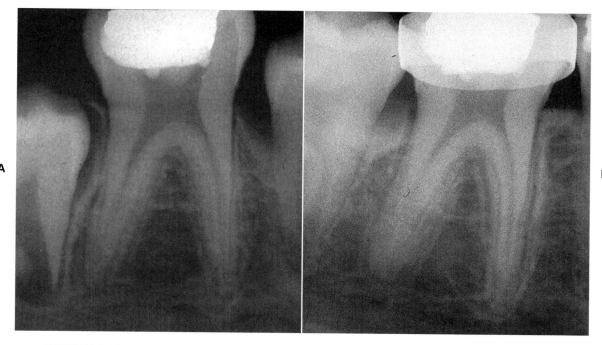

FIGURE 3-10
A, Mechanically exposed pulp horns of a mandibular molar with signs of reversible pulpitis were capped with mineral trioxide aggregate. **B,** On recall, a follow-up radiograph shows no calcific metamorphosis in the pulp chamber and the presence of normal responses during clinical examination.

Hyperplastic Pulpitis

Hyperplastic pulpitis (pulp polyp) is a form of irreversible pulpitis, which results from growth of chronically inflamed young pulp into occlusal surfaces. It is usually found in carious crowns of young patients (Figure 3-11, *A*). Ample vascularity of young pulp, adequate exposure for drainage, and tissue proliferation are associated with formation of hyperplastic pulpitis. Histologic examination of hyperplastic pulpitis shows surface

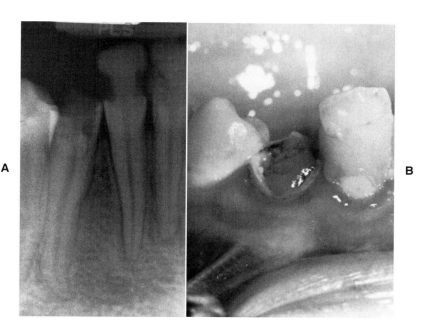

FIGURE 3-11
Pulp polyp, also known as hyperplastic pulpitis. **A,** The involved tooth is usually carious with extensive loss of tooth structure. **B,** The pulp remains vital and proliferaties from the exposure. (Courtesy Dr. Matthew Davis.)

epithelium and underlying inflamed connective tissue (Figure 3-11, *B*). Cells of oral epithelium are implanted and grow over the exposed surface to form an epithelial covering.

Hyperplastic pulpitis is usually asymptomatic. It appears as a reddish cauliflower-like outgrowth of connective tissue into caries that has resulted in a large occlusal exposure. It is occasionally associated with clinical signs of irreversible pulpitis such as spontaneous pain as well as lingering pain to cold and heat stimuli. The threshold to electrical stimulation is similar to that found in normal pulps. The teeth respond within normal limits when palpated or percussed. Hyperplastic pulpitis can be treated by pulpotomy, root canal treatment, or extraction.

HARD TISSUE CHANGES CAUSED BY PULPAL INFLAMMATION

As a result of irritation, two distinct hard tissue changes may be induced: calcification or resorption.

Pulp Calcification

Extensive calcification (usually in the form of pulp stones or diffuse calcification) occurs as a re-

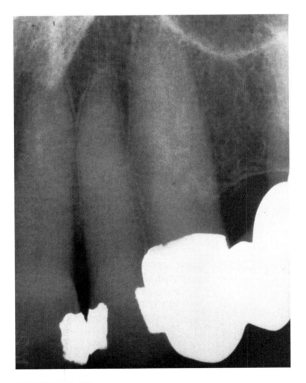

FIGURE 3-12
Calcific metamorphosis. This does not represent pathosis per se and may occur with aging or low-grade irritation.

sponse to trauma, caries, periodontal disease, or other irritants. Thrombi in blood vessels and collagen sheaths around vessel walls are possible nidi for these calcifications.

Another type of calcification is the extensive formation of hard tissue on dentin walls, often in response to irritation or death and replacement of odontoblasts. This process is *calcific metamorphosis* (Figure 3-12). As irritation increases, the amount of calcification may also increase, leading to partial or complete radiographic (but not histologic) obliteration of the pulp chamber and root canal.[51] A yellowish discoloration of the crown is often a manifestation of calcific metamorphosis. The pain threshold to thermal and electrical stimuli usually increases, or often the teeth are unresponsive.

Responses to palpation and percussion are usually within normal limits. In contrast to soft tissue diseases of the pulp, which have no radiographic signs and symptoms, calcification of pulp tissue is associated with various degrees of pulp space obliteration. A reduction in coronal pulp space followed by a gradual narrowing of the root canal is the first sign of calcific metamorphosis. This condition in and of itself is not a pathosis and does not require treatment.

Internal (Intracanal) Resorption

Inflammation in the pulp may initiate resorption of adjacent hard tissues. The pulp is transformed into vascularized inflammatory tissue with dentinoclastic activity; this resorbs the dentinal walls, advancing from the center to the periphery (Figure 3-13).[52] Most cases of intracanal resorption are asymptomatic. Advanced internal resorption involving the pulp chamber is often associated with pink spots in the crown.

Teeth with intracanal resorptive lesions usually respond within normal limits to pulpal and periapical tests. Radiographs reveal a radiolucency with irregular enlargement of the root canal compartment (Figure 3-14). Immediate removal of inflamed tissue and institution of root canal treatment is recommended; these lesions tend to be progressive and eventually perforate to the lateral periodontium. When this occurs, pulpal necrosis ensues, creating major problems in treatment options. Teeth with perforated resorption are difficult to treat nonsurgically.

PULPAL NECROSIS

As stated before, pulp is encased in rigid walls, it has no collateral blood circulation, and its venules and lymphatics collapse under increased tissue pressure; therefore irreversible pulpitis leads to liquefaction necrosis. If exudate produced during

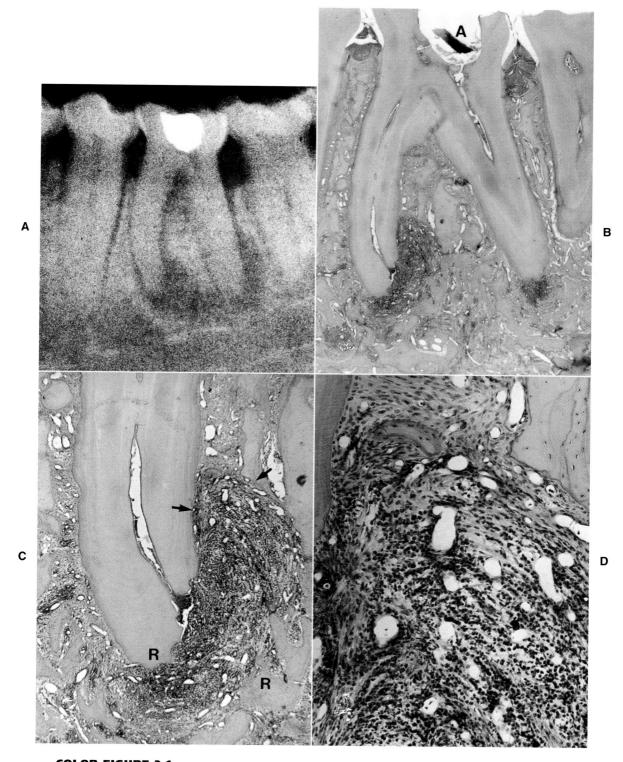

COLOR FIGURE 3-1

A, After coronal exposure in a monkey molar, amalgam was placed to induce pulp necrosis. Seven months later, the radiographic appearance of periapical lesions was evident. This molar and surrounding tissues were removed in block section and prepared for histologic examination. **B,** The first molar shown in **A.** The direction of spread of inflammation is toward the bifurcation. Space occupied by amalgam *(A).* **C,** Inflammation is replacing periodontal and bony structures. Root and bone resorption *(R)* is adjacent to the lesion, which is consistent with chronic apical periodontitis. **D,** Region near arrows in **C.** Note the distinction between the inflammatory lesion below and the intact periodontium above.   *continued*

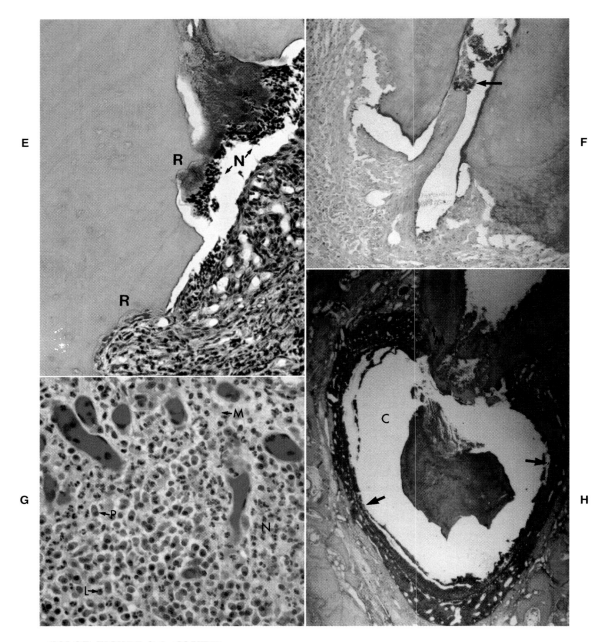

COLOR FIGURE 3-1, CONT'D
E, Apical foramen as shown in **C**. There is funneling resorption of the foramen as well as active root resorption *(R)* . Neutrophils *(N)* are concentrated at the foramen, where irritants are escaping the canal. **F,** Modified bacterial Gram stain shows that bacteria *(arrow)* are confined to the canal space. There are not colonies of bacteria in the periradicular lesion, a common finding. **G,** Periradicular granulomatous inflammation. There is a mix of inflammatory cells: polymorphonuclear leukocytes *(N)*, plasma cells *(P)*, lymphocytes *(L)*, and macrophages *(M)*. **H,** Periradicular cyst. The cyst cavity *(C)* is lined by epithelium *(arrows)* and contains an amorphous material. The empty space is an artifact; fluids within the cavity washed out during histologic processing. *continued*

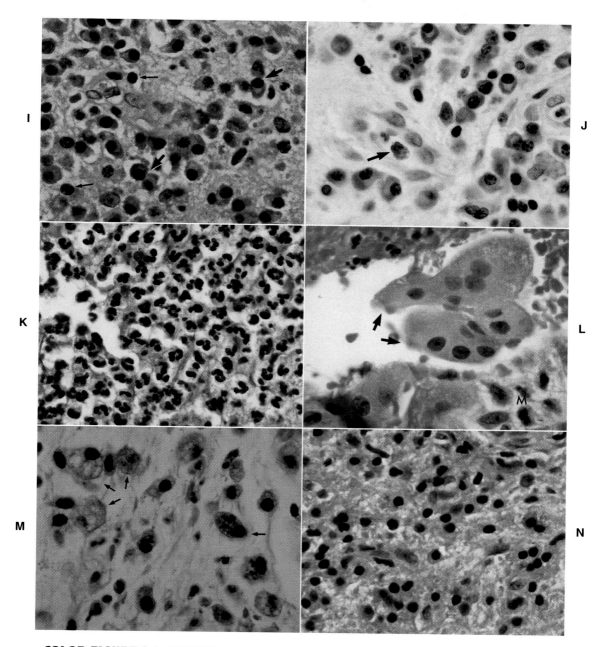

COLOR FIGURE 3-1, CONT'D

I, Lymphocytes *(small arrows)*. Plasma cells *(large arrows)* have an eccentric nucleus with adjacent "clear zone" and a basophilic outer rim of cytoplasm. **J,** Eosinophil *(arrow)* with distinct eosinophilic granules and bilobed nucleus. Plasma cells and lymphocytes are also visible. **K,** Polymorphonuclear leukocytes are concentrated in this field. These have multilobed nuclei; many of these are degenerating and have disrupted cell walls. **L,** Giant cells *(arrows)* with multiple nuclei. Macrophages *(M)* with lighter-stained nuclei and diffuse cytoplasm. **M,** Macrophages *(arrows)* are larger and often have ingested material, as indicated by a "foamy" cytoplasm in these cells. **N,** Lymphocytes, with their densely basophilic nuclei, dominate this field. **(I** to **N** courtesy Dr. C. Kleinegger.)

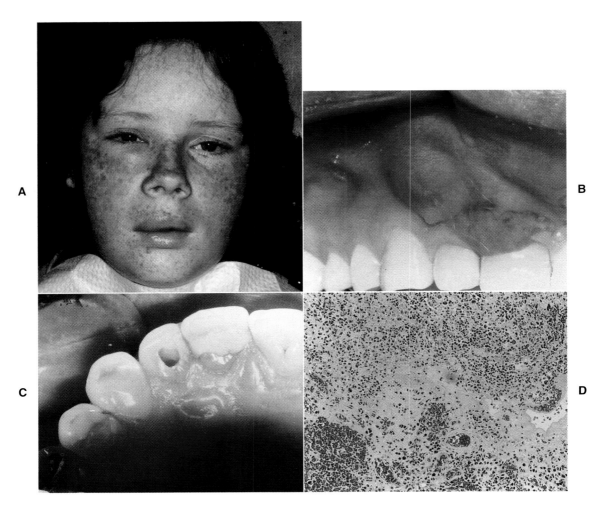

COLOR FIGURE 3-2
A, An acute apical abscess has created severe and diffuse facial swelling. **B,** The vestibular swelling is a result of the necrotic pulp in the right lateral incisor. **C,** An access cavity was made earlier in the lingual surface of this tooth in an attempt to obtain drainage. **D,** Histologic examination of acute apical abscess shows edematous tissue heavily infiltrated by degenerating PMN leukocytes.

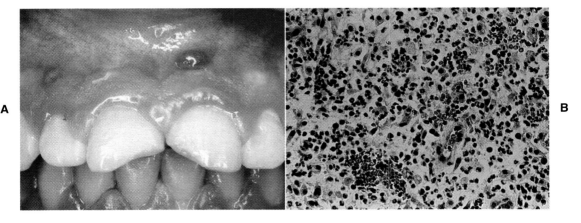

COLOR FIGURE 3-3
A, A sinus tract stoma associated with a necrotic pulp in the left central incisor. **B,** Histologic examination of the peri-radicular tissue associated with this tooth shows numerous lymphocytes, plasma cells, and macrophages (foam cells).

irreversible pulpitis is absorbed or drains through caries or through a pulp exposure into the oral cavity, necrosis is delayed; the radicular pulp may remain vital for long periods. In contrast, closure or sealing of an inflamed pulp induces rapid and total pulpal necrosis and periradicular pathosis.[53] In addition to liquefaction necrosis, ischemic necrosis of pulp occurs as a result of traumatic injury that causes disruption of the blood supply.

Symptoms

Pulpal necrosis is usually asymptomatic but may be associated with episodes of spontaneous pain and discomfort or pain (from the periapex) on pressure. Unlike in teeth with vital pulps, in teeth with necrotic pulps, pain provoked with application of heat is not due to an increase in intrapulpal pressure. This pressure registers zero after heat application to teeth with necrotic pulps.[49] It is commonly believed (but is unlikely) that apply-

ing heat to teeth with liquefaction necrosis causes thermal expansion of gas present in the root canal, which provokes pain.[54] In fact, cold, heat, or electrical stimuli applied to teeth with necrotic pulps usually produces no response.

Tests and Treatment

The presence of various degrees of inflammatory responses ranging from reversible pulpitis to necrosis in teeth with multiple canals is possible and may occasionally cause confusion during testing for responsiveness. Furthermore, effects of necrosis are seldom confined within canals. So, because of the spread of inflammatory reactions to periradicular tissues, teeth with necrotic pulps are often sensitive to percussion. Sensitivity to palpation is an additional indication of periradicular involvement. Root canal treatment or extraction is indicated for these teeth.

Periradicular Pathosis

As a consequence of pulpal necrosis pathologic changes can occur in the periradicular tissues. In

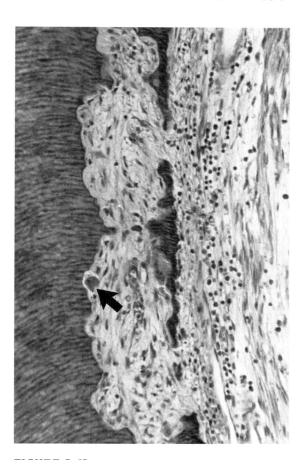

FIGURE 3-13
Internal resorption in canal. Clast cells *(arrow)* actively resorb dentin. This process may be progressive, finally perforating the root.

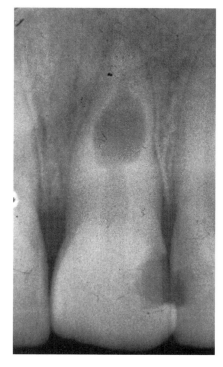

FIGURE 3-14
Hard tissue resorption that causes disappearance of normal radiographic evidence of the root canal *usually* indicates an internal resorption defect.

contrast to pulp, periradicular tissues have an almost unlimited source of undifferentiated cells that participate in inflammation as well as repair. In addition, these tissues have a rich collateral blood supply and lymph drainage. The interaction between the irritants emanating from the canal space and the host defense results in activation of an extensive array of reactions to protect the host. Despite these benefits, some of these reactions are associated with destructive consequences such as periradicular bone resorption. Depending on severity of irritation, duration, and host response, periradicular pathoses may range from slight inflammation to extensive tissue destruction. The reactions involved are highly complex and are usually mediated by nonspecific mediators of inflammation as well as by specific immune reactions (Figure 3-15).[28]

NONSPECIFIC MEDIATORS OF PERIRADICULAR LESIONS

Nonspecific mediators of inflammatory reactions include neuropeptides, fibrinolytic peptides, kinins, complement fragments, vasoactive amines, lysosomal enzymes, arachidonic acid metabolites, and cytokines.[23] Neuropeptides have been demonstrated in inflamed periapical tissues of experimental animals; apparently these substances play a role in the pathogenesis of periradicular pathosis.[26]

Severance of blood vessels in periodontal ligament or bone during canal instrumentation can activate intrinsic as well as extrinsic coagulation pathways. Contact of the Hageman factor with collagen of basement membranes enzymes such as kallikrein or plasmin, or endotoxins from inflamed root canals activates the clotting cascade and the fibrinolytic system. Fibrinopeptides released from fibrinogen molecules and fibrin degradation products released during the proteolysis of fibrin by plasmin contribute to inflammation. Trauma to the periapex during root canal treatment can also activate the kinin system and, in turn, the complement system. C3 complement fragments have been found in periradicular lesions.[55] Products released from the activated systems contribute to the inflammatory process and cause swelling, pain, and tissue destruction.

Mast cells are normal components of connective tissues and are present in normal periodontal

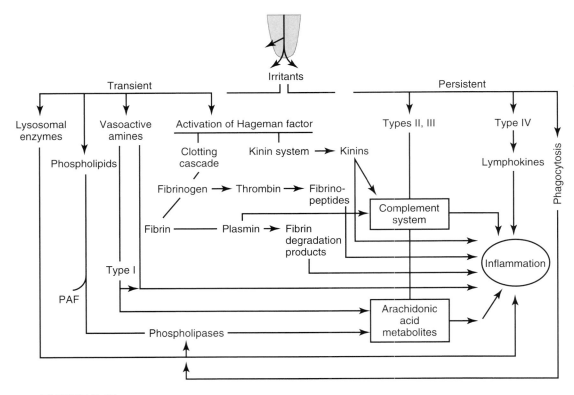

FIGURE 3-15
Pathways of inflammation and bone resorption by nonspecific inflammatory mediators and specific immune reactions.

ligament and in periradicular lesions.[56,57] Physical or chemical injury causes release of vasoactive amines such as histamine, which are chemotactic for leukocytes and macrophages. In addition, lysosomal enzymes cause cleavage of C5 and generation of C5a, a potent chemotactic component, and liberation of active bradykinin from plasma kininogen.[23] Periradicular lesions show increased levels of lysosomal hydrolytic arylsulfatase A and B compared with normal tissues.[58] Significant levels of PGE_2 and leukotriene B_4 have also been found in these lesions.[23] Other studies have confirmed these findings, demonstrating lower levels of PGE_2 associated with either larger periapical lesions[59] or cessation of symptoms subsequent to emergency cleaning and shaping.[60] With immunohistochemical staining PGE_2, $PGF_{2\alpha}$, and 6-keto-$PGF_{1\alpha}$ (a stable metabolite of PGI_2) have been observed in inflamed pulp tissue and periapical lesions.[61,62] Regions staining positively for prostaglandins gradually extended apically into areas not yet inflamed within the pulp tissue. Periapical lesions demonstrated macrophage and fibroblast cell types staining most heavily for the prostaglandins evaluated. Use of indomethacin, a prostaglandin inhibitor, experimentally reduces bone resorption, indicating that prostaglandins are also involved in the pathogenesis of periradicular lesions.[23,63,64]

Various cytokines such as interleukins, tumor necrosis factors, and growth factors are involved in the development and perpetuation of periradicular lesions.[38,65-69] Kawashima and Stashenko[68] examined the kinetics of expression of 10 cytokines in experimentally induced murine periapical le-

sions. Their results showed that a cytokine network is activated in the periapex in response to canal infection and that T helper cell–modulated proinflammatory pathways may predominate during periapical bone resorption.

SPECIFIC MEDIATORS OF PERIRADICULAR LESIONS

In addition to the nonspecific mediators of inflammatory reactions, immunologic reactions also participate in the formation and perpetuation of periradicular pathosis (see Figure 3-15). Numerous potential antigens may accumulate in necrotic pulp, including several species of microorganisms, their toxins, and altered pulp tissue. Root canals are a pathway for sensitization.[23] The presence of potential antigens in the root canals and IgE immunoglobulin, and mast cells in pathologically involved pulp and periradicular lesions indicates that a type I immunologic reaction may occur.[19]

Various classes of immunoglobulins have been found in these lesions.[23,70] These include specific antibodies against a number of bacterial species in infected root canals.[71,72] In addition, different types of immunocompetent cells such as antigen-presenting cells (Ia antigen–expressing nonlymphoid cells), macrophages,[73] PMN leukocytes, and B as well as T cells have been found in human periradicular lesions.[74,75] The presence of immune complexes (Figure 3-16) and immunocompetent cells such as T cells (Figure 3-17) indicates that various types of immunologic reactions (types II through IV) can initiate, amplify, or perpetuate these inflammatory lesions.[23]

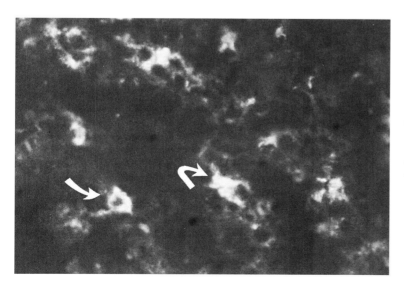

FIGURE 3-16
Using the anticomplement immunofluorescence technique, immune complexes are identified *(arrows)* in human periapical lesions.

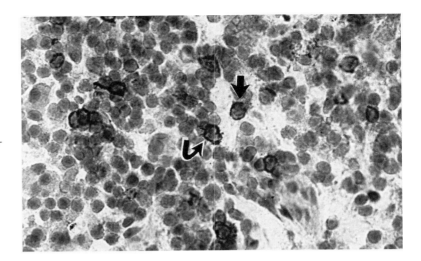

FIGURE 3-17
T lymphocytes *(arrows)* are identified in a human periapical lesion by an immunohistochemical technique.

Classification of Periradicular Lesions

Periradicular lesions have been classified on the basis of their clinical and histologic findings. As with pulpal disease, little correlation exists between the clinical signs and symptoms and duration of lesions compared with the histopathologic findings.[76] Because of these discrepancies and for convenience, these lesions are classified into five main groups: acute apical periodontitis, chronic apical periodontitis, condensing osteitis, acute apical abscess, and chronic apical abscess. Lesions associated with significant symptoms such as pain or swelling are referred to as acute (symptomatic), whereas those with mild or no symptoms are identified as chronic (asymptomatic).

ACUTE APICAL PERIODONTITIS
Etiology

Acute apical periodontitis would be better described as *symptomatic* apical periodontitis. The first extension of pulpal inflammation into the periradicular tissues is called acute apical periodontitis (AAP). Eliciting irritants include inflammatory mediators from an irreversibly inflamed pulp or egress of bacteria toxins from necrotic pulps, chemicals (such as irrigants or disinfecting agents), restorations in hyperocclusion, overinstrumentation, and extrusion of obturating materials. The pulp may be irreversibly inflamed or necrotic.

Signs and Symptoms

Clinical features of AAP are moderate to severe spontaneous discomfort as well as pain on mastication or occlusal contact. If AAP is an extension of pulpitis, signs and symptoms will include responsiveness to cold, heat, and electricity. If AAP is caused by necrosis, teeth do not respond to vitality tests. Application of pressure by fingertip or tapping with the butt end of a mirror handle can cause marked to excruciating pain. "Thickening" of periodontal ligament (PDL) space may be a radiographic feature of AAP (Figure 3-18). However, usually there is a normal PDL space and an intact lamina dura.

Histologic Features

In AAP, PMN leukocytes and macrophages are visible within a localized area at the apex. At times there may be a small area of liquefaction necrosis (abscess). Bone and root resorption may be present histologically; however, resorption is usually not visible radiographically.

Treatment

Adjustment of occlusion (when there is evidence of hyperocclusion), removal of irritants or a pathologic pulp, or release of periradicular exudate usually results in relief.

CHRONIC APICAL PERIODONTITIS
Etiology

Chronic apical periodontitis (CAP) results from pulpal necrosis and usually is a sequel to AAP.

Signs and Symptoms

By definition, CAP is without symptoms or is associated with slight discomfort and would be bet-

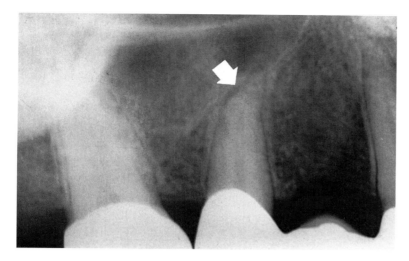

FIGURE 3-18
After cementing a three-unit bridge, the premolar developed clinical signs and symptoms of acute apical periodontitis, and the radiograph shows a thickened periodontal ligament space *(arrow)*.

ter classified as *asymptomatic* apical periodontitis. Because the pulp is necrotic, teeth with CAP do not respond to electrical or thermal stimuli. Percussion produces little or no pain. There may be slight sensitivity to palpation, indicating an alteration of the cortical plate of bone and extension of CAP into the soft tissues. Radiographic features range from interruption of the lamina dura to extensive destruction of periradicular and interradicular tissues (Figure 3-19).

Histologic Features

Histologically, CAP lesions are classified as either *granulomas* or *cysts*. A periradicular *granuloma* consists of granulomatous tissue infiltrated by mast cells, macrophages, lymphocytes, plasma cells, and occasional PMN leukocytes (see Color Figure 3-1 immediately following page 36) Multinucleated giant cells, foam cells, cholesterol clefts, and epithelium are often found.

The *apical (radicular) cyst* has a central cavity filled with an eosinophilic fluid or semisolid material and is lined by stratified squamous epithelium (Figure 3-20). The epithelium is surrounded by connective tissue that contains all cellular elements found in the periradicular granuloma. Therefore an apical cyst is a granuloma that contains a cavity or cavities lined with epithelium (see Color Figure 3-1, *H*). The origin of the epithelium is the remnants of Hertwig's epithelial sheath, the cell rests of Malassez. These cell rests proliferate under an inflammatory stimulus. The actual genesis of the cyst is unclear.

The reported incidence of endodontic lesions is inconsistent. Variations may be due to sampling methods and the histologic criteria used for diagnosis. Nobuhara and del Rio[77] examined peri-

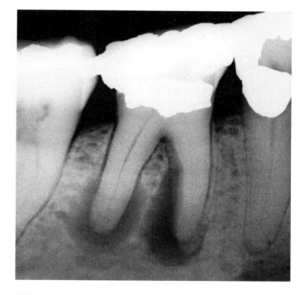

FIGURE 3-19
Chronic apical periodontitis. Extensive tissue destruction in the periapical regions of a mandibular first molar as a result of pulpal necrosis. A lack of symptoms and radiographic lesions is diagnostic.

radicular biopsy specimens of lesions that were refractory to root canal treatment and showed most (59%) to be granulomas, with some (22%) cysts, a few (12%) scars, and a scattering (7%) of other types of lesions.[77] Percentages such as these are misleading. Many lesions are combinations of types and contain granulomatous inflammation, cysts, and areas of scarring; also, the samples usually do not include abscesses, which would not be recovered intact during surgery. Also, the entire lesion is usually not recovered for biopsy; only fragments are obtained during curettage.

Treatment

Removal of inciting irritants (necrotic pulp) and complete obturation usually result in resolution of CAP (Figure 3-21). There is no evidence that apical cysts do not resolve after adequate root canal treatment or extraction.

CONDENSING OSTEITIS
Etiology

Condensing osteitis (focal sclerosing osteomyelitis), a variant of chronic (asymptomatic) apical periodontitis, represents an increase in trabecular bone in response to persistent irritation. The irritant diffusing from the root canal into periradicular tissues

is the main cause of condensing osteitis. This lesion is usually found around the apexes of mandibular posterior teeth, which show a probable cause of pulp inflammation or necrosis. However, condensing osteitis can occur around the apex of any tooth.

Signs and Symptoms

Depending on the cause (pulpitis or pulpal necrosis), condensing osteitis may be either asymptomatic or associated with pain. Pulp tissue of teeth with condensing osteitis may or may not respond to electrical or thermal stimuli. Furthermore, these teeth may or may not be sensitive to palpation or percussion. Radiographically, the presence

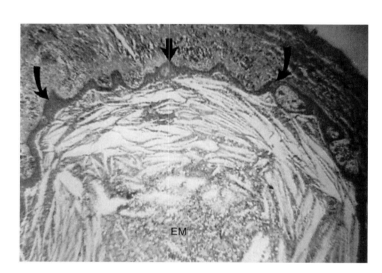

FIGURE 3-20
This region of human apical cyst consists of a central cavity filled with eosinophilic material (EM) and a wall lined with epithelium *(arrows)*. (Courtesy Dr. N. Perrini.)

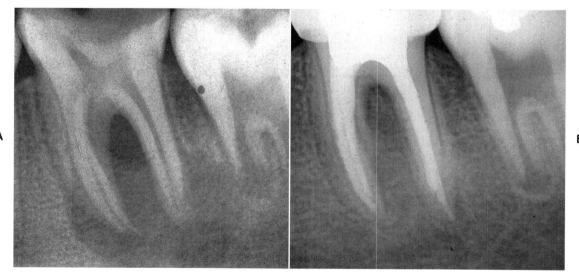

A

B

FIGURE 3-21
A, Preoperative radiograph of a first molar shows pulpal necrosis and chronic apical periodontitis. **B,** A postoperative radiograph 1 year after root canal therapy showing complete resolution of the periradicular pathosis.

of a diffuse concentric arrangement of radiopacity around the root of a tooth is pathognomonic (Figure 3-22). Histologically, there is an increase in irregularly arranged trabecular bone and inflammation.[78]

Root canal treatment, when indicated, may result in complete resolution of condensing osteitis.[79] Condensing osteitis is often confused with the nonpathologic entity, enostosis (sclerotic bone).

ACUTE APICAL ABSCESS
Etiology

Acute (symptomatic) apical abscess (AAA) is a localized or diffuse (see Color Figure 3-2 following page 36) liquefaction lesion that destroys periradicular tissues. It is a severe inflammatory response to microbial and nonbacterial irritants from necrotic pulp.

Signs and Symptoms

Depending on the severity of the reaction, patients with AAA usually have moderate to severe discomfort or swelling. In addition, they occasionally have systemic manifestations of an infective process such as a high temperature, malaise, and leukocytosis. Because this occurs only with pulp necrosis, electrical or thermal stimulation produces no response. However, these teeth are usually painful to percussion and palpation. Depending on the degree of hard tissue destruction caused by irritants, the radiographic features of AAA range from thickening of the PDL space (infrequent) to a frank resorptive lesion (usual).

Histologic Features

Histologic examination in AAA usually shows a localized destructive lesion of liquefaction necrosis containing numerous disintegrating PMN leukocytes, debris, and cell remnants and an accumulation of purulent exudate (Figure 3-23). Surrounding the abscess is granulomatous tissue; therefore the lesion is best categorized as an abscess within a granuloma. Significantly, the abscess often does not communicate directly with the apical foramen; thus an abscess often will not drain through an accessed tooth.

Removal of the underlying cause (necrotic pulp), release of pressure (drainage where possible), and routine root canal treatment lead to resolution of most AAAs.

CHRONIC APICAL ABSCESS (SUPPURATIVE APICAL PERIODONTITIS)

Also classified as suppurative apical periodontitis (SAP), chronic (asymptomatic) apical abscess (CAA) results from a long-standing lesion that has caused an abscess which is draining to a surface.

Etiology

CAA (SAP) has a pathogenesis similar to that of AAA. It also results from pulpal necrosis and is usually associated with CAP that has formed an abscess. The abscess has "burrowed" through bone and soft tissue to form a sinus tract stoma on the oral mucosa (see Color Figure 3-3 following page

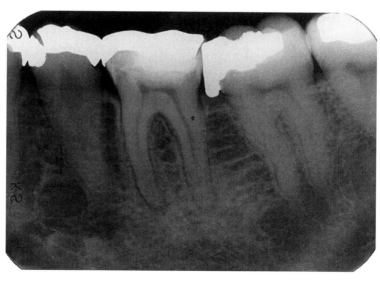

FIGURE 3-22
Condensing osteitis. Inflammation followed by necrosis in the pulp of the first molar has resulted in the diffuse radiopacity of periradicular tissue.

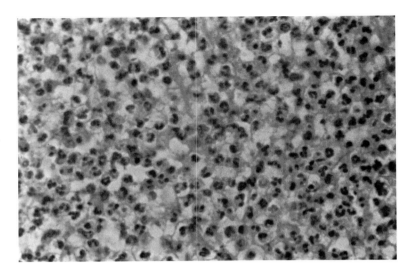

FIGURE 3-23
Histologic examination of acute apical abscess shows edematous tissue heavily infiltrated by many degenerating PMN leukocytes.

36) or sometimes onto the skin of the face. The histologic findings in these lesions are similar to those found in CAP. CAAs may also drain through periodontium into the sulcus and may mimic a periodontal abscess or pocket (see Chapter 26).

Signs and Symptoms

Because drainage exists, CAA is usually asymptomatic except when there is occasional closure of the sinus pathway, which can cause pain. Clinical, radiographic, and histopathologic features of CAA are similar to those described for CAP. An additional feature is the sinus tract, which may be lined partially or totally by epithelium surrounded by inflamed connective tissue.[80]

Healing of Periradicular Lesions Following Root Canal Treatment

Regeneration is a process by which altered periradicular tissues are completely replaced by native tissues to their original architecture and function. Repair is a process by which altered tissues are not completely restored to their original structures. Histologic examination of most tissue sections in experimental animals and humans shows that healing of periradicular lesions after root canal therapy is repair rather than regeneration of the periradicular tissues. Inflammation and healing are not two separate entities and in fact constitute part of one process in response to tissue injury. On the molecular and cellular levels it is impossible to separate the two phenomena. Inflammation dominates the early events after tissue injury,

shifting toward healing after the early responses have subsided. However, for convenience and to simplify the complex inflammatory-resorptive process, they are studied as two separate entities.

EXTENT OF HEALING

The extent of healing is proportional to the degree and extent of tissue injury and the nature of tissue destruction. When injury to periradicular tissues is slight, little repair or regeneration is required. However, extensive damage requires substantial healing (see Figure 3-21). In other words, periradicular repair ranges from a relatively simple resolution of an inflammatory infiltrate in the PDL to considerable reorganization and repair of a variety of tissues.

PROCESS OF HEALING

The sequence of events leading to resolution of periradicular lesions has not been studied extensively. Based on the processes involved in repair of extraction sites (which may not be totally synonymous), after the cause is removed, inflammatory responses decrease and tissue-forming cells (fibroblasts and endothelial cells) increase; tissue organization and maturation ensue.[81] Bone that has resorbed is replaced by new bone; resorbed cementum and dentin are repaired by cellular cementum. The PDL, which is the first tissue affected, is the last to be restored to normal architecture. Histologic examination of periradicular lesions that were healing showed evidence in the form of cementum deposition, increased vascularity, and increased fibroblastic and osteoblastic activity.[82] Recent studies showed that some cytokines play an important role during healing of periradicular lesions.[83,84]

With some lesions it is apparent that not all original structures are restored. Variations are seen in different fiber or bone patterns. These may be seen radiographically with a widened lamina dura or altered bony configuration.

Nonendodontic Periradicular Pathosis

DIFFERENTIAL DIAGNOSIS

A number of radiolucent and radiopaque lesions of nonendodontic origin simulate the radiographic appearance of endodontic lesions. Because of their similarities, dentists must use their knowledge and perform clinical tests in an orderly manner to arrive at a diagnosis and avoid critical mistakes. Pulp vitality tests are the most important aids in differentiating between endodontic and nonendodontic lesions. Teeth associated with radiolucent periradicular lesions have necrotic pulps and therefore generally do not respond to vitality tests. In contrast, lesions of nonpulpal origin usually do not affect the blood or nerve supply to adjacent tooth pulp; therefore the vitality (responsiveness) of these teeth remains unaffected.

Unfortunately, many clinicians use only radiographs for diagnosis and treatment without taking a complete history of the signs and symptoms and performing clinical tests. Many nonendodontic radiolucent lesions (including those caused by pathoses and those with normal morphology) mimic endodontic pathoses and vice versa. Therefore to avoid grievous mistakes, all relevant vitality tests, radiographic examinations, clinical signs and symptoms, and details of the patient history should be used.

NORMAL AND PATHOLOGIC ENTITIES

Most radiographic changes are, in fact, endodontic and arise from pathologic changes in the pulp. However, other radiographic variations, such as anatomic variations as well as benign and malignant lesions, may simulate the appearance of periradicular lesions.[85]

Normal Structures

Such anatomic variations include large marrow spaces adjacent to the apexes of teeth, submandibular fossae, maxillary sinus, apical dental papillae of developing teeth, nasopalatine fora-

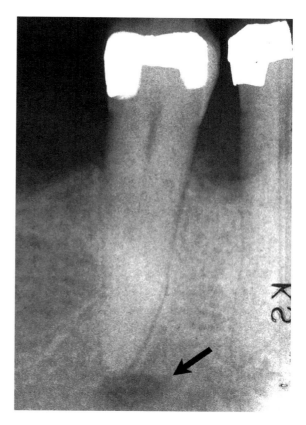

FIGURE 3-24
A mental foramen *(arrow)* simulating a periapical lesion of pulpal origin. Pulp tests are within normal limits, indicating that this radiolucency could not be endodontic pathosis.

men, mental foramen (Figure 3-24), and lingual depressions in the mandible. Associated teeth respond to vitality tests and show no clinical signs and symptoms of any disease process. In addition, by changing the cone angulation, the location of these radiolucent lesions can be moved relative to their original positions and to the root apexes.

Nonendodontic Pathoses

Benign lesions with radiographic appearances similar to those of periradicular lesions include (but are not limited to) the initial stages of periradicular cemental dysplasia (Figure 3-25), early stages of monostotic fibrous dysplasia, ossifying fibroma, primordial cyst, lateral periodontal cyst, dentigerous cyst, nasopalatine duct cyst, solitary bone cyst, central giant cell granuloma, central hemangioma, hyperparathyroidism, myxoma, and ameloblastoma. Usually (but not always) the radiographic lamina dura around the apexes is intact, and responses to pulp tests are normal. The final diagnosis of these lesions is often based on surgical biopsy and histopathologic examination.[86]

Malignant lesions that may simulate endodontic periradicular lesions and are often metastatic include lymphoma (Figure 3-26), squamous cell carcinoma, osteogenic sarcoma, chondrosarcoma, and multiple myeloma. Unlike endodontic lesions, these lesions are usually associated with rapid and extensive hard tissue (bone and tooth) destruction. Ordinarily the teeth in the affected region remain responsive to vitality tests, although occasionally the pulps or sensory nerves are disrupted and are nonresponsive. For a more complete list and description of lesions that may mimic the radiographic appearance of endodontic lesions of pulpal origin an oral pathology text should be consulted.[87]

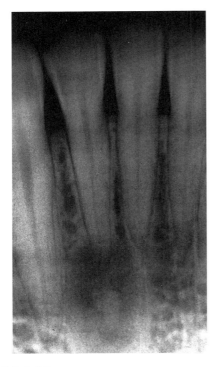

FIGURE 3-25
A periapical radiolucency in the early stages of cementoma can simulate a periapical lesion of pulpal origin. However, the pulps are responding within normal limits.

REFERENCES

1. McKay GS: The histology and microbiology of acute occlusal dentine lesions in human permanent premolar teeth, *Arch Oral Biol* 21:51, 1976.
2. Wirthlin MR: Acid-reaching stains, softening, and bacterial invasion in human carious dentin, *J Dent Res* 49:42, 1970.
3. Brannström M, Lind PO: Pulpal response to early dental caries, *J Dent Res* 44:1045, 1965.
4. Baum LJ: Dental pulp conditions in relation to carious lesions, *Int Dent J* 20:309, 1970.
5. Lin LB, Langeland K: Light and electron microscopic study of teeth with carious pulp exposures, *Oral Surg Oral Med Oral Pathol* 51:292, 1981.
6. Yamasaki M, Kumazawa M, Kohsaka T, et al: Pulpal and periapical tissue reactions after experimental pulpal exposure in rats, *J Endod* 20:13, 1994.
7. Kakehashi S, Stanley HR, Fitzgerald R: The effects of surgical exposures of dental pulps in germ-free and conventional laboratory rats, *Oral Surg Oral Med Oral Pathol* 20:340, 1965.

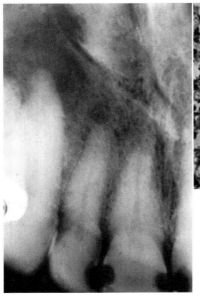

A

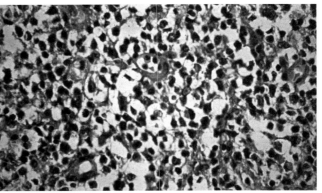

B

FIGURE 3-26
A, A periapical radiolucent lesion of nonpulpal origin. **B,** Positive results of vitality tests and histologic examination of the tissue confirmed a diagnosis of lymphoma. (Courtesy Dr. J Simon.)

8. Moller AJR, Fabricius L, Dahlen G, et al: Influence of periapical tissues of indigenous oral bacteria and necrotic pulp tissue in monkeys, *Scand J Dent Res* 89:475, 1981.

9. Bergenholtz G: Micro-organisms from necrotic pulp of traumatized teeth, *Odont Rev* 25:347, 1974.

10. Sundqvist G: Bacteriological studies of necrotic dental pulps (PhD Thesis), Umea Univ Odontol Dissert 7:1, 1976.

11. Korzen B, Krakow A, Green D: Pulpal and periapical tissue responses in conventional and gnotobiotic rats, *Oral Surg* 37:783, 1974.

12. Bergenholtz G. Inflammatory response of the dental pulp to bacterial irritation, *J Endod* 7:100, 1981.

13. Garberoglio R, Brannström M: Scanning electron microscopic investigation of human dentinal tubules, *Arch Oral Biol* 21:335, 1976.

14. Pashley DH, Kehl T, Pashley E, Palmer P: Comparison of in vitro and in vivo dog dentin permeability, *J Dent Res* 60:763, 1981.

15. Zach L, Cohen G: Biology of high speed rotary operative dental procedures. I. Correlation of tooth volume removed and pulpal pathology (Abstract), *J Dent Res* 37:67, 1958.

16. Hamilton AI, Kramer IRH: Cavity preparation with and without waterspray, *Br Dent J* 123:281, 1967.

17. Takahashi K. Changes in the pulpal vasculature during inflammation, *J Endod* 16:92, 1990.

18. Tschamer H: The histology of pulpal tissue after orthodontic treatment with activators during late adolescence, *Zahnarztl Prax* 25:530, 1974.

19. Bunner M, Johnsen D: Quantitative assessment of intrapulpal axon response to orthodontic movement, *Am J Orthod* 82:244, 1982.

20. Langeland K: Management of the inflamed pulp associated with deep carious lesion, *J Endod* 7:169, 1981.

21. Masillamoni CRM, Masillamoni K, Kettering JD, Torabinejad M: The biocompatibility of some root canal medicaments and irrigants, *Int Endod J* 14:115, 1981.

22. Spangberg GL, Engstrom B, Langeland K: Biological effect of dental materials. 3. Toxicity and antimicrobial effects of endodontic antiseptics in vitro, *Oral Surg Oral Med Oral Pathol* 36:856, 1973.

23. Torabinejad M: Mediators of acute and chronic periradicular lesions, *Oral Surg Oral Med Oral Pathol* 78:511, 1994.

24. Rauschenberger, CR, McClanahan SB, Pederson ED, et al.: Comparison of human polymorphonuclear neutrophil elastase, polymorphonuclear neutrophil cathepsin-G, and alpha 2-macroglobin levels in healthy and inflamed dental pulps, *J Endod* 20:546, 1994.

25. McClanahan SB, Turner DW, Kaminski EJ, et al: Natural modifiers of the inflammatory process in the human dental pulp, *J Endod* 17:589, 1991.

26. Byers MR, Taylor PE, Khayat BG, Kimberly CL: Effects of injury and inflammation on pulpal and periapical nerves, *J Endod* 16:78, 1990.

27. Zachrisson BU, Skogedal O: Mast cells in inflamed human dental pulp, *Scand J Dent Res* 79:488, 1971.

28. Torabinejad M, Eby WC, Naidorf IJ: Inflammatory and immunological aspects of the pathogenesis of human periapical lesions, *J Endod* 11:479, 1985.

29. Goodis H, Saeki K: Identification of bradykinin, substance P and neurokinin A in human dental pulp, *J Endod* 23:201, 1997.

30. Goodis HE, Bowles WR, Hargreaves KM: Prostaglandin E_2 enhances bradykinin-evoked iCGRP release in bovine dental pulp, *J Dent Res* 79:1604, 2000.

31. Lessard G, Torabinejad M, Swope D: Arachidonic acid metabolites in canine tooth pulps and the effects of nonsteroidal anti-inflammatory drugs, *J Endod* 12:146, 1986.

32. Cohen JS, Reader A, Fertel R, et al: A radioimmunoassay determination of the concentrations of prostaglandins E_2 and $F_{2\alpha}$ in painful and asymptomatic human dental pulps, *J Endod* 11:330, 1985.

33. Miyauchi M, Takata T, Ito H, et al: Immunohistochemical demonstration of prostaglandins E_2, F_2, alpha, and 6-keto-prostaglandin F_1 alpha in rat dental pulp with experimentally induced inflammation, *J Endod* 22:600, 1996.

34. Jontell M, Dkiji T, Dahlgren U, Bergenholtz G. Immune defense mechanisms of the dental pulp, *Crit Rev Oral Biol Med* 9:179, 1998.

35. Grutzner EH, Garry MG, Hargreaves KM: Effect of injury on pulpal levels of immunoreactive substance P and immunoreactive calcitonin gene-related peptide, *J Endod* 18:55, 1992.

36. Levin LG, Rudd A, Bletsa A, et al: Expression of IL-8 by cells of the odontoblast layer in vitro, *Eur J Oral Sci* 107:131, 1999.

37. Atsushima K, Ohbayashi E, Takeuchi H, et al: Stimulation of interleukin-6 production in human dental pulp cells by peptidoglycans from *Lactobacillus casei*, *J Endod* 24:252, 1998.

38. Barkhordar RA, Hayashi C, Hussain MZ: Detection of interleukin-6 in human dental pulp and periapical lesions, *Endod Dent Traumatol* 15:25, 1999.

39. Huang GT, Potente AP, Kim JW, et al: Increased interleukin-8 expression in inflamed human dental pulps, *Oral Surg Oral Med Oral Pathol* 88:214, 1999.

40. Rauschenberger CR, Bailey JC, Cootauco CJ: Detection of human IL-2 in normal and inflamed dental pulps, *J Endod* 23:366, 1997.

41. Nakanishi T, Matsuo T, Ebisu S: Quantitative analysis of immunoglobulins and inflammatory factors in human pulpal blood from exposed pulps, *J Endod* 21:131, 1995.

42. Bergenholtz Z, Ahlstedt S, Lindhe J: Experimental pulpitis in immunized monkeys, *Scand J Dent Res* 85:396, 1977.

43. Proctor ME, Turner DW, Kaminski EJ, et al.: Determination and relationship of C-reactive protein in human dental pulps and in serum, *J Endod* 17:265, 1991.

44. Berggreen E, Heyeraas KJ: The role of sensory neuropeptides and nitric oxide on pulpal blood flow and tissue pressure in the ferret, *J Dent Res* 78:1535, 1999.

45. Van Hassel HJ: Physiology of the human dental pulp, *Oral Surg Oral Med Oral Pathol* 32:126, 1971.

46. Heyeraas KJ: Pulpal microvascular and tissue pressure, *J Dent Res* 64:58, 1985.

47. Seltzer S, Bender IB, Ziontz M: The dynamics of pulp inflammation: correlations between diagnostic data and actual histologic findings in the pulp, *Oral Surg Oral Med Oral Pathol* 16:846, 1963.

48. Johnson RH, Dachi SF, Haley JV: Pulpal hyperemia—a correlation of clinical and histologic data from 706 teeth, *J Am Dent Assoc* 81:108, 1976.

49. Bender IB: Pulp biology conference: A discussion, *J Endod* 4:37, 1978.

50. Mumford JM: Pain perception threshold on stimulating human teeth and the histological condition of the pulp, *Br Dent J* 123:427, 1967.

51. Kuyk J, Walton R: Comparison of radiographic appearance of root canal size to its actual diameter, *J Endod* 16:528, 1990.

52. Walton R: Cracked tooth: an etiology for "idiopathic" internal resorption, *J Endod* 12:167, 1986.

53. Walton RE, Garnick J: The histology of periapical inflammatory lesions in permanent molars in monkeys, *J Endod* 12:49, 1986.

54. Mumford JM: Orofacial pain: aetiology, diagnosis and treatment, ed. 3, p 207, New York, 1982, Churchill Livingstone.

55. Pulver WH, Taubman MA, Smith DJ: Immune components in human dental periapical lesions, *Arch Oral Biol* 23:435, 1978.

56. Mathiesen A: Preservation and demonstration of mast cells in human apical granulomas and radicular cysts, *Scand J Dent Res* 81:218, 1973.

57. Perrini N, Fonzi L: Mast cells in human periapical lesions: ultrastructural aspects and their possible physiopathological implications, *J Endod* 11:197, 1985.

58. Aqrabawi J, Schilder H, Toselli P, Franzblau C: Biochemical and histochemical analysis of the enzyme arylsulfatase in human lesions of endodontic origin, *J Endod* 19:335, 1993.

59. Takayama S, Miki Y, Shimauchi H, Okada H: Relationship between prostaglandin E_2 concentrations in periapical exudates from root canals and clinical findings of periapical periodontitis, *J Endod* 12:677, 1996.

60. Shimauchi H, Takayama S, Miki Y, Okada H: The change of periapical exudate prostaglandin E_2 levels during root canal treatment, *J Endod* 23:755, 1997.

61. Miyauchi M, Takata T, Ito H, et al: Immunohistochemical demonstration of prostaglandins $E_{2\alpha}$, $F_{2\alpha}$ and 6-keto-prostaglandin $F_{1\alpha}$ in rat dental pulp with experimentally induced inflammation, *J Endod* 22:600, 1996.

62. Miyauchi M, Takata T, Ito H, et al: Immunohistochemical detection of prostaglandins E_2, $F_{2\alpha}$, and 6-keto-prostaglandin F_α in experimentally induced periapical inflammatory lesions in rats, *J Endod* 22:635, 1996.

63. Oguntebi BR, Barker BF, Anderson DM, Sakumura J: The effect of indomethacin on experimental dental periapical lesions in rats, *J Endod* 15:117, 1989.

64. Anan H, Akamine A, Hara Y, et al: A histochemical study of bone remodeling during experimental apical periodontitis in rats, *J Endod* 17:332, 1991.

65. Safavi KE, Rossomando EF: Tumor necrosis factor identified in periapical tissue exudates of teeth with apical periodontitis, *J Endod* 17:12, 1991.

66. Lim GC, Torabinejad M, Kettering J, et al: Interleukin 1b in symptomatic and asymptomatic human periradicular lesions, *J Endod* 20:225, 1994.

67. Tyler LW, Matossian K Todd R, et al: Eosinophil-derived transforming growth factors (TGF-alpha and TGF-beta 1) in human periradicular lesions, *J Endod* 25:619, 1999.

68. Kawashima N, Stashenko P: Expression of bone-resorptive and regulatory cytokines in murine periapical inflammation, *Arch Oral Biol* 44:55, 1999.

69. Stashenko P, Teles R, D'Souza R: Periapical inflammatory responses and their modulation, *Crit Rev Oral Biol Med* 9:498, 1998.

70. Cortes JO, Torabinejad M, Matiz RAR, Mantilla EG: Presence of secretory IgA in human periapical lesions, *J Endod* 20:87, 1994.

71. Baumgartner JC, Falkler WA Jr: Reactivity of IgG from explant cultures of periapical lesions with implicated microorganisms, *J Endod* 17:207, 1991.

72. Kettering JD, Torabinejad M, Jones SL: Specificity of antibodies present in human periapical lesions, *J Endod* 17:213, 1991.

73. Metzger Z: Macrophages in periapical lesions, *Endod Dent Traumatol* 16:1, 2000.

74. Okiji T, Kawashima N, Kosaka T, et al: Distribution of Ia antigen-expressing nonlymphoid cells in various stages of induced periapical lesions in rat molars, *J Endod* 20:27, 1994.

75. Matsuo T, Ebisu S, Shimabukuro Y, et al: Quantitative analysis of immunocompetent cells in human periapical lesions: Correlations with clinical findings of the involved teeth, *J Endod* 18:497, 1992.

76. Morse D, Seltzer S, Sinai I, Biron G: Endodontic classification, *J Am Dent Assoc* 94:685, 1977.

77. Nobuhara WK, del Rio CE: Incidence of periradicular pathoses in endodontic treatment failures, *J Endod* 19:315, 1993.

78. Maixner D, Green TL, Walton R: Histologic examination of condensing osteitis (Abstract), *J Endod* 18:196, 1992.

79. Hedin M, Polhagen L: Follow-up study of periradicular bone condensation, *Scand J Dent Res* 79:436, 1971.

80. Baumgartner J, Picket A, Muller J: Microscopic examination of oral sinus tracts and their associated periapical lesions, *J Endod* 10:146, 1984.

81. Amler MH: The time sequence of tissue regeneration in human extraction wounds, *Oral Surg Oral Med Oral Pathol* 27:309, 1969.

82. Fouad AF, Walton RE, Rittman BR: Healing of induced periapical lesions in ferret canines, *J Endod* 19:123, 1993.

83. Danin J, Linder LE, Lundqvist G, Andersson L: Tumor necrosis factor-alpha and transforming growth factor-beta$_1$ in chronic periapical lesions, *Oral Surg Oral Med Oral Pathol* 90:514, 2000.

84. Leonardi R, Lanteri E, Stivala F, Travali S: Immunolocalization of CD44 adhesion molecules in human periradicular lesions, *Oral Surg Oral Med Oral Pathol* 89:480, 2000.

85. Morton TH: Differential diagnosis of periapical radiolucent lesions, *Dent Clin North Am* 25:519, 1979.

86. Kerfzoudis N, Donta-Bakoyiannd C, Siskos G: The lateral periodontal cyst: aetiology, clinical significance and diagnosis, *Endod Dent Traumatol* 16:144, 2000.

87. Eversole LR: *Clinical outline of oral pathology,* ed 2, pp 204-259 Philadelphia, 1984, Lea & Febiger.

Diagnosis and Treatment Planning

LEARNING OBJECTIVES

After reading this chapter, the student should be able to:

1 / Define and differentiate subjective symptoms and objective findings.

2 / Interpret the significance of the subjective symptoms and objective findings in the identification of diseases of pulp and periradicular tissues.

3 / State the reasons and procedures used for reviewing the chief complaint, medical and dental histories, and present illness.

4 / Identify findings that affect diagnosis or treatment planning.

5 / Identify the aspects of pain most important in diagnosis.

6 / State the importance of and procedures used for extraoral and intraoral examination of soft and hard tissues.

7 / Discuss the purpose of and procedures used for clinical examinations including visual (mirror and explorer) examination, periodontal evaluation, and mobility.

8 / Describe the importance of and steps involved in performing clinical pulp and periapical tests such as direct dentin stimulation, electrical and thermal pulp tests, percussion, and palpation.

9 / Describe radiographic findings that may indicate pulpal or periapical pathosis.

10 / Describe when caries removal is a diagnostic test, when caries removal is required, and probable pulpal diagnosis according to findings.

11 / Describe the indications and procedures used for test cavity, selective anesthesia, and transillumination tests.

12 / Identify the significant subjective findings and objective tests that are most indicated in differential diagnosis.

13 / State the pulpal and periapical diagnosis, using appropriate terminology, according to the diagnostic findings.

14 / Describe conditions for which root canal treatment is indicated and contraindicated.

15 / Design an appropriate general treatment plan according to the pulpal and periapical diagnosis.

16 / Determine the number of appointments appropriate for different situations.

17 / Recognize and diagnose when it is appropriate to plan adjunctive endodontic treatments such as vital pulp therapy, bleaching, root amputation, endodontic surgery, intentional replantation, autotransplantation, hemisection, apexification, endodontic endosseous implants, orthodontic extrusion, and retreatments.

18 / Identify problems (operative complications, cracked tooth, periodontal problems, isolation difficulties, restorability, strategic value, patient management, medical complications, abnormal root or pulp anatomy, impact trauma, and restricted opening) that require treatment modifications.

OUTLINE

Diagnosis
Chief Complaint
Health History
Subjective Examination
Objective Examination
Radiographic Examination
Special Tests
Selective Anesthesia
Longitudinal Crown Fractures
Difficult Diagnoses
Diagnostic Findings and Terminology

Treatment Planning
To Treat or Not to Treat
Treatment Related to Diagnosis
Number of Appointments
Diagnosis and Treatment Plans
Treatment Choices
Treatment Modifiers

Prognosis

D iagnosis and treatment planning are activities that separate and distinguish the dentist from auxiliary personnel. Expanded-duty personnel may be trained to perform routine endodontic technical procedures. However, only the dentist has training in basic and clinical sciences; this entitles the dentist alone to (1) *perform* all diagnostic tests, (2) *interpret* the test results differentially, (3) *psychologically manage* the patient during testing procedures, and (4) *formulate* an appropriate diagnosis and treatment plan.

Differential diagnosis of orofacial disorders is demanding and may confuse both patient and clinician because there is a tendency to equate a complaint of pain with an endodontic problem. In addition to teeth, other structures and organs such as the periodontium, jaws, sinuses, ears, temporomandibular joints, masticatory musculature, nose, eyes, and blood vessels can induce pain that may mimic dental pain.[1,2] Other pathologic conditions such as neuralgia, multiple sclerosis, myocardial ischemia, or psychiatric disorders may produce the same symptoms. To avoid misdiagnosis (Figure 4-1) and to rule out orofacial pain of nonpulpal or periradicular origin, a step-by-step systematic approach to diagnosis and treatment planning *must* be followed:

1. Ascertain the chief complaint.
2. Take pertinent information related to the patient's medical and dental history.
3. Conduct thorough subjective, objective, and radiographic examinations.
4. Analyze the data obtained.
5. Formulate an appropriate diagnosis and treatment plan.

Endodontics has a wide scope and includes vital pulp therapy, nonsurgical root canal treatment, endodontic surgery, retreatment, hemisection or root amputation, bleaching, intentional replantation, endodontic endosseous implants, apexification or apexogenesis, transplantation, treatment of trauma, periodontal-endodontic pathosis, and orthodontics-endodontics. Obviously, the area most commonly dealt with and the one that receives the most attention is root canal treatment. In addition, the student and general practitioner should have sufficient expertise to perform some other endodontic treatment modalities in clinical practice, but other aspects are complex and should be considered for referral. These aspects are discussed further in this chapter.

This does not mean that the graduating dentist should be knowledgeable about diagnosis and treatment planning in only a limited area of endodontics, that is, root canal treatment. In fact, *the practicing general dentist should be very skilled in diagnosis and treatment planning over a broad base.* The general dentist has initial and repeated contact with the patient. He or she must be able to recognize the pathosis or disorder, diagnose the entity, and suggest the appropriate treatment plan. A further decision then is whether the general dentist has enough experience to treat the condition or whether the patient should be considered for referral.

The dentist with this knowledge is aware of indications and contraindications for treatment and can predict success or failure based on his or her own findings. The choice of who shall perform the treatment is then decided by consultation with the patient and is based on the mode of delivery designed for the best care for that patient. To summarize: The graduating dentist should be proficient in diagnosis and treatment planning and should be treating patients with uncomplicated problems but referring those with complications.

This chapter suggests a systematic approach to diagnosis and treatment planning primarily as related to root canal treatment. Diagnosis, treatment planning, and therapeutic aspects of other entities are found in their respective chapters.

Diagnosis

CHIEF COMPLAINT

The chief complaint is generally the first information obtained. This is the problem expressed in the patient's own words about the condition that prompted him or her to seek treatment. The chief complaint should be recorded as reported in nontechnical language; for example, "I have an infected tooth and a gum boil," or "I have a toothache that may be causing my sinus problem."

To avoid obtaining misleading information, patients should be allowed to verbalize problems in a way that allows them to voice their desire for relief: "Take care of the problem and stop my pain." When the patient is unaware of any problem or has been referred for diagnosis or treatment, these facts should also be recorded (as *"no chief complaint"*) for future reference.

HEALTH HISTORY

Taking a comprehensive health history for new patients and reviewing and updating the data of prior patients constitute the first step in diagnosis. A complete health history for a new patient consists of routine demographic data, medical history, current medications, dental history, chief complaint, and present illness.

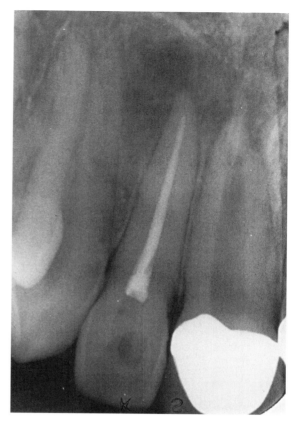

FIGURE 4-1
A reliance on "clinical experience" rather than on adequate tests resulted in the wrong treatment. The dentist relied on a radiograph only (no tests) and concluded that the lateral incisor was the painful problem tooth. After treatment, with no change in the level of pain, the patient was referred for root-end surgery. Examination of preoperative and postoperative radiographs as well as clinical tests showed that treatment had been performed on a tooth with normal pulp. The central incisor was found to have pulp necrosis and an acute apical abscess. Immediate pain relief followed root canal treatment on the correct tooth.

Demographic Data

Demographic data identify the patient's characteristics.

Medical History

Advances in medicine and public awareness of dental maintenance have led to treatment being rendered for patients of all ages, not only the young or those without medical problems. The patient population is, on average, of increasing age and has a higher incidence of pulpal or periradicular pathoses.[3] Older individuals tend to have more medical problems also.

The end result is that there are more older patients who are seen with special problems[4]; these considerations are discussed in more detail in Chapter 31. Consequently, many patients (particularly the elderly) have had systemic diseases, injuries, or surgery or are taking medications that interfere with treatment procedures. In addition, the root canal serves as a conduit between the external environment (oral cavity) and the general system. There is increasing concern (and emerging data) that oral conditions may cause systemic manifestations.[5,6] There is also the possibility and some evidence[7] that intracanal bacteria may be introduced into the general circulation; the significance is at yet unknown but of concern nevertheless.

A thorough medical history not only aids diagnosis but also provides information about a patient's susceptibility and reactions to infection and about bleeding, prescribed medications, and emotional status. Because a medical history is not intended to be a complete clinical examination, extensive medical questionnaires are unnecessary. An abbreviated screening form contains questions about present and past serious illnesses, injuries, and surgery. If there is medical evidence of severe or obscure physical or psychologic disease that might interfere with diagnosis or treatment, further investigation and consultation with other health professionals are indicated.

There are no specific medical conditions that contraindicate root canal treatment other than those that affect any dental procedure. These conditions include irradiation of local tissues or diseases that compromise the immune system, such as acquired immunodeficiency syndrome (AIDS)[8,9] and severe heart disease.[10,11] Other areas of concern that may require special measures are the increasing incidence of latex allergies,[12,13] glucocorticosteroid replacement therapy, hepatitis, delayed hemostasis, certain cardiac conditions, and joint replacement.

Dental History

The dental history is a summary of present and past dental experiences. It provides valuable information about the patient's attitudes toward oral health, care, and treatment. Such information not only has diagnostic importance, but it also affects treatment planning. The questionnaire should ask for information about past and present signs and symptoms. This history is a very important initial step in making a specific diagnosis.

In addition to some obvious findings that are directly related to endodontic problems, the history reveals past dental experience and clues to the patient's psychologic makeup as well as explaining subtle clinical findings. For example, asymptomatic short roots or root resorption may be attributed to orthodontics (Figure 4-2). Pain may develop in a recently restored tooth or after extensive periodontal therapy. This information not only identifies the source of a patient's complaint but also aids in selecting a specific test or treatment modality.

SUBJECTIVE EXAMINATION
Present Illness

Some routine information related to personal data, medical history, and dental history as well as the chief complaint may be obtained by staff. However, the dentist should review and be familiar with the data before proceeding further. Often, the first contact between patient and dentist takes place during collection of data about the present illness.

Most patients with endodontic pathoses are asymptomatic or have mild symptoms. If pulp or periradicular pathosis is suspected because of other findings, the dentist notes the absence of significant symptoms and moves on to objective tests. However, patients may have notable levels of pain and distress. These patients require a careful,

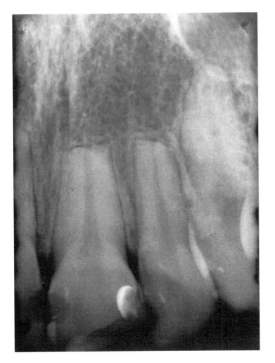

FIGURE 4-2
The presence of short roots, an absence of pathosis in the periapical tissues of the incisors, and a history of orthodontics indicate that resorption is due to tooth movement.

systematic subjective examination with pointed, probing questions. An interesting and often confusing entity is tooth-related pain experienced with changes in ambient pressure. This phenomenon is known as barodontalgia and affects patients who experience a pressure increase or decrease. It has been described in high-altitude flying[14] and scuba diving.[8]

Pain and discomfort associated with pulpal and periradicular diseases do not usually affect a patient's physical state and have little or no effect on vital signs, skin color, or muscle tone. However, severe pulpal or periradicular pain may affect vital signs. Regardless of degree, such pain significantly alters emotional status. Because of apprehension and emotional as well as occasional physical instability, endodontic patients are handled with extra care. Professional appearance, attitude, and a proper atmosphere are the main factors needed to establish good rapport (see Chapter 6). In a friendly and compassionate environment, patients express problems openly. With such a thorough approach, patients often volunteer many details about the location, onset, character, and severity of the pain. After listening with keen interest, the dentist, in a sympathetic and unhurried manner, should ask further questions about the severity, spontaneity, and duration of the pain and the stimuli that induce or relieve it. Medications taken for pain relief and their effectiveness are also important.

Significant Aspects of Pain

Pain of high intensity is usually intermittent, whereas low-intensity pain is often continuous and protracted.[15] In contrast to protracted pain, which is steady and dull, paroxysmal pain consists of a volley of bright jabs. Pain may also be described as pricking, stinging, burning, aching, or throbbing. Often, severe pulpal or periapical pain is synchronized with cardiac systole. Myofascial pain is usually dull, whereas the pain of neuralgia is bright and paroxysmal.[15] Identification of the nature of the pain helps to differentiate dental pain from pain in other tissues. These important considerations are discussed in detail in Chapter 29.

Pain is a complex entity. Many aspects of pain are not particularly diagnostic and do not differentiate dental from nondental problems or indicate the severity. However, some aspects of pain are strongly indicative of pulpal and/or periradicular pathosis and thus of the treatment required. These are the (1) *intensity*, (2) *spontaneity*, and (3) *persistence*.

Intensity. The more intense the pain (i.e., disruptive to a patient's lifestyle), the more likely it is that irreversible pathosis is present. Intense pain is likely to be of recent onset, is unrelieved by analgesics, and has prompted the patient to seek treatment. Long-standing pain is usually not intense. Pain of a mild or moderate nature of long duration is not, by itself, particularly diagnostic endodontically. Intense pain may arise from irreversible pulpitis or from symptomatic (acute) apical periodontitis or abscess.

Spontaneous Pain. Spontaneous pain occurs without an eliciting stimulus. If pain awakens the patient or begins without stimulus, it is spontaneous. As described previously, spontaneous combined with intense pain *usually* indicates severe pulpal and/or periradicular pathosis.

An interesting and very diagnostic occurrence is intense, continuous pain relieved only by cold. Patients with this kind of pain often appear for treatment clutching a glass of ice water that they sip to retain cold on the aching tooth. This pain is pathognomonic of irreversible pulpitis.

Continuous Pain. This lingering type of pain continues and may even increase in intensity after the stimulus is removed. For example, the patient reports prolonged pain after drinking cold liquids. Another describes intense continuous pain after chewing. Continuous pain with thermal stimulus usually indicates irreversible pulpitis. Continuous pain after application of pressure to a tooth indicates periradicular pathosis.

After taking the medical and dental histories and identifying the main subjective signs and symptoms of the patient's present illness (as described previously), the dentist often arrives at a tentative diagnosis.

Tentative Diagnosis

By expanding on the present illness and asking careful subjective questions about the patient's problem, the dentist can often determine the presence or absence of pathologic changes in pulp or periapical tissues. The quality and quantity of present and past pain as well as other important subjective findings often rule out confusing nonendodontic entities. The urgency of treatment is also determined. Careful questioning and interpretation of the patient's responses often offer strong clues to a tentative diagnosis of pulpal or periradicular pathosis. The tentative diagnosis is then confirmed or denied by hands-on oral examination and clinical tests.

OBJECTIVE EXAMINATION

During this stage, extraoral and intraoral tissues are examined, tested, and compared bilaterally for the presence or absence of pathosis.

Extraoral Examination

General appearance, skin tone, facial asymmetry, swelling, discoloration, redness, extraoral scars or sinus tracts, and tender or enlarged facial or cervical lymph nodes are indicators of physical status. A careful extraoral examination helps to identify the cause of the patient's complaint as well as the presence and extent of an inflammatory reaction in the oral cavity (Figure 4-3).

Intraoral Examination

Soft Tissue. This examination includes a thorough visual and digital test of the oral soft tissues. The lips, oral mucosa, cheeks, tongue, palate, and

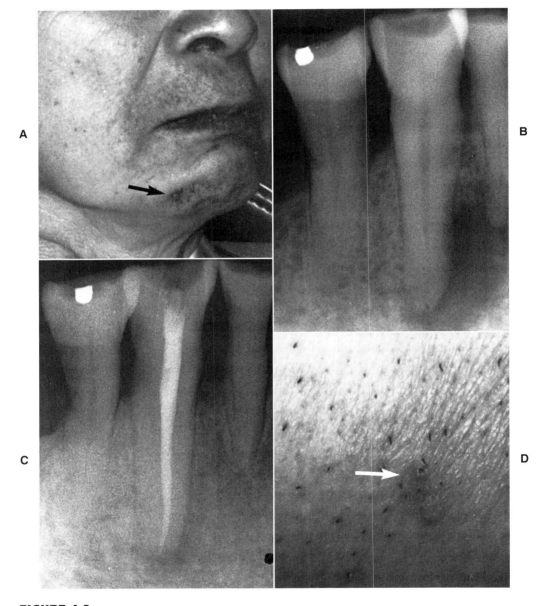

FIGURE 4-3
Extraoral sinus tract. **A,** This surface lesion *(arrow)* was misdiagnosed and treated unsuccessfully by a dermatologist for several months. Fortunately, the patient's dentist then recognized it to be a draining sinus tract with its source being a mandibular anterior tooth. **B,** The pulp was necrotic owing to severe attrition with pulp exposure. **C,** After proper root canal treatment only. **D,** the sinus tract and surface lesion resolved completely *(arrow)*.

muscles are evaluated and abnormalities are noted. Alveolar mucosa and attached gingiva are examined for the presence of discoloration, inflammation, ulceration, and sinus tract formation. A sinus tract stoma parulis usually indicates presence of a necrotic pulp or suppurative apical periodontitis and sometimes a periodontal abscess (Figure 4-4). Gutta-percha placed in the sinus tract occasionally allows localization of the source of these lesions.

Dentition. Teeth are examined for discolorations, fractures, abrasions, erosions, caries, large restorations, or other abnormalities. A discolored crown is often pathognomonic of pulpal pathosis (Figure 4-5) or is the sequela of earlier root canal treatment. Although in some cases the diagnosis is very likely at this stage of examination, a prudent diagnostician should *never* proceed with treatment before performing appropriate confirmatory clinical and radiographic examinations.

Clinical Tests

Clinical tests include use of a mirror and an explorer and periodontal probing as well as indicated pulpal and periapical tests. There are limitations inherent in most of these tests; some cannot be used on each tooth, and the test results themselves may be inconclusive. Therefore, it is risky to rely on a single test; other supplemental confirmatory tests should be performed. These tests are not absolute and tend to be somewhat crude. They require care in performance and caution in

interpretation. Importantly, these are *not* tests of *teeth;* they are tests of a patient's *response* to a variety of perceived stimuli. The testing response process is very complex and involves both the peripheral and central nervous systems as well as occasional complications related to the emotional status of the patient, thus often giving rise to false-negative and false-positive test results. The patient may not understand or may wrongly perceive or misinterpret a stimulus. For these reasons, the series of subjective and objective tests and findings often are inconsistent and results are

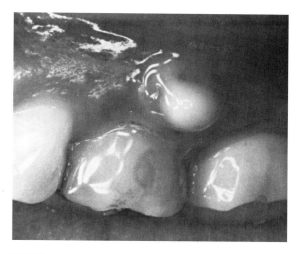

FIGURE 4-4
Intraoral sinus tract. Purulence is expressed from this asymptomatic lesion associated with pulp necrosis of the first molar.

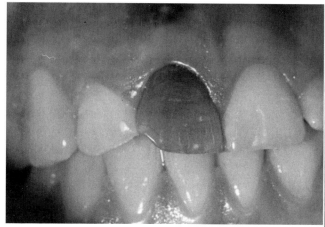

A

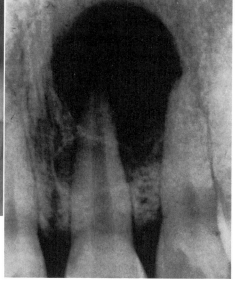

B

FIGURE 4-5
The discolored incisor (**A**) was associated with a necrotic pulp and chronic apical periodontitis (**B**).

confusing for strict interpretation. There is no easy resolution; patience and insight are required, and experience is helpful.

Mirror and Explorer. A mirror and an explorer reveal gross or recurrent caries, pulp exposures, crown fractures, defective restorations, and coronal leakage in teeth with previous root canal therapy. In some instances (i.e., gross coronal decay), the mirror and explorer may provide sufficient information to arrive at a final diagnosis. However, because pathologic changes usually cannot be determined by this method alone, other clinical tests are required.

Control Teeth. An important adjunct to pulp and periapical tests is the use of controls (comparisons). These are healthy teeth that should respond normally. Control teeth have three functions: (1) the patient learns what to expect from the stimulus; (2) the dentist can observe the nature of the patient's response to a certain level of stimulus; and (3) the dentist can determine that the stimulus is capable of invoking a response. For example, posterior teeth in adults, particularly molars, may be unresponsive to thermal tests. This would make cold invalid as a testing modality if ice is placed on a healthy molar and the patient experiences no sensation.

Periapical Tests

Percussion. Percussion may determine the presence of periradicular inflammation. A marked positive response indicates inflammation in the periodontium. Because inflammatory changes in periodontal ligament are not always of pulpal origin and may be induced by periodontal disease, the results should be confirmed by other tests. However, in some cases other tests cannot be performed, and percussion might be the best indicator of significant periradicular pathosis. One difference is that percussion pain related to *periodontal inflammation* is more likely to be in the mild to moderate range. *Periapical inflammation* is probable if the pain is very sharp, causing a withdrawal response.

Percussion is performed by tapping on the incisal or occlusal surface with the end of a mirror handle held parallel or perpendicular to the crown. With severe subjective pain, tapping the teeth is avoided; gentle apical pressure is applied with digital manipulation of the tooth. To establish a basis for comparison, the percussion test should also be performed on control teeth. Another very good test is to have the patient bite hard on an object, such as a cotton swab, with the suspected and a control tooth. This test is confirmatory if the patient reports pain upon mastication (Figure 4-6).

Palpation. Like percussion, palpation determines how far the inflammatory process has extended periapically. A positive response to palpation indicates periradicular inflammation. Palpation is firm pressure on the mucosa overlying the apex (Figure 4-7). Pressure is applied by a fingertip and, like the percussion test, at least one control tooth should be included.

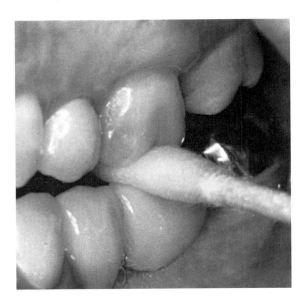

FIGURE 4-6
Biting test. Having the patient bite and grind firmly on a cotton swab is effective in confirming pain on mastication.

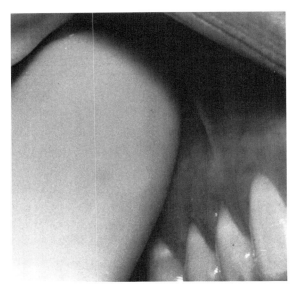

FIGURE 4-7
Palpation. Applying firm pressure with the little finger over the apex of the suspect tooth helps confirm periradicular inflammation.

Pulp Vitality Tests

Direct dentin stimulation, cold, heat, and electricity determine the response to stimuli and occasionally can identify the offending tooth by an abnormal response. Response does not guarantee a pulp's viability or health but at best indicates the *presence of some nerve fibers carrying sensory impulses.* There is wide variation in the pulpal response of both normal and pathologically involved teeth. Because of inherent limitations, these tests should always have adequate controls, and results should be interpreted carefully.

Selecting the Appropriate Pulp Test. The selection depends on the situation. Additional meaningful information is collected when stimuli similar to those that the patient reports will provoke pain are used during clinical tests. When cold (or hot) food or drink initiates a painful response, a cold (or hot) test is conducted in place of other viability tests. Replication of the *same* symptoms in a tooth often indicates the offender. Overall, electrical stimulation is similar to cold (refrigerant) in identifying pulp necrosis; heat is the least reliable stimulus.

Direct Dentin Stimulation. This is probably the most accurate and, in many cases, the best pulp vitality test. Exposed dentin may be scratched with an explorer; however, the *absence* of a response is not as indicative as the *presence* of a response. Caries are probed deeply with an explorer to noncarious dentin; sudden, sharp sensation indicates that the pulp contains vital tissue.

When other tests are inconclusive or cannot be used and a necrotic pulp is suspected, a test cavity is helpful. For example, a tooth with a porcelain-fused-to-metal crown often cannot be tested accurately by standard thermal or electrical tests. After careful subjective examination and an explanation of the nature of the test to the patient, preparation without anesthesia is done with a small and sharp bur. With a vital pulp, the surface of the restoration or the enamel can be penetrated without too much discomfort. If the pulp is vital, there will be a sudden sensation of pain when dentin is reached. In contrast, if discomfort or pain is absent, the pulp is probably necrotic; an access preparation has already been started and the procedure may be continued.

Cold Tests. Three methods are generally used for cold testing: regular ice, carbon dioxide (dry ice), and refrigerant. Carbon dioxide requires special equipment (Figure 4-8), whereas refrigerant in a spray can is more convenient (Figure 4-9). As to effectiveness, regular ice delivers less cold and is not as effective as refrigerant or CO_2 ice. One study found that refrigerant sprayed on a large cotton pellet markedly reduced temperature within the chamber.[16] Overall, refrigerant spray and CO_2 are equivalent for pulp testing.

After the tooth is isolated with cotton rolls and dried, an ice stick or large cotton pellet saturated with refrigerant is applied. This stimulus applied over a vital pulp usually results in sharp, brief pain. This short, sharp response may occur regardless of pulp status (normal or reversible or irreversible pulpitis). However, an intense and prolonged response usually indicates irreversible pulpitis. In contrast, necrotic pulps do not respond. A *false-negative* response is often obtained when cold is applied to teeth with constricted canals (calcific metamorphosis), whereas a *false-positive* response may result if cold water contacts gingiva or is transferred to adjacent teeth with vital pulps.

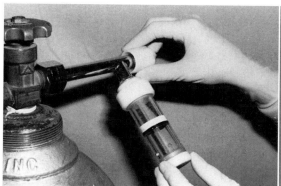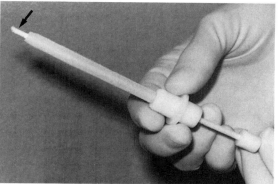

A   B

FIGURE 4-8
Carbon dioxide ice testing. **A,** A carbon dioxide tank and special "ice maker" are required. **B,** A carbon dioxide ice stick is formed *(arrow).* The stick is held in gauze and touched to the facial surfaces of suspect and control teeth. This technique can be used in teeth with various types of restorations. (Courtesy Dr. W. Johnson.)

Cold is more effective on anterior teeth than on more insulated posterior teeth. Therefore, *lack of a response to cold on control posterior teeth indicates another vitality test*. Electric pulp testing is reliable after cold testing; the pulp's responsiveness is unaffected by cold.[17]

Heat Tests. Teeth may be isolated by a rubber dam to prevent false-positive responses. Various techniques and materials are used. Gutta-percha is heated in a flame and applied to the facial surface. The best, safest, and easiest technique is to rotate a dry rubber prophy cup to create frictional heat (Figure 4-10) or to apply hot water. A flame-heated instrument is difficult to control and should be handled with care.

A mechanical, battery-powered device, such as the Touch-n-Heat, is better controlled and will deliver heat safely and effectively. Heat is not used routinely but is helpful when the major symptom is heat sensitivity, and the patient cannot identify the offending tooth. After applying heat, the temperature is gradually increased until pain is elicited. As with cold, a sharp and nonlingering pain response indicates a vital (not necessarily normal) pulp.

Significance of Thermal Tests. An exaggerated and lingering response is a good indication of irreversible pulpitis. Absence of response in conjunction with other tests compared with results on control teeth usually indicates pulpal necrosis. As with cold, calcific metamorphosis may cause a false-negative response. As mentioned earlier, *one test is seldom conclusive for the presence or absence of pulpal or periapical disease*.

Electrical Pulp Testing. Many devices are available commercially for electrical pulp tests. All are powered by batteries and deliver a direct current of high-frequency electricity that is varied. The stimulus is usually applied to the facial surface to determine the presence or absence of sensory nerves and supposedly of a vital pulp.

Electrical pulp testers with digital readouts are popular. These are not inherently superior to other electrical testers but are more user-friendly. All are used in a similar manner. It is very important to clean, dry, and isolate the teeth. Scrub the surface with a cotton roll and isolate it with the same roll, then dry thoroughly with the air syringe. A small amount of toothpaste or other conducting medium (the most effective conducting medium has not been identified) is placed on the electrode. An electrical circuit is established by using a lip clip or having the patient touch the metal handle.[18] The electrode is placed on the facial or lingual surface (Figure 4-11), and the level of current is gradually increased until it surpasses the perception threshold. Sensation may be tingling, stinging, "full," or hot. The presence of a response

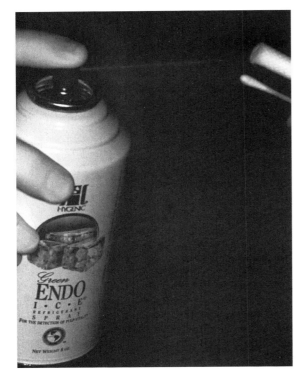

FIGURE 4-9
Refrigerant sprayed on a cotton roll, swab, or pellet (best) is convenient and effective for determining pulp responsiveness.

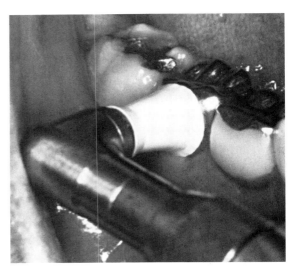

FIGURE 4-10
A prophy cup run at high speed without lubricant generates controlled heat for pulp testing.

usually indicates vital tissue, whereas the absence of such a response usually indicates pulpal necrosis. The electrical pulp tester is not infallible and may produce false-positive or false-negative responses 10% to 20% of the time.[19] Calcific metamorphosis may cause a false-negative response. Warning: *Contrary to popular opinion and persistent notions, different response levels with different teeth as shown by the number on the device do not indicate stages of pulp degeneration.* Electrical testers do not measure the degree of health or disease of a pulp. Because false-positive and false-negative responses are common, reactions to these tests should be interpreted (with some skepticism) only as yes or no responses. Further careful interpretation, comparison, and correlation with other findings and tests must be done; then a tentative determination of vitality or necrosis is appropriate.

Blood Flow Determination. Instruments that detect pulp circulation are part of a developing technology that is likely to produce new approaches for determining the presence of vital pulp tissue in an otherwise nonresponsive tooth. An example is the previously traumatized tooth that has an intact blood supply, but no intact sensory nerves and therefore is unresponsive to stimuli. These very sensitive devices will detect pulp blood components or blood flow in these situations. Sensors are applied to the enamel surface, usually on both the facial and lingual nerves. Blood flow is shown by beams of light (dual wavelength spectrophotometry),[20] pulse oximetry,[21] or laser Doppler flowmetry.[22,23] Blood components are demonstrated by detecting oxyhemoglobin,[24] low concentrations of blood,[25] or pulsations in the pulp. These approaches are still more experimental than clinically practical, and the devices are expensive. As the technology improves and becomes less costly, and more experience is gained, their use as sensitive pulp testers in the future is likely.

Periodontal Examination

Periapical and periodontal lesions may mimic each other and therefore require differentiation (see Chapter 26). It is also important to establish the periodontal health of the tooth or teeth as part of overall treatment planning.

Probing. Probing is an important clinical test that is often overlooked and underused for diagnosing periapical lesions. Bone and periodontal soft tissue destruction are induced by both periodontal disease and periradicular lesions and may not be easily detected or differentiated radiographically.

A periodontal probe determines the level of connective tissue attachment. Also, the probe penetrates into an inflammatory periapical lesion that extends cervically. Probing is a diagnostic aid that has prognostic value. The prognosis for a tooth with a necrotic pulp that induces cervically extending periapical inflammation is good after adequate root canal treatment. However, the outcome of root canal treatment on a tooth with severe periodontal disease usually depends on the success of periodontal treatment. Teeth with marked periodontal disease involvement are poor candidates for endodontic procedures. Probing depths should be recorded for future comparison.

Mobility. The mobility test partially determines the status of both the periodontal ligament and prognosis. Teeth with extreme mobility usually have little periodontal support. Occasionally an extensive periradicular lesion may alter the periodontal support markedly; mobility usually decreases dramatically after successful root canal treatment.

Mobility is determined by placing the index finger on the lingual aspect and applying pressure with the mirror handle on the opposite facial surface. Movement of more than 2 to 3 mm or depression indicates that the tooth is a poor candidate for root canal treatment if the mobility is due primarily to periodontal disease and not to periradicular pathosis.

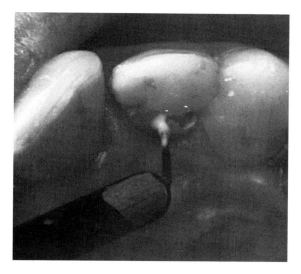

FIGURE 4-11
Electric pulp tester. A special minitip (electrode) with a small spot of conductive medium is useful for electrical pulp testing where tooth structure availability is limited.

RADIOGRAPHIC EXAMINATION

Perhaps radiographs should be termed "the great pretenders." Dentists tend to rely excessively on

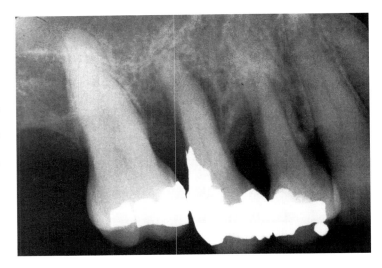

FIGURE 4-12
Horizontal as well as vertical bone loss is evident in this quadrant. All teeth are responsive to vitality tests; therefore, the resorptive defects represent a severe periodontal condition and not pulp or periradicular pathosis. Root canal treatment is not indicated.

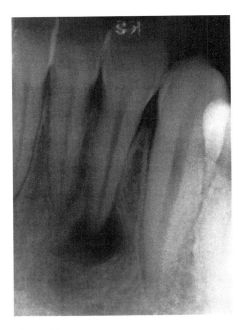

FIGURE 4-13
Characteristic appearance of an endodontic lesion. This radiograph shows loss of lamina dura and a hanging-drop appearance. There was a history of trauma in this patient. A film made at a different angle would show the lesion remaining at the apex. (Courtesy Dr. L. Wilcox.)

radiographs to supply conclusive diagnostic information. Certainly they are useful and necessary as diagnostic and treatment aids. But the use of radiographs to diagnose pulpal or periradicular pathosis has been exaggerated, and many limitations are overlooked. Pathologic changes in the pulp are not visible; likewise, periradicular lesions produce no radiographic changes in the early stages. Evidence of pathosis often appears only

when the inflammatory process spreads to medullary bone, particularly to the cortical plates.[26,27] Radiographs are only two-dimensional; various projections may allow several views of the same structures, permitting three-dimensional interpretation. With these and other limitations, it is evident that good-quality films are only one of the tools used for diagnosis.

Radiographs allow evaluation of tooth-related problems (e.g., carious lesions, defective restorations, and root canal treatments), abnormal pulpal and periradicular appearances, malpositioned teeth, relationship of the neurovascular bundle to the apexes, the general bony pattern, and periodontal disease (Figure 4-12).

Periapical Lesions

Radiolucent and radiopaque entities in the jaws (both normal structures and nonendodontic pathosis) may be confused with endodontic pathosis. Obviously, such confusion may lead to misdiagnosis and incorrect treatment. Periradicular lesions of pulpal origin usually have four characteristics: (1) the lamina dura is lost apically; (2) the lucency remains at the apex regardless of the cone angle; (3) the lucency tends to resemble a hanging drop; and (4) usually a cause of the pulp necrosis is evident (Figure 4-13).

The dentist should remember the most important diagnostic radiographic relationship between the pulp and the periapical tissues: *A well-developed radiolucent periapical lesion is invariably associated with and results from a necrotic pulp!* A sizable radiolucency in the periapical region of a tooth with a vital pulp is *not* of endodontic origin and is either a normal structure or a nonendodontic pathosis.

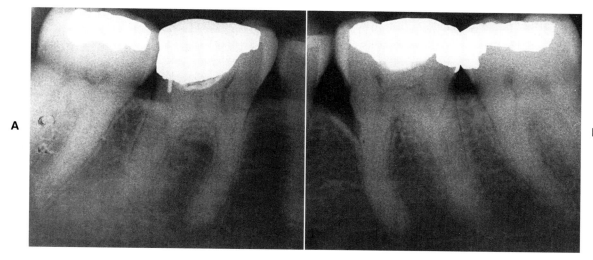

FIGURE 4-14
Condensing osteitis. **A,** Surrounding the distal root apex is diffuse trabeculation. **B,** This contrasts with the contralateral molar, which demonstrates a normal, sparse trabecular pattern.

Radiopaque changes also occur. Condensing osteitis is a reaction to pulp or periradicular inflammation and results in an increase in medullary bone.[28] It has a diffuse circumferential medullary pattern with indistinct borders (Figure 4-14). The well-circumscribed, more homogeneous normal structure that occurs commonly in the mandibular posterior region is enostosis (or sclerotic bone); this is a nonpathologic condition.

New radiographic technology permits early detection of bony changes, allowing new approaches to differential diagnosis. Digital subtraction radiography "reads" subtle early changes with periapical bone resorption.[29] Digital radiometric analysis and computed tomography may distinguish bony pathoses such as granulomas and cysts.[30] Radiovisiography and magnetic resonance imaging demonstrate changes of resorptive lesions over time.[31] However, all these technologies are still neither perfected nor cost effective nor offer significant diagnostic benefits for routine clinical application[32]; undoubtedly these or similar devices will prove useful in the future.

Pulpal Lesions

Few specific pathologic entities that relate to irreversible pulpitis are visible radiographically. An inflamed pulp with dentinoclastic activity may show abnormally altered pulp space enlargement and is pathognomonic of internal resorption (Figure 4-15). Extensive diffuse calcification in the chamber may indicate long-term, low-grade irritation (not necessarily of irreversible pulpitis).

Dentin formation that radiographically "obliterates" the canals (usually in patients with a history of trauma) does not in itself indicate pathosis (Figure 4-16). These teeth ordinarily require no treatment, but when treatment is necessary (see Figure 4-15, *B*), they can be managed with reasonable success.[33]

SPECIAL TESTS

After subjective and objective examinations and clinical tests have been completed, it is usually possible to make an accurate diagnosis and create a reasonable treatment plan. However, if special circumstances prevent making a definitive diagnosis, additional tests such as caries removal, selective anesthesia, and transillumination are options.

Caries Removal

Determining the depth of caries penetration is necessary in some situations for definitive pulp diagnosis. A common clinical situation is the presence of deep caries on radiographs, no significant history or presenting symptoms, and a pulp that responds to clinical tests. All other findings are normal. The final definitive test is complete caries removal to establish pulp status.

Penetration of caries into a symptomatic pulp indicates irreversible pulpitis, requiring root canal treatment. Nonpenetration usually indicates reversible pulpitis (although a percentage of pulps are irreversibly inflamed without exposure); the

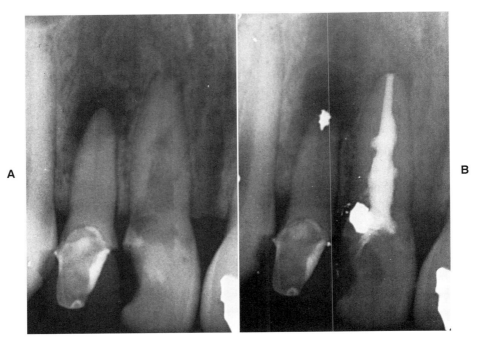

FIGURE 4-15
Differing pulp responses to injury. **A,** Central incisor shows extensive, perforating internal resorption; the lateral incisor has calcific metamorphosis. **B,** Special techniques manage these problems with both surgical and nonsurgical treatment.

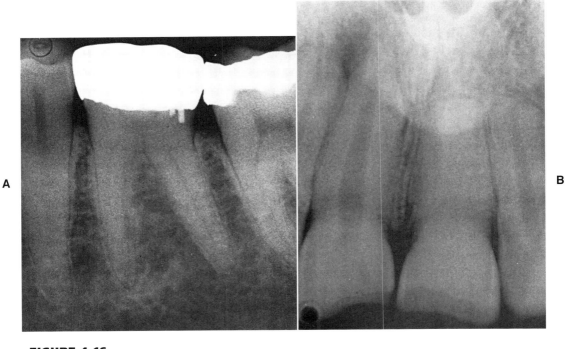

FIGURE 4-16
Calcific metamorphosis. **A,** This lesion has resulted from repeated insults from caries and restorations. **B,** This dentin formation ("obliteration") resulted from trauma and irritation to the pulp. Neither **A** nor **B** is pathosis. Occasionally apical pathosis does develop; this is a treatment challenge. (**B** courtesy Dr. L. Wilcox.)

tooth is then restored atraumatically. The patient is informed of possible future treatments.

Selective Anesthesia

This test is in contrast to the test cavity, which is performed in symptomatic as well as pain-free teeth. The selective anesthesia test is useful in painful teeth, particularly when the patient cannot isolate the offending tooth even to a specific arch. If a mandibular tooth is suspected, a mandibular block will confirm at least the region if the pain disappears after the injection.

Individual tooth anesthesia is most effective in the maxilla. Anesthetic should be administered in an anterior to posterior direction because of the distribution of the sensory nerves. Because an inferior alveolar nerve block anesthetizes all teeth in the quadrant, selective anesthesia is not useful for the mandible. The periodontal ligament injection will often anesthetize multiple teeth[34] and should not be used to identify a suspect tooth. Selective anesthesia is most useful to identify which arch has the tooth that is the source of pain.

Transillumination

This test helps to identify longitudinal crown fractures because a fracture will not transmit the light. Transillumination produces contrasting dark and light at the fracture site.

LONGITUDINAL CROWN FRACTURES

These fractures seem to be increasing in number and are a challenge for both diagnosis and treatment. There are some classic signs occurring often that indicate a cracked tooth. This is a fairly common cause of endodontic pathosis and therefore requires consideration during diagnosis. More detail about diagnosis and management of these fractures is in Chapter 28.

DIFFICULT DIAGNOSES

Some perplexing conditions defy diagnosis even after thorough subjective, objective, and radiographic examinations.[35] Usually these situations do not require immediate treatment and the patient may be scheduled for a return visit for further evaluation or possibly dental and medical consultations. Collection and careful analysis of data by consultation with others are prudent to prevent misdiagnosis and mistreatment of these patients. It is a mistake to feel compelled to treat all patients who express symptoms immediately. Often time or a different approach will permit the correct diagnosis and logical treatment. Also, symptoms that have significant pathosis as their source tend to be isolated to the offending tooth with time. Symptoms unrelated to significant pathosis will generally subside. Patients usually accept this explanation and are willing to wait for a definitive diagnosis.

DIAGNOSTIC FINDINGS AND TERMINOLOGY

Use of a data form to accumulate diagnostic findings serves three purposes: first, it ensures that all pertinent information has been assessed and included; second, it ensures that findings have been recorded and may be analyzed; and third, it allows future reference to findings noted at the initial appointment. Figure 4-17 is an example of such a form.

The findings are arranged in a rational order to arrive at a pulpal or periradicular diagnosis. This process is summarized in Table 4-1. Consistency of all findings does not always exist because of the variations and unpredictability of diagnoses and of patient responses. In addition to diagnosing pathoses and determining what treatment is indicated, the approach used must fit into the patient's overall needs and treatment plan. To accomplish this, the practitioner should know the indications and contraindications for root canal therapy and recognize conditions that make treatment difficult. This knowledge, combined with the diagnosis, determines the treatment plan.

Treatment Planning

Once the nature of the pathosis has been determined, treatment decisions must be made. The major decision is whether root canal treatment is necessary or some other approaches are preferred. Some teeth may require extraction or a temporary measure (i.e., an emergency situation) with definitive root canal treatment at a future appointment. At times the decision as to the treatment approach becomes complicated. For example, with failed root canal treatment, whether to retreat or to manage surgically involves a number of considerations.[36] Many patients with these problems are best referred to an endodontist.

TO TREAT OR NOT TO TREAT

After diagnosis and treatment plan have been formulated, the next step is to discuss these with the patient so he or she will understand the problem and its management. A common question is, "But

1. Subjective Findings	2. Objective Signs and Tests	3. Radiographic Findings

Chief Complaint:

Significant Medical History:

History of Tooth: (Mark all appropriate)
1 Trauma   6 Pulp cap
2 Caries   (direct or
3 Carious exposure   indirect)
4 Mech. exposure   7 Pulpotomy
5 Restoration   8 Root canal
               treatment
         9 _____

Reaction to Thermal Stimulus:
0 None   1 Short
            2 Continuous

Reaction to Mastication:
0 None   1 Mild-moderate
            2 Severe

Nature of Pain: (Mark all appropriate)
0 None   1 Spontaneous
2 Diffuse   3 Localized

Duration of Pain:
4 Short   5 Prolonged

Electrical Pulp Tester

Tooth No.	Response	No Response
_____	_____	_____
_____	_____	_____
_____	_____	_____

Reaction to Thermal Stimulus:
0 None   1 Short   2 Prolonged

Reaction to Direct Dentin Stimulus:
0 None   1 Response

Tender to Palpation of Overlying Mucosa:
0 No   1 Yes

Reaction to Percussion:
0 None   1 Mild-moderate
            2 Severe

Swelling:
       0 Absent   1 Present

Sinus Tract:
       0 Absent   1 Present

Caries Excavation:
0 No exposure   1 Exposure

Periodontal Status of Suspect Tooth:
0 Normal
1 Excessive mobility (1 + 2 + 3 +)
2 Significant periodontitis
    Explain: _____

Periapical Radiographic Findings
0 Normal
1 Thickened periodontal ligament space
2 Apical radiolucency < 10 mm
3 Apical radiolucency > 10 mm
4 Apical root resorption
5 Apical radiopacity
6 Furcal radiolucency

Other Significant Findings Affecting Diagnosis and/or Treatment (Anatomy, isolation, calcification, etc.):
_____
_____
_____

---

4. Diagnosis

1 Normal
2 Reversible pulpitis
3 Irreversible pulpitis
4 Necrotic pulp

5 Not applicable

6 Normal PDL
7 Acute apical periodontitis
8 Chronic apical periodontitis
9 Suppurative apical periodontitis
10 Acute apical abscess
11 Condensing osteitis
12 Other _____

FIGURE 4-17
A sample form used in diagnosis and treatment planning. (Adapted from Krell K, Walton R: Odontalgia: diagnosing pulpal, periapical, and periodontal pain. In Clark J, editor: *Clinical dentistry,* Philadelphia, 1987, Harper & Row.)

doctor, it doesn't hurt. Is it necessary to do this at all, or can't we just wait and see if it does bother me?" One explanation of the necessity for immediate treatment is that progressive disease (pulp and/or periapical) is present, and early management enhances the chances for successful treatment. A good explanation to the asymptomatic patient is that this problem is a time bomb ticking away. The problem is that we cannot know when it will go off, but it probably will do so at an inopportune time. Management is better, easier, and more predictable before such symptoms occur.

TREATMENT RELATED TO DIAGNOSIS

The pulpal diagnosis in general dictates the approach. If the various states of pulp pathosis are listed, that is, normal pulp, reversible pulpitis, irreversible pulpitis, and necrosis, a line is drawn between reversible and irreversible pulpi-

tis. Those entities on the reversible side may or may not require noninvasive treatment; those on the irreversible side require extraction or root canal treatment or at least removal of the inflamed portion of the pulp with pulpotomy or partial pulpectomy.

The periapical diagnosis indicates the specific nature of the procedure to be followed, usually in conjunction with root canal treatment. In other words, a periradicular lesion has developed only because significant, severe pulp pathosis exists. This requires root canal therapy (if appropriate) and sometimes other surgical procedures such as extraction, or incision and drainage.

NUMBER OF APPOINTMENTS

Although traditionally a point of debate, most investigations indicate that, in general, single-appointment root canal treatment is acceptable.[37-39] However, the general dentist should approach

TABLE 4-1				

Diagnostic Terminology

	SYMPTOMS	RADIOGRAPHIC	PULP TESTS	PERIAPICAL TESTS
Pulpal				
Normal	None of significance	No periapical changes	Responds	Not sensitive
Reversible	May or may not have slight symptoms to thermal stimulus	No periapical changes	Responds	Not sensitive
Irreversible	Similar to reversible; also may have spontaneous or severe pain to thermal stimuli	No periapical radiolucent changes; one exception: occasional condensing osteitis	Responds (possibly with extreme pain on thermal stimulus)	May or may not have pain on percussion or palpation
Necrotic	None to thermal stimulus. Other symptoms: see under *Periapical*	See under *Periapical*	No response	Depends on periapical status
Periapical				
Normal	None of significance	No significant change	Response	Not sensitive
Acute apical periodontitis	Significant pain on mastication or pressure	No significant change	Response or no response (depends on pulp status)	Pain on percussion or palpation
Chronic apical periodontitis and apical cyst	None to mild	Apical radiolucency	No response	None to mild on percussion or palpation
Acute apical abscess	Swelling and/or significant pain	Usually a radiolucent lesion	No response	Pain on percussion or palpation
Suppurative apical periodontitis (chronic apical abscess)	Draining sinus or parulis	Usually a radiolucent lesion	No response	Not sensitive
Condensing osteitis	Varies (depends on pulp or periapical status)	Increased trabecular bone density	Response or no response (depends on pulp status)	May or may not have pain on percussion or palpation

this type of treatment with caution and careful patient selection.

Multiple Appointments

There are situations that require more than a single appointment. One is the condition that is complex or time consuming. Related to this and most important is patient management and the tolerance level of patient and operator. If fatigue or frustration on the part of either occurs, the appointment is terminated, a temporary filling is placed, and another appointment is scheduled.

Another situation is the patient with severe periradicular symptoms or persistent canal exudation. These are often emergencies, and the tolerance level of the patient is low. Also, flare-ups between appointments occur more often in these situations.[40] Posttreatment flare-up is considerably more difficult to manage if the canals are obturated.

A third indication may be a diagnosis of pulp necrosis and asymptotic apical pathosis. There is some preliminary evidence (not conclusive) that healing may be better if there are two visits and calcium hydroxide is placed as an intracanal medicament.[41]

Effects on Prognosis and Pain

The long-term prognosis and patient symptoms after treatment are two major concerns related to the number of appointments. As yet, most studies indicate that in the asymptomatic patient, posttreatment pain[37,42,43] is unrelated to whether treatment is completed in single or multiple appointments. Effects on prognosis are uncertain to date. Again, single-appointment root canal treatment should always be approached with some caution and with consideration of each individual case.

When to Conclude the Appointment

The questions to be answered are as follows: What should be completed to minimize interappointment problems? At what point may a temporary filling be placed? Studies have not indicated all factors that dictate what must be accomplished; however, there is no increase in posttreatment symptoms from incomplete cleaning and shaping.[40,44] But, when there is pulpal necrosis, there may be improved healing if débridement is completed and intracanal calcium hydroxide is placed.[45]

DIAGNOSIS AND TREATMENT PLANS

Specific treatment approaches are indicated, depending on the diagnosis and the individual situation. The following general recommendations are made accordingly. *Variations or alterations in specific treatment options are dictated by circumstances.*

Pulpal Diagnosis

Normal or Reversible Pulpitis. Root canal treatment is not indicated (unless elective). In patients with reversible pulpitis, the cause is usually removed and restoration follows (if necessary).

Irreversible Pulpitis. Root canal treatment, pulpotomy, partial pulpectomy, or extraction is required. Ultimately total pulp removal is preferred; attempting to maintain a damaged pulp, for example, by capping a carious exposure, is likely to result in long-term failure.[46] Partial pulp removal is a temporary measure in certain circumstances (emergency or apexogenesis). Total pulpectomy is not always accomplished with the use of broaches alone, which leave shreds of pulp tissue. The pulp is totally removed only when cleaning and shaping are essentially complete. At the initial appointment, if circumstances do not permit complete pulpectomy, pulpotomy or partial pulpectomy is acceptable.[47]

Necrosis. Root canal treatment or extraction is indicated. Necrotic debris may be removed completely on the first visit. Again, this situation includes establishing working lengths and completing cleaning and shaping. Careful instrumentation and copious irrigation are important. If a situation does not permit total débridement, partial débridement is acceptable.

Caustic pungent chemical medicaments are contraindicated; these are of no benefit. If more than minimal preparation has been done (more than 25 file), calcium hydroxide paste may be placed in the canal.

Rarely should these teeth be left open to the oral cavity.[48,49] Occasionally the tooth might be left open if a continuous, copious flow of exudate exists during canal preparation. Adjunctive treatment with pulp necrosis may be necessary, depending on the periradicular diagnosis.

Periradicular Diagnosis

There are more treatment variations related to periradicular status. With significant periradicular pathosis, associated pulp necrosis exists. It should be remembered that the most important factors in the resolution of periradicular pathosis, whether acute or chronic, are débridement and removal of irritants from the pulp space! These are *always* prerequisites. Of course, ultimate success depends on coronal and radicular obturation as well as débridement.[50]

Normal. No special treatment approach is required.

Acute Apical Periodontitis. Because this is a small (but painful) inflammatory lesion, there is no special treatment required. It is critical to remove the inflamed pulp or necrotic debris and other irritants. Pain comes primarily from fluid pressure; some exudate or transudate may be released into the canal space when it is opened or during instrumentation. This may be a small amount and may not be visible clinically, but will aid in pain relief.

Intracanal medicaments do not reduce symptoms. However, to inhibit bacteria with pulp necrosis, calcium hydroxide is placed in the canal(s), and the access is closed with a cotton pellet and a temporary filling. Occlusal reduction in patients with severe percussion sensitivity may ease symptoms.[51]

Chronic Apical Periodontitis. This lesion is associated with pulp necrosis. The size of the lesion generally is not a factor in choosing the treatment approach (Figure 4-18). Calcium hydroxide is placed as an intracanal medicament, and the access opening is sealed with dry cotton and a temporary filling.

Acute Apical Abscess

Débridement. Because this lesion is accompanied by pain and/or swelling, different approaches are necessary. *Most critical is débridement of irritants from the canal space;* therefore, complete or nearly complete cleaning and shaping with copious, careful irrigation are desired.

Drainage. Next in importance is drainage through the tooth or soft tissue. Treatment (incision and drainage, extraction) varies, depending on the presence or absence of swelling, extent of involvement, and other factors. Specific details on managing acute apical abscess are discussed in Chapter 17.

Suppurative Apical Periodontitis (Chronic Apical Abscess)

Because this lesion is asymptomatic owing to intraoral or extraoral drainage of an abscess,[52] no special treatment measures are necessary. Again, the key is débridement; the tract or parulis should resolve spontaneously once irritants from the pulp space are removed (see Figure 4-3). A persistent draining sinus tract indicates a misdiagnosis (is it a periodontal abscess?), a missed canal, or inadequate débridement or obturation. Generally, the sinus tract resolves a few days to a month after débridement and obturation. Calcium hydroxide should be placed in the canal(s) and in the access cavity, which is always closed temporarily between appointments.

Condensing Osteitis. This entity requires no special treatment. Because it occurs with different pulp conditions, treatment will vary. Condensing osteitis resolves in approximately 50% of teeth after *successful* root canal treatment.[53] There is no apparent problem if the condensing osteitis does *not* resolve; no further treatment is required unless there are other findings that indicate failure.

TREATMENT CHOICES
Routine Cases

There are some procedures that the graduating dentist (and general dentist) should be able to perform. According to the *Curriculum Guidelines for Endodontics* (see Chapter 1), sufficient educational experience in specific procedures must be provided to the student. Obviously, there is variation between and even within individual institutions; however, the practicing dentist often acquires additional skills by advanced formal training, experience, or continuing education.

Most uncomplicated root canal treatment procedures can and should be done by the general practitioner. The most important point is to identify the routine nature of each case and plan accordingly. So, what is within the capabilities of the general practitioner, and which patients should be considered for referral? This information is covered in detail in Chapter 5.

Difficult Procedures

Difficult procedures include a wide spectrum of problems. Managing difficulties depends on the knowledge and skills of the general practitioner. Equally important is access to the appropriate instruments and materials. With all these considerations, the practitioner (in collaboration with the patient) decides what to treat. *The decision to treat*

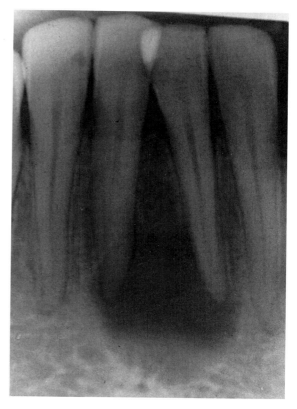

FIGURE 4-18
Because of its size, this lesion is likely to be an apical radicular cyst. The lesion is related to pulp necrosis in the left central incisor. Although superimposed over the apex of the adjacent incisor, the pulp is not affected and therefore does not require treatment. Proper root canal treatment of the left incisor would lead to resolution without surgery.

or refer is based on the individual patient case and not on a predetermined set of criteria.

TREATMENT MODIFIERS
Complications

While progressing through the diagnostic process, the practitioner makes observations that modify the treatment approach. A decision may be made to extract a tooth that is nonrestorable, has severe periodontal involvement, or is noncritical to the overall treatment plan or if the patient is disinterested in comprehensive care. Other conditions that may require modifications include severe caries, failed root canal treatment, operative problems, isolation difficulties (Figure 4-19), abnormal root or pulp anatomy (Figure 4-20), medical complications, and calcifications (Figure 4-21). Any one or a combination of these may designate a patient with a complex problem that should be considered for consultation or referral (see Chapter 5).

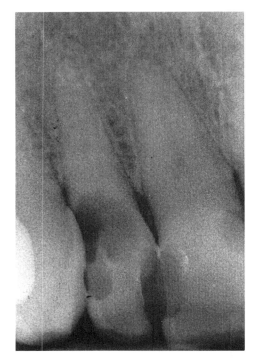

FIGURE 4-19
Isolation problem. Deep subgingival caries require an adjunctive surgical procedure for adequate isolation and restoration.

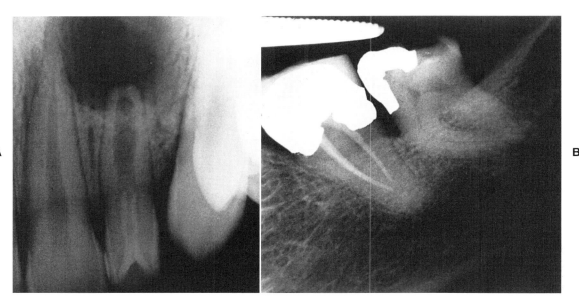

A   B

FIGURE 4-20
Anatomic difficulties. **A,** Dens invaginatus has resulted in communication and resultant necrosis of the pulp. In-complete dentin formation and an irregular internal form make these teeth anatomically difficult to clean, shape, and obturate. The size of the periradicular lesion does not itself contraindicate nonsurgical treatment. **B,** A se-verely curved root and the position make treatment for this third molar difficult.

Adjunctive Procedures

Many procedures often are beyond the training and experience of the general practitioner. These include but are not limited to surgery, complex bleaching, replantation, retreatment, transplantation, apexification, root resection, and management of cracked teeth. The general-ist should understand these techniques and how they mesh with the overall treatment plan and explain them to the patient. These adjunctive

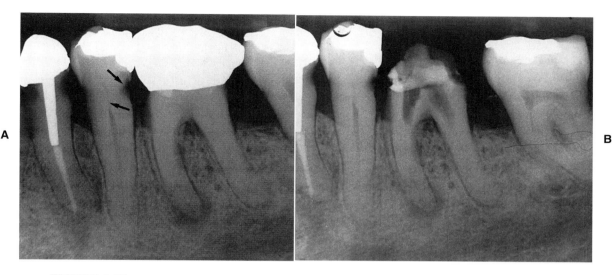

FIGURE 4-21
Anatomic difficulties. **A,** Numerous insults from caries, restorations, and restorative procedures have resulted in calcific metamorphosis in the molar. A very small canal contains necrotic tissue sufficient to cause apical pathosis. Note that cervical caries are also altering the pulpal anatomy on the adjacent premolar *(arrows)*. **B,** Removal of the crown and an extensive search failed to locate the canals. Periradicular surgery with a root end filling will be necessary.

procedures are described in more detail in other chapters.

Prognosis

Patients are entitled to the best dental care. Unfortunately, this is not always available or is not presented during discussion of the treatment plan. The practitioner should calculate a prognosis for each situation, including a *contingency prognosis* if problems are encountered after treatment has begun.

It has been reported (as a summarization of relative success and failure rates) that success rates for treatment by general practitioners are lower than those of specialists or specialty clinics.[10] Although there may be a number of reasons for this, certainly a major one is the tendency of general practitioners to attempt treatments that are inappropriate or beyond their abilities.[54] Thus, to provide the best treatment, the generalist and specialist must communicate, share treatment problems, and exchange ideas for providing the best treatment for their patients.[55]

REFERENCES

1. Drinnan AJ: Differential diagnosis of orofacial pain, *Dent Clin North Am* 22:73, 1978.
2. Moore R, Miller ML, Weinstein P, et al: Cultural perceptions of pain and coping among patients and dentists, *Commun Dent Oral Epidemiol* 14:327, 1986.
3. Eriksen H: Endodontology epidemiologic considerations, *Endod Dent Traumatol* 7:189, 1991.
4. Walton R: Endodontic considerations in the geriatric patient, *Dent Clin North Am* 41:795, 1997.
5. Slavkin H: Does the mouth put the heart at risk? *J Am Dent Assoc* 130:109, 1999.
6. Murray C, Saunders W: Root canal treatment and general health: a review of the literature, *Int Endod J* 33:1, 2000.
7. Debelian G, Olsen I, Tronstad L: Anaerobic bacteremia and fungemia in patients undergoing endodontic therapy: an overview, *Ann Periodontol* 3:281, 1998.
8. Gerner N, Hurlen B, Dobloug J, Brandtzaeg P: Endodontic treatment and immunopathology of periapical granuloma in an AIDS patients, *Endod Dent Traumatol* 4:127, 1988.
9. Cooper H: Root canal treatment on patients with HIV infection, *Int Endod J* 26:369, 1993.
10. Findler M, Galili D, Meidan Z, et al: Dental treatment in very high risk patients with active ischemic heart disease, *Oral Surg Oral Med Oral Pathol* 76:298, 1993.
11. Niwa H, Sato Y, Matsuura H: Safety of dental treatment in patients with previously diagnosed acute myocardial infarction or unstable angina pectoris, *Oral Surg Oral Med Oral Pathol Oral Radiol Endod* 89:35, 2000.
12. Kleier D, Shibilski K: Management of the latex hypersensitive patient in the endodontic office, *J Endod* 25:825, 1999.
13. Dias de Andrade E, Ranali J, Volpato M, et al: Allergic reaction after rubber dam placement, *J Endod* 26:182, 2000.

14. Kollmann W: Incidence and possible causes of dental pain during simulated high altitude flights, *J Endod* 19:154, 1993.

15. Bell WE: *Orofacial pains*, ed 2, Chicago, 1979, Year Book.

16. Jones D: Effect of the type carrier used on the results of dichlorodifluoromethane application to teeth, *J Endod* 25:692, 1999.

17. Pantera E, Anderson R, Pantera C: Reliability of electric pulp testing after pulpal testing with dichlorodifluoromethane, *J Endod* 19:312, 1993.

18. Pantera E, Anderson R, Pantera C: Use of dental instruments for bridging during electric pulp testing, *J Endod* 18:37, 1992.

19. Peterson K, Soderstrom C, Kiani-Anaraki M, Levy G: Evaluation of the ability of thermal and electrical tests to register pulp vitality, *Endod Dent Traumatol* 15:127, 1999.

20. Nissan R, Trope M, Zhang C, Chance B: Dual wavelength spectrophotometry as a diagnostic test of the pulp chamber contents, *Oral Surg Oral Med Oral Pathol* 74:508, 1992.

21. Schnettler J, Wallace J: Pulse oximetry as a diagnostic tool of pulpal vitality, *J Endod* 17:488, 1991.

22. Evans D, Reid J, Strang R, Stirrups D: A comparison of laser Doppler flowmetry with other methods of assessing the vitality of traumatised anterior teeth, *Endod Dent Traumatol* 15:284, 1999.

23. Emshoff R, Kranewitter R, Norer B: Effect of LeFort I osteotomy on maxillary tooth type related blood flow characteristics, *Oral Surg Oral Med Oral Pathol Oral Radiol Endod* 89: 88, 2000.

24. Noblett C, Wilcox L, Johnson W, et al: Detection of pulpal circulation in vitro by pulse oximetry, *J Endod* 2:1, 1996.

25. Diaz-Arnold A, Arnold M, Wilcox L: Optical detection of hemoglobin in pulpal blood, *J Endod* 22:19, 1996.

26. Bender IB: Factors influencing the radiographic appearance of bony lesions, *J Endod* 8:161, 1982.

27. Lee S, Messer H: Radiographic appearance of artificially prepared periapical lesions confined to cancellous bone, *Int Endod J* 19:64, 1986.

28. Maixner D, Green TL, Walton R, Leider A: Histological examination of condensing osteitis (abstract), *J Endod* 18:196, 1992.

29. Tyndall D, Kapa S, Bagnell C: Digital subtraction radiography for detecting cortical and cancellous bone changes in the periapical region, *J Endod* 16:173, 1990.

30. Shrout M, Hall M, Hildebolt C: Differentiation of periapical granulomas and radicular cysts by digital radiometric analysis, *Oral Surg Oral Med Oral Pathol Oral Radiol Endod* 76:356, 1993.

31. Lockhart P, Kim S, Lund N: Magnetic resonance imaging of human teeth, *J Endod* 6:237, 1992.

32. Holtzmann D, Johnson WT, Southard T, et al: Storage-phosphor computed radiography versus film radiography in the detection of pathologic periradicular bone loss in cadavers, *Oral Surg Oral Med Oral Pathol Oral Radiol Endod* 86:90, 1998.

33. Åkerblom A, Hasselgren G: The prognosis for endodontic treatment of obliterated root canals, *J Endod* 14:565, 1988.

34. D'Souza JE, Walton RE, Peterson LC: Periodontal ligament injection: an evaluation of the extent of anesthesia and postinjection discomfort, *J Am Dent Assoc* 114:341, 1987.

35. Krell K, Walton R: Odontalgia: diagnosing pulpal, periapical, and periodontal pain. In Clark J, editor, *Clinical dentistry*, Philadelphia, 1986, Harper & Row.

36. Kvist T, Reit C: Results of endodontic retreatment: A randomized clinical study comparing surgical and nonsurgical procedures, *J Endod* 25:814, 1999.

37. Roane JB, Dryden JA, Grimes EW: Incidence of postoperative pain after single- and multiple-visit endodontic procedures, *Oral Surg Oral Med Oral Pathol* 55:68, 1983.

38. Pekruhn RB: The incidence of failure following single-visit endodontic therapy, *J Endod* 12:68, 1986.

39. Jurcak J, Bellizzi R, Loushine R: Successful single-visit endodontics during Operation Desert Shield, *J Endod* 19:412, 1993.

40. Walton R, Fouad A: Endodontic interappointment flare-ups: prospective study of incidence and related factors, *J Endod* 18:172, 1992.

41. Katebzadeh N, Sigurdsson A, Trope M: Radiographic evaluation of periapical healing after obturation of infected root canals: an *in vivo* study, *Int Endod J* 33:60, 2000.

42. Mulhern JM, Patterson SS, Newton CW, Ringel AM: Incidence of postoperative pain after one-appointment endodontic treatment of asymptomatic pulpal necrosis in single-rooted teeth, *J Endod* 8:370, 1982.

43. Fava L: A comparison of one- versus two-appointment endodontic therapy in teeth with non-vital pulps, *Int Endod J* 22:179, 1989.

44. Maddox D, Walton R, Davis C: Effects of medicaments and other factors on the incidence of post-treatment endodontic pain, *J Endod* 3:447, 1977.

45. Trope M, Delano O, Orstavik D: Endodontic treatment of teeth with apical periodontitis: single vs. multivisit treatment, *J Endod* 25:345, 1999.

46. Banthel C, Rosenkranz B, Leuenberg A, Roulet J-F: Pulp capping of carious exposures: Treatment outcome after 5 and 10 years, *J Endod* 26: 525, 2000.

47. Oguntebi B, DeSchepper E, Taylor T, et al: Postoperative pain incidence related to the type of emergency treatment of symptomatic pulpitis, *Oral Surg Oral Med Oral Pathol* 73:479, 1992.

48. Weine FS, Healy HJ, Theiss EP: Endodontic emergency dilemma: leave tooth open or keep it closed? *Oral Surg Oral Med Oral Pathol* 40:531, 1975.

49. August DS: Managing the abscessed open tooth: instrument or close? Part II. *J Endod* 8:364, 1982.

50. Bystrom A, Happonen RP, Sjögren U, Sundqvist G: Healing of periapical lesions of pulpless teeth after endodontic treatment with controlled asepsis, *Endod Dent Traumatol* 3:58, 1987.

51. Rosenberg P, Babick P, Schertzer L, Leung A: The effect of occlusal reduction on pain after endodontic instrumentation, *J Endod* 24:492, 1998.

52. Calman HI, Eisenberg M, Grodjesk JE, Szerlip L: The external fistula, its diagnosis and importance, *Dent Radiog Photog* 53:26, 1980.

53. Hedin M, Polhagen L: Follow-up study of periradicular bone condensation, *Scand J Dent Res* 79:436, 1971.

54. Molven O: The frequency, technical standard and results of endodontic therapy, *Nor Tannlasg Tidsskr* 86:142, 1976.

55. Scharwatt B: The general practitioner and the endodontist, *Dent Clin North Am* 23:747, 1979.

Mahmoud Torabinejad and Denis E. Simon III

5

When and How to Refer

LEARNING OBJECTIVES

After reading this chapter, the student should be able to:

1 / Understand the importance of referral.

2 / Classify complications of endodontic procedures.

3 / Identify factors complicating diagnosis.

4 / Discuss factors that make root canal treatment difficult.

5 / Describe factors that make determination of prognosis difficult.

6 / Identify situations that might require consultation with a physician or a dental specialist.

7 / Identify which procedures should be within the capabilities of the generalist.

8 / Identify which procedures are ordinarily not within the graduating dentist's realm of training or experience and which patients should be considered for referral.

9 / Recognize reasons for referral after treatment is initiated.

10 / Describe the relationship, responsibilities, and communication modes among the general dentist, patient, and endodontist.

OUTLINE

Identification and Classification of Cases

Case Selection System

Patient Considerations
Health and Medical History
Local Anesthesia
Physical Limitations

Objective Clinical Findings
Diagnosis
Radiographs
Anatomic Complications

Additional Factors
Restorability and Isolation
Existing Restorations
Cracked Tooth
Root Resorption

Endodontic-Periodontic Lesion

Traumatic Injuries

Previous Endodontic Treatment

Procedural Accidents
Separated Instrument or Canal Blockages
Ledging

Perforations

Emergencies
Persistent Signs and/or Symptoms
Persistent Radiographic Pathosis
Persistent Probing Defect or Sinus Tract

Referral During Treatment
Flare-ups
Procedural Accidents
Inability to Locate Root Canals
Financial Considerations

Referral to a Specialist

What Is Expected of a General Practitioner
Instructions to Endodontist
Explanation to Patient

What Is Expected of an Endodontist
Treatment Performed
Feedback to Dentist
Feedback to Patient

A patient deserves the best quality of care possible. Depending on the treatment, the general dentist may be best suited to deliver that care. In some situations, either a general dentist or a specialist may efficaciously perform the procedure. However, in more complex cases, the specialist will provide the best care.[1]

Referrals are part of comprehensive health care management and are appropriate when the patient's needs are beyond the generalist's capabilities.[2] By definition, *standard of care* means that the *quality of endodontic care provided to patients by the general dentist should be similar to that provided by an endodontist.*[3] Because of the subjectivity of criteria used to evaluate degrees of complexity, it is difficult to determine when to proceed versus when to refer. Epidemiologic data show that success rates for root canal treatment are lower for generalists than for specialists.[4] A possible contributing factor for this finding is that general dentists often attempt treatment that is beyond their abilities. An objective measure of when and which patients to refer is very important.

This chapter presents guidelines for determining case complexity using specific risk factors and then rating them systematically. Application of this system allows a general dentist to recognize patients with problems within their scope and treat them accordingly.[5] It should also help general practitioners to avoid mishaps and misunderstandings and ultimately to provide the best treatment for their patients.

Obviously, there are referral considerations other than case complexity. For example, a general dentist may have the training and experience to manage a particular situation but may choose not to do so, preferring to concentrate on other aspects of treatment. Or a dentist may have learned that he or she cannot complete certain procedures quickly enough for cost effectiveness. This chapter does not discuss these considerations.

Identification and Classification of Cases

The decision about what to treat and what to refer depends on different *risk* factors, including the skills of the dentist and the case difficulty.[6] There are three general categories of cases based on their complexity:

1. *Average risk.* An experienced practitioner should expect to achieve a favorable outcome based on the pretreatment evaluation of the risk factors.

2. *High risk.* An experienced practitioner with advanced training may be able to manage these situations, but caution should be observed. These patients may be considered for referral if one or more of the risk factors fall in this range.

3. *Extreme risk.* The preoperative conditions show exceptionally difficult situations; even the most skilled practitioner will be challenged. These patients should be considered for referral.

Complexity may be related to diagnostic, procedural, or prognostic difficulties.

Diagnostic difficulties include confusing test results, nonspecific or unusual patterns of pain from periradicular lesions of nonpulpal origin, endodontic or periodontal lesions, and resorption. Radiographic problems may be either technical or interpretive.

Procedural difficulties may relate to the patient's physical limitations, medical history, or management problems, inadequate anesthesia, isolation difficulties, tooth restorability, or complex tooth anatomy. Additional complications include the presence (or absence) of restorations, the presence of previous obturating materials or posts, traumatic injuries and fractures, endodontic emergencies, and procedural accidents.

Prognostic difficulties are associated with persistent symptoms and or/lesions and failure to heal after prior treatment.

Case Selection System

This system involves the recognition and rating of risks associated with endodontic therapy. Every case has certain unique difficulties that deserve observation and rating before the dentist makes the ultimate decision to treat or refer a patient. This program presents a means of evaluating each case based on degree of difficulty by considering *risk* factors related to the patient and the tooth and parameters affecting treatment and prognosis. Determining the various factors yields a systematic, measurable rating.

Each factor is given a numerical value. These values are *average risk* (rate 1), *high risk* (rate 2), and *extreme risk* (rate 3). If all ratings fall in the *average* category, a general practitioner usually can treat the patient. If one or more factors fall in the *high-risk* category, the patient may be treated by an experienced generalist or referred. Patients with one or more factors in the *extreme* range should be *considered for referral* to an endodontist. For example, a relatively straightforward root canal treatment

for a central incisor may be best managed by referral if the patient has a very limited oral opening and film placement would be difficult, or if the canal space is calcified as a result of trauma or other complicating factors.

Figure 5-1 is a *working model reproduction* of the *Endodontic Case Difficulty Assessment Form* selection system. Consideration involves a checklist that rates all factors systematically. At first, the process seems cumbersome; however, *repeated* usage and familiarity will *reduce risk* for both patient and dentist. This should allow the dentist to provide optimum quality care.

Patient Considerations

HEALTH AND MEDICAL HISTORY

General practitioners may treat medical complications that affect diagnosis and/or treatment and patients who require premedication. However, severity must be evaluated. In patients with more serious disorders, an endodontist may best provide treatment. Specialist care is generally more expedient and offers better prevention and management of complications during treatment. Diabetes and anticoagulant therapy are examples of a systemic condition and a medication that may affect the decision of whether to refer. Consultation with the patient's physician before deciding whether to refer is advisable when the medical history indicates a potential problem.

LOCAL ANESTHESIA

Some patients report an "allergy" to local anesthetics. However, a true allergic reaction to commonly used local anesthetics, particularly the amides, is almost nonexistent.[7] Tachycardia is often confused with an allergy. A patient may report adverse reactions to an anesthetic with epinephrine. This is probably apprehension and not truly an "allergy."

A major dilemma is highly inflamed pulp, particularly in mandibular molars.[8] Difficulty with anesthesia may transform a cooperative patient into a budding dental phobic. When difficulty is encountered in obtaining profound anesthesia, referral should be considered. Endodontists are accustomed to dealing with these situations.

PHYSICAL LIMITATIONS

Physical limitations may present problems for providing proper treatment. If the patient cannot be suitably reclined or if the mouth opening is such that access is compromised, referral should be considered. Even endodontists are challenged,

Endodontic Case Difficulty Assessment Form

Patient Information

Name _____

Address _____

City/State/Zip _____

Phone _____

PATIENT CONSIDERATIONS

Medical History

cardiovascular diseases
cerebral vascular considerations
bleeding disorders
renal dysfunction
medical prostheses
abnormalities in host defense
diabetes
mental impairment
acute systemic disease
pregnancy
need for pre-medications
other systemic conditions

Local Anesthetic Considerations

vasoconstrictor contraindication
anesthetic allergy
history of difficulty in obtaining profound anesthesia

Personal Factors and General Considerations

limited ability to open mouth
gagger
fear of dentistry
motivation to preserve dentition
physical impairment—difficulty holding film
limitation to be reclined
size of mouth

OBJECTIVE CLINICAL FINDINGS

Diagnosis

inconclusive or contradictory findings

Radiographic Findings

difficulty in obtaining films of diagnostic value

Pulpal Space

calcification
chamber
orifice
canal
number of canals

Root Morphology

curvature
dilaceration
long
recurvature
length
long
short

Apical Morphology

open

Malpositioned Teeth

buccal version
rotated or tipped
too far distally

ADDITIONAL CONDITIONS

Restorability

isolation challenge
caries
need for crown lengthening

Existing Restoration

porcelain crown
PBM/PFM
gold castings
impaired access to root canal
abutment
long axis of crown vs. long axis of root
size of crown
crown anatomy vs. original anatomy
post and core (Rate 2 or 3 only)

Fractured Tooth

crown
root

Resorptions

internal
external
apical

Endo-Perio Lesion

tooth mobility
attached gingiva minimal/inadequate
furcation involved
periodontal prognosis
root section or hemisection consideration

Trauma

avulsion
luxation

Previous Endodontic Treatment

Rate 2 or 3 only

Perforations

Rate 3 only

Disposition

Treat in Office   Yes ☐   No ☐

Refer patient to: _____

Date: _____

FIGURE 5-1

Endodontic case difficulty assessment form. (Reprinted with permission from the American Association of Endodontists.)

but they may have encountered the problem and devised a solution. A second molar in one patient may be easier to manipulate than a premolar in another patient. The area should be inspected carefully; if problems are detected before the rubber dam is placed, the patient should be referred.

Objective Clinical Findings

DIAGNOSIS

Appropriate treatment follows accurate diagnosis. Many procedures are done inappropriately (or not done) because of diagnostic errors. The endodontist is experienced, and the generalist may be unfamiliar with that particular problem. *Referred pain is a prime example of a condition that often presents the practitioner with a significant diagnostic challenge.* Unless a definitive diagnosis is obtained, no treatment should be rendered, and the patient referred.

RADIOGRAPHS

Diagnostic and treatment films of good quality are critical (Figure 5-2). Patient characteristics

and oral anatomy (e.g., shallow palatal vault or large and narrow dental arches) may hinder this task. Also, some apprehensive patients are prone to gag or cannot maintain film position. When case rating is considered, possible difficulties in obtaining diagnostic or treatment films must be kept in mind.

ANATOMIC COMPLICATIONS

A number of anatomic factors are related to developmental and acquired tooth morphology.

Pulp Chamber

As the tooth ages, pulp chamber space decreases. Chamber size and pulp stones, as well as the extent of calcifications in the canal system, must be considered (Figure 5-3).

Calcific Metamorphosis

In addition to chamber calcification, the canals may show calcific metamorphosis from dentin deposition (Figure 5-4).[8] Considered are the visibility of the canals, the canal orifices, and the general

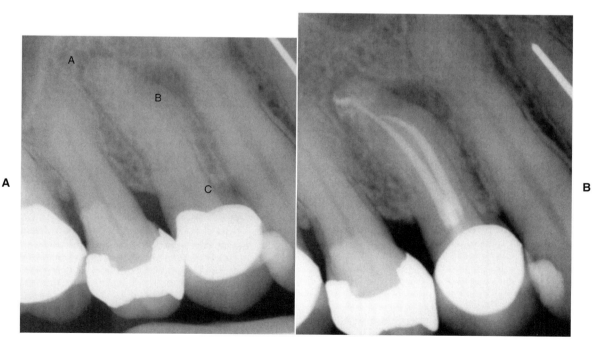

FIGURE 5-2
A, Periapical radiolucency (*A*) and mesial radiolucency in the apical third (*B*). The canals are calcified, the root is narrow, and there is a hint of a significant mesial concavity in the coronal third (*C*). The tooth is also crowned, thereby increasing access complexity. This case is considered as high risk. **B,** Postoperatively, the mesial radiolucency resulted from the buccal root exiting several millimeters shorter than the palatal root with a significant distal curvature. The practitioner must manage the unexpected should problems arise during treatment.

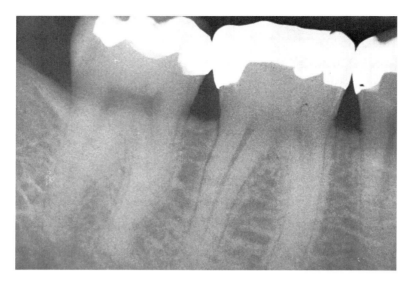

FIGURE 5-3
Pulp chamber and root canals show calcific metamorphosis; this situation is rated as extreme risk.

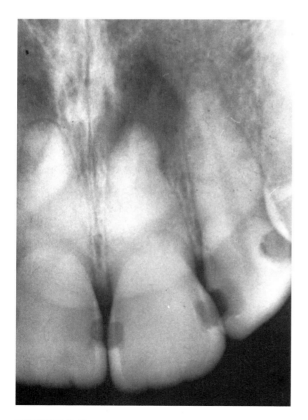

FIGURE 5-4
Apical pathosis—the canal is not visible (calcific metamorphosis); this situation is rated as extreme risk.

decrease in canal size as evident on radiographs[9] (Figure 5-5).

Number of Canals

A good rule is to always expect "extra" canals or roots unless the preoperative film clearly shows a distinct number of canals; the reality is that more may exist (Figures 5-6 and 5-7). There are difficulties with multiple canals. For example, many mandibular incisors have two root canals and mandibular premolars may have multiple canals.[10,11] A significant percentage of mandibular first molars have two canals in the distal root, and mesiobuccal roots of maxillary molars often have two canal systems.[12]

Root Curvature

Canals are rarely straight, although roots may appear so on a facial radiograph. Curvature factors include the direction, severity, and number of curves (Figure 5-8). Especially common are "recurvatures" of the mesial roots of mandibular molars, in which the apices bend toward each other. Another treatment challenge is the bayonet curve (Figure 5-9). This should be considered extremely difficult (rate 3).

Root Length

Long root canal systems are a challenge to treat. Very short roots also pose unique problems.

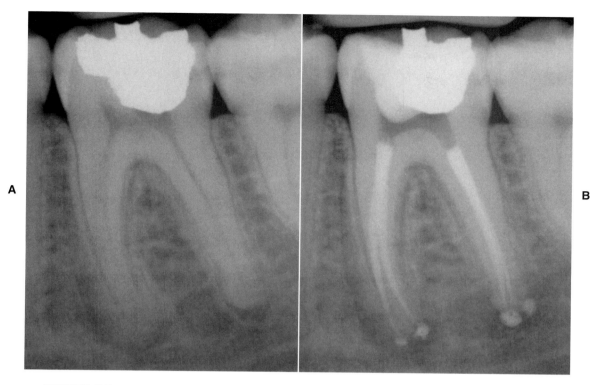

A   B

FIGURE 5-5
A, Calcific metamorphosis in the mesial root plus chamber narrowing and orifice angulation, which compromise the access into the mesial canals. **B,** The postoperative radiograph reveals four canals, gradual curvature of mesial canals, and apical delta with accessory canals in the distal root. Slight sealer overextensions should not adversely affect healing. This tooth should be treated by an experienced practitioner, but with caution.

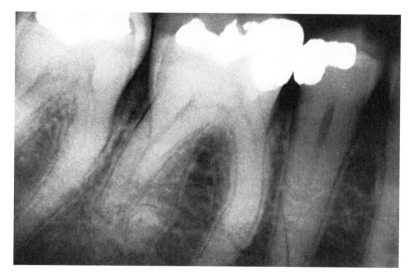

FIGURE 5-6
Mandibular molars with an "extra" distolingual root; this situation is rated as high risk.

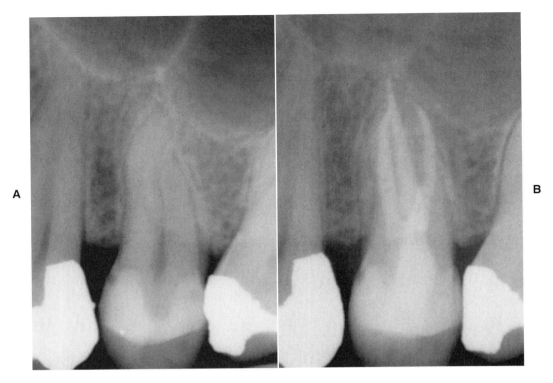

FIGURE 5-7
A, Unusual anatomy. Note the abrupt curvature in the middle and apical third, suggesting a third canal. **B,** Post-operative image. The difficulty of this situation should be a consideration for referral to a specialist.

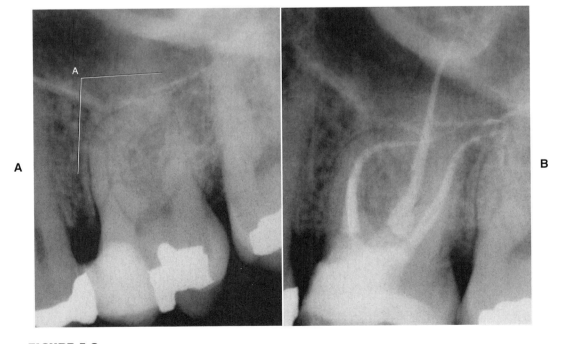

FIGURE 5-8
A, Extreme curvature of the mesiobuccal root of tooth 14. This nearly 90° curve (*A*) would place this situation in the extreme risk category and the patient should be considered for referral. **B,** Note the curvature of the disto-buccal root in the postoperative radiograph.

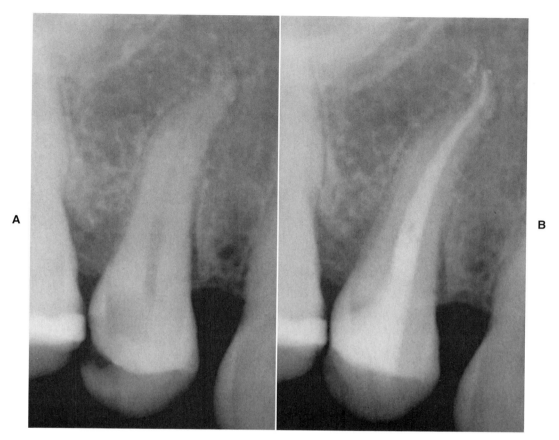

FIGURE 5-9
A, Dilaceration in the apical third. The degree and location of curvature strongly suggest caution and a consideration for referral. **B,** Note in the postoperative radiograph that the apical third curvature has been maintained.

Degree of Apical Closure

The size of the apical opening correlates with the difficulty of the situation. Recently erupted teeth with immature apices are complicated to treat and often require special procedures. Outcome and duration of treatment are unpredictable; these teeth are difficult to manage (see Chapter 22). Problems with teeth in which the initial apical foramen is between file sizes 50 and 70 are categorized as *high risk.*

Tooth Location and Malpositioning

Generally, second and third molars, especially maxillary molars, are difficult to reach, particularly in a patient with a limited opening. Buccally positioned maxillary second molars are associated with a variety of treatment problems. Rotated, tipped, or crowded teeth may also complicate isolation and access as well as inhibit adequate cleaning and shaping or obturation (Figure 5-10).

Additional Factors

RESTORABILITY AND ISOLATION

Severe caries or other damage may render the tooth too difficult to isolate or to restore; extraction may be the best alternative. In some instances crown lengthening may be necessary to create biologic width. Referral to a periodontist for such treatment should be considered. Also, an endodontist may combine crown lengthening with root canal treatment in the same appointment (Figure 5-11).

EXISTING RESTORATIONS

Many teeth requiring root canal treatment have castings.[13] Access through gold is easier than that through nonprecious metals. Porcelain is somewhat fragile, creating difficulties in access and preparation. If the tooth is a bridge abutment, the angulation and length of span must be considered. Often, restoration anatomy does not duplicate the

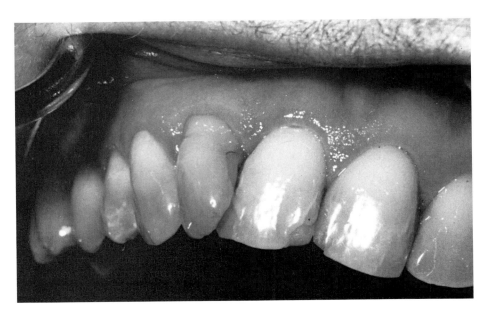

FIGURE 5-10
Rotated lateral incisor may create isolation and access problems; this situation is rated as high risk.

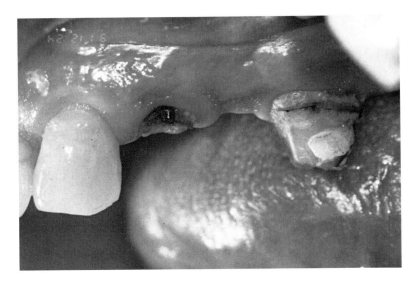

FIGURE 5-11
Mesial abutment requires crown lengthening for root canal treatment as well as for the creation of biologic width for restoration.

original crown anatomy, and the pulp chamber is difficult to locate. When the chamber and orifices are not visible in the preoperative film or the anatomy of the underlying tooth is questionable, the rating is *high risk* (see Figure 5-2).

Other considerations include the size of the crown and the presence of precision attachments as well as parallelism between the long axis of the crown and the long axis of the root. These consid-

erations are particularly important in premolars, maxillary lateral incisors, and mandibular incisors. These teeth are narrow and there is little room for error.

CRACKED TOOTH

Cracked or fractured teeth are often difficult to diagnose and treat. Symptoms can vary from vague

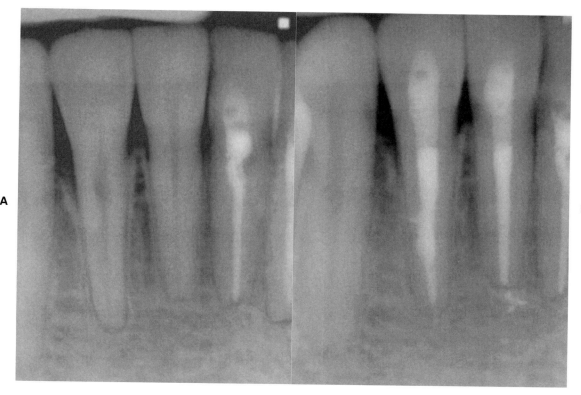

FIGURE 5-12
A, Complexity caused by trauma. Previous treatment of 23 and 24. Tooth 25 is symptomatic, with percussion sensitivity and nonresponsiveness to pulp testing. Tooth 26 shows internal resorption that is asymptomatic. Care must be taken to completely clean and shape the canal system, as is demonstrated in the postoperative image. **B,** This situation exhibits a high degree of difficulty.

pain while chewing to extreme pulpalgia. Definitive diagnosis must be achieved before treatment; then the prognosis must be determined based on the degree of fracture (see Chapter 28).

ROOT RESORPTION

Resorption can be either internal (intracanal) or external (extracanal).

All instances of perforating (pulp-periodontal communication) resorption are complex. External resorption may take one of the following forms:

1. *Inflammatory* resorption is related to pulp necrosis. A periradicular lesion may cause apical resorption. Lateral resorption usually results from impact trauma.
2. *Replacement* resorption occurs after impact injuries (luxation or avulsion). This resorption is associated with fusion, then replacement, of tooth structure with bone.
3. *Idiopathic* (unknown) or *known etiology* is unrelated to pulpal or periradicular pathosis (e.g., resorption due to orthodontic treatment).

Patients with tooth resorption, whether internal or external, are high risk, and should be referred for evaluation and treatment (Figure 5-12).

Limited internal (intracanal) resorption may not present treatment complications, but external apical resorption may drastically alter the geometry of the root canal. A structure that was once round may now be irregular and difficult to clean and seal. Extensive apical resorption may be best managed by referral.

Endodontic-Periodontic Lesion

Another diagnostic dilemma arises with patients with periodontal problems who also have pulpal problems. If there is doubt about whether the problem is endodontic or periodontal (or has another cause), the patient should be referred. Differential diagnosis of periodontal and endodontic lesions is discussed in Chapter 26. Marginal periodontitis is best evaluated by a periodontist. An endodontist or a periodontist or both can best differentiate endodontic from periodontal

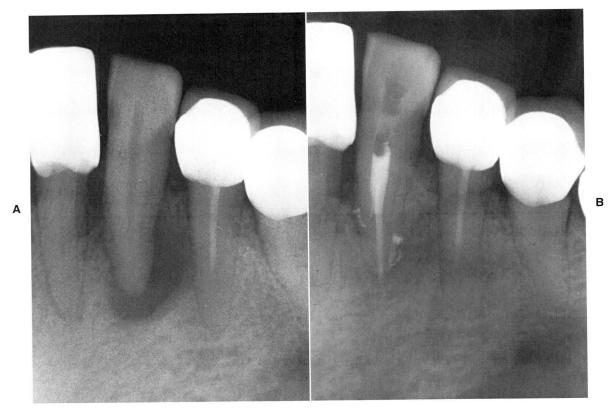

FIGURE 5-13
Combined endodontic-periodontal problem. **A,** This tooth may have been considered hopeless from a periodontal perspective. **B,** However, correct diagnosis and root canal treatment resolved most of the periradicular pathosis, although the periodontal component persists.

pathosis (Figure 5-13). Referral is best for patients needing surgical procedures such as hemisection or root resection.

Traumatic Injuries

Trauma to the dentition has two treatment components: primary and secondary management. *Primary* management is the first contact the injured patient has with a dentist; *secondary* management is the follow-up care. Primary care is required for patients with severe trauma such as luxations, displaced root fractures, and avulsions; the general dentist may render treatment immediately after the injury. Primary care includes patient management, repositioning, replantation, splinting, and suturing of soft tissue lacerations.

For secondary follow-up care the patient should be referred to an endodontist, who can determine an appropriate schedule for long-term management, recall, or treatment as necessary. Some changes may have a delayed onset. Examples of complications range from reversible pulpal inflammation to pulpal necrosis. These phenomena may or may not be obvious owing to variability in pulp response to testing, lack of symptoms, and so on. More subtle changes may include resorption (both external and internal), calcific metamorphosis, tooth discoloration, and obscure root fractures. Because many changes occur gradually, these patients must be followed over a prolonged period of time, preferably by an endodontist.

Previous Endodontic Treatment

Teeth are more difficult to retreat than to treat originally. Thus, rating of these cases is limited to rate 2 or rate 3 (Figure 5-14). These situations require a variety of approaches, including conventional retreatment, surgery, or combined treatment. Endodontists are more skilled than general practitioners in diagnosing and managing the myriad of problems presented and are more experienced in crown and post removal. Because of the complexity of retreatment, most patients should be referred. Generally, because endodontists commonly retreat teeth that have had previously unsuccessful root canal treatment, they have not only the experience but also an armamentarium useful for both nonsurgical and surgical approaches. Retreatments are becoming more commonplace as a result of procedural accidents of various types, described herein.

Procedural Accidents

SEPARATED INSTRUMENT OR CANAL BLOCKAGES

A separated instrument or other blockage may have a significant effect on prognosis. Consultation with an endodontist may be advisable. Different approaches are possible, and probably require an endodontist's expertise.

LEDGING

If a canal is ledged far from the working length, prognosis is compromised. The generalist should refer the patient to an endodontist. Canals that have not been ledged too far from the working length can be obturated, and the patient can be followed by the general practitioner. If retreatment or surgery is subsequently needed, the patient should be referred.

Perforations

Cases involving root or crown perforations can only be rated as rate 3. Patients with these conditions should be referred to an endodontist. Depending on the size, location, and strategic importance of the tooth, several options are available. These treatment approaches, as well as long-term assessment, are generally beyond the expertise of a general practitioner.

Emergencies

Emergencies are not addressed on the rating form, but are a significant part of decision making in the daily practice of general dentistry. General practitioners should be able to diagnose and treat most uncomplicated preoperative, interappointment, and postobturation emergencies. However, more severe problems are difficult to manage. For example, if the generalist cannot control the patient psychologically or is unable to obtain profound anesthesia, the patient should

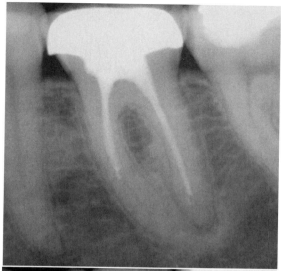

A

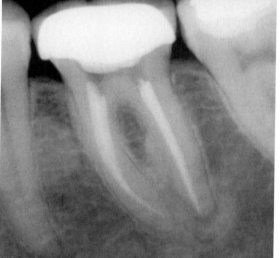

B

FIGURE 5-14
A, Previously attempted root canal treatment with very short obturation. The mesial root appears ledged. The tooth is percussion sensitive; also note the apical radiolucency of the distal root. Such retreatment cases should be considered as high or extreme risk. **B,** Only an experienced practitioner should manage this patient; referral is recommended.

be referred. If pain or swelling continues after emergency treatment and the general practitioner cannot assist the patient, an endodontist should be consulted or the patient should be referred.

PERSISTENT SIGNS AND/OR SYMPTOMS

If pain and/or swelling persist or develop after treatment, the patient should be referred or an endodontist should be consulted. The symptoms may have several causes: lack of débridement, lack of obturation, missed canals, root fractures, and so on. Extraction, retreatment, or surgical intervention may be required.

PERSISTENT RADIOGRAPHIC PATHOSIS

If periradicular lesions persist or develop after root canal treatment, consultation may be indicated. The endodontist may retreat, perform surgery, or advise the generalist on appropriate measures to resolve the problem.

PERSISTENT PROBING DEFECT OR SINUS TRACT

If a probing defect of pulpal origin or a sinus tract does not resolve after treatment, the patient should be referred. In addition, a new defect or sinus tract indicates treatment failure; referral should be considered.

Referral During Treatment

Timing of referral is important. *A poor practice is to initiate treatment with the idea that if problems arise, a referral can be made at the time.* Patients prefer to have a procedure started and completed by the same dentist. This saves appointment time for both patient and dentist. In addition, an initial referral prevents potential procedural errors by the general practitioner. The most important consideration is the effect on prognosis of a midtreatment referral. Preferably, the endodontist performs the entire procedure without having to correct iatrogenic problems. Also, with midtreatment referral, the patient may lose confidence in the original dentist. Another major problem is economics; monetarily, someone loses. The endodontist certainly is entitled to a full fee (or often *more* than a full fee; a treatment is generally more difficult if started by someone else). If the patient is responsible for two fees for the same tooth, ill will is created. It is far better for the general dentist to study the case and recommend referral than to "bail out" in the middle of treatment.

However, during treatment unanticipated problems may arise that require referral; a call to the endodontist and an explanation to the patient are in order. Reasons for possible midtreatment referral include flare-up (pain and/or swelling), procedural accidents, inability to achieve adequate anesthesia, and other factors that hinder completion of root canal therapy.

FLARE-UPS

Usually most pain or swelling occur before initial treatment. After emergency measures, pain usually substantially decreases in 24 to 48 hours. Flare-ups are not common.[14] Occasionally, however (particularly with an acute apical abscess), symptoms do not subside or arise de novo. The generalist may elect to treat such flare-ups with appropriate local procedures and therapy (analgesics and occasionally antibiotics for severe cellulitis). These flare-ups, however, are considerations for referral. There are rare situations in which severe endodontic infection results in a potentially life-threatening crisis. When the problem is out of control or is not responding to treatment, there must be a call for help!

PROCEDURAL ACCIDENTS

Procedural accidents occur during treatment. Again, the specialist's experience allows a better assessment of the probable outcome as well as the means of addressing the problem.

INABILITY TO LOCATE ROOT CANALS

Enhanced lighting and magnification improve the chances of locating canals. However, the greatest aid is experience. Rather than gouging or perforating while attempting to find a canal, referral should be considered. The endodontist may also have difficulty in locating canals. *Locating canals is easier if the chamber has not already been altered.*

FINANCIAL CONSIDERATIONS

Monetary considerations are important. Complicated problems, particularly those that involve prolonged treatment periods of months or years tend to be financial losses for the general dentist.

Referral to a Specialist

Communicating to the patient the need for referral for consultation and diagnosis or treatment must be done skillfully to avoid misunderstanding. The patient must realize that the most important consideration is optimal care. The reasons and timing of referral vary. Factors to be considered are the expertise of the dentist, treatment complexity, specialist availability, and other management factors. The patient is reminded that the specialist is generally able to handle problems more skillfully. Most patients understand and accept referral.

After briefly explaining the treatment needed and the options, a simple explanation is in order: "Mrs. Jones, because of the type of treatment, you need to obtain the best possible results. I would like you to see Dr. Smith, who routinely treats root canal problems. Dr. Smith is an expert in this field, and it would be to your advantage to go to a specialist. When Dr. Smith has completed treatment, you will return to me so that I can restore your tooth permanently."

Patients occasionally are reluctant to venture into another new office experience; empathy and words of encouragement help this transition. Explaining the treatment complexity (if such is the case) is helpful in supporting the reason for referral.

Sometimes a generalist and endodontist may meet, each bringing all records and diagnostic aids, for a "team planning session." Patients appreciate that their health care providers collaborate for optimum diagnosis and treatment planning. Overall, clear and prompt communication enhances comprehensive patient care and reduces patient misunderstandings and dissatisfaction.[15] Both referring dentist and endodontist have specific responsibilities in a referral case.

What is Expected of a General Practitioner

INSTRUCTIONS TO ENDODONTIST

Explicit written instructions and appropriate radiographs (original or duplicate) should be sent to the endodontist. Preferably this is done by mail because there is less opportunity for error. A call from one office to the other is acceptable, but there is more chance for misunderstanding when communication is verbal. It is undesirable to give the information verbally only to the patient and expect the patient to relay the information accurately to the endodontist. Also it is inadvisable to make patients deliver radiographs and instructions in writing to the specialist. Of course, at times this may be necessary, for example, in an emergency situation.

Generally, the patient is instructed to make his or her own appointment. As an alternative, the receptionist contacts the endodontist's office to arrange an appointment before the patient leaves. This ensures better patient compliance in seeking further care. The receptionist should explain the need for an appointment and should supply enough information for proper scheduling.

When appropriate, particularly if a key tooth is involved, the endodontist should be informed (in writing) how the tooth is to be restored and briefed on the overall treatment plan. If there are complications, this information gives the endodontist ideas about alternative approaches.

EXPLANATION TO PATIENT

After patient and generalist discuss the treatment planning, there is an explanation of "what is going to happen." The patient should understand that often the first appointment is for examination and consultation; procedures are performed when the endodontist and patient agree on a treatment plan.

Information is supplied about what to expect at the endodontic office. This information need not be detailed; that is the responsibility of the endodontist. Patients are concerned and need reassurance that the procedure will not be unpleasant and that no significant problems are likely to occur. However, there should be no overstating or overselling of the procedure. Guaranteeing a successful outcome by the endodontist is unfair and gives the patient false expectations.

What is Expected of an Endodontist

Specialists serve both the patient and referring dentist. Their responsibilities are to both; they should deliver appropriate treatment and communicate with the practitioner as well as the patient.

TREATMENT PERFORMED

Usually the procedure is limited to that requested by the referring dentist. Occasionally, different determinations are made, such as diagnostic or treatment difficulties or periodontal problems. The endodontist should first contact the referring dentist before proceeding and should inform the patient about the new treatment plan.

FEEDBACK TO DENTIST

When treatment is complete, the referring dentist should receive written confirmation from the endodontist that includes a radiograph of the obturation. A note is included about how the tooth was treated, anticipated recalls, prognosis (both short-term and long-term), unusual findings or circumstances, and, at times, suggestions about the permanent restoration and when it should be placed. Other findings related to adjacent structures or to the treated tooth are also included (for example, recurrent caries on other teeth, periodontal problems, or defective restorations).

FEEDBACK TO PATIENT

Before and during treatment, the endodontist explains all of the important aspects of the procedure and the anticipated outcome. After completion of treatment, the patient is informed about prognosis, appropriate follow-up care, and the need to return to the referring dentist for continued care and any possible additional future procedures. At this final appointment, the receptionist may call the generalist's office to arrange the next visit.

REFERENCES

1. Molven O: The frequency, technical standard and results of endodontic therapy, *Nor Tannlasg Tidsskr* 86:142, 1976.
2. Scharwatt BR: The general practitioner and endodontist, *Dent Clin North Am* 23:747, 1974.
3. Cohen S, Schwartz S: Endodontic complications and the law, *J Endod* 13:191, 1987.
4. Ericksen H: Endodontology-epidemiologic consideration, *Endod Dent Trauma* 7:189, 1991.
5. Rosenberg RJ, Goodis HE: Endodontic case selection—to treat or to refer, *J Am Dent Assoc* 123:57, 1992.
6. Caplan D, Reams G, Weintraub J: Recommendations for endodontic referral among practitioners in a dental HMO, *J Endod* 25:369, 1999.
7. DiPrio JT, Talbert RL, Yee GC, Posey LM, editors: *Pharmacotherapy, a pathophysiologic approach*. New York, 1989, Elsevier, p. 642.
8. Seltzer S, Bender IB: *The dental pulp: biologic considerations in dental practice*, ed 3, St Louis, 1990, Ishiyaku Euro-America, p. 127.
9. Kuyk J, Walton R: Comparison of radiographic appearance of root canal size to its actual diameter, *J Endod* 16:528, 1990.
10. Benjamin KA, Dowson J: Incidence of two root canals in human mandibular incisor teeth, *Oral Surg Oral Med Oral Pathol Oral Radiol Endod* 58:589, 1984.
11. Vertucci FJ: Root canal morphology of mandibular premolars, *J Am Dent Assoc* 97:47, 1978.
12. Vertucci FJ: Root canal anatomy of human permanent teeth, *Oral Surg Oral Med Oral Pathol Oral Radiol Endod* 58:589, 1984.
13. Burns R, Herbranson E: Tooth morphology and cavity preparation. In Cohen S, Burns RC, editors, *Pathways of the pulp*, ed 8, St Louis, 2001, Mosby.
14. Walton R, Fouad A: Endodontic inter-appointment flare-ups: a prospective study of incidence and related factors, *J Endod* 18:172, 1992.
15. Kramer S: Communications regarding referrals, *Risk Manage Rep* I(IV):4, 1989.

Stephen Cohen and Mahmoud Torabinejad

6

Patient Education

LEARNING OBJECTIVES

After reading this chapter, the student should be able to:

1 / Describe endodontic procedures in terms understandable to a layperson.

2 / Explain to the patient in understandable terms why and when root canal treatment is or is not indicated.

3 / Make clear to the patient that there are alternatives to endodontic treatment.

4 / Describe briefly the steps involved in root canal treatment.

5 / Explain to the patient the number of appointments needed, potential postoperative discomfort, potential complications, and cost of treatment.

6 / Discuss the importance of a timely restoration after treatment, the need for recall examinations, and signs or symptoms of endodontic treatment failure.

7 / Explain to the patient the reasons for retreatment.

8 / Explain what is involved in retreatment and the alternatives to retreatment.

9 / Explain why referral to an endodontist is necessary in certain cases.

10 / Provide the information needed for clear informed consent for endodontic procedures.

11 / Describe and discuss the verbal and nonverbal signals that support a patient's willingness to listen to the doctor.

OUTLINE

Nonverbal Messages
   Professional Appearance and Manner
   Sense of Sincere Caring
Listening
   How Patients Process Information
   Doctor-Patient Interaction
Informed Consent
Dentist-Patient Dialogue
Art of Communication

The word *doctor* is derived from the Latin "to teach." Complete treatment of any patient involves educating the patient about the treatment to be rendered and the options available. An open exchange is part of the education of the patient; it establishes communication between doctor and patient and creates an open clinician-patient relationship. Such a relationship fosters trust and relieves anxiety.

Not every patient is interested in learning about treatment; occasionally patients may tell the dentist that they do not care to know. However, because there is always at least one treatment alternative, the clinician must attempt to communicate information about treatment options. No single approach can be used to communicate this necessary information to patients. To do this appropriately, the doctor must be sensitive not only to what the patient says but also to facial expressions and body language of each patient. The words "root canal treatment" cause dread in many patients. This sometimes unarticulated fear interferes with patients' understanding about the treatment to be provided. The doctor's reassurance becomes the foundation for the patient's receptivity to information about root canal treatment.

Nonverbal Messages

The expression "We do not get a second chance to make a first impression" holds especially true for the doctor-patient relationship. When a doctor greets a new patient, the patient forms an impression from several nonverbal messages, including the following:

PROFESSIONAL APPEARANCE AND MANNER

The patient observes whether the doctor and the staff are dressed appropriately and whether the dental environment (i.e., the reception area and the treatment room) are clean, modern, and tasteful.

SENSE OF SINCERE CARING

If the staff and the doctor make the patient feel as if he or she is the most important person at that moment, it helps to establish a sense of trust and rapport that provides the foundation for effective communication.

Listening

Commonly, patients are fearful of the prospect of having root canal treatment; often they are anxious to discuss their anxieties. If staff and doctor make it evident that they are truly listening without distraction to everything the patient is saying, the patient feels as if he or she is really being heard. This, too, provides further support for effective communication. The doctor and staff must immediately create an environment in which the patient experiences them as caring professionals. This will lessen the fear and anxiety that are often impediments to effective communication in the treatment room. Commonly, patients have had prior personal experience or have heard of an experience from others that fosters a stereotypical image of root canal treatment as painful. A sense of dread can significantly impair a patient's ability to listen well and to hear what the doctor is trying to communicate.

The doctor should confront this unspoken anxiety immediately by asking the patient, "Do you have any concerns about root canal treatment?" This gives the patient an opportunity to express any concerns and fears about anticipated pain. Because of what is known about pain control today, the doctor can, even *before* the dental examination and diagnostic testing, provide the patient an almost ironclad assurance that root canal treatment will be relatively painless. The doctor should state this fact calmly and confidently and allow the patient to respond with any questions.

A typical inquiry may be, "But will it hurt *after* the root canal treatment?" A truthful and reassuring response is that some mild to moderate transient discomfort is common after anesthesia subsides, but this can be managed with analgesics, such as nonnarcotic pain control medications (e.g., nonsteroidal antiinflammatory drugs). Furthermore, the postoperative experience should not interfere with normal business and social activities. If any pain occurs that is stronger than expected, the patient should be assured and reassured that he or she can reach the doctor for prompt relief at any time any day. This verbal reassurance should be reinforced by written instructions that are easily understood by a layperson.[1] Because of the increasing diversity of our society, reflected in part by the prevalence of English as a second language for many people, printed instructions in other languages (e.g., Spanish, Chinese, etc.) is a helpful adjunct. When the issue of pain has been fully discussed and the patient's fears allayed, the foundation for imparting information about root canal treatment has been established.

HOW PATIENTS PROCESS INFORMATION

Each patient processes information in his or her own way. Some respond to information they read. For this kind of information, brochures are pub-

lished by the American Association of Endodontists, and a slide series is available through the American Dental Association. These materials cover virtually the full range of endodontic procedures. Other patients respond to information they hear. The doctor (not the staff) must patiently explain the significant facts about root canal treatment. Because individuals retain information differently, it is prudent to explain the procedures in detail and to encourage all patients to read the appropriate brochures as well. This provides a higher level of assurance that the patient understands the doctor's examination and recommended treatment. However, it is important for the clinician to use more subtle, nonverbal signals to support continued communication. These more subtle nonverbal signals include the following.

DOCTOR-PATIENT INTERACTION
Body Positions

The position of a doctor standing above a seated patient (or a patient lying back in a chair) tends to infantilize the patient. Rather, the patient should be seated at the same level as the doctor. This establishes the patient as an equal and supports responsible communication.

Eye Contact

The doctor must maintain frequent eye contact with the patient. Eye contact during transmission of information connects doctor and patient and engenders confidence.

Body Language

The doctor should be attentive to the patient's body language as well as to his or her own. The defensive position of crossed arms or legs indicates that the patient is not open to receiving information. In contrast, the more relaxed position of holding the hands in the lap with uncrossed legs suggests that the patient is listening well and understands what is being said.

Informed Consent

Not all patients really want to know the details of root canal treatment. Many doctors have heard patients say, "As long as it doesn't hurt, I don't care what you do." In an earlier time these patients would have been treated without further discussion. However, today the doctor is required to inform a patient fully before proceeding with treatment. For patients who do not want to know

I understand that root canal treatment is a procedure undertaken to retain a tooth that may otherwise *require* extraction. Although root canal therapy has a very high degree of clinical success, it is a biologic procedure and results cannot be guaranteed.

I also understand that occasionally a tooth that has had nonsurgical root canal therapy may require retreatment. In addition, approximately 10 percent of teeth that have had nonsurgical root canal treatment may require an additional procedure, root-end surgery, at a later time. Even after root canal therapy, retreatment, and/or surgery, a small percentage of teeth (5 percent) nevertheless require extraction.

I understand that the final restoration for this tooth should usually be completed within 1 month.

Signed: PATIENT or PARENT: _____

Date: _____

FIGURE 6-1
Informed consent form.

about root canal treatment, the following procedure is recommended:

- The patient is asked to sign and date a written informed consent form (Figure 6-1 and Box 6-1). The dental assistant should note in the treatment record that the patient declined to receive information about endodontic therapy.
- The patient is reminded that if he (or she) changes his (or her) mind, he (or she) is free to ask questions at any time.
- Fees for service are clearly explained (and must be understood by the patient) before treatment is initiated.[2]

Dentist-Patient Dialogue

Most patients are curious about and interested in their treatment. For these patients, the following information should be discussed, not in a rote

---

BOX 6-1

Legal Aspects of Informed Consent   **Edwin Zinman**

A patient has a legal right to refuse a dentist's recommended treatment. Accordingly, should a dentist proceed to treat a patient without the patient's consent, the dentist would be liable for battery. This is true even if the dentist meant well and performed the treatment in what was regarded as the patient's best interest. For instance, an unexpected pulpal exposure may create the need for root canal treatment. Before proceeding, the dentist must obtain the patient's consent for treatment even if endodontics is a foregone conclusion, because the patient has the right to do with his or her own body as he or she sees fit.

Emergency care also requires consent. Therefore rather than *immediately* extracting a salvageable tooth in a patient who has severe pain, the dentist should first relieve the pain so that the patient can make an intelligent and informed decision about the proper course of treatment. Many patients who seek immediate pain relief by extraction regret having foregone root canal treatment. It is better to attenuate the pain with local anesthetic, pulpal extirpation, analgesics, or other pain-relieving methods to allow the patient to weigh intelligently the choice between tooth salvation or extraction unfettered by painful distraction.

The legal doctrine of informed consent requires that the patient be advised of the benefits, risks, reasonable alternatives, and consequences of doing nothing. Otherwise the patient may claim that he or she did not appreciate all of the ramifications of endodontic therapy, precluding a reasonably intelligent informed choice of treatment. In root canal treatment the choices are as follows:

A. Benefits
1. Preservation of an existing tooth and avoidance of restorative replacement with a crown, bridge, or implant
2. Preservation of underlying alveolar support including a stronger abutment tooth

B. Risks
1. Failure in some instances, necessitating retreatment, root canal surgery, or possible extraction
2. Paresthesia, particularly if the tooth is close to the mental foramen
3. Infection
4. Fractured endodontic instruments, necessitating retrieval
5. Perforation

C. Alternatives
1. Extraction
2. Waiting for further symptoms or signs if diagnosis is only a differential or screening diagnosis and not final

D. Consequences of doing nothing
1. Abscess
2. Pain
3. Further loss of bone
4. Severe infection
5. Extraction

manner, but in anticipation of the questions commonly asked. Here are examples of typical questions, with the answers the dentist might give.

- *What is endodontics?* Teeth are composed of a hard structure surrounding a soft, living tissue (Figure 6-2). This is called the pulp (sometimes called "the nerve"), which contains blood vessels, fibers, and nerves. Endodontics (root canal treatment) is the diagnosis and treatment of inflamed or diseased pulps.

- *Why does the pulp ("nerve") become inflamed or diseased?* Some of the main causes of pulp problems include tooth decay, the treatment of tooth decay (fillings, crowns, and so on), trauma, and advanced gum disease (Figures 6-3 and 6-4).

- *How can you tell if the pulp is inflamed or diseased?* Some of the symptoms of an inflamed pulp include prolonged toothache when you have hot or cold liquids in your mouth, spontaneous (unprovoked) toothache, pain with chewing or biting, and pain when you lie down. Some of the signs of diseased pulp include evidence of decay or evidence of a shadow (abscess) at the end of the root, drainage, or swelling (Figure 6-5).

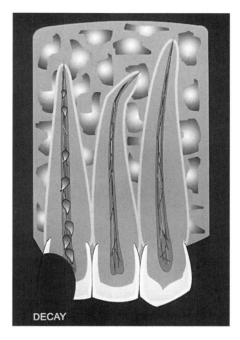

FIGURE 6-3
The crown may be damaged by decay, which has reached the pulp (nerve), causing severe damage.

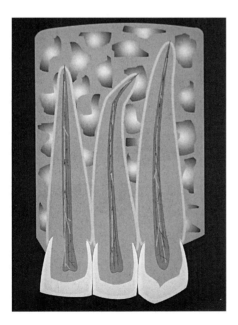

FIGURE 6-2
This and the following diagrams (Figures 6-3 through 6-16) provide a format and description suitable for patient education. This diagram schematically demonstrates normal, healthy structures.

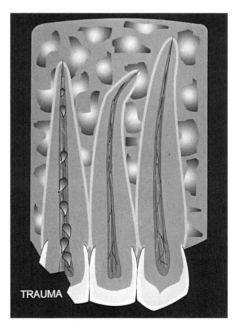

FIGURE 6-4
A blow may fracture the crown, exposing and damaging the pulp (nerve).

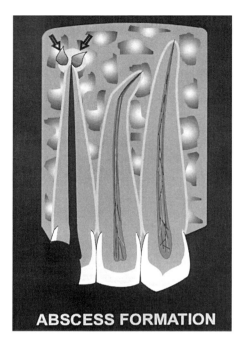

FIGURE 6-5
After severe injury, the pulp may die. Bacteria then enter the space. Irritants from the pulp go into bone and cause an area of disease, with resorption (erosion) of bone and ligament at the end of the root. This may form an abscess *(arrows)*.

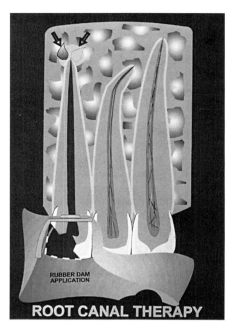

FIGURE 6-6
After local anesthesia (novocaine), the first step is to apply a rubber dam with a metal clamp.

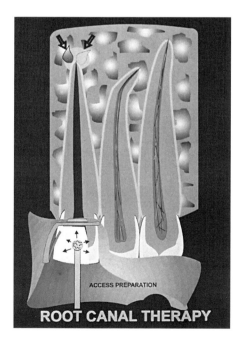

FIGURE 6-7
An opening is made into the crown with a bur (drill).

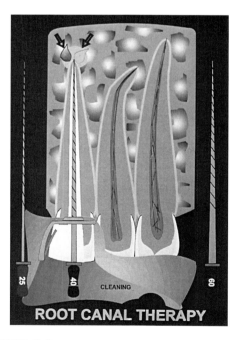

FIGURE 6-8
Small metal instruments (files) plane (rasp) the insides of the canal. This process cleans and enlarges the canal. Different numbers indicate different sizes of files.

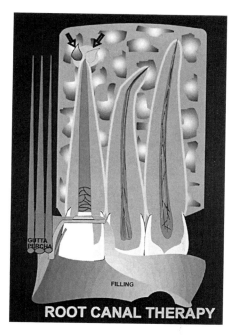

FIGURE 6-9
An inert rubber-like material called *gutta-percha* is packed tightly into the canal; this seals the end of the root and fills and seals the length of the canal.

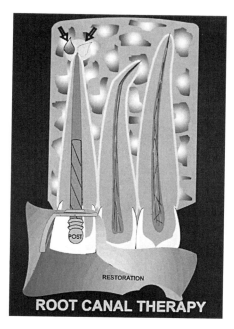

FIGURE 6-10
Different types of restorations (fillings) are required. Some require placement of a post into the canal to hold the restoration in place.

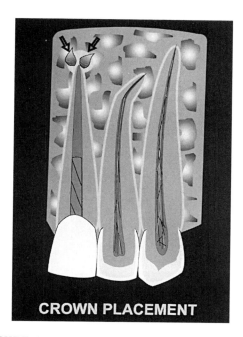

FIGURE 6-11
A crown (cap) is cemented over the post and tooth.

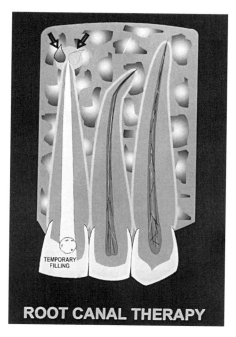

FIGURE 6-12
If the patient will need more than one treatment or when root canal treatment is completed, a temporary filling is usually placed.

■ *How do you do root canal treatment?* After the tooth is numb, I apply a rubber sheet to isolate the tooth and make an opening into the center of the tooth to reach the pulp (nerve). With very small instruments I remove the pulp and sculpt the space it occupied. I sterilize, fill, and seal the root canal inner space with a rubber-like material that will prevent bacteria from entering this space (Figures 6-6 to 6-9). To restore the missing parts or broken piece of the tooth, a post may be placed inside the tooth (Figure 6-10). The tooth may also require a crown (Figure 6-11).

■ *How many visits will it take to complete this treatment?* Today, treatment for most teeth often can be completed in one visit, which will take 1 to 1½ hours. Treatment for other teeth may require two visits, and a few might even require more. If more than one visit is needed, I will place a temporary filling in the tooth (Figure 6-12).

■ *If I have root canal treatment, how likely is it that I'll keep my tooth?* When root canal treatment is done thoroughly, there is a very good chance of success (Figure 6-13); however, some treatment may fail no matter how well the treatment is done (Figure 6-14). In these instances, retreatment or endodontic surgery may rem-

edy the lingering problem. These treatments are usually best done by a specialist.

■ *What is endodontic surgery?* Endodontic surgery corrects the problem from the end of the root (Figure 6-15). Under local anesthesia the gum tissue is gently lifted so that the dentist can find the end of the root (Figure 6-15, *A* and *B*). Then the inflamed tissue is removed around the end of the root and a filling is placed there to prevent the problem from recurring. To secure the gum tissue, several stitches are placed (Figure 6-15, *C*). A few days later, the stitches are removed. This procedure usually leads to complete healing (Figure 6-15, *D*).

■ *Will this tooth in the front of my mouth turn dark after root canal treatment?* Years ago some teeth like this eventually darkened over time. Based on what we do today, it is unlikely that you will see any change in color. However, if this should occur, we can often bleach the tooth back to a normal shade. Bonding veneers and crowns are additional choices for the few teeth that might darken.

■ *Will the root canal treatment be painful?* Almost never. Years ago it really was not always possible to control pain (Box 6-2). Today, with a better understanding of local anesthesia,

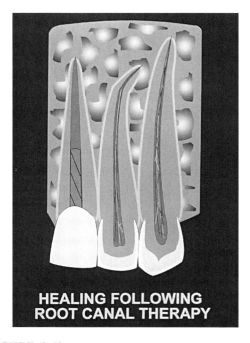

FIGURE 6-13
If the canals are cleaned, filled, and sealed, the bone lost at the root tip will heal with new bone and ligaments.

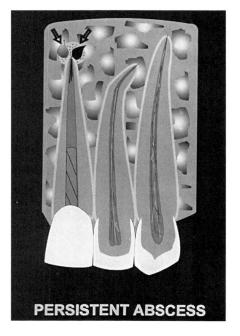

FIGURE 6-14
If there are defects or problems with the treatment, the area of disease will spread and an abscess may form. This usually requires retreatment of the root canal.

profound anesthesia is more predictable. After the anesthetic dissipates, there will probably be transient soreness for a few days, which can be controlled with nonnarcotic pain pills. However, if there should be

unexpected strong pain, you can call and talk with me directly any time, any day.

■ *If I don't have root canal treatment, what are my other choices?* It depends on the nature of the problem. Generally speaking, other choices

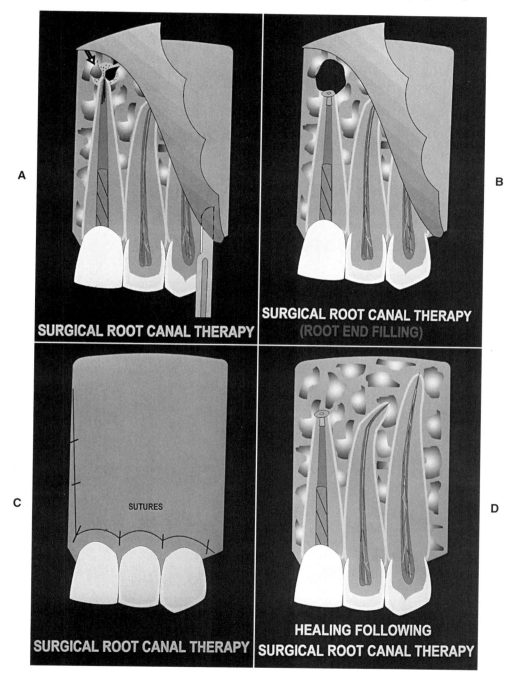

A   SURGICAL ROOT CANAL THERAPY

B   SURGICAL ROOT CANAL THERAPY (ROOT END FILLING)

C   SUTURES   SURGICAL ROOT CANAL THERAPY

D   HEALING FOLLOWING SURGICAL ROOT CANAL THERAPY

FIGURE 6-15
Some treatment failures or other situations may require surgery. **A,** After anesthesia, the gum tissue is raised to expose the root end. **B,** The root end is cut off, and a filling is placed to seal the end. **C,** Several sutures (stitches) are placed to hold down the gum to allow healing. **D,** If the problem is resolved, the bone will heal around the root tip.

BOX 6-2

History of Pain Control   Dr. William Johnson

Profound local dental anesthesia has been one of the "Holy Grails" for dentists for centuries. In the 1840s, Drs. William Morton and Horace Wells (both dentists) introduced general anesthesia to the medical profession in the forms of nitrous oxide ("laughing gas") and ether; this ushered in the concept of truly painless dentistry. These events were so significant, that to this day "Ether Dome," a part of Massachusetts General Hospital,—the only national park located within a hospital—still exists exactly as it was over 160 years ago. Ether Dome has only two honorary seats in its amphitheater—both for dentists! Cocainization (applying cocaine on "the gums") began in 1884 with Karl Koller, a Viennese physician. This concept was made safer and more effective with the introduction of novocaine (procaine) by the unheralded Dr. Alfred Einhorn, a biochemist working for Bayer Company in

Berlin in 1905. Almost at the same time (1906) Dr. Noguie of Paris introduced to the dental profession the concept of conduction anesthesia. Novocaine was not widely used until a U.S. Army dentist, Dr. Harvey S. Cook, developed a cartridge delivery system. In the 1930s, Dr. Leonard Monheim advocated local dental anesthesia.

From this modest beginning, newer, safer, and more effective local anesthetics were introduced by Dr. Nils Lofgren (lidocaine), better anesthetic syringes (aspirating) were introduced, and better, stronger, and more flexible needles were introduced.

Today, profound local anesthesia is *expected* by patients. If this brief history were more widely known, patients and dentists might show a deeper sense of gratitude to the courageous people who made effective dental anesthesia possible.

---

are doing nothing at present (postponement) or extracting the tooth (probably requiring a bridge or implant to fill the space). (NOTE: If the patient is suffering, a delay in treatment is not reasonable, so the choice is between endodontics and extraction.) Some situations present additional choices, such as apical surgery or replantation.

- *Can you explain the steps involved in bridge construction?* Yes. After extraction of the involved tooth and healing of the wound, the adjacent teeth are prepared (ground down), which can result in pulpal (nerve) inflammation. Finally, a bridge is constructed consisting of two crowns and a fake tooth (Figure 6-16).
- *After root canal treatment, will I have a dead tooth?* No. Years ago this is what it was called. Today we know that the tooth is still quite alive after root canal treatment because it has a blood supply to the ligament that keeps the tooth firmly in its socket. Because there is a blood supply, the tooth continues to receive nutrition and remains quite healthy.
- *Will I need to get my tooth filled after the root canal treatment?* Yes. If your care requires a specialist who treats complicated situations (an endodontist), I will refer you. If the procedure is straightforward and uncomplicated, I can do this quite well myself. In either case, the treatment should be promptly completed by final restoration.
- *After the root canal treatment and the final restoration ("filling"), will I have to do anything*

more? Yes, I will want to examine the tooth 6 months to 1 year later to assess long-term healing. When you return for follow-up, I will take an x-ray, check your gum tissue, and reexamine the final restoration. The tooth should feel comfortable to you. The tooth must also be firm, functional, and appear normal on the x-ray film. Even though the tooth feels comfortable to you, if I do not see complete repair on the film, I may refer you to an endodontist for further consultation and possibly additional treatment.

- *Why does my tooth have to be retreated? Dr. Doe just did the root canal treatment 2 years ago.* I'll have to call Dr. Doe to find out what problems he encountered when he did the root canal treatment. (NOTE: If the root canal treatment is incomplete [i.e., the canal filling is several millimeters too short from the apex, or if a root canal is completely unfilled], the patient must be given this information in an informative—but not alarming—manner. The purpose of this portion of patient education is to inform and not alarm the patient. It is an egregious error to use harsh and judgmental terms before knowing all the facts.) This information will help me decide what should be done to try to correct this failure.
- *How much will root canal treatment cost? The* fee for this treatment is $_____. Alternative: I will ask my financial secretary to explain the fees for complete treatment. Customarily there is a set fee, whether it takes one, two, or more appointments to complete it.

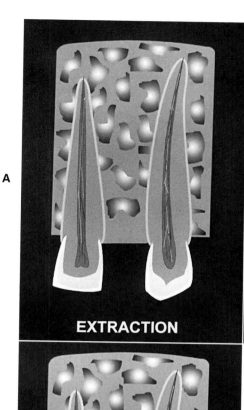

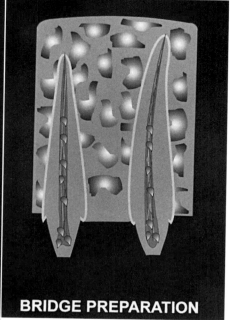

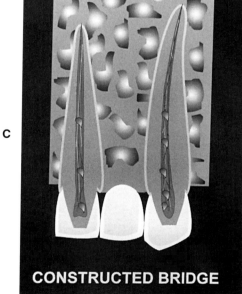

FIGURE 6-16
Replacing a missing tooth. **A,** If a tooth is lost, a space remains; this space is unsightly and can cause problems. **B,** The teeth on each side are cut down. **C,** The bridge is made and cemented. A replacement tooth is attached to the crowns on each side.

Art of Communication

In the treatment room there is an extended dialogue of informing (giving information) and listening (receiving information). Both patient and doctor are informing. The doctor informs the patient about treatment, prognosis, alternatives, follow-up, and so on. Patients inform the doctor about who they are, what they want, what they fear, and

so on. Both are also listening. The doctor listens for the subtext that will lead to better care. The patient listens for information and reassurance.

A doctor both heals and cures; the healing begins with the first opportunity for an extended dialogue that we call patient education. Patient education must be preceded by doctor education, not just the technical information learned in dental school but also the process of self-discovery that leads to an open heart and compassion. When patients make a true connection with the dentist, they are able and willing to learn; only then does the dentist truly earn the title "Doctor."

REFERENCES

1. Alexander RE: Patient understanding of postsurgical instruction forms, *Oral Surg Oral Med Oral Pathol Oral Radiol* 87:153, 1999.
2. Christensen G: Educating patients, *J Am Dent Assoc* 130:731, 1999.

Local Anesthesia

LEARNING OBJECTIVES

After reading this chapter, the student should be able to:

1 / Explain why apprehension and anxiety, fatigue, and tissue inflammation create difficulties in obtaining profound anesthesia.

2 / Define pain threshold and the factors affecting pain threshold.

3 / Describe patient management techniques that will facilitate obtaining adequate anesthesia.

4 / List techniques that are helpful in giving "painless" injections.

5 / Describe the "routine" approach to conventional local anesthesia: when and how to anesthetize.

6 / Describe circumstances that create difficulties in obtaining profound anesthesia using conventional techniques.

7 / Describe when to use supplemental methods of obtaining pulpal anesthesia if standard block or infiltration methods fail.

8 / Review techniques of intraosseous, periodontal ligament, and intrapulpal injections.

9 / Discuss how to obtain anesthesia for specific pulpal and periradicular pathoses: irreversible pulpitis, symptomatic teeth with pulpal necrosis, asymptomatic teeth with pulpal necrosis, and surgical procedures.

OUTLINE

Factors Affecting Endodontic Anesthesia
Apprehension and Anxiety
Fatigue
Tissue Inflammation
Previous Unsuccessful Anesthesia

Initial Management
Psychologic Approach
"Painless" Injections
When to Anesthetize
Adjunctive Pharmacologic Therapy

Conventional Anesthesia

Mandibular Anesthesia
Anesthetic Agents
Related Factors
Alternative Techniques

Maxillary Anesthesia
Anesthetic Agents
Related Factors
Alternative Techniques

Anesthesia Difficulties

Supplemental Anesthesia
Indications
Anesthetic Agents
Intraosseous Anesthesia
Periodontal Ligament Injection
Intrapulpal Injection
Alternative Primary Techniques

Anesthetic Management of Pulpal or Periradicular Pathoses
Irreversible Pulpitis
Symptomatic Pulp Necrosis
Asymptomatic Pulp Necrosis

Anesthesia for Surgical Procedures
Incision for Drainage
Periradicular Surgery

When a tooth which is loose or painful is to be extracted, the nose of the patient should be rubbed with brown sugar, ivy and green oil; he is advised to hold his breath, a stone is then placed between his teeth, and he is made to close his mouth. The fluid which causes the pain is then seen to flow from the mouth in such quantity as frequently to fill three pots; after having cleansed the nose with pure oil, rinsed the mouth with wine, the tooth is no longer painful, and may easily be extracted.

SCRIBONIUS, 47 AD

Т his historical anecdote illustrates Scribonius' description of a method of obtaining "anesthesia." He was convinced that he could perform painless extractions using what was apparently a rather crude technique of pressure anesthesia. Our concern for the patient continues: How are adequate levels of anesthesia attained to keep our patients relatively comfortable during endodontic procedures? Obtaining profound anesthesia for the endodontic patient is difficult and challenging. Many patients recount vivid (and often valid) accounts of painful experiences. Although routine anesthetic techniques are usually effective for restorative dentistry, endodontic procedures present special situations that require additional techniques and special approaches.

Factors Affecting Endodontic Anesthesia

Emotional considerations as well as tissue changes impair the effectiveness of local anesthesia.[1] A patient who is psychologically distraught with an inflamed pulp will have a decreased pain threshold; that is, less stimulus is required to produce pain.[2]

In addition, the trigeminal nerve, which supplies primary sensory innervation to oral structures, is a complex entity. Knowledge of its more common anatomical features will aid in successful anesthesia.

APPREHENSION AND ANXIETY

Many endodontic patients have heard horror stories about root canal treatment. The cause may not be the treatment but the experience of a painful or "infected" tooth. They vividly recall the pain, swelling, and sleepless nights associated with the tooth before treatment. The procedure itself is generally less threatening—a survey of endodontic patients completing therapy indicated that 96 percent would agree to have future root canal treatment.[3] Therefore because they fear the unknown and have heard unfavorable stories, patients will be apprehensive or anxious. This emotion plays a role in their perceptions and also affects how they react to pain.[4,5] Many patients effectively mask this apprehension!

FATIGUE

Over a course of days many patients with a toothache have not slept well, not eaten properly, or otherwise not functioned normally. In addition, many are apprehensive or anxious about the appointment. The end result is a patient with a decreased ability to manage stress and with less tolerance for pain.

TISSUE INFLAMMATION

Inflamed tissues have a decreased threshold of pain perception.[6] This is the "hyperalgesia" phenomenon. In other words, a tissue that is inflamed is much more sensitive and reactive to a lower stimulus.[7] Therefore an inflamed tissue responds painfully to a stimulus that otherwise would be unnoticed or perceived only mildly. Because root canal treatment procedures generally involve inflamed pulpal or periradicular tissues, this phenomenon has obvious importance. A related complication is that inflamed tissues are more difficult to anesthetize.[8]

A good example of the phenomenon of increased sensitivity (a form of hyperalgesia) is sunburn. Exposed tissues that have been burned are irritated and inflamed. The skin has now become quite sensitive (decreased pain threshold) to contact and is painful. This same principle also applies to inflamed pulpal and periradicular tissues.[9]

PREVIOUS UNSUCCESSFUL ANESTHESIA

Unfortunately, profound pulpal anesthesia is not always obtained with conventional techniques. Previous difficulty with teeth becoming anesthetized is associated with a likelihood of subsequent unsuccessful anesthesia.[10] These patients are likely to be apprehensive (decreased pain threshold) and generally identify themselves by comments such as "Novocaine never seems to work very well on me" or "A lot of shots are always necessary to deaden my teeth." The practitioner should anticipate difficul-

ties in obtaining anesthesia in such patients. Often, psychologic management and supplemental techniques are required.

Initial Management

The early phase of treatment is most important. If the patient is managed properly and anesthetic techniques are done smoothly, the pain threshold elevates. The result is more predictable anesthesia and a less apprehensive, more cooperative patient.

PSYCHOLOGIC APPROACH

The psychologic approach involves the four Cs: control, communication, concern, and confidence. *Control* is important and is achieved by obtaining and maintaining the upper hand. *Communication* is accomplished by listening and explaining what is to be done and what the patient should expect. *Concern* is shown by verbalizing awareness of the patient's apprehensions. *Confidence* is expressed in body language and in professionalism, giving the patient confidence in the management, diagnostic, and treatment skills of the dentist. Management of the four Cs effectively calms and reassures the patient, thereby raising the pain threshold.

"PAINLESS" INJECTIONS

Patients generally have a fear of dental injections.[3,11] A good practice-builder and a method of winning confidence and cooperation is to master injection techniques that are nearly painless.[12] Assuredly, patients will inform their friends and family that their dentist does not "hurt when he/she gives me a shot." Although most injections cannot be totally pain-free, there can be a minimum of discomfort. This also relaxes the patient and effectively raises the pain threshold and the tolerance level.

Obtaining Patient Confidence: Patient confidence is critical. Before any injection is given, establishing communication, exhibiting empathy, and informing patients of an awareness of their apprehension as well as their dental problem will markedly increase confidence levels.[13] Most important, having the patient's confidence will give control of the situation to the dentist; this is a requisite!

Topical Anesthetic: Use of a topical anesthetics is popular as an adjunct to painless injections.[14] Some investigators have shown topical anesthetics to be effective, whereas others have not.[15,16] The most important aspect of using topical anesthesia is not primarily the actual decrease in mucosal sensitivity but rather the demonstrated concern that everything possible is being done to prevent pain. Also operating is the power of suggestion that the topical anesthetic will reduce the pain of injection.[17] When a topical anesthetic gel is used, a small amount on a cotton-tipped applicator is placed on the dried mucosa for 1 to 2 minutes before the injection.[18]

A relatively new device is an intraoral adhesive, 20% lidocaine patch. When in place for 5 minutes, it was shown to reduce the pain of needlestick.[19]

Solution Warming: A common belief is that an anesthetic solution warmed to or above body temperature is better tolerated and results in less pain during injection. However, in a clinical trial, investigators found that patients could not differentiate between prewarmed and room temperature anesthetic solutions.[20] Therefore warming anesthetic cartridges is not necessary.

Needle Insertion: Initially, the needle is inserted *gently* into the mucosal tissue. This will be almost unnoticed by the patient, regardless of the needle gauge.

Small-Gauge Needles: A common concept is that smaller needles cause less pain, but this is not true for dental needles. Patients cannot differentiate between 25-, 27-, or 30-gauge needles during injections.[21] These sizes also have similar deflection patterns and resistance to breakage.[22,23] As a recommendation, a 27-gauge needle is suitable for most conventional dental injections.

Slow Injection: Slow injection is a very effective means of decreasing pressure and patient discomfort during injection. *Slow* deposition of solution permits its gradual distribution into the tissues. This is particularly important in the maxillary anterior region (a very sensitive area) and in regions where tissue is tightly bound (posterior palate and nasopalatine area). As a general rule, solution deposition should take approximately 1 minute per cartridge.

Two-Stage Injection: A two-stage injection consists of initial very slow administration of approximately a quarter-cartridge of anesthetic under the mucosal surface; this will be nearly painless. After regional numbness occurs, additional anesthetic is given to the full depth at the target site, usually with minimal pain. The two-stage injection is indicated for apprehensive and anxious patients or pediatric patients but may be used for anyone. It is also useful in any region including the inferior alveolar nerve block.

WHEN TO ANESTHETIZE

Preferably, anesthesia should be given at each appointment. There is a common belief that instru-

ments may be used in canals with necrotic pulps and periradicular lesions painlessly without anesthesia. Occasionally, there may be vital tissue in the apical few millimeters of the canal. This inflamed tissue contains nerves and is sensitive.[24] Not only is this vital tissue contacted during instrumentation, but also pressure is created. These may cause discomfort if the patient is not anesthetized.

There is an antiquated notion that canal length can be determined in a nonanesthetized patient by passing an instrument into a necrotic canal until the patient shows an "eye blink response." Unfortunately, patient perceptions and responses are too variable for accuracy. Pain may be felt when the instrument is far short of the apex, or some patients may have no sensation even when the instrument is several millimeters beyond the apex. Use of nonanesthesia for length determination cannot replace radiographs or an apex locator for accuracy. Another misconception is that after the canals have been cleaned and shaped, it is not necessary to anesthetize the patient at the obturation appointment. However, during obturation pressure is created and small amounts of sealer may be extruded beyond the apex. This may be quite uncomfortable. Many patients (as well as the dentist) are more at ease if regional hard and soft tissue anesthesia is present.

ADJUNCTIVE PHARMACOLOGIC THERAPY

Sedation (intravenous, oral, or inhalation) may enhance local anesthesia, particularly in patients who want to cooperate but are extremely apprehensive. A discussion on agents that control anxiety is included in Chapter 30.

Conventional Anesthesia

Success of local anesthesia is variable. Two surveys of patients and dentists indicated that some patients were not adequately anesthetized during restorative treatment.[10,25] Overall, of 10 patients treated, 3 may feel pain during the procedure. This is a significant number! A number of factors affect anesthesia, such as the type of procedure (endodontic, extraction, restorative, periodontal, and so on), arch location (maxillary or mandibular), anxiety level, and the presence of inflamed tissue.

Many clinical studies have subjectively evaluated local anesthetic agents and techniques. A measurement of pulpal anesthesia before beginning a procedure is obtained with an electric pulp tester or with application of carbon dioxide (dry ice) or spray refrigerant. No pulpal response after administration of anesthetic means probable profound anesthesia in asymptomatic teeth with vital pulps.[26,27] Experimental studies have investigated the use of local anesthesia; these are discussed in the following sections. Conventional injection techniques are detailed in other textbooks.

Mandibular Anesthesia

ANESTHETIC AGENTS

The most commonly used agent is 2% lidocaine with 1:100,000 epinephrine. This agent is indicated for procedures in this chapter unless specified otherwise.

Lidocaine is a safe and effective drug.[28,29] Vasoconstrictors are generally safe. In a few circumstances (patients taking tricyclic antidepressants or nonselective -adrenergic blocking agents, or patients with moderate to severe cardiovascular disease), there is the potential for problems.[30]

RELATED FACTORS

Although the most common method of mandibular anesthesia is the inferior alveolar nerve block, this injection also has the greatest number of failures.[25,31] What are the expected signs of successful or unsuccessful anesthesia after administering one cartridge?

Lip Numbness: Numbness usually occurs in 5 to 7 minutes.[32-37] What does lip numbness mean? It indicates only that the injection blocked the nerves to the soft tissues of the lip, not necessarily that pulpal anesthesia has been obtained.[32-37] If lip numbness is not obtained, the block has been "missed." If this occurs frequently, the technique should be reviewed.

Onset of Pulpal Anesthesia: Pulpal anesthesia usually occurs in 10 to 15 minutes.[32-37] In some patients onset occurs sooner and in others it is delayed.[32-37]

Duration: Duration of pulpal anesthesia in the mandible is very good.[32-37] Therefore if successful, anesthesia usually (but not always) persists for approximately 2½ hours.

Success: The incidence of successful mandibular pulpal anesthesia tends to be more frequent in molars and premolars and least frequent in anterior teeth.[27,33-37] Not all patients achieve pulpal anesthesia after what appears to be a clinically successful (lip and chin numb) inferior alveolar nerve block; other approaches are required in these patients.

ALTERNATIVE TECHNIQUES

Increasing the Volume: Increasing the volume of anesthetic from one to two cartridges does not increase the success rate of pulpal anesthesia with the inferior alveolar nerve block.[33]

Alternative Solutions: Mepivacaine 2% with 1:20,000 levonordefrin, 4% prilocaine with 1:200,000 epinephrine, or solutions without vasoconstrictors (3% mepivacaine plain and 4% prilocaine plain) are alternatives to 2% lidocaine with 1:100,000 epinephrine for pulpal anesthesia with effects that last at least 1 hour.[34,37,38]

Alternative Injection Locations: Neither the Gow-Gates nor the Akinosi technique is superior to the standard inferior alveolar injection.[39-42] These techniques are not replacements but are useful when standard approaches cannot be used (for example, trismus).

Infiltration Injections: Labial or lingual infiltration injections used alone are not effective for pulpal anesthesia in anterior or posterior teeth.[43-45]

Long-Acting Anesthetics: Clinical trials of bupivacaine and etidocaine have been conducted in oral surgery, endodontics, and periodontics.[46-51] These agents provide a prolonged analgesic period and are indicated when postoperative pain is anticipated. However, not all patients want prolonged lip numbness.[47] For those patients, analgesics may be prescribed. Compared with lidocaine, bupivacaine has a somewhat slower onset but almost double the duration of pulpal anesthesia in the mandible (approximately 4 hours).[52]

Accuracy of Needle Placement: Accurate anatomic positioning is no guarantee of a successful block.[53,54] Interestingly, even locating the inferior alveolar nerve with ultrasound before the injection did not improve success.[55] The anesthetic solution may not completely diffuse into the nerve trunk to reach and block all nerves even if deposited at the correct site.[56]

Accessory Innervation: Anatomic evidence suggests that accessory innervation exists from branches of the mylohyoid nerve.[57,58] An experimental study using a mylohyoid injection lingual and inferior to the retromolar fossa in addition to an inferior alveolar nerve block showed no enhancement of pulpal anesthesia.[59] The contribution of the mylohyoid nerve to pulpal sensitivity is probably insignificant.

Cross-Innervation: Cross-innervation from the contralateral inferior alveolar nerve has been implicated in failure to achieve anesthesia in anterior teeth after an inferior alveolar injection. Cross-innervation does occur in incisors but is not the primary cause of anesthetic failure.[43]

Pain and Inflammation: Most studies have evaluated anesthesia in the absence of symptoms and inflammation; results differ if these conditions are present.[8,60] Patients who have symptomatic pulpal or periapical pathosis (or who are anxious) present additional anesthesia problems.[10,26,38]

Maxillary Anesthesia

ANESTHETIC AGENTS

Unless otherwise specified, the conventional solution is used, that is, 2% lidocaine with 1:100,000 epinephrine.

RELATED FACTORS

Anesthesia is more successful in the maxilla than in the mandible. The most common injection for the maxillary teeth is infiltration. Several events can be expected with this technique when one cartridge is used.

Lip Numbness: Lip numbness usually occurs within a few minutes. Lip or cheek numbness does not correspond entirely to the duration of pulpal anesthesia because the pulp does not remain anesthetized as long as these soft tissues.[61,62]

Success and Failure: Infiltration results in a high incidence of successful pulpal anesthesia. Therefore it is more successful than the inferior alveolar nerve block.[62-65]

Onset of Pulpal Anesthesia: Pulpal anesthesia usually occurs in 3 to 5 minutes. Occasionally, onset is slower in first molars.[62-65]

Duration: A problem with maxillary infiltration is duration.[62-65] In about a third of patients, pulpal anesthesia of the anterior teeth declines after about 30 minutes, with most losing anesthesia by 60 minutes.[64-65] In premolars and first molars, about a third of patients have no pulpal anesthesia at 45 minutes, with half losing anesthesia by 60 minutes.[62-65] Frequently, additional local anesthetic must be administered depending on the duration of the procedure and the tooth group affected.

ALTERNATIVE TECHNIQUES
Volumes of Solution

For infiltrations, increasing the volume (two cartridges instead of one) increases the duration of pulpal anesthesia.[63] A suggestion for anterior teeth and premolars is to give two cartridges initially, or to give one initially and inject another approximately 30 minutes later. In first molars, administration of two cartridges initially will speed onset and prolong duration.[63]

Alternative Solutions

In maxillary infiltrations, prilocaine, mepivacaine, and lidocaine (all with vasoconstrictors) act similarly.[64,65] Solutions without vasoconstrictors (3% mepivacaine plain and 4% prilocaine plain) provide a short duration of pulpal anesthesia, averaging 15 to 20 minutes.[64,65]

Long-acting anesthetics do not provide prolonged pulpal anesthesia in a maxillary infiltration (as they do in a mandibular block).[61,62]

Other Techniques

The *posterior superior alveolar (PSA) block* anesthetizes the second and third molars and usually the first molar.[66] On occasion, an additional mesial infiltration injection is necessary to anesthetize the first molar. Generally, the PSA injection is indicated when all molar teeth require anesthesia. When one tooth is treated, infiltrations are preferred.

The *infraorbital block* results in lip numbness but does not predictably anesthetize incisor pulps.[67,68] It usually anesthetizes the premolars, but duration is less than one hour.[67,68] Essentially, the infraorbital injection is similar to infiltration over the premolars.

The *second division block* usually anesthetizes pulps of molars and some second premolars but does not predictably anesthetize anterior tooth pulps.[69] The high tuberosity technique is preferred to the greater palatine approach because it is easier and less painful.[69]

Pain and Inflammation

Again, results will differ from the normal when anesthesia is given to patients with either or both of these conditions.

Anesthesia Difficulties

What follows is a classic scenario. The diagnosis is irreversible pulpitis. The dentist administers the standard block or infiltration. The patient reports classic signs of anesthesia (lip numbness and a dull feeling of the tooth or quadrant). After isolation, access preparation is begun. When the bur is in enamel, the patient feels nothing. Once the bur enters dentin or possibly not until the pulp is exposed, the patient feels sharp pain. Obviously, pulpal anesthesia is not profound; additional anesthetic is required. Why does the problem occur? There are three main reasons and theories.

1. The anesthetic solution may not penetrate to the sensory nerves that innervate the pulp, especially in the mandible. A local anesthetic, articaine, was synthesized to provide good lipid solubility and protein

binding, with presumably more predictable anesthesia. However, articaine's action has proved to be similar to that of other local anesthetics.[70]

2. Local tissue or nerve changes occur because of inflammation. One popular theory is that the lowered pH of inflamed tissue reduces the amount of the base form of the anesthetic available to penetrate the nerve membrane.[18] Consequently, there is less of the ionized form within the nerve to achieve anesthesia. This theory has no experimental support and is an unlikely cause of anesthesia difficulties. It does not explain the major problem, which is the mandibular molar with pulpitis that is not anesthetized by an inferior alveolar injection. The injection site is distant from the area of inflammation; changes in tissue pH would be unrelated to the anesthesia problem. A more plausible explanation is the **hyperalgesia theory:** nerves arising in inflamed tissue have altered resting potentials and decreased excitability thresholds; these changes are not restricted to the inflamed pulp itself but affect the entire neuronal membrane, extending to the central nervous system.[8,9] Local anesthetic agents are not sufficient to prevent impulse transmission, owing to these lowered excitability thresholds.[8]

3. Patients in pain often are apprehensive, which lowers their pain threshold. A vicious cycle may be established: Initial apprehension leads to decreased pain threshold, which leads to anesthesia difficulties, which leads to increased apprehension, which results in loss of control and confidence, and so on. Therefore if this cycle becomes evident, the practitioner should stop treatment immediately and regain control or schedule another appointment or consider referral to an endodontist. Most patients will endure some pain during the initial stages of root canal treatment if they have confidence in the dentist. However, they will not tolerate being hurt repeatedly!

Supplemental Anesthesia

INDICATIONS

A supplemental injection is used if the standard injection is not effective. It is useful to repeat an injection only if the patient is not exhibiting the "classic" signs of soft tissue anesthesia. Generally, if the classic signs are present, reinjection is ineffective. For example, after the inferior alveolar (IA) injection, the patient develops lip, chin, and tongue numbness and quadrant "deadness" of the teeth. However, he or she cannot tolerate pulp or dentin invasion with a bur. To think that reinjection using the IA approach will be successful is wishful thinking; failure the first time is usually followed by failure on the second attempt. The dentist should go directly to a supplemental technique. Three such injections are (1) the intraosseous (IO), (2) the periodontal ligament (PDL), and (3) the intrapulpal (IP). The PDL and IO injections are the preferred approaches with the IP injection being reserved for special situations.

ANESTHETIC AGENTS

With any of the three supplemental techniques, a conventional anesthetic agent is indicated. Therefore 2% lidocaine with 1:100,000 epinephrine is used unless an alternative is suggested.

INTRAOSSEOUS ANESTHESIA

The IO injection is a supplemental technique that has been shown to be effective through substantial research and clinical usage. It is particularly useful in conjunction with a conventional injection when it is likely that supplemental anesthesia will be necessary, e.g., pulpitis in mandibular posterior teeth.[71-73] The IO injection allows placement of a local anesthetic directly into the cancellous bone adjacent to the tooth. There is an intraosseous system of two components (Figure 7-1). One part is a slow-speed handpiece-driven perforator, which drills a small hole through the cortical plate. The anesthetic solution is delivered into cancellous bone through a matching 27-gauge ultrashort injector needle (Figure 7-2).

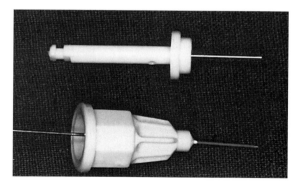

FIGURE 7-1
Components for intraosseous injection. The perforator (*top*) is a small, sharp, latch-type drill to make an opening through soft tissue and bone. The needle (*bottom*) is a short and small gauge to insert and inject directly through the opening.

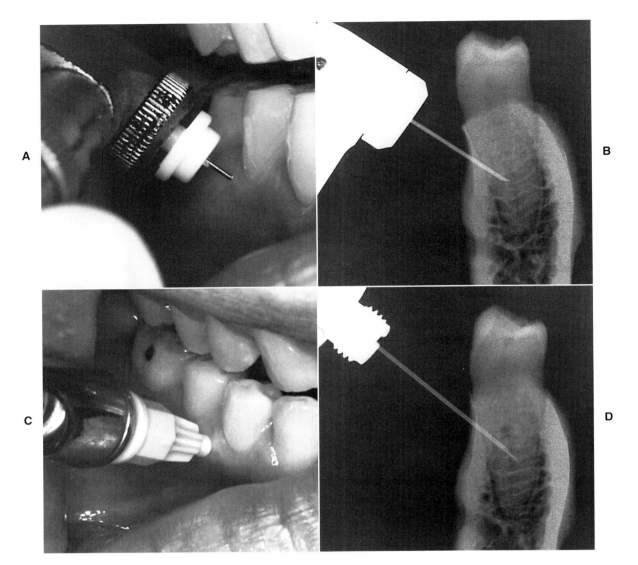

FIGURE 7-2
Intraosseous injection technique. **A,** Location and angulation of the perforator. **B,** Perforator "breaks through" cortical bone into medullary space. **C,** Needle is inserted directly into opening. **D,** Anesthetic is injected into medullary bone, where it diffuses widely to block dental nerves.

Technique

The area of perforation and injection is on a horizontal line of the buccal gingival margins of the adjacent teeth and a vertical line that passes through the interdental papilla distal to the tooth to be injected. A point approximately 2 mm below the intersection of these lines is selected as the perforation site. The soft tissue is first anesthetized by infiltration. The perforator is placed through the gingiva perpendicular to the cortical plate. With the point gently resting against bone, the handpiece is activated in a series of short bursts, using light pressure, until there is a "break through" into cancellous bone (taking approximately 2 to 5 seconds).[74-77]

Holding the standard syringe in a "pen-gripping" fashion, the needle is aligned with and inserted into the perforation. Approximately half a cartridge of anesthetic solution is SLOWLY delivered over a 1- to 2-minute time period with light pressure! If back-pressure is encountered, the needle is rotated approximately a quarter turn and deposition is reattempted. If this attempt is unsuccessful, the needle should be removed and checked for blockage. If the needle is not blocked, it is reinserted or the site is opened with a new perforator and the injection is repeated.

A recent, useful innovation is an interosseous injection system using a plastic sleeve that remains in the perforation. This serves as a guide for the needle and may remain in place throughout the procedure if reinjection is necessary.

Perforator "Breakage": Rarely, the metal perforator "separates" from the plastic shank. The perforator is easily removed with a hemostat; there are no reports of a perforator breaking into parts.[73,75-80]

Injection Discomfort: When the IO injection is used as a primary injection, neither perforation, needle insertion, nor solution deposition is painful for most patients.[75,77] However, when the IO injection is used as a supplemental injection in a patient with irreversible pulpitis, moderate pain may occur.[71,72]

Selection of Perforation Site: Distal perforation and injection to the tooth will result in the best anesthesia.[75-82] An exception would be in second molars where a mesial site is preferred.[75-77] When necessary, a lingual approach may also be successful.

Onset of Anesthesia: The onset of anesthesia is rapid.[75-82] There is no "waiting period" for anesthesia.

Success: For use as a primary injection, success rates are good; lower success rates are seen with 3% mepivacaine.[75,77]

For use as a supplemental injection after the IA block, excellent success has been reported for 2% lidocaine with 1:100,000 epinephrine, 2% mepivacaine with 1:20,000 levonordefrin, and 1.5% etidocaine with 1:200,000 epinephrine.[76,79,82] However, because of adverse cardiovascular reactions with the long-acting anesthetics (etidocaine and 0.5% bupivacaine with 1:200,000 epinephrine), these agents should not be used.[83] Mepivacaine 3% is successful, but the duration of pulpal anesthesia is shorter.[81]

For use as a supplemental injection with irreversible pulpitis, high success rates (around 90%) have been reported.[72,73] Mepivacaine has a 80% success rate, which increases to 98% with a second IO injection.[71]

Failure: If the anesthetic solution squirts out of the perforation, there will be failure (a rare occurrence).[71] Reperforation or choosing another perforation site would then be necessary.

Duration: With a *primary* IO injection, duration of pulpal anesthesia declines steadily over an hour.[75,77] There is an even shorter duration with 3% mepivacaine or 1.5% etidocaine with 1:200,000 epinephrine compared with 2% lidocaine with 1:200,000 epinephrine.[77,84] With a *supplemental* IO injection after the IA block, duration of pulpal anesthesia is very good.[76,79,82] A solution of 3% mepivacaine will result in a shorter duration.[81] For irreversible pulpitis, the IO injection should provide anesthesia for the entire débridement appointment.[71-73]

Postoperative Problems: With primary and supplemental techniques, patients report no pain or mild pain. Less than 5% will develop exudate and/or localized swellings at the perforation site, possibly from overheating of the bone during perforation.[75-80]

Systemic Effects: With both primary and supplemental techniques using 1.8 ml of 2% lidocaine with 1:100,000 epinephrine, most patients perceive an increased heart rate.[75-78,85] With 0.9 ml of 2% lidocaine with 1:100,000 epinephrine, 1.8 ml of etidocaine with 1:200,000 epinephrine, or 1.8 ml of 2% mepivacaine with 1:20,000 levonordefrin, there is a similar increased heart rate.[78,79,82] When these agents are used, the patient should be informed of this tachycardia to lessen his or her anxiety. No significant heart rate increase occurs with 3% mepivacaine plain.[81,85]

Medical Contraindications: Patients with cardiovascular disease or those taking tricyclic antidepressants or nonselective β-adrenergic blocking agents should not receive IO injections of epinephrine- or levonordefrin-containing solutions.[85] Mepivacaine 3% plain is preferred.

PERIODONTAL LIGAMENT INJECTION

The PDL injection is also a useful technique if a conventional injection is unsuccessful. The PDL (or intraligamental) injection technique has generated considerable research and has spawned the marketing of a variety of special syringes. The technique (regardless of the device used) is clinically effective and is a valuable adjunct.[38,86,87] It is particularly useful if a rubber dam is in place; the needle may be inserted between the tooth and rubber dam margin.

Technique: The procedure (Figure 7-3) is not difficult but does require practice and familiarity. A standard syringe or pressure syringe is equipped with a 30-gauge ultrashort needle or a 27-or a 25-gauge short needle. The needle is inserted into the mesial gingival sulcus at a 30-degree angle to the long axis of the tooth. The needle is supported by the fingers or hemostat and is positioned with maximum penetration (wedged between root and crestal bone). Heavy pressure is SLOWLY applied on the syringe handle for approximately 10 to 20 seconds (conventional syringe), or the trigger is

SLOWLY squeezed once or twice with resistance (pressure syringe). *Back-pressure is important.* If there is no back-pressure (resistance)—that is, if the anesthetic readily flows out of the sulcus—the needle is repositioned, and the technique repeated until back-pressure is attained. The injection is then repeated on the distal surface. Only a small volume (approximately 0.2 ml) of anesthetic is deposited on each surface.

Mechanism of Action: The PDL injection forces anesthetic solution through the cribriform plate (Figure 7-4) into the marrow spaces and into the vasculature in and around the tooth (Figures 7-5 and 7-6).[88-90] The primary route is not the periodontal ligament; the mechanism of action is not related to direct pressure on the nerves.[91,92]

Injection Discomfort: When the PDL injection is used as a primary injection, needle insertion and injection are usually only mildly uncomfortable in posterior teeth; in anterior teeth, the PDL injection may be quite painful.[93-95] Patients must be informed of this possibility.

Onset of Anesthesia: Onset of anesthesia is rapid; there is no waiting period to begin the clin-

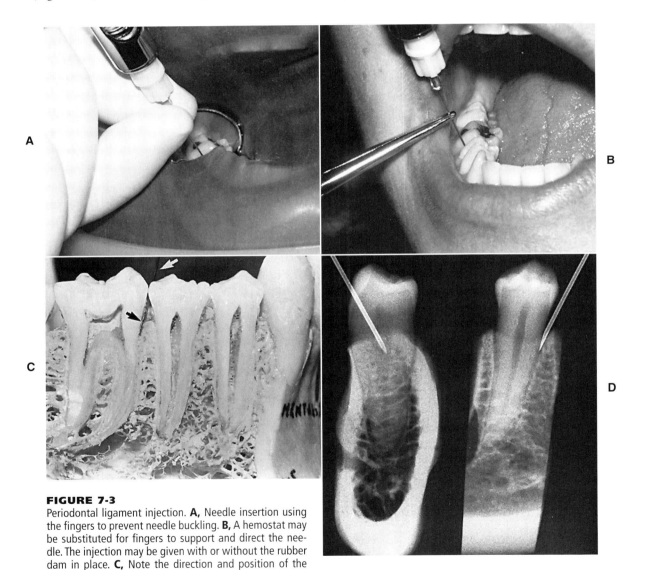

FIGURE 7-3
Periodontal ligament injection. **A,** Needle insertion using the fingers to prevent needle buckling. **B,** A hemostat may be substituted for fingers to support and direct the needle. The injection may be given with or without the rubber dam in place. **C,** Note the direction and position of the needle (*arrows*). The tip of the needle will be wedged between the crestal bone and the root surface. **D,** Angle of the needle relative to the long axis of the tooth (*left*). With approximately a 30-degree orientation, the needle tip will be positioned close to the midline of the root.

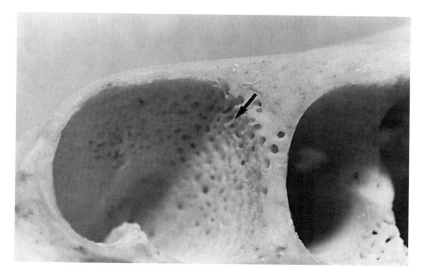

FIGURE 7-4
An extraction socket of a second molar. The bone of the cribriform plate is very porous, particularly in the cervical region *(arrow)*. During the periodontal ligament injection, this is the region of passage of most anesthetic solution into the medullary space.

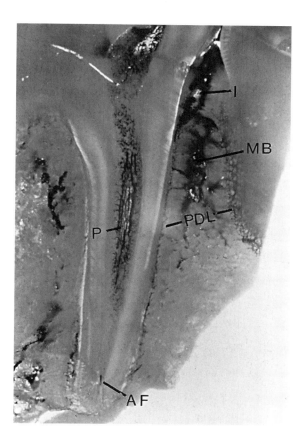

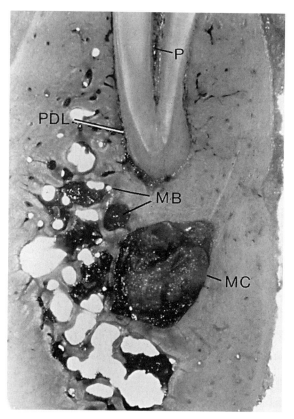

FIGURE 7-5
A single periodontal ligament injection of carbon dye adjacent to a dog's tooth demonstrates the distribution of dye particles. Particles are concentrated at the injection site *(I)* as well as in the medullary bone *(MB)*, the apical foramen *(AF)*, and the pulp *(P)* of the injected tooth. Dye particles have been spread through the periodontal ligament *(PDL)* of both the injected and the adjacent teeth.

FIGURE 7-6
A single injection of dye was made in the distal periodontal ligament. This frontal section, including the tooth apex and surrounding structures, shows that dye distributes to the pulp *(P)*, periodontal ligament space *(PDL)*, medullary bone *(MB)*, and mandibular canal *(MC)*. The widespread distribution of solutions from the periodontal ligament injection may anesthetize the adjacent teeth.

ical procedure.[86,87,93-96] If anesthesia is still not adequate, reinjection is indicated.

Success: For use as a primary injection, good success rates have been reported for restorative procedures and extractions. More difficulty in achieving adequate pain control occurs in endodontic treatment. One study showed higher success rates in posterior teeth than in anterior teeth.[94]

For use as a supplemental injection (standard techniques have failed to provide adequate anesthesia), good success rates (83 to 92%) are achieved.[38,86,87,96] Reinjection increases the success rate.[86,87]

Duration: The duration of profound pulpal anesthesia (either primary or supplemental) is approximately 10 to 20 minutes.[92-94] The operator must work quickly and be prepared to reinject.

Postoperative Discomfort: When PDL injection is used as a primary technique, postoperative discomfort (mostly mild pain) usually occurs.[93-95] The duration of discomfort ranges from 14 hours to 3 days.[93-95] The discomfort is related to damage from needle insertion rather than to the pressure of depositing the solution.[95] Many patients report that their tooth feels "high in occlusion."[93,94]

Selective Anesthesia: It has been suggested that the PDL injection may be used in the differential diagnosis of poorly localized, painful irreversible pulpitis.[97] However, adjacent teeth are often anesthetized with PDL injection of a single tooth.[92-95] Therefore this injection is *not* useful for differential diagnosis.

Systemic Effects: PDL injection of epinephrine-containing solutions may cause systemic changes (a transient decrease in blood pressure and increase in heart rate).[98] Generally, in most dental patients effects are minimal, but tachycardia may be noticed, requiring explanation.

Other Factors: Different needle gauges (25-, 27-, or 30-gauge) are effective.[86] Special pressure syringes have been marketed (Figure 7-7); these have not proved to be more effective than a standard syringe.[86,87,95] Anesthetic solutions without vasoconstrictors (3% mepivacaine plain) or with reduced vasoconstrictor concentrations (bupivacaine or etidocaine with 1:200,000 epinephrine) are not very effective, producing a limited duration of anesthesia.[93,99,100]

Safety to the Periodontium: Clinical and animal studies have demonstrated the relative safety of the PDL injection.[92-94,101-104] Minor local damage is limited to the site of needle penetration (Figure 7-8); this subsequently undergoes repair. In rare instances, periodontal infections have occurred.[94] Histologic areas of root resorption after PDL injections have also been reported, which also heal with time.[105,106] There are no studies on the effects of injecting into an area of periodontal disease, but an adverse effect is unlikely.

Safety to the Pulp: Clinical and animal studies have shown no adverse effects on the pulp after PDL injections.[92-94,105,107,108] However, physiologic changes in the pulp do occur, including a rapid and prolonged marked decrease in blood flow caused by epinephrine.[109] This vascular impairment has no demonstrated damaging effect, even in conjunction with restorative procedures.[110] The PDL injection probably would not result in severe pulpal injury, although this has not been studied with extensive (crown) preparations or in teeth with caries.

Safety to Primary Teeth: Minor enamel hypoplasia of succedaneous teeth has been seen after PDL injections in primary teeth.[111] However, this effect was caused by the cytotoxicity of the local anesthetic rather than by the actual injection. Therefore the PDL injection may be used for anesthetizing primary teeth.[91]

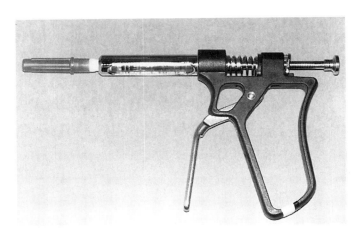

FIGURE 7-7
Example of a special syringe used for the periodontal ligament injection. Although these devices are capable of injecting with more pressure, they have not been shown to be superior to the standard syringe.

INTRAPULPAL INJECTION

Indications: On occasion, the IO and PDL injections, even when repeated, do not produce profound anesthesia; pain persists when the pulp is entered. This is an indication for an IP injection. However, the IP injection should not be used without first administering an IO or PDL injection. The IP injection is very painful without some other supplemental anesthesia.

Advantages and Disadvantages: Although the IP injection is popular, it has disadvantages as well as advantages, making it the third supplemental injection of choice. The major drawback is that the needle is inserted directly into a vital and very sensitive pulp; the injection may be exquisitely painful. Also, the effects of the injection are unpredictable if it is not given under pressure. Duration of anesthesia, once attained, is short (15 to 20 minutes). Therefore the bulk of the pulp must be removed quickly and at the correct working length to prevent recurrence of pain during instrumentation. Another disadvantage is that obviously the pulp must be exposed to permit direct injection; often problems with anesthesia occur before exposure.

The advantage is the predictability of profound anesthesia if the IP injection is given under back-pressure. Onset will be immediate, and no special syringes or needles are required, although different approaches may be necessary to attain the desired pressure.

Mechanism of Action: Strong back-pressure has been shown to be the major factor in producing anesthesia.[112,113] Depositing anesthetic passively into the chamber is not adequate; the solution will not diffuse throughout the pulp. Therefore the anesthetic agent is not solely responsible for intrapulpal anesthesia, being dependent on pressure.

Technique: Again, the patient must be informed that a "little extra" anesthetic will ensure comfort; there will be "a sharp sensation."

One technique creates back-pressure by stoppering the access with a cotton pellet to prevent backflow (Figure 7-9).[113,114] Other stoppers, such as gutta-percha, waxes, or pieces of rubber, have been used. If possible, the roof of the pulp chamber should be penetrated by a half-round bur; the needle will then fit snugly in the bur hole.

Another approach is an injection into each canal after the chamber is unroofed. A standard syringe is usually equipped with a bent short needle. With fingers supporting the needle shaft to prevent buckling, the needle is positioned in the access

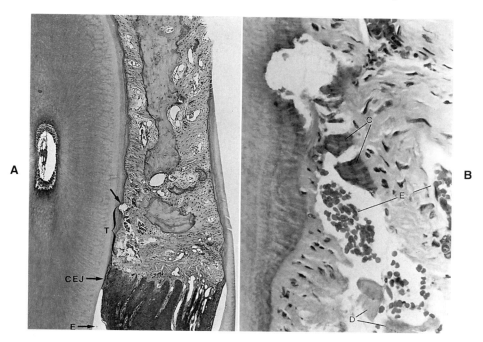

FIGURE 7-8
Photomicrographs of the injection site at the time of injection. **A,** Areas visible are the enamel space *(E)* and the cementoenamel junction region *(CEJ)*. The needle tract *(T)*, which ends in a gouge in cementum *(arrow)*, is apparent in the connective tissue. No tissue changes are evident outside the penetration site, including the more apical tissues. **B,** Region *T* in part **A**. Needle tract and adjacent tissues contain small chips of cementum *(C)*, erythrocytes *(E)*, and debris *(D)*, which presumably have been carried in by the needle.

opening and then moved down the canal, while slowly expressing the anesthetic, to the point of wedging. Maximum pressure is then applied *slowly* on the syringe handle for 5 to 10 seconds. If there is no back-pressure, anesthetic flows out of the access opening. The needle is wedged deeper or withdrawn and replaced with a larger gauge needle (or stoppered with a cotton pellet), and the injection is repeated. This may be necessary in each canal.

ALTERNATIVE PRIMARY TECHNIQUES

Electronic dental anesthesia and transcutaneous electronic nerve stimulation are two fairly recent techniques that have been promoted as means of attaining anesthesia without injection. Both involve electronic devices. These devices use electrical stimulation (of low or high frequency) applied to tissues surrounding the teeth. Although some

studies have shown good results, others have shown little effect on pain suppression when these techniques are used as the sole means of anesthesia.[115-118] Additional investigations are needed to clarify the mechanisms of action as well as clinical effectiveness for endodontic procedures before they can be recommended.

Anesthetic Management of Pulpal or Periradicular Pathoses

IRREVERSIBLE PULPITIS

With irreversible pulpitis, the teeth most difficult to anesthetize are the mandibular molars followed by (in order) mandibular and maxillary premolars, maxillary molars, mandibular anterior teeth, and maxillary anterior teeth. The vital inflamed pulp must be invaded and removed.

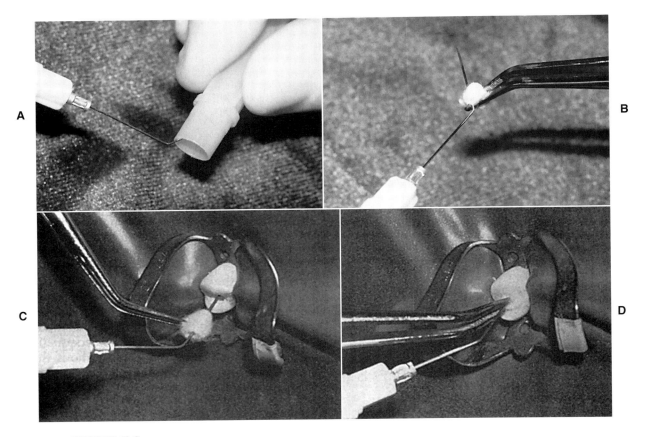

FIGURE 7-9
Intrapulpal injection technique. **A,** A 45-degree bend is placed on the needle using the needle cap. **B,** For stoppering the injection site, a cotton pellet is pulled over the needle. **C,** The needle is placed in the opening in the roof of the chamber (forewarn the patient of discomfort!). **D,** The cotton pellet is packed *tightly* into the access opening, and the syringe handle is pushed *slowly*. The patient often feels sharp pain with resistance on the syringe handle; this resistance usually indicates successful anesthesia.

Also, pulpal tissue has a very concentrated sensory nerve supply, particularly in the chamber. These factors, combined with others related to inflammatory effects on sensory nerves and failures occurring with conventional techniques, make anesthetizing patients with painful irreversible pulpitis a challenge.

Different clinical situations present surprises. In some cases, inflamed vital tissue exists only in the apical canals; the tissue in the chamber is necrotic and does not respond to pulp testing. Obviously, in this situation the chamber is entered with no problem, but when the operator attempts to place a file to length, severe pain results. IO or PDL injections are helpful and an IP injection may be used. However, irreversible pulpitis must be differentiated from a symptomatic apical pathosis because, in the latter condition, IO, PDL, and IP injections are contraindicated.

General Considerations: Conventional anesthesia, using primary techniques, is administered. After signs of soft tissue anesthesia occur, the pain abates and the patient relaxes. Frequently, however, upon access opening or when the pulp is entered, pain results because not all sensory nerves have been blocked. A useful procedure is to pulp test the tooth with cold or an electric pulp tester before the access is begun.[38,70,71] If the patient responds, an IO or PDL injection is given. However, no response does not ensure complete anesthesia.[26,38,70,71] The patient is always informed that the procedure will be immediately discontinued if pain is experienced or if there is a "premonition" of impending pain. Appropriate supplementary injections are then used. Occasionally, all attempts fail; in this case, it is best to place a temporary restoration and schedule another appointment or refer the patient to an endodontist.

Mandibular Posterior Teeth: A conventional inferior alveolar injection is administered, usually in conjunction with a long buccal injection. Because of the high failure rate of anesthesia for these teeth, an IO or PDL injection is routinely administered before access is begun.[38,70,71] If pain is felt, the IO or PDL injection may be repeated or an IP injection is given if the pulp is exposed. Usually, once the pulp is removed, further pain is minimal owing to the longer duration of mandibular anesthesia.[33-37,52]

Mandibular Anterior Teeth: An inferior alveolar injection is given. If pain is felt, an IO injection is administered. If this is unsuccessful, an IP injection is added.

Maxillary Posterior Teeth: Approaches are the same as those outlined under "General Considerations" *except* that the initial dose is doubled (3.6 ml) for buccal infiltration. The injection site may be a PSA block for molars. Infiltration of 0.5 ml of anesthetic over the palatal apex enhances pulpal anesthesia.[119] If pain is felt during the access, an IO or PDL injection is administered. Seldom is an IP injection needed.

The duration of anesthesia in the maxilla is less than that in the mandible.[62-65] Therefore if pain is experienced during instrumentation, additional primary or supplemental injections are necessary.

Maxillary Anterior Teeth: Anesthetic is administered initially as a labial infiltration and, occasionally, as a palatal infiltration for the retainer. Rarely is an IO injection needed; the PDL injection also is not very effective.[94] The duration of anesthesia may be less than 1 hour, requiring additional infiltration.[62-65]

SYMPTOMATIC PULP NECROSIS

This diagnosis indicates pain and/or swelling and therefore periradicular inflammation. Because the pulp is necrotic and apical tissues are inflamed, anesthesia problems are different. These teeth may be painful when manipulated during treatment.

For the mandible, an inferior alveolar nerve block and long buccal injection are administered. For maxillary teeth, if no swelling is present, anesthesia is given with a conventional infiltration or block. If soft tissue swelling is present (cellulitis or abscess), a regional block plus infiltration on either side of the swelling is administered. Access is begun *slowly*. Usually the pulp chamber is entered without discomfort if the tooth is not torqued excessively. File placement and débridement also can be performed without much pain if instruments are used gently.

Occasionally, conventional injections do not provide adequate anesthesia. IO, PDL, or IP injections are *contraindicated*. Although effective for vital pulps, these injections are painful and ineffective with apical pathosis. Rather, the patient should be informed that profound anesthesia is not present owing to inflammation in the bone. As an alternative with maxillary molars, a PSA injection or second division nerve block (high tuberosity injection) may be given. In anterior teeth and premolars, an infraorbital injection is administered to provide some degree of bone and soft tissue anesthesia.

In patients with severe preoperative pain without drainage from the tooth (or when no swelling can be incised), a long-acting anesthetic (such as bupivacaine or etidocaine) may help control postoperative pain in mandibular teeth. However, the duration of analgesia is usually not so long to preclude use of oral analgesics.

ASYMPTOMATIC PULP NECROSIS

Asymptomatic teeth are the easiest to anesthetize. Although it may be tempting to proceed without anesthesia, vital sensitive tissue may be encountered in the apical portion of canals.

The conventional injections are usually administered: inferior alveolar nerve block and long buccal injection for mandibular teeth and infiltration (or PSA block) in the maxilla. Usually the patient remains comfortable. Rarely, there may be some sensitivity during canal preparation that requires an IO or PDL injection. IP injection is not indicated because bacteria and debris may be forced periradicularly. In the maxilla an additional infiltration may be necessary during longer procedures.

Anesthesia for Surgical Procedures

INCISION FOR DRAINAGE

Patients tolerate the procedure better when some anesthesia is present before incision and drain placement are begun. However, profound anesthesia is difficult, which should be explained to the patient. In the mandible, inferior alveolar plus long buccal injections (for posterior teeth) or labial infiltration (for anterior teeth) are administered. In the maxilla, infiltration is given at several sites peripheral to the swelling. As an alternative, a PSA or second-division block may suffice for molars and an infraorbital injection for anterior teeth and premolars. For palatal swellings, a small volume of anesthetic is infiltrated over the greater palatine foramen (for posterior teeth) or over the nasopalatine foramen (for anterior teeth). With swelling over either foramen, lateral infiltration is indicated. An adjunctive measure is to spray ethyl chloride on the area just before incision.

Injection directly into a swelling is contraindicated. These inflamed tissues are hyperalgesic and difficult to anesthetize. Traditional beliefs are that the anesthetic solution may be affected by the lower pH and is rendered less effective and that direct injection will "spread the infection"; neither belief is proved. Nevertheless, although these ideas may have some merit, reasons for avoiding injection into a swelling are the pain from the pressure and ineffectiveness. Theoretically, the area of swelling (cellulitis) has an increased blood supply; thus anesthetic is transported quickly into the systemic circulation, diminishing the anesthetic effect. Also, edema and purulence may dilute the solution.

PERIRADICULAR SURGERY

Additional considerations in periradicular surgery involve anesthesia of both soft tissue and bone. Also, inflammation is usually present. In the mandible the inferior alveolar injection is reasonably effective. Additional infiltration injections in the vestibule are useful to achieve vasoconstriction, particularly in the mandibular anterior region. In the maxilla, infiltration injections are generally effective; usually larger volumes are necessary to provide anesthesia over the surgical field.

If the area of operation is inflamed or the patient is apprehensive, anesthesia may not be totally successful. After the flap is reflected, if anesthesia is inadequate, attempts to enhance or regain anesthesia (through additional infiltrations or injecting the sensitive area) are not particularly effective.

As a prophylactic measure, an IO or PDL injection is administered at the site, after the above injections and before the surgery. This seems to enhance depth of anesthesia and may provide better hemostasis.

Use of a long-acting anesthetic has been advocated.[46,47] In the mandible, this is reasonably effective. In the maxilla, long-acting agents have a shorter duration of anesthesia and decreased epinephrine concentrations, which result in more bleeding during surgery.[51,120] After periradicular surgery, administration of a long-acting anesthetic has been suggested.[18] However, postsurgical pain is usually not severe and can be managed by analgesics.[120]

REFERENCES

1. Walton R, Torabinejad M: Managing local anesthesia problems in the endodontic patient, *J Am Dent Assoc* 123:97, 1992.
2. Walton R: Managing endodontic anaesthesia problems, *Endod Pract* 1:15, 1998.
3. LeClaire A, Skidmore A, Griffin J Jr, Balaban F: Endodontic fear survey, *J Endod* 14:560, 1988.
4. Dworkin S: Anxiety and performance in the dental environment: an experimental investigation, *J Am Soc Psychol Dent Med* 14:88, 1967.
5. Murray J: Psychology of the pain experience. In Weisenberg M, editor: *Pain: clinical and experimental perspectives*, St Louis, 1975, Mosby.
6. Seltzer S: *The character of pain: pain control in dentistry*, Philadelphia, 1978, JB Lippincott.
7. Rood J, Pateromichelakis S: Inflammation and peripheral nerve sensitization, *Br J Oral Surg* 19:67, 1981.
8. Wallace J, Michanowicz A, Mundell R, Wilson E: A pilot study of the clinical problem of regionally anesthetizing the pulp of an acutely inflamed mandibular molar, *Oral Surg Oral Med Oral Pathol* 59:517, 1985.

9. Byers M, Taylor P, Khayat B, Kimberly C: Effects of injury and inflammation on pulpal and periapical nerves, *J Endod* 16:78, 1990.
10. Weinstein P, Milgrom P, Kaufman E, et al: Patient perceptions of failure to achieve optimal local anesthesia, *Gen Dent* May-June, 218, 1985.
11. Kleinknecht R, Klepac R, Alexander L: Origins and characteristics of fear of dentistry, *J Am Dent Assoc* 86:842, 1973.
12. Milgrom P, Coldwell S, Getz T, et al: Four dimensions of fear of dental injections, *J Am Dent Assoc* 128:756, 1997.
13. Fieset L, Milgrom P, Weinstein P: Psychophysiological responses to dental injections, *J Am Dent Assoc* 11:4, 1985.
14. Meechan J: Intra-oral topical anaesthetics: a review, *J Dent* 28:3, 2000.
15. Rosivack R, Koenigsberg S, Maxwell K: An analysis of the effectiveness of two topical anesthetics, *Anesth Prog* 37:290, 1990.
16. Gill C, Orr D: Double blind crossover comparison of topical anesthetics, *J Am Dent Assoc* 98:213, 1979.
17. Martin M, Ramsay D, Whitney C, et al: Topical anesthesia: differentiating the pharmacological and psychological contributions to efficacy, *Anesth Prog* 41:40, 1994.
18. Malamed S: *Handbook of local anesthesia*, ed 4, St Louis, 1997, Mosby.
19. Hersh E, Houpt M, Cooper S, et al: Analgesic efficacy and safety of an intraoral lidocaine patch, *J Am Dent Assoc* 127:1626, 1996.
20. Peterson D, Kein D: Pain sensation related to local anesthesia injected at varying temperatures, *Anesth Prog* 25:14, 1978.
21. Fuller N, Menke R, Meyers W: Perception of pain to intraoral penetration of three needles, *J Am Dent Assoc* 99:822, 1979.
22. Cooley R, Robison S: Comparative evaluation of the 30-gauge dental needle, *Oral Surg Oral Med Oral Pathol* 48:400, 1979.
23. Robison S, Mayhew R, Cowan R, Hawley R: Comparative study of deflection characteristics and fragility of 25-, 27-, and 30-gauge short dental needles, *J Am Dent Assoc* 109:920, 1984.
24. Lin L, Shovlin F, Skribner J, Langeland K: Pulp biopsies from the teeth associated with periapical radiolucency, *J Endod* 10:436, 1984.
25. Kaufman E, Weinstein P, Milgrom P: Difficulties in achieving local anesthesia, *J Am Dent Assoc* 108:205, 1984.
26. Dreven L, Reader A, Beck M, et al: An evaluation of an electric pulp tester as a measure of analgesia in human vital teeth, *J Endod* 13:233, 1987.
27. Certosimo A, Archer R: A clinical evaluation of the electric pulp tester as an indicator of local anesthesia, *Oper Dent* 21:25, 1996.
28. Dionne R: Lidocaine and cancer: risk or rumor? *Compend Contin Educ Dent* 19:1118, 1998.
29. Lustig J, Zusman S: Immediate complications of local anesthetic administered to 1007 consecutive patients, *J Am Dent Assoc* 130:496, 1999.
30. Yagiela J: Adverse drug interactions in dental practice: interactions associated with vasoconstrictors, *J Am Dent Assoc* 130:701, 1999.
31. Potocnik I, Bajrovic F: Failure of inferior alveolar nerve block in endodontics, *Endod Dent Traumatol* 15:247, 1999.
32. Ågren E, Danielsson K: Conduction block analgesia in the mandible, *Swed Dent J* 5:81, 1981.
33. Vreeland D, Reader A, Beck M, et al: An evaluation of volumes and concentrations of lidocaine in human inferior alveolar nerve block, *J Endod* 15:6, 1989.
34. Hinkley S, Reader A, Beck M, Meyers W: An evaluation of 4% prilocaine with 1:200,000 epinephrine and 2% mepivacaine with 1:20,000 levonordefrin compared with 2% lidocaine with 1:100,000 epinephrine for inferior alveolar nerve block, *Anesth Prog* 38:84, 1991.
35. Chaney M, Kerby R, Reader A, et al: An evaluation of lidocaine hydrocarbonate compared with lidocaine hydrochloride for inferior alveolar nerve block, *Anesth Prog* 38:212, 1992.
36. Nist R, Reader A, Beck M, Meyers W: An evaluation of the incisive nerve block and combination inferior alveolar and incisive nerve blocks in mandibular anesthesia, *J Endod* 18:455, 1992.
37. McLean C, Reader A, Beck M, Meyers W: An evaluation of 4% prilocaine and 3% mepivacaine compared with 2% lidocaine (1:100,000 epinephrine) for inferior alveolar nerve block, *J Endod* 19:146, 1993.
38. Cohen H, Cha B, Spangberg L: Endodontic anesthesia in mandibular molars: a clinical study, *J Endod* 19:370, 1993.
39. Gow-Gates G: Mandibular conduction anesthesia: a new technique using extra-oral landmarks, *Oral Surg Oral Med Oral Pathol* 36:321, 1973.
40. Akinosi J: A new approach to the mandibular nerve block, *Br J Oral Surg* 15:83, 1977.
41. Goldberg S, Reader A, Beck M, Meyers W: Comparison of Gow-Gates and Akinosi techniques in human mandibular anesthesia, *J Endod* 15:173, 1989 (abstract).
42. Montagnese T, Reader A, Melfi R: A comparative study of the Gow-Gates technique and a standard technique for mandibular anesthesia, *J Endod* 10:158, 1984.
43. Yonchak T, Reader A, Beck M, Meyers W: Bilateral IAN blocks and infiltrations in human mandibular anterior anesthesia, *J Endod* 16:192, 1990 (abstract).
44. Clark K, Reader A, Meyers W, et al: Lingual infiltration and combination IAN/infiltrations in mandibular anterior anesthesia, *J Endod* 18:192, 1992 (abstract).
45. Haas D, Harper D, Saso M, Young E: Comparison of articaine and prilocaine anesthesia by infiltration in maxillary and mandibular arches, *Anesth Prog* 37:230, 1990.
46. Davis W, Oakley J, Smith E: Comparison of the effectiveness of etidocaine and lidocaine as local anesthetic agents during oral surgery, *Anesth Prog* 31:159, 1984.
47. Rosenquist J, Rosenquist K, Lee P: Comparison between lidocaine and bupivacaine as local anesthetics with diflunisal for postoperative pain control after lower third molar surgery, *Anesth Prog* 35:1, 1988.
48. Dunsky J, Moore P: Long-acting local anesthetics: a comparison of bupivacaine and etidocaine in endodontics, *J Endod* 10:6, 1984.

49. Moore P, Dunsky J: Bupivacaine anesthesia a clinical trial for endodontic therapy, *Oral Surg Oral Med Oral Pathol* 55:176, 1983.

50. Linden E, Abras H, Matheny J, et al: A comparison of postoperative pain experience following periodontal surgery using two local anesthetic agents, *J Periodontol* 57:637, 1986.

51. Crout R, Koraido G, Moore P: A clinical trial of long-acting local anesthetics for periodontal surgery, *Anesth Prog* 37:194, 1990.

52. Fernandez C, Reader A, Nist R, et al: Evaluation of bupivacaine in human mandibular anesthesia, *J Dent Res* 70:444, 1991.

53. Berns J, Sadove M: Mandibular block injection: a method of study using an injected radiopaque material, *J Am Dent Assoc* 65:735, 1962.

54. Galbreath J, Eklund M: Tracing the course of the mandibular block injection, *Oral Surg Oral Med Oral Pathol* 30:571, 1970.

55. Hannan L, Reader A, Nist R, et al: The use of ultrasound for guiding needle placement for inferior alveolar nerve blocks, *Oral Surg Oral Med Oral Pathol Oral Radiol Endod* 87:658, 1999.

56. Strichartz G: Molecular mechanisms of nerve block by local anesthetics, *Anesthesiology* 45:421, 1976.

57. Frommer J, Mele F, Monroe C: The possible role of the mylohyoid nerve in mandibular posterior tooth sensation, *J Am Dent Assoc* 85:113, 1972.

58. Wilson S, Johns P, Fuller P: The inferior and mylohyoid nerves: an anatomic study and relationship to local anesthesia of the anterior mandibular teeth, *J Am Dent Assoc* 108:350, 1984.

59. Clark S, Reader A, Beck M, Meyers W: Anesthetic efficacy of the mylohyoid nerve block and combination inferior alveolar nerve block/mylohyoid nerve block, *Oral Surg Oral Med Oral Pathol Oral Radiol Endod* 87:557, 1999.

60. Bunczak-Reeh M, Hargreaves K: Effect of inflammation of the delivery of drugs to dental pulp, *J Endod* 24:822, 1998.

61. Danielsson K, Evers H, Nordenram A: Long-acting local anesthetics in oral surgery: an experimental evaluation of bupivacaine and etidocaine for oral infiltration anesthesia, *Anesth Prog* March/April, 65, 1985.

62. Gross R, Reader A, Beck M, Meyers W: Anesthetic efficacy of lidocaine and bupivacaine in human maxillary infiltrations, *J Endod* 14:193, 1988 (abstract).

63. Mikesell A, Reader A, Beck M, Meyers W: Analgesic efficacy of volumes of lidocaine in human maxillary infiltration, *J Endod* 13:128, 1987 (abstract).

64. Mason R, Reader A, Beck M, Meyers W: Comparison of epinephrine concentrations and mepivacaine in human maxillary anesthesia, *J Endod* 15:173, 1989 (abstract).

65. Katz S, Reader A, Beck M, Meyers W: Anesthetic comparison of prilocaine and lidocaine in human maxillary infiltrations, *J Endod* 15:173, 1989 (abstract).

66. Loetscher C, Melton D, Walton R: Injection regimen for anesthesia of the maxillary first molar, *J Am Dent Assoc* 117:337, 1988.

67. Berberich G, Reader A, Beck M, Meyers W: Evaluation of the infraorbital nerve block in human maxillary anesthesia, *J Endod* 16:192, 1990 (abstract).

68. Karkut B, Reader A, Nist R, et al: Evaluation of the extraoral infraorbital nerve block in maxillary anesthesia, *J Dent Res* 72:274, 1993 (abstract).

69. Broering R, Reader A, Beck M, Meyers W: Evaluation of second division nerve blocks in human maxillary anesthesia, *J Endod* 17:194, 1991 (abstract).

70. Malamed S, Gagnon S, Leblanc D: Efficacy of articaine: a new amide local anesthetic, *J Am Dent Assoc* 131:635, 2000.

71. Reisman D, Reader A, Nist R, et al: Anesthetic efficacy of the supplemental intraosseous injection of 3% mepivacaine in irreversible pulpitis, *Oral Surg Oral Med Oral Pathol Oral Radiol Endod* 84:676, 1997.

72. Nusstein J, Reader A, Nist R, et al: Anesthetic efficacy of the supplemental intraosseous injection of 2% lidocaine with 1:100,000 epinephrine in irreversible pulpitis, *J Endod* 24:487, 1998.

73. Parente, SA, Anderson RW, Herman WW, et al: Anesthetic efficacy of the supplemental intraosseous injection for teeth with irreversible pulpitis, *J Endod* 24:826, 1998.

74. *Stabident Instruction Manual*, Miami, 2000, Fairfax Dental Inc.

75. Coggins R, Reader A, Nist R, et al: Anesthetic efficacy of the intraosseous injection in maxillary and mandibular teeth, *Oral Surg Oral Med Oral Pathol Oral Radiol Endod* 81:634, 1996.

76. Dunbar D, Reader A, Nist R, et al: Anesthetic efficacy of the intraosseous injection after an inferior alveolar nerve block, *J Endod* 22:481, 1996.

77. Replogle K, Reader A, Nist R, et al: Anesthetic efficacy of the intraosseous injection of 2% lidocaine (1:100,000 epinephrine) and 3% mepivacaine in mandibular first molars, *Oral Surg Oral Med Oral Pathol Oral Radiol Endod* 83:30, 1997.

78. Reitz J, Reader A, Nist R, et al: Anesthetic efficacy of the intraosseous injection of 0.9 ml of 2% lidocaine (1:100,000 epinephrine) to augment an inferior alveolar nerve block, *Oral Surg Oral Med Oral Pathol Oral Radiol Endod* 86:516, 1998.

79. Guglielmo A, Reader A, Nist R, et al: Anesthetic efficacy and heart rate effects of the supplemental intraosseous injection of 2% mepivacaine with 1:20,000 levonordefrin, *Oral Surg Oral Med Oral Pathol Oral Radiol Endod* 87:284, 1999

80. Reitz J, Reader A, Nist R, et al: Anesthetic efficacy of a repeated intraosseous injection given 30 min following an inferior alveolar nerve block/intraosseous injection, *Anesth Prog* 45:143, 1999.

81. Gallatin E, Stabile P, Reader A, et al: Anesthetic efficacy and heart rate effects of the intraosseous injection of 3% mepivacaine after an inferior alveolar nerve block, *Oral Surg Oral Med Oral Pathol Oral Radiol Endod* 89:83, 2000.

82. Stabile P, Reader A, Gallatin E, et al: Anesthetic efficacy and heart rate effects of the intraosseous injection of 1.5% etidocaine (1:200,000 epinephrine) after an inferior alveolar nerve block, *Oral Surg Oral Med Oral Pathol Oral Radiol Endod* 89:407, 2000.

83. Bacsik CJ, Swift JQ, Hargreaves KM: Toxic systemic reactions of bupivacaine and etidocaine hydrochloride, *Oral Surg Oral Med Oral Pathol Oral Radiol Endod* 79:18, 1995.

84. Hull TE, Rothwell BR: Intraosseous anesthesia comparing lidocaine and etidocaine, *J Dent Res* 77, Abstract 733, 1998.

85. Replogle K, Reader A, Nist R, et al: Cardiovascular effects of intraosseous injections of 2% lidocaine with 1:100,000 epinephrine and 3% mepivacaine, *J Am Dent Assoc* 130:649, 1999.

86. Walton R, Abbott B: Periodontal ligament injection: a clinical evaluation, *J Am Dent Assoc* 103:103, 1981.

87. Smith G, Walton R, Abbott B: Clinical evaluation of periodontal ligament anesthesia using a pressure syringe, *J Am Dent Assoc* 107:953, 1983.

88. Smith G, Walton R: Periodontal ligament injections: distribution of injected solutions, *Oral Surg Oral Med Oral Pathol* 55:232, 1983.

89. Dreyer W, van Heerden J, Joubert J: The route of periodontal ligament injection of local anesthetic solution, *J Endod* 9:471, 1983.

90. Walton R: Distribution of solutions with the periodontal ligament injection: clinical, anatomical, and histological evidence, *J Endod* 12:492, 1986.

91. Tagger M, Tagger E, Sarnat H: Periodontal ligament injection: Spread of solution in the dog, *J Endod* 20:283, 1994.

92. Moore K, Reader A, Meyers W, et al: A comparison of the periodontal ligament injection using 2% lidocaine with 1:100,000 epinephrine and saline in human mandibular premolars, *Anesth Prog* 34:181, 1987.

93. Schleder J, Reader A, Beck M, Meyers M: The periodontal ligament injection: a comparison of 2% lidocaine, 3% mepivacaine, and 1:100,000 epinephrine to 2% lidocaine with 1:100,000 epinephrine in human mandibular premolars, *J Endod* 14:397, 1988.

94. White J, Reader A, Beck M, Meyers W: The periodontal ligament injection: a comparison of the efficacy in human maxillary and mandibular teeth, *J Endod* 14:508, 1988.

95. D'Souza J, Walton R, Peterson L: Periodontal ligament injection: an evaluation of extent of anesthesia and postinjection discomfort, *J Am Dent Assoc* 114:341, 1987.

96. Eriksen H, Aamdal H, Kerekes K: Periodontal anesthesia: a clinical evaluation, *Endod Dent Traumatol* 2:267, 1986.

97. Simon D, Jacobs L, Senia S, Walker W: Intraligamentary anesthesia as an aid in endodontic diagnosis, *Oral Surg Oral Med Oral Pathol* 54:77, 1982.

98. Pashley D: Systemic effects of intraligamental injections, *J Endod* 12:501, 1986.

99. Johnson G, Hlava G, Kalkwarf K: A comparison of periodontal intraligamental anesthesia using etidocaine HCl and lidocaine HCl, *Anesth Prog* 32:202, 1985.

100. Gray R, Lomax A, Rood J: Periodontal ligament injection: alternative solutions, *Anesth Prog* 37:293, 1990.

101. Walton R, Garnick J: The periodontal ligament injection: histologic effects on the periodontium in monkeys, *J Endod* 8:22, 1981.

102. List G, Meister Jr F, Nery E, Prey J: Gingival crevicular fluid response to various solutions using the intraligamentary injection, *Quintessence Int* 19:559, 1988.

103. Brannström M, Nordenvall K, Hedstrom K: Periodontal tissue changes after intraligamentary anesthesia, *J Dent Child* 11/12:417, 1982.

104. Galili D, Kaufman E, Garfunkel A, Michaeli Y: Intraligamental anesthesia: a histological study, *Int J Oral Surg* 13:511, 1984.

105. Roahen J, Marshall J: The effects of periodontal ligament injection on pulpal and periodontal tissues, *J Endod* 16:28, 1990.

106. Pertot W, Dejou J: Bone and root resorption. Effects of the force developed during periodontal ligament injections in dogs, *Oral Surg Oral Med Oral Pathol* 74:357, 1992.

107. Peurach J: Pulpal response to intraligamentary injection in cynomolgus monkey, *Anesth Prog* 32:73, 1985.

108. Torabinejad M, Peters D, Peckham N, et al: Electron microscopic changes in human pulps after intraligamental injection, *Oral Surg Oral Med Oral Pathol* 76:219, 1993.

109. Kim S: Ligamental injection: A physiological explanation of its efficacy, *J Endod* 12:486, 1986.

110. Plamondon T, Walton R, Graham G, et al: Pulp response to the combined effects of cavity preparation and periodontal ligament injection, *Oper Dent* 15:86, 1990.

111. Brannström M, Lindsko S, Nordenvall K: Enamel hypoplasia in permanent teeth induced by periodontal ligament anesthesia of primary teeth, *J Am Dent Assoc* 109:735, 1984.

112. Birchfield J, Rosenberg P: Role of the anesthetic solution in intrapulpal anesthesia, *J Endod* 1:26, 1975.

113. VanGheluwe J, Walton R: Intrapulpal injection—factors related to effectiveness, *Oral Surg Oral Med Oral Pathol Oral Radiol Endod* 83:38, 1997.

114. Smith G, Smith S: Intrapulpal injection: distribution of an injected solution, *J Endod* 9:167, 1983.

115. Clark M, Silverstone J, Lindenmuth J, et al: An evaluation of the clinical analgesia/anesthesia efficacy on acute pain using the high frequency neural modulator in various dental settings, *Oral Surg Oral Med Oral Pathol* 63:501, 1987.

116. Gerschman J, Giebartowski J: Effect of electronic dental anesthesia on pain threshold and pain tolerance levels of human teeth subjected to stimulation with an electric pulp tester, *Anesth Prog* 38:45, 1991.

117. Rooney J, Tronstad L: Effect of transcutaneous electrical nerve stimulation on pain perception threshold and pain tolerance level of human teeth subjected to electrical stimulation, *Endod Dent Traumatol* 2:109, 1986.

118. Donaldson D, Quarnstrom F, Jastak J: The combined effect of nitrous oxide and oxygen and electrical stimulation during restorative dental treatment, *J Am Dent Assoc* 118:733, 1989.

119. Guglielmo A, Nist R, Reader A: Palatal and buccal infiltrations in maxillary first molar anesthesia, *J Dent Res* 72:274, 1993 (abstract).

120. Meechan J, Blair G: The effect of two different local anaesthetic solutions on pain experience following apicoectomy, *Br Dent J* 175:410, 1993.

8

Gerald L. Scott

Isolation

LEARNING OBJECTIVES

After reading this chapter, the student should be able to:

1 / Describe the reasons for rubber dam isolation during endodontic procedures.

2 / List a rubber dam clamp selection for anterior, premolar, and molar teeth.

3 / Identify those clamps that have several applications. (Which two are "universal?")

4 / Describe techniques for application of clamp/rubber dam in single-tooth isolation.

5 / Describe techniques to stop salivary or hemorrhage "seepage" into the operative field.

6 / Recognize situations in which special isolation approaches are necessary.

7 / Describe the technique to use in those special situations.

8 / Describe surgical techniques to use as adjuncts to attain required isolation.

9 / Identify patients with difficult isolation situations who should be considered for referral.

OUTLINE

Reasons for Use of the Rubber Dam
Protection
Facilitate and Increase Efficiency
Minimize Cross-Infection
Legal Considerations
Additional Considerations

Preparation for Placement
Areas of Potential Leakage
Coronal Considerations
Gingival Preparation
Replacement of Missing Crown Structure

Equipment
Rubber Dam Material
Frames
Combinations
Clamps (Retainers)
Additional Instruments
Clamp Substitutes

Application of the Rubber Dam
Hole Placement
Clamp Selection
Placement Techniques
Rubber Dam Positioning
Disinfection of Operating Field

Aids for a Leaking Dam
Prevention
Corrective Methods

Modifications for Difficult Isolation Situations
Unusual Crown to Root Alignment
Little Remaining Tooth Structure
Root Caries
Unusual Tooth Position
Unusual Tooth Shape
Bridges or Orthodontic Appliances
Porcelain Restoration
Multiple Tooth Isolation
Emergency Situations

When and What to Refer
Problems with Inadequate Isolation
Other Situations

Isolation requires proper placement of the rubber dam. This device will isolate the pulp space from saliva and hemorrhage and protect tissues from irrigating solutions, other chemicals, and instruments.

The rubber dam was first introduced in 1863 by Sanford Barnum, a New York dentist. His invention was a way to achieve isolation for the placing of gold foil. Shortly thereafter his colleague, C. E. Francis, pleaded, "Gentlemen of the profession—learn to use Barnum's rubber dam, and when you thoroughly understand its true value, you will bless the name of the worthy dentist whose ingenuity gave us so valuable a boon."[1] Surveys indicate that rubber dam usage is inconsistent, with many dentists seldom or never using the rubber dam for endodontic procedures.[2] Some use it occasionally, and about half use a rubber dam for isolation almost always.[3] This indicates a need for better understanding of the rationale for its use.[4]

Reasons for Use of the Rubber Dam

PROTECTION

The rubber dam prevents aspiration or accidental swallowing of endodontic instruments and irrigants. It also affords protection from injury caused by rotary and hand instruments.[5] The patient should not be exposed to these avoidable risks.

The dentist and assistant are also protected. Aerosol spray from the handpiece and air-water syringe are potentially harmful. Use of the rubber dam minimizes this risk; the aerosol will deflect off the clean rubber dam rather than mixing with saliva and oral debris.[6,7] Contamination of the environment is also reduced because the dental team has less direct contact with the patient's oral tissues and fluids.

FACILITATE AND INCREASE EFFICIENCY

The rubber dam (1) improves visibility; (2) prevents salivary leakage, thus providing a dry field; (3) prevents fogging of the mirror; (4) relaxes the patient, who need not fear swallowing instruments nor suffer the unpleasant taste of chemicals or irrigants; and (5) minimizes conversation and the need (perceived or actual) for frequent rinsing.

MINIMIZE CROSS-INFECTION

There is increasing concern about transmission of infectious diseases [especially acquired immunodeficiency syndrome (AIDS), tuberculosis, and hepatitis); use of the rubber dam may reduce the risk of spreading these diseases.[8] The rubber dam, although helpful, must not be considered total protection; other preventive measures are essential as well.

LEGAL CONSIDERATIONS

All dental schools in the United States require use of the rubber dam during endodontic procedures. *Its routine usage during root canal treatment is a standard of care.* In fact, expert testimony is not required to justify claims of negligence when an instrument is swallowed or aspirated. Liability is so evident that a jury is deemed competent enough to determine negligence. Although the reasons for rubber dam application are primarily facilitative and biologic, legal ramifications make its use mandatory.[9]

ADDITIONAL CONSIDERATIONS

The necessity for rubber dam isolation is apparent. It is important to recognize early those situations in which isolation will be difficult or time-consuming; this is part of treatment planning. Before treatment is initiated, isolation must be carefully considered. Occasionally, it is best for patients with difficult isolation situations to be referred to an endodontist because special techniques may be required.

Preparation for Placement

Root canal treatment begins with consideration of several factors before actual rubber dam placement.

AREAS OF POTENTIAL LEAKAGE

Areas having a potential for leakage include subgingival caries and defects such as fractures, defective restorations, and open margins.

CORONAL CONSIDERATIONS

Margins of existing restorations are evaluated both radiographically and clinically. Defective restorations may allow leakage between the oral cavity and pulp space. The entire restoration, or at least the defective portion, must be removed early and before the access preparation is completed.

The extent and presence of caries should also be an early determination. Caries may communicate with the oral cavity and pulp chamber. Gen-

erally all caries are removed to prevent leakage during and after treatment.

GINGIVAL PREPARATION

When restorations or carious lesions extend subgingivally or when crown destruction is excessive, sound tooth structure may require exposure by gingivectomy or crown lengthening.

Gingivectomy: Gingival tissue is removed to expose an intact surface to allow clamp placement. When gingivectomy is necessary to restore normal gingival architecture for restoration, it is best done before root canal treatment is initiated. This simplifies isolation and aids in determining restorability.

Crown Lengthening: Crown lengthening is a more involved procedure that requires flap reflection and contouring of bone and gingiva.[10] Healing requires approximately 6 weeks; the tooth should not be clamped during that time. Root canal treatment and crown lengthening are often best accomplished at the same appointment. Because of the treatment complexity, these patients may benefit by being referred.

REPLACEMENT OF MISSING CROWN STRUCTURE

The perfect access preparation for maximal visibility and ease of straight-line access is through a crown sectioned in the cervical third, thus opening the chamber wide. Therefore adding restorative materials or placing bands or temporary crowns only hinders treatment. However, pretreatment occasionally requires a provisional restoration before rubber dam placement.

Temporary Restoration: A reinforced cement, such as IRM (Cavit is not acceptable), is suitable. This is indicated in regions that are difficult to isolate (such as subgingival interproximal caries) but where crown lengthening or gingivectomy is not required. The cement should maintain proximal contact or, if little tooth structure remains, be contoured to help prevent interproximal food impaction.

Buildups: These procedures are usually not necessary. However, when gingival procedures or temporary restorations to facilitate isolation are not feasible, amalgam, glass ionomer, or composite buildups may suffice.[11-13] Special retentive approaches are required.[14]

Disadvantages to buildup procedures are that they are time-consuming, may hinder visibility and access to the canal space, and usually must be redone before the permanent restoration is placed. Generally, there is no need for such procedures.

Bands: Copper and orthodontic bands have been advocated as an isolation aid and as a means of protecting weakened cusps.[15] Bands are time-consuming to adapt properly, generally leak, often come loose, and usually cause gingival irritation. Therefore they are rarely indicated. If cusps have been undermined or are otherwise weakened, it is preferable to reduce their height by several millimeters and then, if necessary, onlay with the temporary material.

Temporary Crowns: Temporary crowns are also of dubious value in aiding isolation. There are suggestions that temporary crowns be cemented and then access made through the occlusal surface. Temporary crowns have the same disadvantages as bands (described above). Two additional disadvantages outweigh any transient benefits provided by temporary crowns. First, they are often displaced by the force of the clamp or tension of the rubber dam. Second, there is loss of orientation and impaired visibility. Therefore accurate access preparation, canal locating, and overall treatment through a temporary crown are more difficult.

Temporary crowns may be used between appointments after the canal space or chamber has been sealed off with another temporary material and after the rubber dam has been removed. The temporary crown is then adjusted and cemented temporarily and removed at the next appointment. Before the root canal treatment begins, it is usually preferable to remove a temporary crown that has been placed earlier.

Equipment

RUBBER DAM MATERIAL

Rubber dams are available in several colors and four thicknesses or weights. There is also a nonlatex dam (nonallergenic) material. Although color choice is largely personal preference, the light-colored (yellow) dam has advantages. It allows better illumination and is transparent enough to facilitate film placement when making radiographs. Of the four thicknesses (light, medium, heavy, and extra heavy), the light and medium are preferred. The light is easier to slide between the teeth and puts the least amount of tension on the clamp. However, it is difficult to tuck and does not seal as well. Medium weight is slightly more difficult to apply but fits better at the gingival margin and provides better soft tissue retraction. Thickness does not have a consistent effect on tear resistance properties.[16] Experience, different isolation conditions, and personal preference will dictate rubber dam selection for each situation.

FRAMES

Four frames are commonly used for endodontic procedures. The Young's frame is metal (radiopaque) and must be removed while taking radiographs. The Nygaard-Ostby and the Star Visi-frames are radiolucent and need not (should not) be removed while radiographs are being made. The Nygaard-Ostby frame attaches the rubber dam on all four sides and requires more care in hole placement, because it is more difficult to adjust the height of the superior border of the dam. The Plast-Frame is autoclavable plastic and can be folded to one side for radiographs. All four frames comfortably hold the dam away from the patient's face and require no napkin under the dam.

COMBINATIONS

Recently frame and rubber dam combinations have been introduced (Figure 8-1). One has a pliable oval plastic frame around the perimeter of the rubber dam and is available in three sizes. Another has a plastic tube inserted in prepared holes in the rubber dam material and comes in one size. A third is autoclavable. All appear to provide adequate protection, are easy to apply, do not inter-

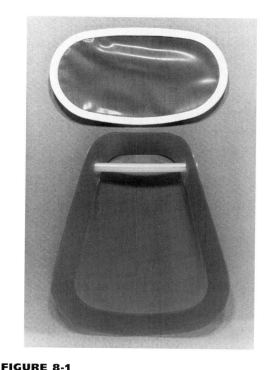

FIGURE 8-1
Two rubber dam and frame combinations: Quickdam and HandiDam. These are easily applied and disposable, but are more costly.

fere with making radiographs, and eliminate bulky and cumbersome frames.

CLAMPS (RETAINERS)
Styles and Shapes

Many different styles and shapes designed for different situations are available. One manufacturer lists an assortment of more than 50 clamps. A large number of clamps is neither necessary nor desirable for isolation. A complete selection includes (1) anterior teeth: Ivory 9 or Ash 9; (2) premolars: SSW 20, 27, Ivory 0, 2, 9, 1, and IA; and (3) molars: SSW 18, Ivory 14, 14A, and 56, and Ash 8. Five clamps that will manage most root canal treatment isolation situations are shown in

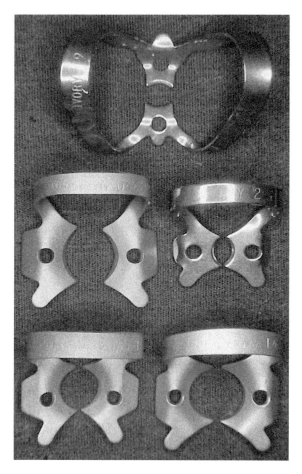

FIGURE 8-2
Top, Butterfly design clamp Ivory 9 for anterior teeth and premolars. *Middle left,* Hu-Friedy 56 for molars. *Middle right,* Ivory 2 for molars when a smaller beaked, deeper-reaching clamp is necessary. *Lower left,* Hu-Friedy 14. *Lower right,* Hu-Friedy 14 A for molars of different sizes. Nos. 56 and 9 can be used in most situations. Note the nonglare finish on Hu-Friedy clamps.

Figure 8-2. Winged clamps are preferred for efficient dam application. Recently, a series of clamps with a dull finish has been introduced to reduce light reflection. Plastic, disposable clamps are also available.

Universal Clamp Designs

Two designs (Figure 8-2), the "butterfly" Ivory 9 and the Ivory 56, are suitable for most isolations. The butterfly design (no. 9) has small beaks and is deep reaching and is useful for most anterior and premolar teeth. The no. 56 is used for molars. Both usually provide isolation, particularly in difficult situations.

Small radius beaks can be positioned farther apically on the root; this will stretch the dam cervically in the interproximal space. With teeth that are smaller or abnormally shaped, a clamp (no. 14, 9, or 2) with smaller radius beaks is necessary.

Additional Designs: Clamps that may be necessary when little coronal tooth structure remains have beaks that are inclined apically. These are termed *deep-reaching* clamps (Figure 8-3).

For stability, four-point contact between the tooth and beaks of the clamp is necessary and dic-

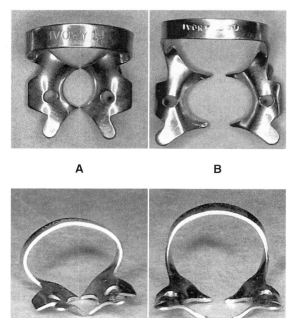

A	B
C	D

FIGURE 8-3
Two styles of deep-reaching clamps: **A** and **B,** Ivory 14; **C** and **D,** 14A. These are often more stable when coronal tooth structure is missing.

tates the size selected. Fatigued anterior and premolar clamps may be used for unusual molar applications (Figure 8-4). Clamps may also be modified by grinding to adapt to unusual situations.[17] Plastic clamps are more easily modified.

ADDITIONAL INSTRUMENTS

Punch: Any punch is acceptable. The punch should be sharp to make a clean hole and not tear or nick the dam.

Forceps: Any forceps are acceptable. One type has projections extending from the beaks to allow better control in clamp placement. Also, the projections allow greater pressure gingivally and provide more maneuverability for seating the front or rear of the clamp.

Tucking Instruments: A plastic instrument or spoon excavator slides the dam off the wings of the clamp and then inverts the edge of the dam. A stream of air will dry the area and helps to invert the dam.

Dental Floss: Dental floss is used to pass the dam between both contacts. With single tooth isolation, at least the mesial and often the distal surface should be flossed through the contact. Checking contacts for tightness before dam placement is advisable. Floss may be used to ligate the necks of the teeth to hold the dam if a clamp cannot be used.

Saliva Ejector: A saliva ejector enhances patient comfort. The tip may be positioned under the dam, or the patient may maneuver it under the dam as needed.

CLAMP SUBSTITUTES

In some circumstances, floss holds the dam in place by ligating the tooth. In these cases, multiple isolation is usually needed (Figure 8-5). Floss can also be used with a bead from a necklace, a rubber polishing disc, or a rubber anesthetic plunger.[18] Floss is threaded through the hole in the bead or rubber disc or around the plunger, leaving enough to ligate when the bead is placed on the lingual surface (Figure 8-6). Wedjets (Hygenic Corp.) are also a means of holding the rubber dam in position.[19] Ortho separators may also

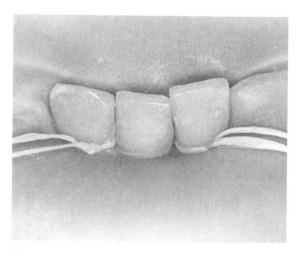

FIGURE 8-5
Multiple isolation secured with floss, useful when a clamp cannot be placed.

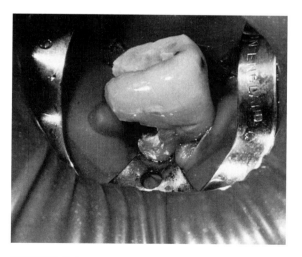

FIGURE 8-4
A butterfly design clamp (Ivory 9) may be used on a posterior tooth. This unusual clamp selection allows isolation gingival to the caries.

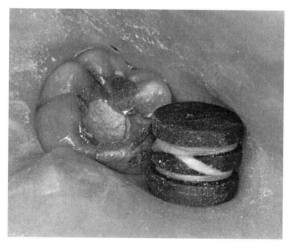

FIGURE 8-6
Rubber dam secured with bead (anesthetic cartridge stopper) and floss ligation.

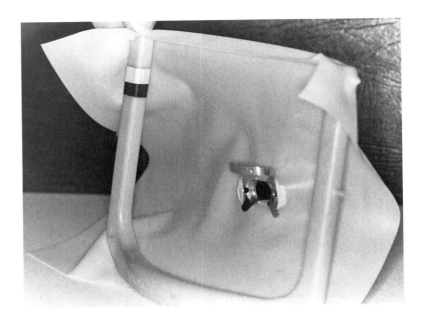

FIGURE 8-7
Rubber dam and clamp properly attached to a frame before placement as a unit. Note that the dam is stretched tightly across the top and bottom with slack in the middle for ease of placement.

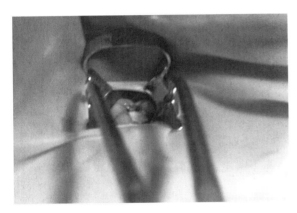

FIGURE 8-8
Rubber dam, clamp, and frame being placed as a unit; this is usually faster and more effective than other techniques.

be placed around the neck of the tooth to hold the dam in position.

Application of the Rubber Dam

HOLE PLACEMENT

The hole is located so that the dam covers the entire mouth and extends up to the nose. The dam should cover the nose to reduce inhalation of aerosol particles and to control objectionable odors. Some patients are uncomfortable with the dam over their nose. Placing the hole 1 inch off the center of the dam toward the quadrant being isolated will usually suffice.

A simple method of hole placement is as follows: (1) engage the dam on the frame, (2) center the dam over the patient's mouth, (3) push the dam over the tooth to be isolated, (4) mark the dam, and (5) remove and punch the dam.

CLAMP SELECTION

The appropriate clamp with four-point contact is selected. To prevent swallowing or aspiration if displacement occurs, floss is attached to the clamp bow. A floss tie is unnecessary if the clamp and dam are placed together.

PLACEMENT TECHNIQUES

After the necessary preparation procedures detailed earlier have been completed, the dam is placed using one of the following three methods.

Method 1: Placement as a unit. Placement of rubber dam, clamp, and frame as a unit is preferred. This is most efficient and is applicable in most cases.

1. Place the dam on the frame so that it is stretched tightly across the top and bottom but has slack in the middle (Figure 8-7).
2. Punch the hole in the dam and attach clamp wings to the dam.
3. Place the dam, frame, and clamp as a unit to engage the tooth near the gingival margin (Figure 8-8). Finger pressure is usually necessary on the forceps or the clamp because of resistance from the rubber as it is stretched.

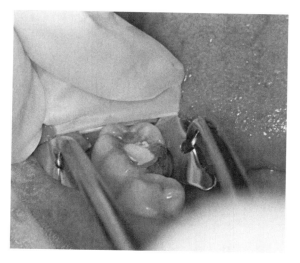

FIGURE 8-9
Placement of clamp and rubber dam for better visibility of the neck of the tooth. The rubber dam is attached to the clamp bow and is held out of the way for unobstructed vision while the clamp is positioned. Then the rubber dam is stretched around the clamp and the neck of the tooth.

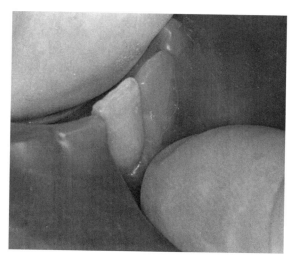

FIGURE 8-10
The rubber dam is stretched over the tooth before clamp placement.

4. Slide the dam off the clamp wings to allow the dam to constrict around the tooth neck. Draw the dam through the contacts with floss.
5. Adjust the dam on the frame for patient comfort.

Method 2: Placement of clamp and dam and then the frame (Figure 8-9). This method is seldom used but may be necessary when an unobstructed view is required while the clamp is positioned.

Method 3: Placement of the rubber dam and frame and then the clamp. This is the preferred method for applying a butterfly clamp. Better visualization is possible when the hole is stretched over the tooth and gingiva first (Figure 8-10) and then the clamp is placed (Figure 8-11).

RUBBER DAM POSITIONING

After placement, the rubber dam is adjusted on the frame so that the mouth is completely covered. Tension is adjusted to minimize bunching and to retract soft tissue without dislodging the clamp (Figure 8-12).

DISINFECTION OF THE OPERATING FIELD

Various chemicals and techniques have been tried to remove and destroy bacterial contaminants from the tooth surface, clamp, and sur-

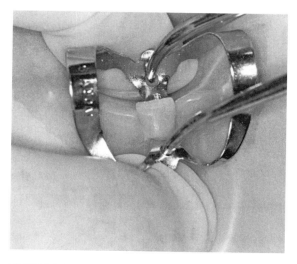

FIGURE 8-11
The clamp is placed to hold the prepositioned and pre-stretched rubber dam (see Figure 8-10).

rounding rubber dam. These include alcohol, quaternary ammonium compounds, sodium hypochlorite, organic iodine, mercuric salts, and hydrogen peroxide. An effective technique is as follows: (1) plaque is removed by rubber cup and pumice; (2) the rubber dam is placed; (3) the tooth surface, clamp, and surrounding rubber dam are scrubbed with 30% hydrogen peroxide; and (4) the surfaces are swabbed with 5% tincture of iodine or with sodium hypochlorite.[20]

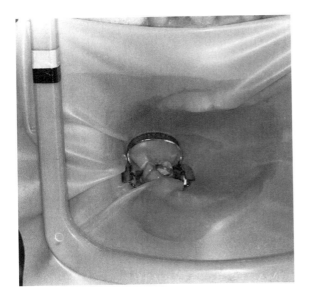

FIGURE 8-12
Final position of the adjusted rubber dam, clamp, and frame. Floss should be drawn through the contacts. The tooth, clamp and surrounding dam may now be cleaned and disinfected. The dam edge may be folded away from the nose.

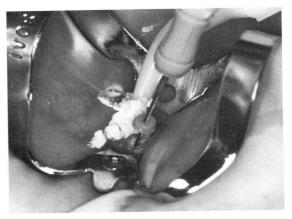

FIGURE 8-13
Silicone sealant (OraSeal) is injected in an area of leakage. The material is then pressed and adapted into place with a wet cotton pellet.

Aids for a Leaking Dam

PREVENTION

Proper tooth and site preparation, clamp selection, hole positioning, placement on the tooth, and final sealing with floss all reduce leakage problems.[21]

CORRECTIVE METHODS

If seepage occurs, one of the following techniques will usually correct the problem:

Cavit: Cavit is somewhat useful. Cavit is placed at the site and compacted with a large wet cotton pellet. A major disadvantage is that, with longer procedures, Cavit usually will crack and leak, requiring replacement.

Sealants: Special sealants are applied topically (Figure 8-13), or, if leakage is anticipated, they may be applied to the undersurface of the dam before placement.[22]

Rubber base adhesive: This is easily painted on the dam in an area of minor seepage.[23]

Floss ligation: Floss around the cervical region helps to keep the dam inverted. Ligation is useful during isolation of multiple teeth but is time consuming.

Additional corrective methods: Use of cyanoacrylate, a prosthetic block-out putty, Stomadhesive, or a denture adhesive-zinc oxide mixture has also been proposed for correction of seepage.[19,24,25]

Modifications for Difficult Isolation Situations

UNUSUAL CROWN TO ROOT ALIGNMENT

Sometimes the crown is misaligned with the root or has been modified by large restorations. To enhance proper angulation or orientation to the chamber, access preparation in those situations should be done *before* rubber dam placement. First, the location and long axis of the tooth are determined by visualizing and palpating the root prominence. Second, as a guide for the bur, a pencil line is drawn on the crown aligned with the long axis of the root.[10] The rubber dam is placed when the chamber (or canal) is located.

LITTLE REMAINING TOOTH STRUCTURE

Teeth with severe loss (particularly subgingival) of coronal tooth structure compromise rubber dam placement. One of the following can be used to ensure adequate isolation.

1. Use of a deep-reaching ("A" style or small beak) clamp often solves the problem and is the first method attempted (Figure 8-14).
2. Adjacent teeth are clamped, giving multiple isolation. This is slightly less effective

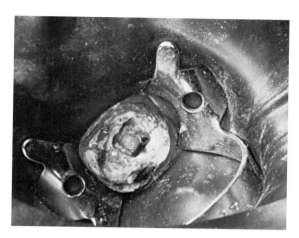

FIGURE 8-14
A deep-reaching clamp secures the rubber dam on a tooth with little clinical crown.

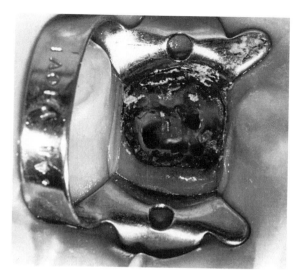

FIGURE 8-15
Clamp beaks may be placed on anesthetized gingiva if the coronal tooth structure is not sufficient to secure the clamp. This does no permanent damage to the gingiva.

than single-tooth isolation and usually requires the use of other aids such as floss ligation and/or sealants.

3. The clamp beaks may be placed on anesthetized gingiva (Figure 8-15). There must be sufficient gingival purchase to prevent the clamp from cutting through the gingival sulcus and, in essence, performing a crude, unplanned gingivectomy. Plastic clamps create less gingival trauma. Patients experience minimal discomfort after clamp placement on the gingiva.
4. Gingivectomy or flap reflection or crown lengthening can be performed before isolation.
5. Build-up procedures are generally not recommended.

ROOT CARIES

Subgingival caries are a challenge.[26] Placement of the clamp and dam cervical to the caries (see Figure 8-4) should be attempted, but may be unsuccessful. Caries removal is necessary and often requires a temporary restoration. The challenge is to avoid introducing restorative material into the canal space. One technique is to remove caries first followed by access. Then a tight-fitting file is placed into the canal apical to the defect. A temporary or permanent restoration is placed. When

set, the blocking instrument is removed, leaving the canal patent.

UNUSUAL TOOTH POSITION

Teeth that are inclined because of crowding or that have tipped owing to tooth loss present isolation problems. Isolation can usually be accomplished by careful clamp selection. Other methods include clamping the adjacent tooth (multiple isolation) or ligation with floss, floss and bead, or Wedjets.

UNUSUAL TOOTH SHAPE

Occasionally coronal configuration makes tooth clamping difficult. Beak placement below the height of contour may not be possible if teeth are not fully erupted. Crown reduction for full coverage usually removes the gripping area. Remedies, in order of preference are the following:

1. Deep-reaching clamp
2. Gingival clamping
3. Acid etch composite on buccal and/or lingual surface to retain clamp or dam[27]
4. Grooves on buccal and lingual surfaces for clamp retention
5. Orthodontic separators over the necks of the teeth
6. Gingivectomy or crown lengthening

BRIDGES OR ORTHODONTIC APPLIANCES

These are usually approached in the same manner as single-tooth isolation. Because of openings, it may be necessary to punch two holes, cut a slit between the holes, and then use a sealant; this is the easiest technique (Figure 8-16). More elaborate methods have been designed—for example, cutting a slit and then suturing the dam closed under the pontics or by ligating interproximally.[28] However, such procedures are complicated and rarely necessary.

PORCELAIN RESTORATION

Placing a clamp on porcelain may cause crazing, although not consistently.[29,30] It is best to avoid clamping such restorations if the quality of porcelain condensation is uncertain. Damage is avoided by clamping the adjacent tooth or by using floss or floss and bead ligation. An alternative is to stretch an unpunched dam over the tooth and secure the dam with the appropriate clamp. Then with a hot instrument a hole is melted over the access preparation. The access must be done before rubber dam placement.

MULTIPLE TOOTH ISOLATION

When more than one tooth requires treatment, isolation is accomplished with multiple clamps (Figure 8-17) or with clamps and floss ligation or other combinations (Figure 8-18). For anterior teeth (or tooth), all teeth would have to be isolated and the rubber dam would be stretched and clamped over the first premolars.

EMERGENCY SITUATIONS

Occasionally a patient has such intense pain that he or she cannot tolerate the clamp. Multiple isolation is usually preferred by clamping another tooth. An alternative is floss, floss and bead, or Wedjets ligation with either single or multiple isolation.

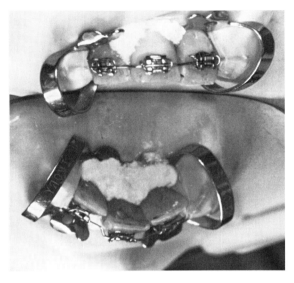

FIGURE 8-16
Isolation with an orthodontic appliance. A slit is made between the two end punch holes. Seepage is then prevented by silicone sealant placement. This could also be treated by removing the arch wire and using single-tooth isolation. (Courtesy Dr. M. Davis.)

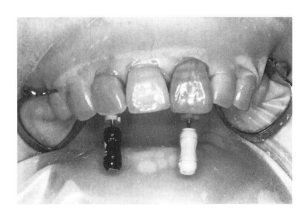

FIGURE 8-17
Example of multiple isolation when several teeth are undergoing treatment. This may also need to be used when a clamp cannot be conveniently placed, such as on a crown-prepared tooth.

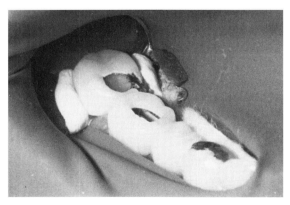

FIGURE 8-18
To isolate this double-abutted bridge, a combination of techniques is used. One large rubber dam opening is necessary. OraSeal is packed around the clamp. A cotton roll on the lingual aspect reduces seepage. (Courtesy Dr. C. Koloffon.)

When and What to Refer

If isolation is not obtainable, patients should be considered for referral.

PROBLEMS WITH INADEQUATE ISOLATION

Patients with the following conditions should be considered for referral: (1) gross and persistent bacterial contamination of the pulp space and possibly the periapex; (2) excessive time required for treatment; (3) frustration and delays when leakage occurs or with dam displacement; and (4) anxiety or discomfort for the patient when isolation fails or when solutions violate the oral cavity.

OTHER SITUATIONS

Patients with the following should be considered for referral: (1) badly broken-down teeth with minimal coronal tooth structure remaining. These are a challenge—attempting multiple-tooth isolation leads to seepage; (2) bridge abutments with problem seepage; (3) full crown preparations that are difficult to clamp, when multiple isolation is difficult; (4) malpositioned teeth with unique isolation problems; and (5) the most distal tooth in the arch if it cannot be clamped.

Individual capabilities (experience, training, and interest) determine which patients the practitioner might treat and which should be referred. In assessing these capabilities from a legal perspective, courts have set the standard of care as that provided by the specialist, not the general dentist. Consideration of the patient's time and comfort are also important factors. Finally, nothing is more upsetting to a full schedule or more frustrating to both practitioner and patient than difficulties encountered during treatment. Lowering the practitioner's stress levels is an additional incentive for considering referral.

REFERENCES

1. Francis C: The rubber dam, *Dental Cosmos* 7:185, 1866.
2. Joynt R, Davis E, Schreier P: Rubber dam usage among practicing dentists, *Oper Dent* 14:176, 1989.
3. Marshall K: The use of rubber dam in the UK, *Br Dent J* 168:286, 1990.
4. Marshall K: Isolation and tissue control: the role of rubber dam, *Endod Pract* 1:40, 1998.
5. Huggins D: The rubber dam: insurance policy against litigation, *J Indiana Dent Assoc* 65:23, 1986.
6. Miller R, Micik R: Air pollution and its control in the dental office, *Dent Clin North Am* 22:453, 1978.
7. Wong R: The rubber dam as a means of infection control in an era of AIDS and hepatitis, *J Indiana Dent Assoc* 67:41, 1988.
8. Cochran M, Miller C, Sheldrake M: The efficacy of the rubber dam as a barrier to the spread of micro-organisms during dental treatment, *J Am Dent Assoc* 119:141, 1989.
9. Cohen S, Schwartz S: Endodontic complications and the law, *J Endod* 13:191, 1987.
10. Gutmann J, Dumsha T, Lovdahl P, Hovland EJ: *Problem solving in endodontics*, ed 2, St Louis, 1992, Mosby.
11. Morgan L: Solving endodontic isolation problems with interim buildups of reinforced glass ionomer cement, *J Endod* 16:450, 1990.
12. Kahn H: Coronal build-up of the degraded tooth before endodontic therapy, *J Endod* 8:83, 1982.
13. Estafan DJ, Harris R, Estafan A: A simplified approach to isolating a single tooth before endodontic therapy, *J Am Dent Assoc* 130:846, 1999.
14. Greene R, Sikora F, House J: Rubber dam application to crownless and cone-shaped teeth, *J Endod* 10:82, 1984.
15. Linden R: Using a copper band to isolate severely broken teeth before endodontic procedures, *J Am Dent Assoc* 130:1095, 1999.
16. Svec T, Powers J, Ladd G, Meyer T: Tensile and tear properties of dental dam, *J Endod* 22:253, 1996.
17. Weisman M: A modification of the no. 3 rubber dam clamp, *J Endod* 9:30, 1983.
18. Ireland I: The rubber dam: its advantages and application, *Tex Dent J* 24:6, 1962.
19. Aesaert, G: The use of rubber dam in difficult clinical situations, *Endod Pract* 3:6, 2000.
20. Hermsen K, Ludlow M: Disinfection of rubber dam and tooth surfaces before endodontic therapy, *Gen Dent* 35:355, 1997.
21. Fors V, Berg J, Sandberg H: Microbiological investigation of saliva leakage between the rubber dam and tooth during endodontic treatment, *J Endod* 12:396, 1986.
22. Glick D: Use of a protective emollient as an endodontic aid, *Oral Surg Oral Med Oral Pathol* 24:250, 1967.
23. Bramwell D, Hicks M: Solving isolation problems with rubber dam adhesive, *J Endod* 12:363, 1986.
24. Roahen J, Lento C: Using cyanoacrylate to facilitate rubber dam isolation of teeth, *J Endod* 18:517, 1992.
25. Weisman M: Remedy for dental dam leakage problems, *J Endod* 17:88, 1991.
26. Iglesias A, Urrutia C: Solution for the isolation of the working field in a difficult case of root canal therapy, *J Endod* 21:394, 1995.
27. Wakabayashi H, Ochi K, Tachibana H, et al: A clinical technique for the retention of a rubber dam clamp, *J Endod* 12:422, 1986.
28. Liebenberg W: Manipulation of rubber dam septa: an aid to the meticulous isolation of splinted prostheses, *J Endod* 21:208, 1995.
29. Madison S, Jordon R, Krell K: The effects of rubber dam retainer on porcelain fused-to-metal restorations, *J Endod* 12:183, 1986.
30. Zerr, M, Johnson W, Walton R: Effect of rubber dam retainers on porcelain-fused-to-metal, *Gen Dent* 44:132, 1996.

9

Richard E. Walton

Endodontic Radiography

LEARNING OBJECTIVES

After reading this chapter, the student should be able to:

1 / Describe the importance of radiographs in endodontic diagnosis and treatment.

2 / Discuss special applications of radiography to endodontics.

3 / Discuss reasons for limiting the number of exposures.

4 / Identify normal anatomic features in the maxilla and mandible on radiographs.

5 / Describe radiographic characteristics to differentiate between endodontic and nonendodontic (normal and pathologic) radiolucencies and radiopacities.

6 / Describe the reasons for varying horizontal and vertical cone angulations on working radiographs to create image shift.

7 / Describe how to determine the third dimension on angled radiographs (i.e., facial-lingual structures [SLOB] rule).

8 / Describe structural elements of the tooth as visualized on both facial and angled projections.

9 / Discuss how to detect the presence and to locate undiscovered canals or roots on angled working radiographs.

10 / Describe techniques for making "working" radiographs (i.e., film placement and cone alignment with rubber dam in place).

11 / Describe specific details of film placement and cone alignment for each tooth on working radiographs.

12 / Describe the limitations of rapid processing of working films.

13 / Describe the radiographic technique for locating a "calcified" canal.

14 / Discuss the limitations of radiographic interpretation.

15 / Describe some new technologies and their application to endodontic radiography now and in the future.

OUTLINE

Importance of Radiography in Endodontics
Diagnosis
Treatment
Recall
Special Applications
Radiographic Sequence
Diagnostic Radiographs
Working Films
Obturation
Recall
Exposure Considerations
Cone-Image Shift
Principles
Indications and Advantages
Disadvantages
Endodontic Radiographic Anatomy
Interpretation
Limitations
Differential Diagnosis
Endodontic Pathosis
Nonendodontic Pathosis
Anatomic Structures
Special Techniques
Bitewing Projections
Film-Cone Placement
Rapid Processing
Viewers
New Technology

We are sick of the roentgen ray . . . you can see other people's bones with the naked eye, and also see through eight inches of solid wood. On the revolting indecency of this there is no need to dwell. But what we seriously put before the attention of the Government . . . that it will call for legislative restriction of the severest kind. Perhaps the best thing would be for all civilized nations to combine to burn all works on the roentgen rays, to execute all the discoverers, and to corner all the tungstate in the world and whelm it in the middle of the ocean.

EDITORIAL IN *PALL MALL GAZETTE*
LONDON, 1896

Obviously (and fortunately), the concern expressed by the editorial in this London publication did not become the popular view of radiography. Radiographs are essential; they are a second set of "eyes" for the dentist. This is particularly true in endodontics, in which so many diagnostic and treatment decisions are based on radiographic findings. Because most structures of concern are not visible to the naked eye, there is considerable dependence on radiographs, which are an obvious necessity and a blessing. But they also may be somewhat of a liability from the standpoint of both safety and time, and unfortunately they are often overinterpreted.

A radiographic exposure is an irreversible procedure, and therefore only necessary exposures are made. With the increasing emphasis and justifiable concern for radiation safety, overall radiation exposure must be minimized.[1] However, the amount of radiation dosage to oral and other tissues has been calculated to be very low and cause minimal (but some) risk.[2,3]

Another concern is the time required to make and process individual radiographs—time is money. Therefore, in the interests of both safety and time, only the radiographs necessitated by the procedure should be made.

This chapter will discuss radiography as applied to endodontic procedures. Radiography as a discipline in dentistry has increased in importance with advances in technology and has recently been granted specialty status, thereby replacing endodontics as the youngest dental specialty.[4] Technology has exploded in recent years, with new devices and approaches that require special training and experience. How these new devices and approaches apply to diagnosis and treatment in endodontics will be discussed later in this chapter.

Importance of Radiography in Endodontics

Radiographs perform essential functions in three areas. However, they have limitations that require special approaches. A single radiograph is but a two-dimensional shadow of a three-dimensional object. For maximum information, the third dimension must be visualized and interpreted.[5] The three general areas of application are diagnosis, treatment, and recall; each requires its own special approach.

DIAGNOSIS

Diagnostic radiology involves not only identifying the presence and nature of pathosis but also determining root and pulp anatomy and characterizing and differentiating other normal structures.

Identifying Pathosis: Radiographs must be studied carefully by someone with a working knowledge of the changes that indicate pulpal, periapical, periodontal, or other bony lesions. Many changes are obvious, but some are subtle.

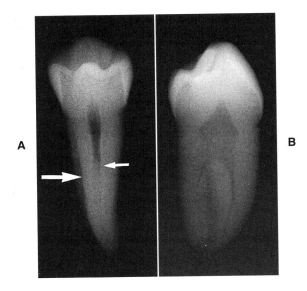

FIGURE 9-1

A, The facial projection of this premolar gives some limited information about pulp/root morphology. "Fast break" *(small arrow)* usually indicates canal bifurcation. A double root prominence on the mesial surface *(large arrow)* indicates two bulges and a concavity; its absence on the distal surface indicates a flat or convex root surface. **B,** The same premolar from the proximal view. The presence of two definitive canals, each in its own "root bulge," is confirmed.

Determining Root and Pulpal Anatomy: Determining the anatomy involves not only identifying and counting the roots and canals but also determining curvatures, canal relationships, and canal location.[6-8] Identification also involves characterizing the cross-sectional anatomy of individual roots and canals (Figure 9-1).

Characterizing Normal Structures: Numerous radiolucent and radiopaque structures often lie in close proximity. Frequently, these structures are superimposed over and obscure crowns and roots.[9] These must be distinguished and differentiated from pathosis and from dental anatomy.

TREATMENT

"Working" radiographs are made while the rubber dam is in place, creating problems in film placement and cone positioning. These radiographs are exposed *during* the treatment phase and have special applications.

Determining Working Lengths

Distance from a reference point to the radiographic apex is determined precisely. This establishes the distance from the apex at which the canal is to be prepared and obturated.[10]

Moving Superimposed Structures: Radiopaque anatomic structures often overlie and obscure roots and apexes. By using special cone angulations, these radiopaque structures can be "moved" to give a clear image of the apex.

Locating Canals: Canal location is obviously essential to success. Standard and special techniques allow the practitioner to determine the position of canals not located during access.

Differentiating Canals and Periodontal Ligament Spaces: Canals end in the chamber and at the apex. A periodontal ligament space ends on a surface and in a furcation (molars) and demonstrates an adjacent lamina dura (Figure 9-2).

Evaluating Obturation: Length, density, configuration, and the general quality of obturation in each canal are determined.

RECALL

Ultimate success is verified at specified intervals of months or years after treatment. Because failures often occur without signs or symptoms, radiographs are essential to evaluate periapical status.[11]

Identifying New Pathosis: The presence and nature of lesions that have arisen after treatment are best detected on radiographs. These lesions may be periapical, periodontal, or nonendodontic. Importantly, such lesions frequently present with no overt signs or symptoms and are detectable only on radiographs (Figure 9-3).

Evaluating Healing: Pretreatment lesions should be resolving or should have resolved. In a successful (healed) treatment, restitution of generally normal structures should be evident on recall radiographs (Figure 9-4).

SPECIAL APPLICATIONS

Radiographs should be used to their maximum advantage. There are alternative techniques that greatly enhance the ability to make an accurate and definitive diagnosis and to control treatment procedures. Although the techniques may be applied to disciplines other than endodontics, the following apply and are essential to diagnosis and treatment.

Cone-Image Shift: Varying either the vertical or, particularly, the horizontal cone angulation from parallel alters images and enhances interpretation.[5,12] These shifts reveal the third dimension and superimposed structures. Shifts also permit identification and positioning of objects that lie in the facial-lingual plane.

Working Films

Essential for aid in treatment, working films are exposed when necessary but with discretion.

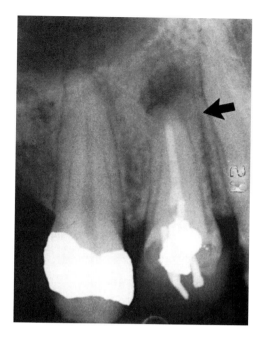

FIGURE 9-3
Failed root canal treatment because of missed root or canal. This mesial angled radiograph clearly shows the untreated lingual root *(arrow)*. (Courtesy Dr. L. Wilcox.)

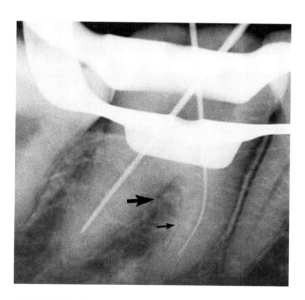

FIGURE 9-2
This distal angulation shows the root surface outline *(large arrow)* and a periodontal ligament space *(small arrow)* with an adjacent lamina dura. The file is in the mesiobuccal canal (same lingual, opposite buccal [SLOB] rule).

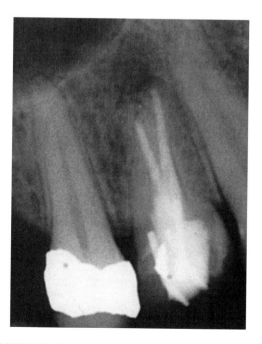

FIGURE 9-4
Same tooth as shown in Figure 9-3. Recall radiograph after 9 months shows almost complete regeneration of bone, indicating a healing lesion. A permanent restoration must be placed as soon as possible. (Courtesy Dr. L. Wilcox.)

Radiographic Sequence

Radiographs are made in a recommended order and number for each procedure. The minimum number are described here; special situations require extra exposures.

DIAGNOSTIC RADIOGRAPHS
Number

The number of exposures depends on the situation. For diagnosis in most cases, only a single exposure is necessary. A properly positioned film and cone (usually a parallel projection is best) permits visualization at least 3 to 4 mm beyond the apex. The initial diagnostic film is used primarily to detect pathosis and to provide general information on root and pulp anatomy. Usually it is not necessary at this time to make additional films for identification of extra canals; this will be accomplished later with shifted working length radiographs.

Frequently, several films are available for study, for example, if a full mouth survey has been taken. If other films are at hand, each will give a slightly different view of the same tooth (Figure 9-5). *Examine that tooth on each film in which it appears.*

Angulation

Unquestionably, the most accurate radiographs are made using a paralleling technique.[13] The advantages are, first, less distortion and more clarity and, second, reproducibility of film and cone placement with preliminary and subsequent radiographs. Reproducibility is important when assessing whether changes occurring in the periapex indicate healing or nonhealing. Paralleling devices enhance reproducibility.

There may be special situations in which the paralleling technique is not feasible, such as a low palatal vault, maxillary tori, exceptionally long roots, or an uncooperative or gagging patient; these may necessitate an alternative techniques. A second choice is the modified paralleling technique, and least accurate is the bisecting angle.

WORKING FILMS

Special situations require special considerations. Although the basic principles of doing everything possible to obtain the best quality radiograph are followed, there are definite limitations in making working films. These require cooperation by the patient if they hold the film in position.

These radiographs are usually neither parallel nor bisecting angle. The technique used is called *modified paralleling.*[14] Essentially, the film is not parallel to the tooth, but the central beam is oriented at right angles to the film surface. In endodontic working films, a further modification is made by varying the horizontal cone angle. Specific details of film and cone placement and film interpretation are discussed later in this chapter.

Working Length: Generally, establishment of working length should require only a single exposure. If a root contains or may contain two superimposed canals, either a mesial or distal angle projection is absolutely necessary; the straight facial view is not particularly helpful.[15] Additional working length films may be required later for confirmation of working lengths to detect the presence or lengths of newly discovered canals

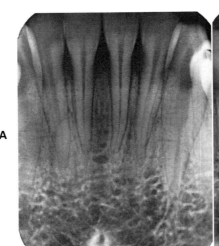
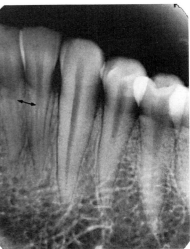

FIGURE 9-5
A, Facial projection of incisors suggests a single canal and a single root. **B,** Distal (canine) projection gives a different perspective. The canals of the lateral and central incisors are seen to bifurcate in the middle third of the root *(arrow)* and reunite in the apical third.

A

B

(Figure 9-6), or for reexposure if an apex has been cut off in the first radiograph.

Master Cone: The same principles used with working length films apply. With proper technique, only one radiograph is necessary to evaluate the length of the master gutta-percha cone.

Exposure and Film: As with diagnostic films, adequate clarity (and decreased exposure) is achieved by using an E film at intermediate kilovoltage.[16] Clarity is particularly important when trying to visualize the tips of files or small apexes to determine working lengths. The F film, very recently introduced, requires 20% to 25% less exposure than E film. There are no studies yet as to quality and usefulness of this new film type.

Other Considerations: Additional working films are often required. For example, they are useful as aids in locating a canal or in determining the occurrence of procedural accidents (perforations, separated instruments, or ledges). Varia-

tions in cone positioning and angulation are made as required.

OBTURATION

The same basic principles used for diagnostic radiographs apply. At least a parallel projection should be made. It may be desirable to supplement this with an angled film to visualize separate superimposed canals for separate evaluation of each. The exposure factors used for diagnostic radiographs are duplicated for obturation. However, the radiograph gives only a rough indication of obturation length and quality.[17,18]

RECALL

The same principles used for diagnostic and obturation radiographs (parallel projection and exposure factors) apply to recall radiographs. There

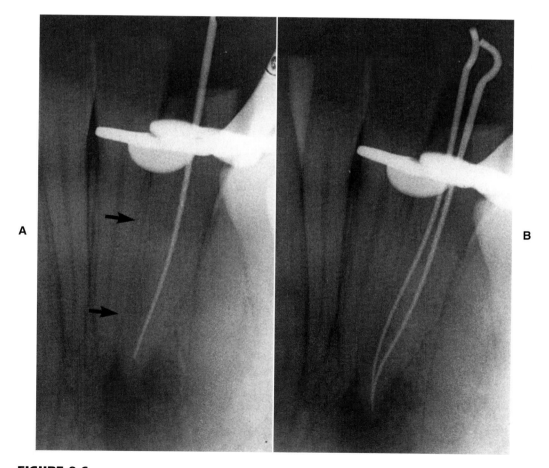

FIGURE 9-6
Identifying and locating a canal. This incisor was rotated, requiring mesially angled working radiographs. **A,** The file is off-center as indicated by the mesial root surface *(arrows)*. Therefore, the file is in the facial canal. **B,** A search to the lingual locates the lingual canal. There is a common canal apically.

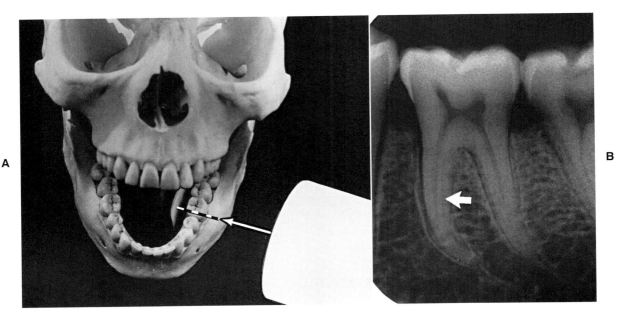

FIGURE 9-7
A, The film is positioned parallel to the plane of the arch. The cone has the central ray *(arrow)* directed toward the film at right angles. This is the basic cone-film relationship used for horizontal or vertical angulations. **B,** There is a clear outline of the first molar but limited information about superimposed structures (canals that lie in the buccolingual plane). The *arrow* points to a periodontal ligament space adjacent to a superimposed root bulge, not to a second canal. (From Walton R: *Dent Radiogr Photogr* 46:51, 1973.)

is one exception. If treatment is deemed to be questionable or a failure, additional angled radiographs are often required to search for a previously undetected canal or other abnormality.

Exposure Considerations

Proper x-ray machine settings and careful film processing are important for maximal quality and interpretative diagnostic and working radiographs. Both D (Ultraspeed) and E (Ektaspeed) films have been used and compared. Although D film has been shown to have slightly better contrast, overall suitability is equivalent between the two film types.[19] The newer Ektaspeed Plus film produces an image similar in quality to Ultraspeed film, but requires only half the radiation of Ultraspeed.[20]

The optimal setting for maximal contrast between radiopaque and radiolucent structures is 70 kV. Exposure time and milliamperage should be set individually on each machine. Therefore, the preferred film types are E and Ektaspeed Plus to minimize x-irradiation, at 70 kV to maximize clarity.

Cone-Image Shift

The cone-image shift reveals the third dimension.

PRINCIPLES
Image Shift

Superimposed Structures. The cone-image shift technique separates and identifies the facial and lingual structures.[5] An example is the mesiobuccal root of a maxillary molar that contains two superimposed canals. The cone shift separates and permits visualization of both canals.

Facial-Lingual Determination. Principles of relative movement of structures and film orientation are applied to the differentiation of object position (Figures 9-7 and 9-8).

SLOB Rule

As the cone position moves from parallel, whether toward the horizontal or toward the vertical, the objects on the film shift away from the direction of the cone (or in the direction of the central beam). In other words, when two objects and the film are in a fixed position and the radiation source (cone) is moved, images of both objects move in the opposite direction (Figure 9-9). The facial (buccal) object shifts farthest away; the lingual object shifts less. The resulting radiograph shows a lingual object that moved relatively in the same direction as the cone and a buccal object that moved in the opposite direction.[21] This prin-

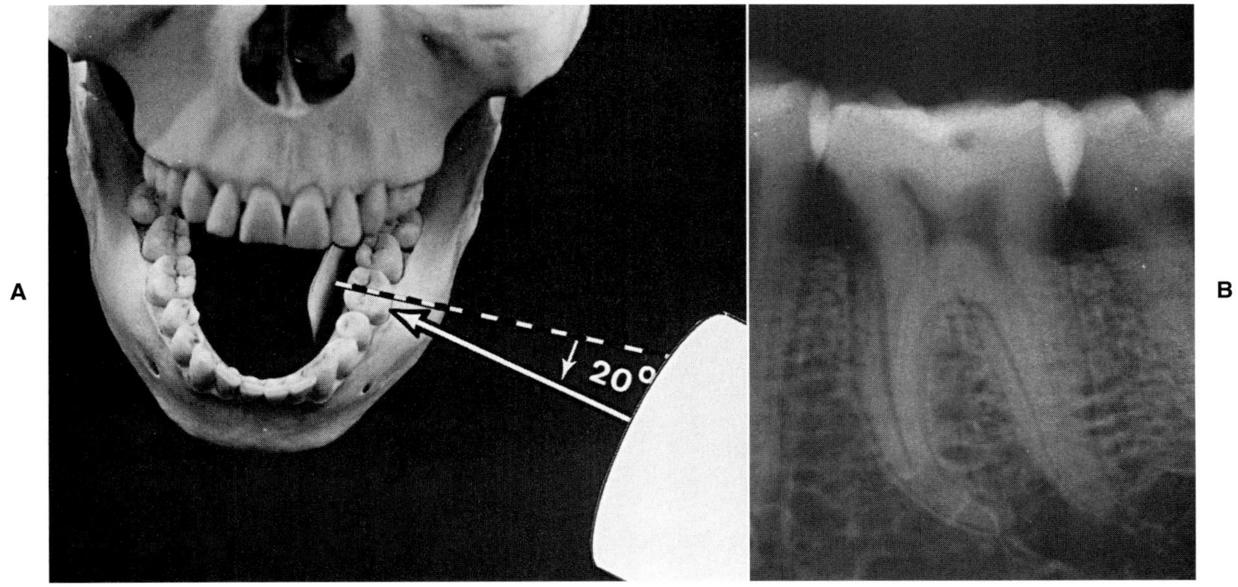

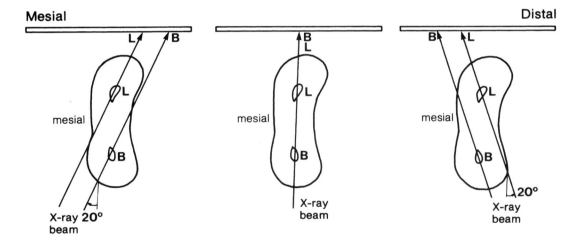

FIGURE 9-8
A, The horizontal angulation of the cone is 20 degrees mesial from the parallel, right angle position (mesial projection). **B,** The resultant radiograph demonstrates the morphologic features of the root or canal in the third dimension. For example, two canals are now visible in the distal root of the first molar. (From Walton R: *Dent Radiogr Photogr* 46:51, 1973.)

FIGURE 9-9
Central (x-ray) beam passing directly through a root containing two canals will superimpose the canals on the film. When the cone is shifted to the mesial or distal aspect, the lingual object will move in the same direction as the cone; the buccal object will move in the opposite direction (SLOB rule). (Courtesy Dr. A. Goerig.)

ciple is the origin of the acronym SLOB (same lingual, opposite buccal) (Figure 9-10).

One way to visualize this is to close one eye and hold two fingers directly in front of the open eye so that one finger is superimposed on the other. By moving the head one way and then the other, the position of the fingers relative to each other shifts.

The same effect is produced with two superimposed roots (the fingers) and the way in which they move relative to the radiation source (the eye) and the central beam (the line of sight). When the cone-shift technique is used, it is critical to determine what is facial and what is lingual. Otherwise, serious errors may occur.

INDICATIONS AND ADVANTAGES

Separation and Identification of Superimposed Canals: This is necessary in all teeth that may contain two canals lying in a faciolingual plane.

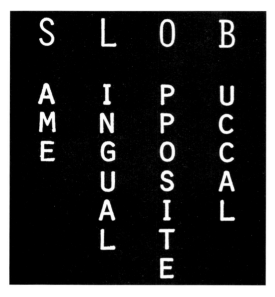

FIGURE 9-10
The SLOB rule.

Movement and Identification of Superimposed Structures: Occasionally, a radiopaque object may overlie a root. An example is the zygomatic process, which often obscures the apexes of maxillary molars.[7] Because this dense structure lies facial to the roots, a mesial shift of the cone "pushes" the zygoma distally (Figure 9-11). In addition, a decrease in vertical angulation of the cone "pushes" the zygoma superiorly.

Determination of Working Length: Individual superimposed canals may be traced from orifice to apex (Figure 9-12).

Determination of Curvatures: The SLOB rule applies. Depending on the direction of movement of the curvature relative to the cone, it can be determine whether this curvature is facial or lingual. The severity of the curvature can also be determined.

Determination of Facial-Lingual Locations: The SLOB principle is applied to locating something on a root surface or within a canal. One example might be the site of a perforation: to which surface does it extend, facial or lingual? Two radiographs at different horizontal angles readily disclose this (Figure 9-13).

Identification of Undiscovered Canals

The SLOB procedure applies during access. An anatomic axiom is that *if a root contains only a single*

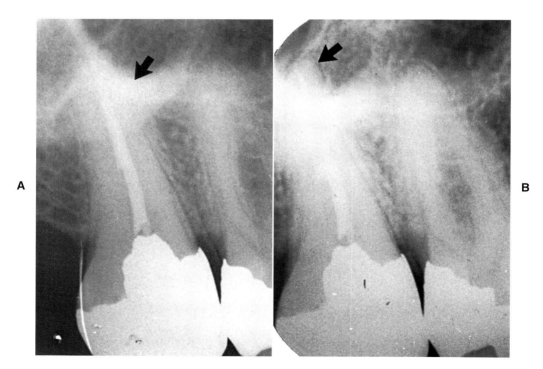

FIGURE 9-11
A, Malar process of maxillary zygoma *(arrow)* obscures the apex and blocks the view of the obturation. **B,** Slight mesial shift of the cone "pulls" the lingually positioned root apex *(arrow)* to the mesial for visibility.

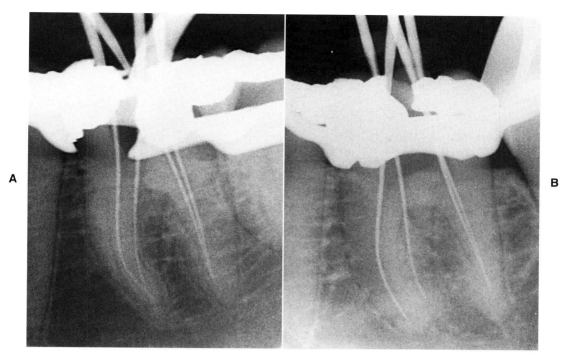

FIGURE 9-12
A, Mesial projection gives limited information about morphologic features and relationship of four canals. **B,** Correct distal projection for mandibular molars "opens up" roots. Mesial canals are easily visualized for their entire length. The distal canal is a single wide canal because instruments are close and parallel.

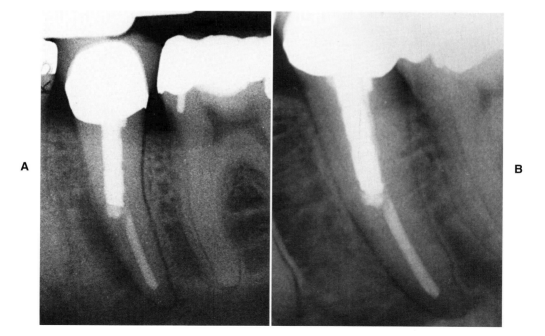

FIGURE 9-13
A, A perforation of the post preparation is indicated by the mesial lesion, although the perforation is not visible on this facial projection. The perforation will be visible toward the buccal or lingual aspect; this will be revealed on an additional angled radiograph. **B,** The tip of the post has moved slightly distal on this mesial projection; the perforation is therefore located toward the buccal aspect (SLOB rule).

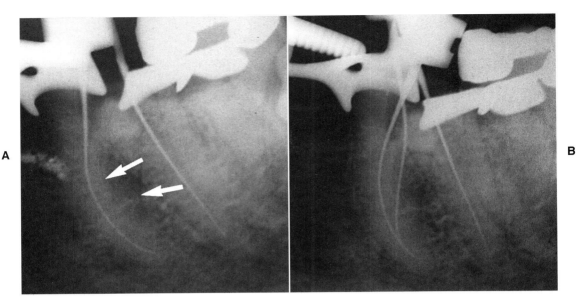

FIGURE 9-14
Technique for locating a canal missed during access preparation and searching of the chamber. **A,** Distal radiograph with a single file in the mesial root shows the file skewed buccally. Therefore, another canal would be located toward the lingual aspect. The vertical radiolucent lines *(arrows)* are periodontal ligament spaces of the mesial root. **B,** A careful search toward the lingual aspect reveals the canal.

canal, that canal will be positioned close to the center of the root. If a single canal is discovered initially on access preparation, an instrument is placed in the canal. Then a radiograph *must* be made either mesial or distal because another canal may be present. If the instrument is skewed considerably off center, another canal must be present (Figure 9-14). The location of the missed canal is determined by applying the SLOB rule.

Location of "Calcified" Canals: This procedure also applies during access preparation. Another endodontic anatomic axiom is that *a root always contains a canal.* The canal may be very tiny, or it may be difficult or impossible to find or negotiate, but it is present. Also, canals are frequently not visible on radiographs. A single canal will lie in the center of the root. Therefore, when searching for an elusive canal by penetrating progressively deeper with a bur, occasionally two working radiographs must be made. One is made from the straight facial view and the other from either the mesial or distal view. The straight facial radiograph gives the mesial-distal location of the bur penetration; the mesial or distal angled radiograph indicates the facial-lingual angulation of the bur. The direction is adjusted accordingly toward the center of the root where the canal surely lies (Figure 9-15).

DISADVANTAGES

The cone-image shift has inherent problems and therefore on occasion should not be used, or the angulation of the cone should be minimized.

Decreased Clarity: The clearest radiograph with the most definition is a parallel or modified parallel projection.[22] When the central beam changes direction relative to object and film (passing through the object and striking the film at an angle), the object becomes blurred. Distinctions between radiolucent and radiopaque objects show less contrast. This blurred or fuzzy appearance increases as the cone angle increases; other structures are more likely to be superimposed. Therefore, for maximum clarity, the cone angle should deviate only to the extent necessary to obtain sufficient shift for interpretive purposes.

Superimposition of Structures: Objects that ordinarily have a natural separation on parallel radiographs may, with cone shift, move relative to each other and become superimposed. One example is the roots of a maxillary molar. A parallel radiograph generally shows three separate roots and separate apexes. A mesial or distal angled radiograph moves the palatal root over the distobuccal or mesiobuccal root, decreasing the ability to distinguish the apexes clearly (Figure 9-16). Another example is an increase in the vertical angulation

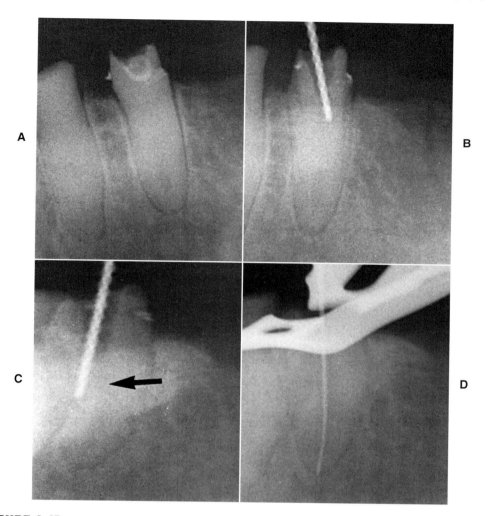

FIGURE 9-15
Location of a canal that has undergone severe calcific metamorphosis. Initial searching is done without a rubber dam. **A,** A small, receded canal and missing crown make orientation and canal search difficult. **B,** Facial radiograph taken during access shows that preparation is mesial to the canal. (Remember, the canal occupies the center of the root.) **C,** Mesial radiograph shows that access is also misdirected to the buccal aspect; the canal will be centered *(arrow)*. Therefore, the subsequent search must be to the distal and lingual aspects. **D,** On redirecting the bur, the single canal is discovered in the center of the root. Now the rubber dam is placed.

of the cone in the maxillary incisor region; this may "pull" the apexes "into" the radiodense anterior nasal spine.

Endodontic Radiographic Anatomy

INTERPRETATION

Radiographs can be termed "the great pretenders"—they often are as misleading as they are helpful.[23,24] There is a definite tendency to try to extract more information from a radiograph than is present. The practitioner must remember that only hard tissues, not soft tissues, are visible.

LIMITATIONS

Studies of interpretation of bony lesions have shown that considerable bone must be resorbed before the lesion is clearly visible.[25,26] This, of course, varies with root location and thickness of the overlying cortical bone. In most regions, a periradicular lesion tends to be most evident radiographically if cortical bone has resorbed.

A

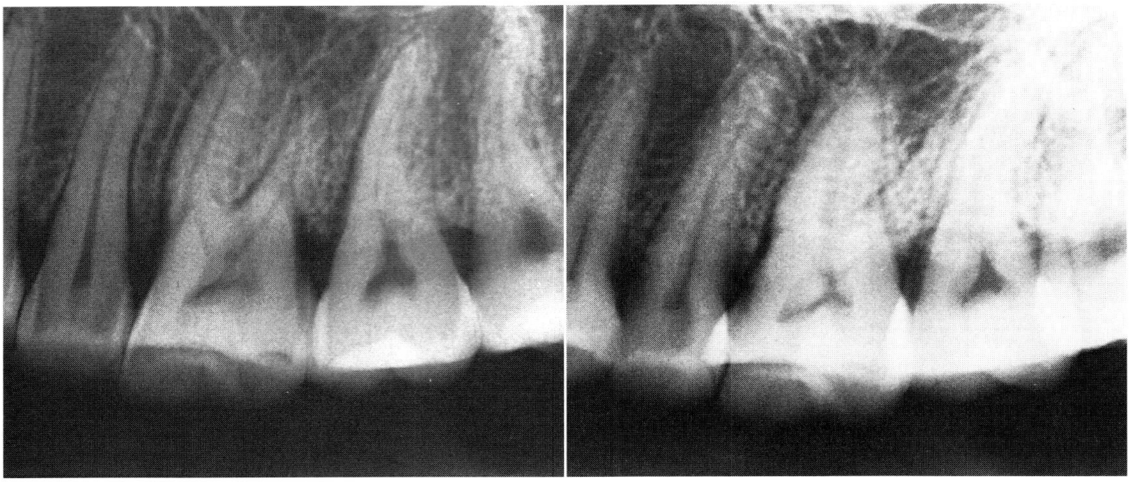

B

FIGURE 9-16
A, Facial parallel projection shows maximum clarity on the first molar. **B,** Mesial shift of 30 degrees reduces contrast and the distinction between radiopaque and radiolucent objects. Also, roots are now superimposed, making interpretation more difficult.

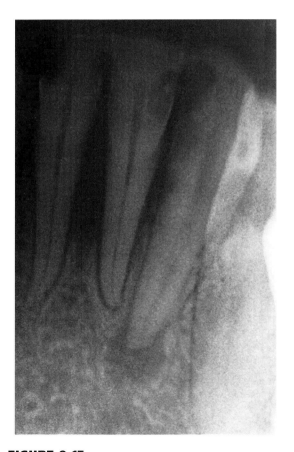

FIGURE 9-17
Characteristics of apical radiolucency strongly suggest endodontic pathosis. Lamina dura is not present, and the lesion has a "hanging drop of oil" appearance. The cause of pulpal necrosis is also evident.

However, resorption of only medullary bone may be sufficient for visualization.[27,28] In either case, a periradicular inflammatory lesion must be well developed and fairly extensive before an obvious radiolucency can be seen.

Differential Diagnosis
ENDODONTIC PATHOSIS
Radiolucent Lesions

These have four distinguishing characteristics that aid in differentiating them from nonendodontic pathoses (Figure 9-17):

1. Apical lamina dura is absent, having been resorbed.
2. A "hanging drop of oil" shape is characteristic of the radiolucency. This is a generalization because these lesions may have a variety of appearances.
3. The radiolucency "stays" at the apex regardless of cone angulation.
4. A cause of pulpal necrosis is usually (but not always) evident.

The ultimate differentiation is not the radiograph but the pulp test. If a developed, sizable radiolucency is an endodontic lesion, it *must* result from a necrotic (and therefore nonresponsive) pulp.

Radiopaque Lesions

These lesions are better known as condensing osteitis or, synonymously, focal sclerosing osteomy-

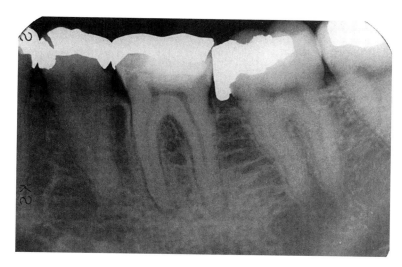

FIGURE 9-18
Condensing osteitis. There is diffuseness and a concentric arrangement of increased trabeculation around the apex. Close inspection shows a radiolucent lesion at the apexes also.

elitis. Such lesions have an opaque diffuse appearance; histologically they represent an increase in trabecular bone.[29] The radiographic pattern is one of diffuse borders and a roughly concentric arrangement around the apex (Figure 9-18). Pulpal necrosis and a radiolucent inflammatory lesion may or may not be present. Frequently, condensing osteitis and apical periodontitis are present together. The pulp is often vital and inflamed.

NONENDODONTIC PATHOSIS

Radiolucent Lesions: These are varied but infrequent. Bhaskar, in his oral pathology handbook,[30] lists 38 radiolucent lesions of the jaws, 35 of which are nonendodontic and have a variety of configurations and locations. Importantly, many are positioned at or close to the apexes and radiographically mimic endodontic pathosis. Again, the pulp test provides the cardinal differentiation—nonendodontic lesions are associated with a responsive tooth.

Radiopaque Lesions: Frequently interpretive errors are made in identifying radiopaque structures located in the apical region of the mandibular posterior teeth. Unlike condensing osteitis, these are not pathologic and have a more well-defined border and a homogeneous structure. They are not associated with pulpal pathosis (Figure 9-19).

ANATOMIC STRUCTURES

Several anatomic entities are superimposed on or may be confused with endodontic pathosis. Although most radiology courses cover identification of these structures, it is not uncommon for a practitioner to fail to identify these normal structures when there is an existing or suspected endodontic problem. Common sources of confusion are the

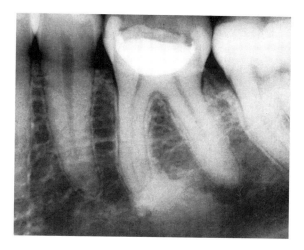

FIGURE 9-19
Enostosis (or sclerotic bone) is represented by the dense, homogeneous, defined radiopacity. This is not a pathosis and is common in the posterior mandible near the apexes, although it may occur in any region. This radiodense area would have appeared on earlier radiographs.

areas created by sparse trabecular patterns, particularly in the mandible. Another problem area is the apical region of the maxillary anterior teeth. One must remember to look *through* these radiolucencies for an apical lamina dura.

Mandible: The classic example of a radiolucency that may overlie an apex is the mental foramen over a mandibular premolar.[31] This is easily identified by noting movement on angled radiographs and by identifying the lamina dura (Figure 9-20).[32]

Maxilla: This region contains several structures (both radiolucent and radiopaque) that may be confused with endodontic pathosis. Examples are the maxillary sinus, incisive canals, nasal fossa,

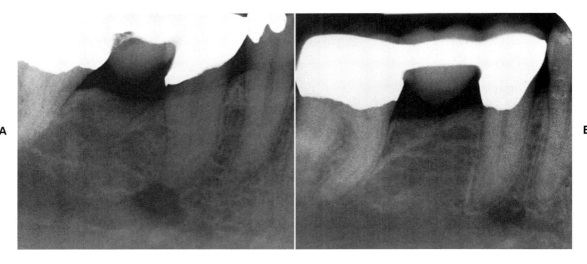

A

B

FIGURE 9-20
A, Radiolucent area over the apex could be mistaken for pathosis. **B,** Pulp testing (vital response) and a more distal angulation show the radiolucency to be a buccally placed (SLOB rule) mental foramen.

FIGURE 9-21
Bitewing radiograph shows important features clearly: relationship of bone to gingival extent of caries *(arrow)* as well as depth of caries and restorations relative to the pulp *(arrows).* (Courtesy Dr. C. Koloffon.)

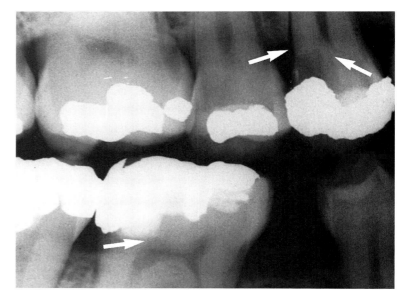

zygomatic process, and anterior nasal spine. Again, characteristics of the structure as well as pulp responsiveness to tests are important in differentiation.

Special Techniques

BITEWING PROJECTIONS

Although not truly a "special technique," bitewing projections are often helpful in diagnosis and treatment planning. The relationships of

film, cone, and tooth give a more consistent parallel orientation (Figure 9-21).

FILM-CONE PLACEMENT
Film Selection

Posterior packet film should be used for every projection in all patients except children. The anterior (narrow) films are unnecessary and in fact are frequently not wide enough to pick up an apex on an angled radiograph. Use of wider packet film obviously requires special placement for anterior pro-

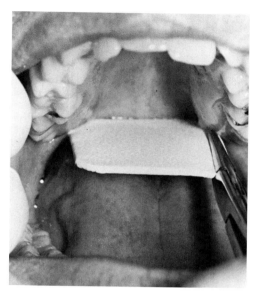

FIGURE 9-22
Narrow palate requires placement of posterior packet film distally. Note that the superior edge of the film is distal to the tuberosities.

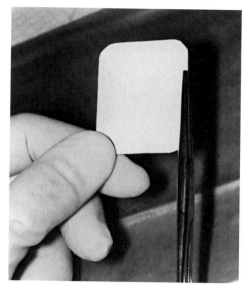

FIGURE 9-23
A hemostat is used for grasping the film and as a cone positioning ¬nd orientation device.

jections (Figure 9-22). The film type recommended for diagnostic radiographs is E (Ektaspeed) film.[16]

Film Holders

There are devices or special adaptations of paralleling devices that can be used for endodontic working films.[33] However, with some practice, nothing is more effective than a hemostat for ease and adaptability. The hemostat also is conveniently placed and sterilized in a kit with other instruments. The hemostat handle aligns the cone in both the vertical and horizontal planes (Figure 9-23). Having the patient hold the film with direct finger pressure is discouraged. This is awkward and frequently results in a bent film with a distorted radiographic image (Figure 9-24). The film surface must remain flat!

The hemostat-held film is placed by the operator. Then the patient holds the hemostat in the same position. The cone is aligned parallel to the hemostat in the frontal plane (vertical angulation) (Figure 9-25) and at 90 degrees to the handle (horizontal plane) (Figure 9-26). Because the handle is at an angle of 90 degrees to the film surface, the central beam strikes the film at the same 90-degree angle. This is the modified parallel technique because the film is often not parallel to the tooth. However, with the modified parallel technique, distortion is minimal and is not significant in working radiographs.[14]

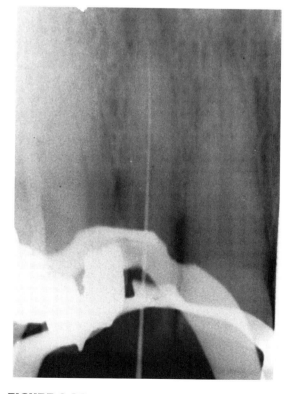

FIGURE 9-24
Pressure on film often causes bending, producing a distorted image. This bent film "stretches" the apical half of the root, making accurate interpretation and length determination impossible.

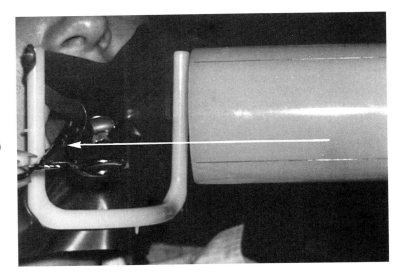

FIGURE 9-25
Vertical angulation of the cone is set by aligning the long axis of the cone *(arrow)* with the end of the hemostat handle.

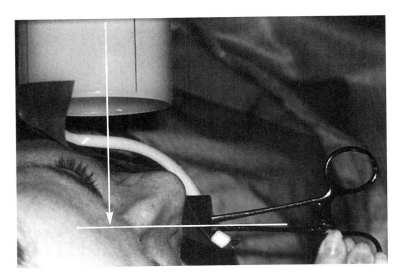

FIGURE 9-26
Horizontal angulation is determined by looking down from the top of the patient's head. The position is set by aligning the long axis of the cone (central beam) 90 degrees *(arrow)* to the long axis of the hemostat handle *(line)*. Mesial and distal horizontal angulations are then varied accordingly.

Film Placement

Usually films are positioned in the standard periapical projection. However, there are exceptions. Because of the film width and the relative narrowness of the arches, maxillary and mandibular anterior projections require film placement farther posteriorly.

In the maxillary posterior region, particularly when imaging molars, the film is placed on the side of the median raphe opposite the teeth to be radiographed. This has the effect of positioning the top of the film in a more superior position relative to the apexes (Figure 9-27).

In the mandibular posterior region, the film is positioned toward the midline (under the tongue). Also, if the mouth is closed slightly, the mylohyoid muscle relaxes and permits the film to drop inferiorly.

The rubber dam frame is not removed during film placement. A lower corner or edge of the rubber dam is released to allow insertion and positioning of hemostat and film (see Figure 9-25).

Cone Alignment

Indicated cone positions (Figures 9-28 and 9-29) (facial, mesial, or distal) are as follows.

Facial. Maxillary anterior teeth rarely have more than a single root and a single canal; only a facial (straight-on) projection is required. This is also true for maxillary molars unless a second mesiobuccal (mesiolingual) canal is detected and negotiated during access. The straight facial projection provides maximum resolution and clarity (which is difficult at best with maxillary molars).

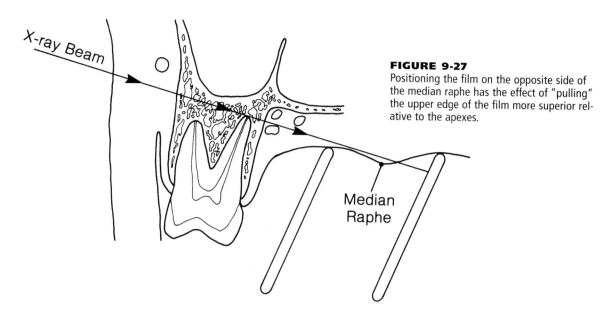

FIGURE 9-27
Positioning the film on the opposite side of the median raphe has the effect of "pulling" the upper edge of the film more superior relative to the apexes.

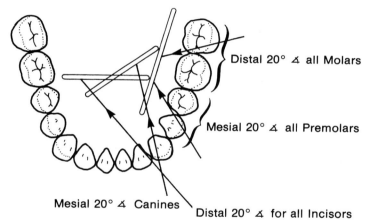

FIGURE 9-28
Correct film-cone placement on the mandible.

FIGURE 9-29
Correct film-cone placement on the maxilla.

Mesial. The mesial projection is indicated for maxillary and mandibular premolars and for mandibular canine teeth. A mesial projection is used for maxillary molars with a mesiolingual canal.

Distal. The distal projection is used for mandibular incisors and mandibular molars. The distal is preferred to the mesial projection for mandibular molars because of the relative position of the canals. Generally, the distal angle more effectively "opens up" the mesial root.

To summarize, angled working radiographs are made for maxillary premolar and molars with a mesiolingual canal and for all mandibular teeth. The maxillary projections are mesial and the mandibular projections are: incisor—distal; canine–mesial; premolar—mesial; and molar—distal. An acronym for the cone angles on the mandible is DMMD.

RAPID PROCESSING

Different techniques and special solutions are available for fast processing (less than 1 minute) of working films and may be of benefit for speed viewing. If these rapid processing techniques are used, films may not retain their quality with time unless they are thoroughly fixed and washed.[34] Therefore, if a film is to be processed rapidly, a double-packet film should be used, with the duplicate processed in the routine manner.

VIEWERS

There are several types of radiographic viewers, both commercial and adapted. Commercial view-ers magnify the image and block out peripheral light (Figure 9-30). This enhances the readability and interpretation of the film.[35] Other techniques or adaptations are also useful, such as a standard magnifying glass and small slide viewers.

New Technology

New approaches to radiography have been and are being developed. These are unique; some will improve existing techniques in addition to decreasing the radiation dose to patients. This new technology includes digital radiography, digital subtraction radiology, and tomography.[36-38]

These systems are of considerable interest, offering the advantages of reduced radiation to the patient, increased speed of obtaining the image, ability to be transmitted, computer storage and enhancement, and a system that does not require a darkroom or x-ray processor.[39] However, these systems generally show no superiority to conventional radiographs for diagnosis or for working films.[40-43] Furthermore, computer-image enhancement does not seem to improve diagnostic interpretation significantly.[44,45]

Ease of use and cost are factors that currently preclude routine use of these systems in the general dental office. Endodontists, however, require

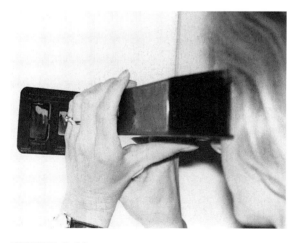

FIGURE 9-30
Magnifier-viewer blocks out peripheral light for better contrast. Contained within is a lens that magnifies the image four times.

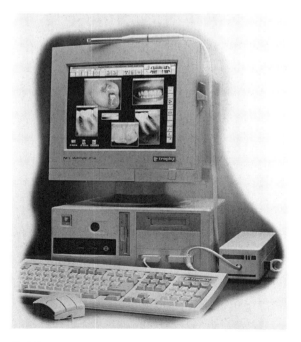

FIGURE 9-31
A digital imaging workstation for the dental operatory. The system integrates filmless digital images with an intraoral camera into a standard PC. (Courtesy Trophy USA.)

many working films and are finding the speed and versatility of digital radiography to be useful. As costs decrease and technology improves, there is no doubt that these or similar devices will come into more common usage by all groups of practitioners. This includes some very elaborate equipment that combines digital radiography and intraoral photography (Figure 9-31).

REFERENCES

1. Bengtsson G: Maxillo-facial aspects of radiation protection focused on recent research regarding critical organs, *Dentomaxillofac Radiol* 7:5, 1978.
2. Torabinejad M, Danforth R, Andrews K, Chan C: Absorbed radiation by various tissues during simulated endodontic radiography, *J Endod* 15:249, 1989.
3. Danforth R, Torabinejad M: Estimated radiation risks associated with endodontic radiography, *Endod Dent Traumatol* 6:21, 1990.
4. Berry J: Oral and maxillofacial radiology arrives; first new dental specialty in 36 years, *Am Dent Assoc News* 30:1, 1999.
5. Walton R: Endodontic radiographic techniques, *Dent Radiog Photog* 46:51, 1973.
6. Serman N, Hasselgren G: The radiographic incidence of multiple roots and canals in human mandibular premolars, *Int Endod J* 25:234, 1992.
7. Skidmore AE: The importance of preoperative radiographs and the determination of root canal configuration, *Quintessence Int* 10:55, 1979.
8. Sion A, Kaufman B, Kaffe I: The identification of double canals and double rooted anterior teeth by Walton's projection, *Quintessence Int* 15:747, 1984.
9. Tamse A, Kaffe I, Fishel D: Zygomatic arch interference with correct radiographic diagnosis in maxillary molar endodontics, *Oral Surg Oral Med Oral Pathol* 50:563, 1980.
10. Stein TJ, Corcoran JF: Radiographic "working length" revisited, *Oral Surg Oral Med Oral Pathol* 74:796, 1992.
11. Zakariasen K, Scott D, Jensen J: Endodontic recall radiographs: how reliable is our interpretation of endodontic success or failure and what factors affect our reliability? *Oral Surg Oral Med Oral Pathol* 57:343, 1984.
12. Slowey R: Radiographic aids in the detection of extra root canals, *Oral Surg Oral Med Oral Pathol* 37:762, 1974.
13. Bhakdinaronk A, Manson-Hing LR: Effect of radiographic technique upon prediction of tooth length in intraoral radiography, *Oral Surg Oral Med Oral Pathol* 51:100, 1981.
14. Forsberg J: Radiographic reproduction of endodontic "working length" comparing the paralleling and the bisecting-angle techniques, *Oral Surg Oral Med Oral Pathol* 64:353, 1987.
15. Klein R, Blake S, Nattress B, Hirschmann P: Evaluation of x-ray beam angulation for successful twin canal identification in mandibular incisors, *Int Endod J* 30:58, 1997.
16. Powell-Cullingford A, Pitt Ford T: The use of E-speed film for root canal length determination, *Int Endod J* 26:268, 1993.
17. Kersten H, Wesselink P, VanVelzen T: The diagnostic reliability of the buccal radiograph after root canal filling, *Int Endod J* 20:20, 1987.
18. Eckerbom M, Magnusson T: Evaluation of technical quality of endodontic treatment—reliability of intraoral radiographs, *Endod Dent Traumatol* 13:259, 1997.
19. Kleier D, Benner S, Averbach R: Two dental X-ray film compared for rater preference using endodontic views, *Oral Surg Oral Med Oral Pathol* 59:201, 1985.
20. Brown R, Hadley J, Chambers D: An evaluation of Ektaspeed Plus film versus Ultraspeed film for endodontic working length determination, *J Endod* 24:54, 1998.
21. Richards AG: The buccal object rule, *Dent Radiogr Photogr* 53:37, 1980.
22. Biggerstaff RH, Phillips JR: A quantitative comparison of paralleling long-cone and bisection-of-angle periapical radiography, *Oral Surg Oral Med Oral Pathol* 41:673, 1976.
23. Goldman M, Pearson AH, Darzenta N: Endodontic success—who's reading the radiograph? *Oral Surg Oral Med Oral Pathol* 33:432, 1972.
24. Reit C, Hollender L: Radiographic evaluation of endodontic therapy and the influence of observer variation, *Scand J Dent Res* 91:205, 1983.
25. Bender I, Seltzer S: Roentgenographic and direct observation of experimental lesions of bone, *J Am Dent Assoc* 62:153, 1961.
26. Schwartz S, Foster J: Roentgenographic interpretation of experimentally produced bony lesions. Part I, *Oral Surg Oral Med Oral Pathol* 32:606, 1971.
27. Pitt Ford T: The radiographic detection of periapical lesions in dogs, *Oral Surg Oral Med Oral Pathol* 57:662, 1984.
28. Lee S, Messer H: Radiographic appearance of artificially prepared periapical lesions confined to cancellous bone, *Int Endod J* 19:64, 1986.
29. Maixner D, Green T, Walton R, Leider A: Histologic examination of condensing osteitis, *J Endod* 18:196, 1992 (abstract).
30. Bhaskar SN: *Radiographic interpretation for the dentist*, ed 6, St Louis, 1981, Mosby.
31. Phillips JL, Weller RN, Kulild JC: The mental foramen: Part II. Radiographic position in relation to the mandibular second premolar, *J Endod* 18:271, 1992.
32. Fishel D, Buchner A, Hershkowith A, Kaffe I: Roentgenologic study of the mental foramen, *Oral Surg Oral Med Oral Pathol* 41:682, 1976.
33. Gound T, DuBois L, Biggs S: Factors that affect rate of retakes for endodontic treatment radiographs, *Oral Surg Oral Med Oral Pathol* 77:514, 1994.
34. Pestritto ST: Comparison of diagnostic quality of dental radiographs produced by five rapid processing techniques, *J Am Dent Assoc* 89:353, 1974.
35. Brynolf I: Improved viewing facilities for better roentgenodiagnosis, *Oral Surg Oral Med Oral Pathol* 32:808, 1971.
36. Hedrick R, Dove SB, Peters D, McDavid W: Radiographic determination of canal length: direct digital radiography versus conventional radiography, *J Endod* 20:320, 1994.
37. Pascon E, Introcaso J, Langeland K: Development of predictable periapical lesion monitored by subtraction radiography, *Endodont Dent Traumatol* 3:192, 1987.

38. Kullendorf B, Grondahl K, Rohlin M, Nilsson M: Subtraction radiology of interradicular bone lesions, *Acta Odontol Scand* 50:259, 1992.
39. Baker W, Loushine R, West L, et al: Interpretation of artificial and in vivo periapical bone lesions comparing conventional viewing versus a video conferencing system, *J Endod* 26: 39, 2000.
40. Borg E, Kallqvist A, Grondahl K, et al: Film and digital radiography for detection of simulated root resorption cavities, *Oral Surg Oral Med Oral Pathol* 86:110, 1998.
41. Holtzmann D, Johnson W, Southard T, et al: Storage-phosphor computed radiography versus film radiography in the detection of pathologic periradicular bone loss in cadavers, *Oral Surg Oral Med Oral Pathol* 86:90, 1998.
42. Sullivan J, Di Fiore P, Koerber A: RadioVisiography in the detection of periapical lesions, *J Endod* 26:32, 2000.
43. Burger C, Mork T, Hutter J, Micoll B: Direct digital radiography versus conventional radiography for estimation of canal length in curved canals, *J Endod* 25:260, 1999.
44. Kullendorff B, Petersson K, Rohlin M: Direct digital radiography for the detection of periapical bone lesions: a clinical study, *Endod Dent Traumatol* 13:183, 1997.
45. Scarfe W, Czerniejewski W, Farman A, et al: In vivo accuracy and reliability of color-coded image enhancements for the assessment of periradicular lesion dimensions, *Oral Surg Oral Med Oral Pathol Oral Radiol Endod* 88:603, 1999.

Endodontic Instruments

LEARNING OBJECTIVES

After reading this chapter, the student should be able to:

1 / Define a basic set of instruments appropriate for these procedures: diagnosis, emergency treatment, canal preparation, obturation, and bleaching.

2 / Describe the general physical properties of endodontic instruments and show how these characteristics are related to their use.

3 / Describe the design (longitudinal, cross-sectional, and tip configuration) of the more common canal preparation instruments and their mode of use.

4 / Explain the basis for sizing and taper (standardization) of hand-operated instruments.

5 / Describe proper use of instruments to prevent breakage within the canal.

6 / Recognize visible changes in instruments that will predispose to breakage.

7 / Describe techniques used for sterilization and disinfection of instruments.

8 / Select appropriate sterilization methods for each instrument type.

9 / Identify procedures and chemicals that might cause deterioration of files and how to recognize that deterioration.

10 / Describe and differentiate between conventional files and files of alternative designs.

11 / Define the differences between stainless steel and nickel titanium intracanal instruments including both physical properties and usage characteristics.

12 / Describe the action and use of rotary instruments for both cleaning and shaping canals.

| OUTLINE |

Physical Characteristics
Instrument Fabrication
Hand-Operated Instruments
Physical Properties
Standardization
Variations
Engine-Driven Instruments

Intracanal Usage
Hand Instruments
Rotary Instruments

Obturation
Lateral Condensation
Vertical Condensation

Adjunctive Instruments
Diagnostic Instruments
Instruments Unique to Root Canal Treatment

Sterilization and Disinfection
Sterilization
Disinfection

Instruments for Different Procedures
Examination
Cleaning and Shaping
Obturation
Emergency
Bleaching

I n considering endodontic instruments, those that are hand-operated (such as files and reamers) are the most important. However, other specialized instruments, such as explorers and excavators, have been designed to adapt to root canal treatment requirements. Originally, instruments for root canal treatment were few in number and crude in design.[1] The earliest hand-operated devices had long handles that were best suited for preparation of anterior teeth. As root canal treatment diversified, smaller "finger" instruments were developed for posterior teeth. In addition to being more adaptable, these provided improved tactile sense for the operator.[2] New designs in endodontic instruments have been introduced, and will continue to evolve.

This chapter reviews the types of metals used as well as important aspects of the physical properties and usage characteristics of endodontic instruments. A basic armamentarium will be described for each procedure as well as systems for effective sterilization. Detailed information about all aspects of manufacturing and testing of intracanal instruments is beyond the scope and intent of this chapter. However, certain essential facts, as identified in the learning objectives, will be presented to enable effective use (and not abuse) of these instruments.

The nomenclature follows the recommendations of the International Organization for Standardization (ISO):

1. *Hand-operated* include K-type reamers and files, broaches, Hedstrom-type files, and so on.
2. *Engine-driven* are hand types that have a latch that inserts into a slow-speed handpiece. These include rotary (Gates-Glidden and Peeso) engine-driven reamers and files and reciprocating files or reamers.
3. *Ultrasonic* and *sonic* are diverse in design. Some resemble barbed broaches, some resemble files, and others are diamond-coated wires. All insert into a dedicated vibratory handpiece that energizes the instrument. These are further described in Chapter 13.
4. *Nickel titanium has been adapted both for hand instruments and rotary applications.* Several designs have developed. Both hand- and engine-driven instruments have various configurations. The cross section of the instruments takes many shapes.

In addition to canal preparation, other hand-operated instruments are adapted for other aspects of root canal treatment, for example, canal identification and obturation.

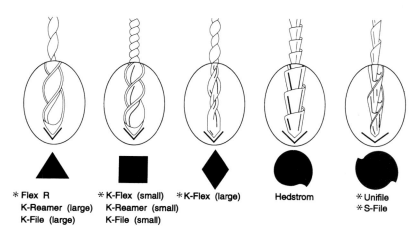

FIGURE 10-1
Longitudinal and cross-sectional shapes of various hand-operated instruments. (Those marked with an asterisk are brand names.) Note that small sizes of K-reamers, K-files, and K-Flex* have a different shape than the larger sizes.

*Flex R
K-Reamer (large)
K-File (large)

*K-Flex (small)
K-Reamer (small)
K-File (small)

*K-Flex (large)

Hedstrom

*Unifile
*S-File

Physical Characteristics

To débride a region of the canal space completely, the instrument must contact and plane all walls.[3] Despite continual improvements in design and physical properties, there are still no instruments that totally clean and shape all root canal spaces. Irregular canal spaces do not correspond to and cannot always be well prepared by an instrument with a regular (round) shape. In addition, stainless steel instruments are relatively inflexible, which renders them not particularly adaptable to canal curvatures. Nickel-titanium instruments are more flexible and adapt more readily to fine, curved canals[4] but have no advantage over stainless steel files in irregular canal spaces.[5-7] These incongruencies between reality and ideal shape require judicious and skillful use of canal preparation instruments to maximize débridement and to avoid procedural errors.

INSTRUMENT FABRICATION

A hand-operated reamer or file begins as a round wire that is modified to form a tapered instrument with cutting edges. The instrument is used with a twisting (reaming) or pulling (filing) motion in an attempt to produce clean, smooth, symmetrical canal walls. However, the prepared canal is rarely round when viewed in cross section.

Several factors inherent in the stainless steel wire that hand-operated instruments are made from have to be considered. How is adequate flexibility maintained without instrument fatigue? How much abuse can these files endure before fatigue and failure ensue? How does the operator know when the file has been fatigued to a critical point? And finally, how does an operator maintain an efficient cutting edge while at the same time avoid cutting new, nonanatomic canal spaces?

With nickel-titanium files, these same questions must be addressed. These instruments have different physical properties and different usage characteristics. Importantly, they can also fatigue and separate when used incorrectly or overused.

HAND-OPERATED INSTRUMENTS

Several cross-sectional shapes of files are commercially available (Figure 10-1). Two techniques for manufacturing these instruments have been developed.

Machined

This technique involves machining (grinding) the instrument directly on a lathe; an example is the Hedstrom-type file (Figure 10-2). All nickel-titanium instruments are machined.

Some manufacturers produce K-type files using the machined (lathe-grinding) process (Figure 10-3). This change from the grinding and twisting manufacturing process results in different physical and working properties from the original K-type file.[8,9] For instance, the machined file has less rotational resistance to breakage than a ground-twisted file of the same size.[9]

Ground-Twisted

Another technique consists of first grinding, then twisting. Raw wire is ground into tapered geometric blanks; (square, triangular, and rhomboid) (Figure 10-4). The blanks are then twisted counterclockwise to produce helical cutting edges. These are K-type files and reamers. K-type files have more twists per millimeter of length than the corresponding size of K-type reamer. Both have a pyramidal tip (75 $\pm$ 15 degrees) that is produced by grinding after twisting.

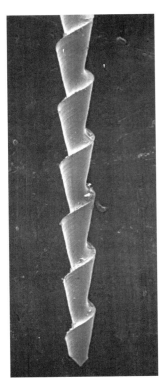

FIGURE 10-2
Hedstrom file, machined by rotating a wire on a lathe. Note the spiral shape. These are efficient cutters (on the pull stroke) but are more susceptible to separation when locked and twisted.

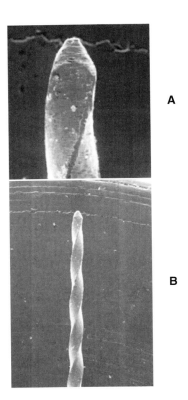

FIGURE 10-3
A and **B**, A machined K-type file. Note that the transition angle at the leading cutting edge of the tip is rounded, rendering it noncutting.

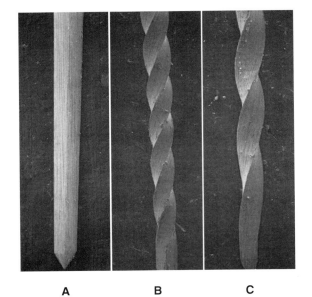

FIGURE 10-4
Ground-twisted instruments. **A**, A square file blank ground from wire. After twisting counterclockwise, the appearance of a file (more flutes) (**B**) and reamer (fewer flutes) (**C**).

Clinical Use

Besides their configuration, the difference between files and reamers is their intended use. Files are manipulated with a rasping, or push-pull planing, motion. This motion is more efficient when there are many flutes or spirals on the instrument shaft making contact with the canal walls; the flutes are at right angles to the long axis. Reamers are twisted and withdrawn; therefore, cutting takes place during rotation. This motion is most efficient with a cutting edge that more closely parallels the instrument shaft. Reamer configuration is created by imparting fewer twists, resulting in increased flute spacing; this tends to prevent clogging of the cutting edge.[10] Files can be both filed and reamed; reamers can only be reamed. Because they are less versatile, reamers are seldom used.

PHYSICAL PROPERTIES

Materials researchers and manufacturers have certain theories or hypotheses about file properties, such as "Flexibility is increased by increasing the length or decreasing the cross-sectional diameter" and "The more acute the cutting angle, the more efficient a blade is in removing a substance."[11,12] These theories are more applicable to the laboratory than to the clinical situation. Because of bench-top research, certain important limits to specific physical properties have been identified and incorporated into a series of standards for the manufacture of hand-operated instruments. However, clinical behavior may not directly relate to such in vitro testing.

Standards for K-type files and reamers were first published in 1976 as American Dental Association (ADA) specification No. 28.[13] These standards were developed specifically for hand-operated instruments used in the canal. Therefore, standards were established for *fracture resistance* by twisting, *stiffness* of the files and reamers, and *corrosion resistance*. In addition to physical characteristics, these standards established *dimensions* as well as acceptable tolerances in manufacturing.

Flexibility, sharpness, and corrosion resistance are properties related to metal and design. Traditional metals have included stainless or carbon steel. Compared to stainless steel, many carbon steel instruments have been shown to cut somewhat more efficiently[14]; they are similar in other respects. However, carbon steel is little used because it is more susceptible to corrosion by autoclaving and irrigating solutions.[15]

By changing the cross-sectional design from square to triangular or rhomboid and decreasing the number of flutes per millimeter, greater flexibility is gained. Blank nickel-titanium wire is even more flexible. Nickel-titanium alloy possesses a modulus of elasticity that is one-fourth to one-fifth that of stainless steel, allowing a wide range of elastic deformation.[16] An advantage of this increased flexibility is that a file follows the canal curvature with less deformation (transportation) during enlargement. A disadvantage of the increased flexibility is the inability to precurve the file for introduction into canals of posterior teeth when there is a decreased interocclusal opening. Another disadvantage is that cutting efficiency of nickel-titanium files may be reduced with clinical usage compared with stainless steel because of the greater elasticity. Therefore to best utilize the properties offered with nickel-titanium files, engine-driven configurations have been developed. All of the present nickel-titanium instruments incorporate a U shaped groove with a flat land area. When the instrument is rotated, the flutes will plane the canal wall while the land area keeps the instrument centered, primarily in fine, curved canals.

STANDARDIZATION

Original (conventional style) K-type files were available in only six sizes with no uniformity among different brands as to taper or tip configuration. ADA specification No. 28 established standards for instrument taper, tip geometry, and size criteria for 19 different sizes of instruments as well as acceptable tolerance of manufacturing error.[13] Also implemented was a color code for instrument handles for identification and an additional file size (No. 06).[17] In 1982, ADA specification No. 58 standardized and established the minimal physical criteria for Hedstrom files.[18] The most recent revisions of ADA specifications No. 28 and No. 58 were published in 1989. These further clarified minimal physical criteria and added newer criteria for plastic handle retention on files.[19] To date, no standards have been developed for nickel-titanium or the lathe-cut K-type instruments.

Despite specific size and shape requirements, hand-operated instruments do not demonstrate reliable and consistent dimensional standardization.[20]

Lengths

Files and reamers are available in three shaft lengths: 21, 25, and 31 mm. Shorter instruments afford improved operator control and easier access to posterior teeth, to which limited opening impairs access. The 25- and 31-mm instruments are used for longer roots.

Sizing

Dimensions of K-type files and reamers are designated according to the diameters of the instrument at specified positions along its length (as stated in ADA specification No. 289) (Figure 10-5). File tip diameters increase in 0.05-mm increments up to the size 60 file (0.60 mm at the tip), and then by 0.10-mm increments up to size 140. The diameter at the tip of the point is known as D_0. The spiral cutting edge of the instrument must be at least 16 mm long, and the diameter at this point is D_{16}. The file diameter increases at a rate of 0.02 mm per running millimeter of length.

Another "standard" introduced by one of the nickel-titanium rotary series (Profile) is a 29% constant increase in tip diameters between sizes; each file tip increases by a constant percentage rather than the random increases seen in ISO sizing.

The nickel titanium rotary instruments have other variable tapers of 0.04 and 0.06. For every millimeter of length, the diameter increases by 0.04 or 0.06 mm. These greater tapers make these more aggressive in creating marked flaring preparation.

Tip Design

Originally the tip angle of K-type files and reamers was approximately 75 degrees plus or minus

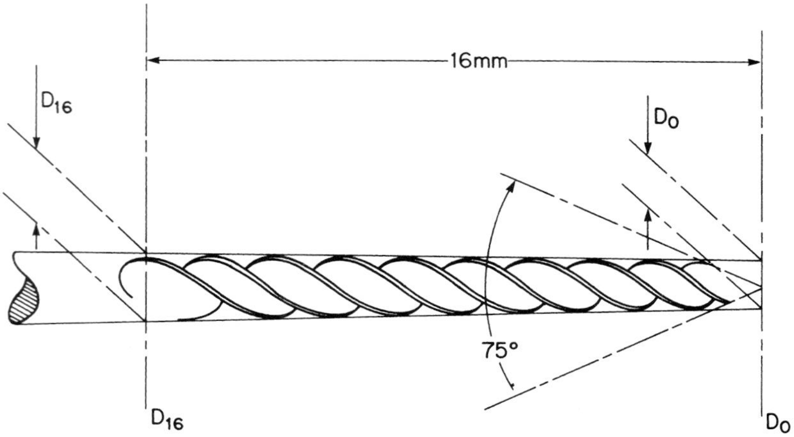

FIGURE 10-5
The specifications for standardization of files and reamers.

15 degrees (see Figure 10-1). This design was intended to provide cutting efficiency without an excessively sharp transition angle. Newer designs have different tip angles and designs in an attempt to minimize canal alterations. Some machined K-files incorporate a so-called nonaggressive tip or noncutting tip (see Figure 10-3) to provide less dentin cutting by reducing the sharp tip transition angle. The flexible file type (Flex-R) has a conical noncutting file tip with a tip angle of 70 degrees and a guiding collar angle of 35 degrees. The intent is to guide the file through the curve rather than cutting only the outer canal wall.[21,22]

Another modification in file design is the Lightspeed. Unlike other instruments that have several millimeters of cutting or planing area, this nickel-titanium instrument has a cutting area of about 3 mm. The tip is noncutting and looks similar to a small Gates-Glidden drill. (A further description of the Lightspeed instrument is found under "Unique Designs").

Torsional Limits

Torsional limit is the amount of rotational torque that can be applied to a "locked" instrument to the point of breakage (separation). Obviously, an instrument should have sufficient strength to be rotated and worked vigorously without separating in the canal. Standards for steel hand-preparation instruments were established for rotational limits (point of breakage) at various forces. Smaller instruments (less than size 20) can withstand more rotations without breaking than larger (greater than size 40) instruments.

Machined K-type files have different physical and working properties than ground-twisted files. There is no difference in torsional strength between ground-twisted and machined files. However, machined files are weaker, demonstrating

less plastic deformation before failure occurs.[8] Therefore, this tendency toward less visible deformation before separation requires more caution with the use of machined files to avoid instrument failure.[9]

Under test conditions, the nickel-titanium files (all are machined) have increased resistance to fracture compared with stainless steel files.[23] Only Lightspeed instruments have incorporated a designated separation point at 18 mm to allow for retrieval of broken instruments. The ADA and ISO are presently working on new torsional[24] standards for all nickel-titanium and stainless steel rotary instruments.[24] Nickel titanium metal may have advantages over stainless steel, although these advantages have not been conclusively demonstrated in clinical usage or in clinical trials.[6,16]

Color Coding

Color coding of file handles designates size. Color coding of the newer nontraditional instruments varies according to the manufacturer.

VARIATIONS

Broaches: Barbed broaches are stainless steel instruments with plastic handles. The tapered wire broach is barbed by scoring and prying a tag of metal away from the long axis of the wire (Figure 10-6). Barbs entangle and remove canal contents. This instrument should be neither bound in the canal nor aggressively forced around a canal curvature. Either action may cause the barbs to engage the canal wall, preventing the broach from being removed intact or fracturing. Barbed broaches should not be reused. Single barbed broaches are available in presterilized bubble packaging.

Unique Designs: An innovative nickel-titanium instrument, the Lightspeed (Figure 10-7), has been

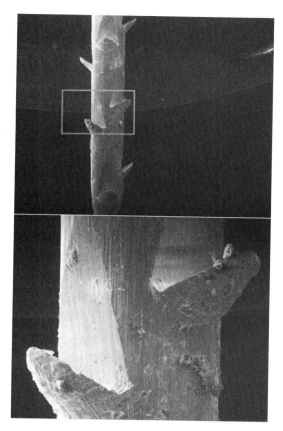

FIGURE 10-6
Barbed broach showing the barbs pulled away from the instrument shaft.

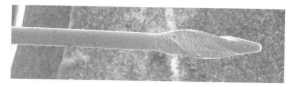

FIGURE 10-7
Innovative file design of the rotary nickel-titanium Lightspeed instrument. The end of the instrument does the work; the noncutting tip and the small flexible shaft tend to stay centered during preparation of the canal.

recently introduced that incorporates three distinct features: a noncutting pilot tip, a small fluted area, and a small flexible shaft. Both hand-operated and engine-driven instruments are available. These instruments tend to stay centered in curved canals if used properly.[25] Although interesting, these have not been shown to be superior to conventional hand instruments and are prone to separation if overused.[26,27]

ENGINE-DRIVEN INSTRUMENTS

Rotary Instruments: Some preparation techniques require slow-speed rotary instruments to facilitate preparation, primarily in establishing straight-line access (Figure 10-8), although engine-driven reamers and files for cleaning and shaping are also marketed. Most common are Gates-Glidden drills and Peeso reamers. Table 10-1 shows the comparative ISO sizes of both Gates-Glidden drills and Peeso reamers.

Gates-Glidden drills and Peeso reamers are made from either carbon or stainless steel. Carbon

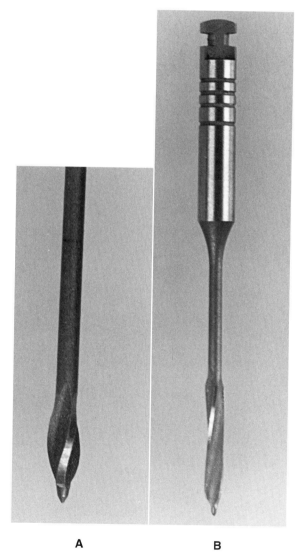

A   B

FIGURE 10-8
A, Gates-Glidden drill. Note the noncutting tip and the elliptical shape. **B,** Peeso reamer. Note the noncutting "safe" tip and parallel sides. These are stiffer and more aggressive than the Gates-Glidden drill. Both can be used for straight-line access preparation.

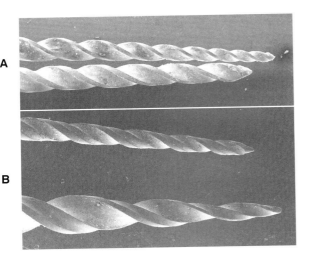

FIGURE 10-9
Nickel-titanium rotary files of varying design. **A,** 0.04 and greater tape (GT) titanium files (Profile). **B,** Quantec files by Analytic; note the aggressive taper of the file on the bottom.

TABLE 10-1		

Rotary Flaring Instruments

SIZE	GATES-GLIDDEN DRILLS	PEESO REAMERS
No. 1	0.4 mm	0.7 mm
No. 2	0.6 mm	0.9 mm
No. 3	0.8 mm	1.1 mm
No. 4	1.0 mm	1.3 mm
No. 5	1.2 mm	1.5 mm
No. 6	1.4 mm	1.7 mm

steel has inferior properties, particularly less strength, and therefore should not be used. Corrosion is not a problem with stainless steel, but dulling occurs with sterilization procedures and repeated usage.

Gates-Glidden Drills: These drills are elliptically (flame) shaped burs with a latch attachment. Gates-Glidden drills are used to open the orifice. They also achieve straight-line access by removing the dentin shelf and rapidly flaring the coronal and middle third of the canal.

Gates-Glidden drills are designed to break high in the shank region. This allows easier removal of the broken instrument from a tooth; fracture near the cutting head may block a canal. No ADA specification exists for torsional failure of rotary intracanal instruments, but Gates-Glidden devices usually do fracture where intended.[28,29] Importantly, these drills must be continuously rotated. If they stop, the head may lock in the canal, with torsional failure and fracture. Gates-Glidden drills are available in 15-and 19-mm lengths. The shorter instruments are helpful in posterior teeth, where access to the canal orifice is limited.

Peeso Reamers: These reamers are also used as adjunctive devices in canal preparation. They are basically similar to Gates-Glidden drills but have parallel cutting sides rather than an elliptical shape. These instruments are available with or without safe tips. Peeso reamers have been suggested as a means of improving straight-line access, although they are less well controlled than Gates-Glidden drills.[30] Both types are aggressive and can rapidly overenlarge the canal.

Engine-Driven Reamers: These instruments are used for cleaning and shaping. The traditional types are of stainless steel. Because of their relative stiffness, they are difficult to control and generally create irregular, poorly débrided preparations, particularly in curved canals. These aggressive instruments also generate large amounts of debris, which packs apically. Their use is not recommended.

Engine-Driven Nickel-Titanium Files: Nickel-titanium engine-driven files allow greater control in tiny, curved canals. These instruments do not have a cutting end and have less tendency to transport the apical preparation.[31,32] The files are available in a variety of shapes and designs (Figure 10-9). Utilization of these instruments by dental students in technique laboratories have demonstrated fewer preparation errors than with use of stainless steel instruments in the same courses.[33-35]

Intracanal Usage

HAND INSTRUMENTS

Broaches: Removal of pulp requires a broach that will not bind and yet is large enough to ensnare the tissue. Binding should be minimized because of possible breakage.

Reamers and Files: Two types of motion (Figure 10-10) are common in root canal preparation, reaming and filing.[36] Reaming consists of rotating the instrument clockwise and scribing an arc from one cutting edge to the next. For example, a triangular reamer has three 60-degree cutting edges and therefore requires 120 degrees of rotation (one-third of a turn), whereas a file with a 90-degree angle necessitates only a quarter turn before withdrawal. Rhomboidal files require a 180-degree turn to make an edge-to-edge arc.

Filing requires a series of repetitive motions. First, the instrument is advanced to its full

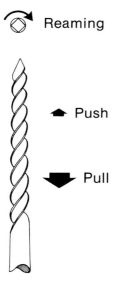

Reaming

← Push

← Pull

FIGURE 10-10
Filing and reaming motions. Tooth structure is removed primarily on the pull stroke with filing and on rotation with reaming.

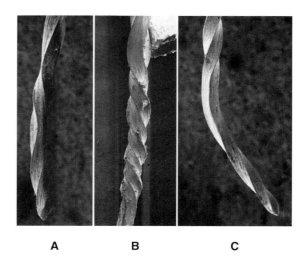

A   B   C

FIGURE 10-11
Defects created during instrumentation. Each file shown must be discarded because of possible breakage. **A,** Unwinding of the flutes. **B,** "Roll-up" of the flutes. **C,** Unwound and bent instrument.

length into the canal space using a passive "twiddling" (teasing without planing) motion. Next, the file is rotated (a quarter turn or more) and then withdrawn from the canal space while the tip is pushed against a canal wall, much as a paintbrush is applied to a wall when painting. The twiddling, reaming, and withdrawal motions are repeated with the file tip pushed against a different portion of the canal wall on each outstroke until all walls have been planed (circumferential filing).

Hedstrom and similar design (S or U) files are used only with a filing motion because they have less torsional resistance to breakage. In other words, Hedstrom-type files are more prone to separation because of the decreased cross-sectional diameter of equivalent-sized instruments. Also, their design does not facilitate reaming.

Avoidance of Instrument Separation: Separation of hand files in the canal is prevented by regularly inspecting the instrument for defects (Figure 10-11) such as (1) unwinding of the flutes (twisting clockwise and opening of the flutes); (2) roll-up of the flutes (excessive continued clockwise twisting after unwinding); (3) tip distortion (the tip has been bent excessively); and (4) corrosion. If an instrument exhibits *any* signs of wear, it should be discarded immediately. Prevention is the key to avoiding untimely instrument separation.

ROTARY INSTRUMENTS

All of the engine-driven nickel-titanium files rely on rotational motion only and therefore have a reaming action.

Avoidance of Instrument Separation

The manufacturer of the nickel-titanium 0.04 and 0.06 mm taper rotary files suggest using them in high-torque slow-speed handpieces that rotate at 150 to 300 rpm. The number of canals that can be prepared with a nickel-titanium instrument varies from 4 to 16, depending on the size and curvature of the canals and pressure used with the files. The smaller and more curved the canal, the more wear and tear on the instrument. All manufacturers suggest discarding the files if any deformation occurs. Recent studies have suggested that lower speeds reduce the likelihood of instrument fracture.[37-39] Figure 10-12 shows instrument fatigue and "roll-up" and breakage of nickel-titanium instruments after use in canals.

The Lightspeed nickel-titanium instruments are also used in high-torque slow-speed handpieces at 750 to 2000 rpm. Within this limit, faster rotational speed does not appear to increase the likelihood of fracture.[40] The manufacturer suggests discarding each file after 10 uses.

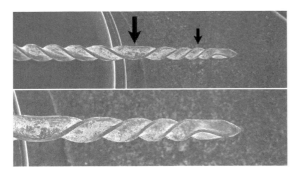

FIGURE 10-12
Overused rotary nickel-titanium files exhibiting "roll-up" *(small arrow),* and "unwinding" *(large arrow).*

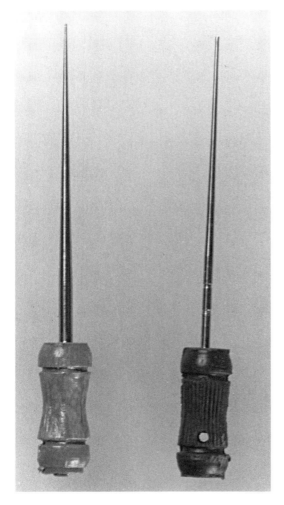

FIGURE 10-13
Fine finger spreader *(left)* and fine finger plugger *(right).* Both are used similarly for lateral condensation. Spreaders are pointed and pluggers are flat at the tip.

Obturation

Several filling techniques are available. The instruments used for the two most practiced techniques, lateral and vertical condensation, are described here.

LATERAL CONDENSATION

The instruments used for lateral condensation are spreaders and small pluggers (Figure 10-13). They are used for condensing and adapting gutta-percha and creating space for accessory cones. They are either handled, having a shank attached to a metal handle, or finger-type, having only a plastic handle (Figure 10-14). The handled instruments are stiff because they are generally made of annealed stainless steel. Finger spreaders and pluggers are not annealed and therefore are dead soft, giving them more flexibility. Handled instruments do not negotiate curved canals. Finger spreaders and pluggers are best suited for obturating curved canals.

Finger spreaders and pluggers have different tips (see Figure 10-13). Pluggers are flat, whereas spreaders are pointed. Finger spreaders and pluggers behave similarly and are used interchangeably in lateral condensation.

The taper of spreaders varies among instruments. Highly tapered spreaders increase in diameter at a greater rate than do standardized instruments, which increase 0.02 mm per mm of length. The greater the taper, the more the canal space

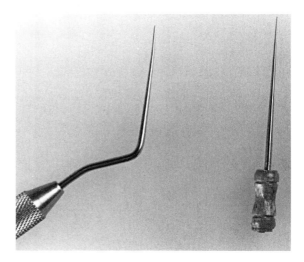

FIGURE 10-14
D11 handled spreader *(left)* and a fine finger spreader *(right).* Both are designed for lateral condensation. The finger spreader (or plugger) is more versatile and safer.

must be enlarged or flared to facilitate spreader penetration.

Both stainless steel and nickel-titanium spreaders are available. The obvious advantage of nickel-titanium spreaders over stainless steel spreaders is greater spreader penetration in highly curved canals.[41] Nickel-titanium spreaders also create less stress in curved canals compared with stainless steel spreaders.[42] The disadvantage of nickel-titanium spreader is the inability to pre-curve it for patients with limited interocclusal space.

VERTICAL CONDENSATION

In this obturation technique the filling material is alternately softened (with heat) and then vertically compacted with pluggers. The softened gutta-percha filling material is pushed into the interstices of the canal, but this technique offers less apical control of the material than lateral condensation.

Vertical condensation instruments can be divided into two categories: those that are heated to transfer heat to the gutta-percha, and those that condense the gutta-percha (pluggers) (Figure 10-15). Heat transfer instruments have handles, as do most pluggers. Finger pluggers may be used in lieu of handled instruments in small curved canals.

Adjunctive Instruments

DIAGNOSTIC INSTRUMENTS

The conventional explorer, periodontal probe, and mouth mirror are pulpal, periradicular, and periodontal diagnostic aids that have special endodontic applications (Figure 10-16).

INSTRUMENTS UNIQUE TO ROOT CANAL TREATMENT

Explorers are double-ended instruments with long tapered tines at either a right or an obtuse angle. This design facilitates the location of canal orifices. They are very stiff and should not be inserted into canals or used for condensing gutta-percha. Explorers should never be heated.

The *spoon excavator* is another long-shank instrument. The excavator is used to remove caries, deep temporary cement, or coronal pulp tissue. The endodontic excavator has a right or left orientation similar to that of operative hand excavators.

The *Glick No. 1* instrument is used for placement of temporary restorations with the paddle end and removal (and then condensation) of excess gutta-percha with the heated plugger end.

The rod-shaped plugger is graduated in 5-mm increments.

Lentulo spiral drills are twisted wire instruments used in the slow-speed handpiece (Figure 10-17). They have been used to spin pastes, sealer, cements, or calcium hydroxide into the canal. They must be used with care to avoid "throwing" quantities of unset material out of the apex. In fact, there is no reason to use lentulo drills other than

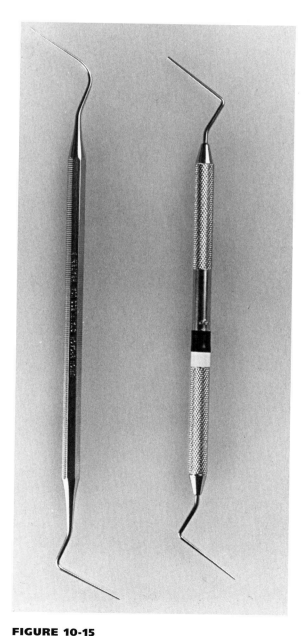

FIGURE 10-15
Heat transfer *(left)* and condenser (heater-plugger) *(right)* for vertical condensation of gutta-percha.

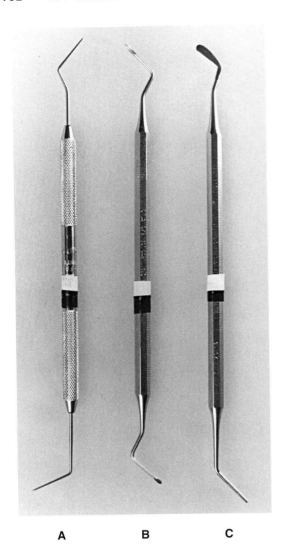

A   **B**   **C**

FIGURE 10-16
Specialized endodontic instruments. **A,** D16 explorer. **B,** 31L spoon excavator. **C,** Glick No. 1. The plugger end *(bottom)* is for heating and removal of gutta-percha; the paddle *(top)* is for placing temporary materials.

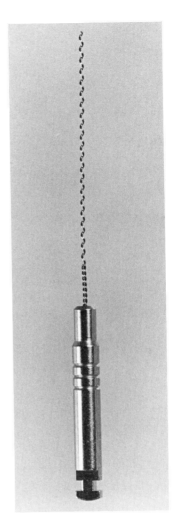

FIGURE 10-17
Lentulo spiral drill is used to spin calcium hydroxide into canals.

to place calcium hydroxide paste. The drill must be rotated so that it will not "screw" itself into the canal; they may lock and separate.

Sterilization and Disinfection

Endodontic instruments are contaminated with blood, soft and hard tissue remnants, and bacteria and bacterial byproducts. Thus they must be cleaned often and disinfected during the procedure and then sterilized. Also, because the instruments may be contaminated when new, they must

be sterilized before initial use. Different techniques are available.

Small kits such as those used for examination may conveniently be bagged, sterilized, and stored in the package until needed. Larger kits for treatment may be more rapidly and easily handled in cassettes for sterilization and storage.

STERILIZATION

Cold- or heat-labile instruments such as some rubber dam frames may be immersed for a sufficiently long period of time in solutions such as glutaraldehyde. Generally, 24 hours are required to achieve cold sterilization. Immersion may be effective for disinfection but will fail to kill all organisms. Because this method of sterilization is not presently verifiable with biologic indicators, it is least desirable in the office and should be reserved for instruments that cannot withstand heat.

Pressure Sterilization

A common method of sterilizing all files and common hand instruments is the steam or chemical autoclave. Instruments that have been wrapped in gauze should be autoclaved for 20 minutes at 121° C and 15 psi.[43] This will kill all bacteria, spores, and viruses. Various sodium nitrite dips will retard rust. These "milk baths" help spare the carbon steel Gates-Glidden drills.

Pressure sterilizers using a chemical rather than water have the advantage of causing less rusting. However, both steam and chemical autoclaving will dull the edges of all cutting instruments owing to expansion with heat and contraction with cooling, resulting in permanent edge deformation.

Dry Heat Sterilization

Dry heat is superior for sterilizing sharp-edged instruments such as scissors to best preserve their cutting edge. The time cycle for dry heat sterilization is temperature dependent. After the temperature reaches 160° C, the instruments should be left undisturbed for 60 minutes. The disadvantage of this method is the substantial time required, both for sterilization and subsequently for cooling. If the temperature falls below 160° C, the full 60-minute heat cycle must be repeated.[43]

DISINFECTION

Surface disinfection during canal débridement is accomplished by using a banker's sponge soaked in 70% isopropyl alcohol or proprietary quaternary ammonium solutions. Files can be thrust briskly in and out of this sponge to dislodge debris and contact the disinfectant. This procedure cleans but does not sterilize the instrument.

Instruments for Different Procedures

EXAMINATION

A kit for examination and diagnosis includes (1) a front surface mouth mirror, (2) a periodontal probe, (3) an explorer, such as the double-ended No. 5 explorer, and (4) cotton forceps.

CLEANING AND SHAPING

Instruments used for access and cleaning and shaping include (1) a 5- to 6-ml Luer-Lok syringe with a 27-gauge needle, (2) locking cotton pliers, (3) rotary instruments (Gates-Glidden drills), (4) a plastic instrument (Glick No. 1) for temporary placement, (5) broaches and files, (6) a lentulo spiral drill; and 7) a millimeter rule.

OBTURATION

Instruments used for obturation include (1) spreaders or pluggers, (2) Glick No.1 for heat transfer and temporary placement, (3) locking cotton pliers, and (4) 5/7 plugger or pluggers used for vertical condensation.

EMERGENCY

The instruments necessary for emergency treatment are dictated by the diagnosis. For instance, irreversible pulpitis requires pulpotomy or pulpectomy. An acute apical abscess may require incision and drainage.

Basic instrumentation for most emergency procedures includes (1) an examination kit, (2) an anesthetic armamentarium, (3) canal preparation (cleaning and shaping) system, and (4) occasionally, an incision for drainage kit. Incision and drainage instruments include (1) scalpel handle and blade; (2) periosteal elevator; (3) rubber dam drain; (4) needle holder; and (5) irrigating syringe with an 18-gauge needle, sterile saline, and suction tip.

BLEACHING

Bleaching usually is done with the instruments included with the cleaning and shaping tray. A walking bleach technique requires only the plastic instrument to place the sodium perborate mixture in the chamber and then to temporize.

REFERENCES

1. Weinberger B: *An introduction to the history of dentistry,* St Louis, 1948, Mosby.
2. Luks S: The myth of standardized instruments, *NY J Dent* 43:109, 1973.
3. Walton RE: Histologic evaluation of different methods of enlarging the pulp canal space, *J Endod* 2:304, 1976.

4. Short JA, Morgan LA, Baumgartner JC: A comparison of canal centering ability of four instrumentation techniques, *J Endod* 23:503, 1997.

5. Luiten DJ, Morgan LA, Baugartner JC, Marshall JG: A comparison of four instrumentation techniques on apical canal transportation, *J Endod* 21: 26, 1995.

6. Peters O, Schönenberger K, Laib A: Effects of four Ni-Ti preparation techniques on root canal geometry assesed by micro computed tomography, *Int Endod J* 34:221, 2001.

7. Rhodes JS, Pitt Ford TR, Lynch JA, et al: A comparison of two nickel-titanium instrumentation techniques in teeth using microcomputed tomography, *Int Endod J* 33:279, 2000.

8. Seto BG, Nicholls JI, Harrington GW: Torsional properties of twisted and machined endodontic files, *J Endod* 16:355, 1990.

9. Southard DW, Oswald RJ, Natkin E: Instrumentation of curved molar root canals with the Roane technique, *J Endod* 13:479, 1987.

10. Felt RA, Moser JB, Heuer MA: Flute design of endodontic instruments: its influence on cutting efficiency, *J Endod* 8:253, 1982.

11. Miserendino LJ, Moser JB, Heuer MA, Osetek EM: Cutting efficiency of endodontic instruments. Part 1: a quantitative comparison of the tip and fluted regions, *J Endod* 11:435, 1985.

12. Miserendino LJ, Moser JB, Heuer MA, Osetek EM: Cutting efficiency of endodontic instruments. Part II: analysis of tip design, *J Endod* 12:8, 1986.

13. American Dental Association Council on Dental Materials: New American Dental Association specification No. 28 for endodontic files and reamers, *J Am Dent Assoc* 93:813, 1976.

14. Oliet S, Sorin SM: Cutting efficiency of endodontic reamers, *Oral Surg Oral Med Oral Pathol* 36:243, 1973.

15. Mueller HJ: Corrosion determination techniques applied to endodontic instruments—irrigating solutions systems, *J Endod* 8:246, 1982.

16. Walia HM, Brantley WA, Gerstein H: An initial investigation of the bending and torsional properties of Nitinol root canal files, *J Endod* 14:346, 1988.

17. American Dental Association Council on Dental Materials, Instruments and Equipment: Revised ADA specification No. 28 for endodontic files and reamers, *J Am Dent Assoc* 104:506, 1982.

18. American National Standards Institute-American Dental Association: Specification No. 58 for root canal files, type H (Hedstrom), *J Am Dent Assoc* 104:88, 1982.

19. American Dental Association Council on Dental Materials, Instruments and Equipment: Revised ANSI/ADA specification No. 28 for root canal files and reamers, type K and no. 58 for root canal files, type H (Hedstrom), *J Am Dent Assoc* 118:239, 1989.

20. Stenman E, Spangberg LS: Root canal instruments are poorly standardized, *J Endod* 19:327, 1993.

21. Felcher T, Stiles M, Walton R: A comparison of endodontic file tip designs as to their effect in instrumentation of curved canals (Abstract 1899), *J Dent Res* 66(Spec Issue):344, 1987.

22. Powell SE, Simon JH, Maze BB: A comparison of the effect of modified and nonmodified instrument tips on apical canal configuration, *J Endod* 12:293, 1986.

23. Yared GM, Bou Dagher FE, Machtou P: Cyclic fatigue of profile rotary instruments after clinical use, *Int Endod J* 33:204, 2000.

24. American Dental Association Council on Scientific Affairs: Proposed American National Standard/American Dental Association specification no. 95, root canal enlargers, pp 1-16, Chicago, 2000, American Dental Association.

25. Glosson CR, Haller RH, Dove SB, del Rio CE: A comparison of root canal preparations using Ni-Ti hand, Ni-Ti engine-driven, and K-Flex endodontic instruments, *J Endod* 21:146, 1995.

26. Ramirez-Salomon M, Soler-Bientz R, de la Garza-Gonzalez R, Palacios-Garza CM: Incidence of Lightspeed separation and the potential for bypassing, *J Endod* 23:586, 1997.

27. Pruett JP, Clement DJ, Carnes DL, Jr: Cyclic fatigue testing of nickel-titanium endodontic instruments, *J Endod* 23:77, 1997.

28. Luebke NH, Brantley WA: Physical dimensions and torsional properties of rotary endodontic instruments. 1. Gates Glidden drills, *J Endod* 16:438, 1990.

29. Luebke NH, Brantley WA: Torsional and metallurgical properties of rotary endodontic instruments. 2. Stainless steel Gates Glidden drills, *J Endod* 17:319, 1991.

30. Luebke NH, Brantley WA, Sabri ZI, Luebke JH: Physical dimensions, torsional performance, and metallurgical properties of rotary endodontic instruments. 3. Peeso drills, *J Endod* 18:13, 1992.

31. Coleman CL, Svec TA: Analysis of Ni-Ti versus stainless steel instrumentation in resin simulated canals, *J Endod* 23:232, 1997.

32. Kuhn WG, Carnes DL, Jr, Clement DJ, Walker WA: Effect of tip design of nickel-titanium and stainless steel files on root canal preparation, *J Endod* 23:735, 1997.

33. Himel VT, Ahmed KM, Wood DM, Alhadainy HA: An evaluation of Nitinol and stainless steel files used by dental students during a laboratory proficiency exam, *Oral Surg Oral Med Oral Pathol Oral Radiol Endod* 79:232, 1995.

34. Pettiette MT, Metzger Z, Phillips C, Trope M: Endodontic complications of root canal therapy performed by dental students with stainless-steel K-files and nickel-titanium hand files, *J Endod* 25:230, 1999.

35. Baumann MA, Roth A: Effect of experience on quality of canal preparation with rotary nickel-titanium files, *Oral Surg Oral Med Oral Pathol Oral Radiol Endod* 88:714, 1999.

36. Webber J, Moser JB, Heuer MA: A method to determine the cutting efficiency of root canal instruments in linear motion, *J Endod* 6:829, 1980.

37. Gabel WP, Hoen M, Steiman HR, et al: Effect of rotational speed on nickel-titanium file distortion, *J Endod* 25:752, 1999.

38. Gambarini G: Rationale for the use of low-torque endodontic motors in root canal instrumentation, *Endod Dent Traumatol* 16:95, 2000.

39. Dietz DB, Di Fiore PM, Bahcall JK, Lautenschlager EP: Effect of rotational speed on the breakage of nickel-titanium rotary files, *J Endod* 26:68, 2000.

40. Poulsen WB, Dove SB, del Rio CE: Effect of nickel-titanium engine-driven instrument rotational speed on root canal morphology, *J Endod* 21:609, 1995.

41. Berry KA, Loushine RJ, Primack PD, Runyan DA: Nickel-titanium versus stainless-steel finger spreaders in curved canals, *J Endod* 24:752, 1998.

42. Joyce AP, Loushine RJ, West LA, et al: Photoelastic comparison of stress induced by using stainless-steel versus nickel-titanium spreaders in vitro, *J Endod* 24:714, 1998.

43. Council on Dental Therapeutics: Sterilization or disinfection of dental instruments. In *Accepted dental therapeutics*, ed 40, p 136, Chicago, 1984, American Dental Association.

11

Richard E. Walton and Frank J. Vertucci

Internal Anatomy

LEARNING OBJECTIVES

After reading this chapter and the Appendix, the student should be able to:

1 / Recognize errors that may cause difficulties or failures in root canal treatment owing to lack of knowledge of pulp anatomy.

2 / List ways that help to determine the type of pulp canal system.

3 / Draw common shapes of roots in cross section and common canal configurations in these roots.

4 / Describe the most common root and pulp anatomy of each tooth.

5 / List, for each tooth type, the average length, number of roots, and most common root curvatures.

6 / Characterize the more frequent variations in root and pulp anatomy of each tooth.

7 / Explain why standard periapical radiographs do not present the complete picture of root and pulp anatomy.

8 / Draw a representative example of the most common internal and external anatomy of each tooth and root in the following planes: (1) sagittal section of mesiodistal and faciolingual planes and (2) cross section through the cervical, middle, and apical thirds.

9 / Suggest methods for determining whether roots and canals are curved as well as the severity of the curvature.

10 / State the tenet of the relationship of pulp-root anatomy.

11 / List each tooth and the root(s) that require a search for more than one canal.

12 / List and recognize the significance of iatrogenic or pathologic factors that may cause alterations in pulp anatomy.

13 / Define the pulp space and list and describe its major components.

14 / Describe variations in the pulp system in the apical third, including the apical foramen region.

15 / Describe how to determine clinically the distance from the occlusal-incisal surface to the roof of the chamber.

16 / Discuss location, morphology, frequency, and importance of accessory (lateral) canals.

17 / Describe relationships between anatomic apex, radiographic apex, and actual location of the apical foramen.

18 / Describe common variations in pulp anatomy resulting from developmental abnormalities and state their significance.

19 / Describe why many root curvatures are not apparent on standard radiographs.

OUTLINE

Methods of Determining Pulp Anatomy
Textbook Knowledge
Radiographic Evidence
Exploration

General Considerations
Root and Canal Anatomy
Identification of Canals and Roots

Alterations in Internal Anatomy
Age
Irritants
Calcifications
Internal Resorption

Components of Pulp System
Pulp Horns
Pulp Chamber
Root Canals
Accessory Canals
Apical Region

Variations of Root and Pulp Anatomy
Dens Invaginatus (Dens in Dente)
Dens Evaginatus
High Pulp Horns
Lingual Groove
Dilaceration
Other Variations

In terms of success of treatment, knowledge of pulp anatomy cannot be overstated. As a cause of treatment failures, lack of a working knowledge of pulp anatomy ranks second only to errors in diagnosis and treatment planning. It is critical to know the normal or usual configuration of the pulp and to be aware of variations. Special techniques are required to determine the internal anatomy of the tooth under treatment.

Knowledge of the pulp anatomy must be three-dimensional. The pulp cavity must be mentally visualized both longitudinally (from coronal aspect to apical foramen) and in cross section. In addition to general morphologic features, irregularities and "hidden" regions of pulp are present within each canal. To clean and shape the pulp system maximally, intracanal instruments must reach as many of these regions as possible to plane the walls to loosen tissue and tissue remnants.[1] Lack of attention to this important principle may lead to treatment failure.

Methods of Determining Pulp Anatomy

TEXTBOOK KNOWLEDGE

Knowledge of anatomy gained from textbooks is the most important and most useful method. Common and frequent variations *must* be memorized for each tooth. This means having a working knowledge of the number of roots, number of canals per root and their location, longitudinal and cross-sectional shapes, most frequent curvatures (particularly in the faciolingual plane), and root outlines in all dimensions.[2-6] It is useful to know the approximate percentage of each.

Anatomic features are diagrammed in the Appendix.

RADIOGRAPHIC EVIDENCE

Certainly radiographs are useful, but they are somewhat overrated for this purpose, particularly conventional periapical films.[7] The standard parallel facial projection gives just two dimensions; a common error is to examine only this view, overlooking the important third dimension (Figure 11-1). In addition, radiographs tend to make the canals look relatively uniform in shape and taper. In fact, the aberrations often found are generally not visible (Figure 11-2).

Standard projections indicate general anatomic features. Special radiographic techniques disclose

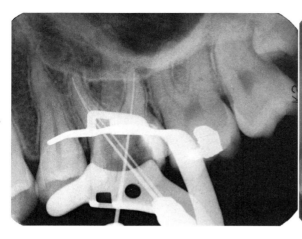
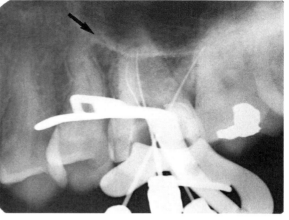

A   B

FIGURE 11-1
A, Facial projection. Both the second premolar and the first molar appear to have fairly straight roots and an uncomplicated anatomy. **B,** Mesial angled projection. The more proximal view shows severe "bayonet" dilaceration of the second premolar with marked buccal curve in the apex *(arrow).* Sharp curves of molar roots and two definitive canals in the mesiobuccal root are now evident. Both are difficult problems to treat.

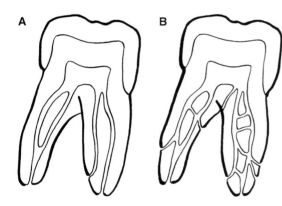

FIGURE 11-2
A, The impression of pulp anatomy received from viewing a radiograph. **B,** The reality: internal anatomy actually has many aberrations and intercommunications. (Courtesy Dr. A. Goerig.)

missed canals and determine curvatures.[8,9] These techniques are discussed in detail in Chapter 9.

EXPLORATION

Additional determinations of pulp anatomy are made during access preparation and when searching for canals. These methods also have limitations because canals often are neither readily apparent nor easily discovered with instruments.[10]

General Considerations

A basic tenet in pulp-root anatomy is *the shape of the pulp system reflects the surface outline of the crown*

and root.[11,12] In other words, because the pulp tends to form the surrounding dentin uniformly on opposite walls, the pulp is generally a miniature version of the tooth and conforms to the tooth surface.[13]

ROOT AND CANAL ANATOMY

Although root shape in cross section is variable, there are seven general configurations: *round, oval, long oval, bowling pin, kidney bean, ribbon,* and *hourglass* (Figure 11-3). Shape and location of canals are governed by root shape (in cross section). Different shapes may appear at any level in a single root. For example, a root may be hourglass-shaped in cross section at the cervical third, taper to a deep oval in the middle third, and blend to oval in the apical third; the number and shape of canals in each level will vary accordingly.[14] Importantly though, a canal is seldom round at any level. To assume that it is may result in improper canal preparation.

IDENTIFICATION OF CANALS AND ROOTS

Obviously, to clean, shape, and obturate a canal, it must be located.[15] In roots that *may* contain two canals, a basic rule is to *assume that the root contains two canals until proved otherwise.* Rather than memorize roots that often contain two canals, it is easier to remember those few that are unlikely to have two canals. Maxillary teeth contain roots that rarely have two canals: anterior root, premolars with two or three roots, and distobuccal and lingual roots of molars. All other maxillary roots

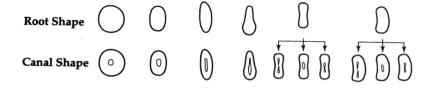

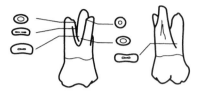

FIGURE 11-3
Common variations in root or pulp cross-sectional anatomy. Note that the pulp outline tends to reflect the root outline. Deep concave roots have a greater variety of pulp anatomies.

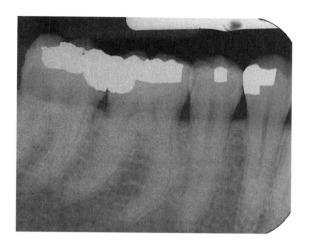

FIGURE 11-4
Note the disclike configuration of the pulp chamber in the first molar because of the predominance of dentin formation in the roof and floor of the chamber. These chambers are difficult to locate during access preparation.

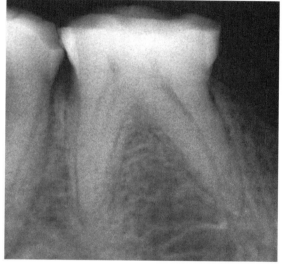

FIGURE 11-5
Severe attrition has resulted in tertiary dentin formation on the roof and floor of the chamber.

and all mandibular roots require a careful search for two (or possibly more) canals.

Alterations in Internal Anatomy

Again, initial pulp shape reflects root shape. However, because pulp and dentin react to their environment, changes in shape occur with increasing tooth age and in response to irritation.

AGE

Although dentin formation tends to occur with age on all surfaces, it occurs predominately in certain areas. For example, in molars, the roof and

floor of the chamber show more dentin formation, eventually making the chamber almost disclike in configuration (Figure 11-4). Treatment implications (difficulty in locating chamber and canals) are obvious.

IRRITANTS

Anything that exposes dentin to the oral cavity can potentially stimulate increased dentin formation at the base of tubules in the underlying pulp.[13] Causes of such dentin exposure include caries, periodontal disease, abrasion, erosion, attrition, cavity preparations, root planing, and cusp fractures (Figure 11-5). Vital pulp therapy such as pulpotomy, pulp capping, or placement of irritating materials in a deep cavity may cause an increase in dentin formation, occlusion, calcific metamorphosis, resorption, or other unusual configurations in the chamber or canals. These tertiary (irregular secondary) dentin formations tend to occur directly under the involved tubules (Figure 11-6).

It is imperative that the clinician study radiographs and visually examine the tooth being treated to identify factors that may cause alterations in anatomy. Failure to do so may result in serious errors, lost time, and inadequate treatment.

CALCIFICATIONS

Calcifications take two basic forms within the pulp: pulp stones (denticles) and diffuse calcifications. Although pulp stones are usually found in the chamber and diffuse calcifications within the radicular pulp, the reverse may also occur. These calcifications may form either normally or in response to irritation. Pulp stones are often seen on radiographs[16]; diffuse calcifications are visible only histologically.

Pulp stones in the chamber may reach considerable size and can markedly alter the internal chamber anatomy (Figure 11-7). Although they do not totally block a canal orifice, they often make the process of locating an orifice challenging. These large pulp stones may be attached or free and are often removed during access preparation. Although pulp stones are not common in canals, if present, they are usually attached or embedded in the canal wall in the apical region. Rarely do they form a barrier to instrument passage.

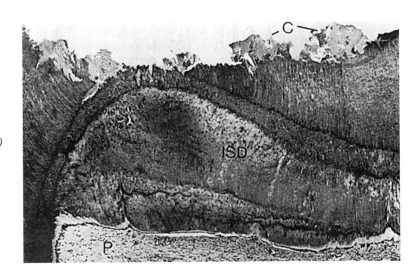

FIGURE 11-6
As shown on this micrograph, tertiary or irregular secondary dentin *(ISD)* has formed in large amounts in the pulp *(P)* directly under the caries *(C)*. At times this may significantly alter internal anatomy. (Courtesy Dr. W. Dowden.)

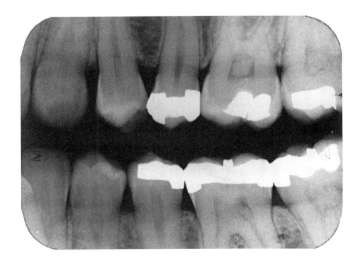

FIGURE 11-7
Calcifications (pulp stones [or denticles]) are visualized in the chambers. Their discrete appearance surrounded by radiolucent spaces shows these calcifications to be natural and not formed in response to irritation. (Courtesy Dr. T. Gound.)

INTERNAL RESORPTION

Such resorptions are uncommon and when present are usually not extensive. They also are a response to irritation that is sufficient to cause inflammation. Most resorptions are small and are not detectable on radiographs or during canal preparation. When visible radiographically, they are usually extensive and often perforate. Internal resorptions usually create operative difficulties (Figure 11-8).

Components of Pulp System

The pulp cavity is divided into a coronal (the pulp chamber) and a radicular portion (the root canal). Other features include *pulp horns, canal orifices, accessory (lateral) canals,* and the *apical foramen* (Figure 11-9). The internal anatomy of these pulp components is altered by secondary dentin or cementum formation.

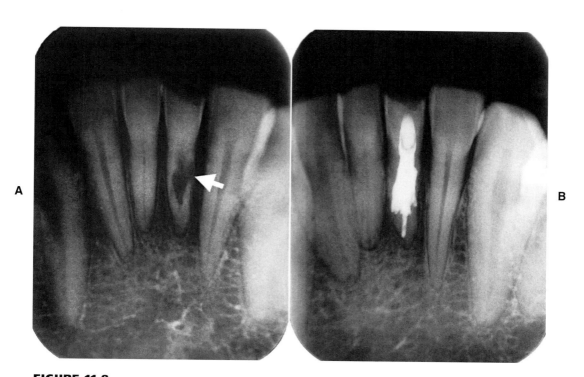

FIGURE 11-8
A, Extensive internal resorption defect *(arrow).* **B,** Four years after treatment. Special cleaning, shaping, and obturating techniques (lateral condensation plus thermoplasticized) were required, resulting in successful treatment.

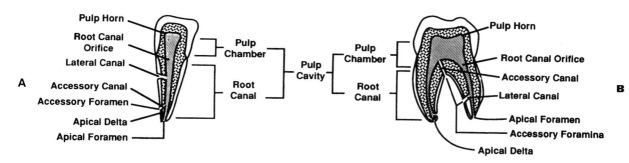

FIGURE 11-9
Major anatomic components of the pulp cavity. **A,** Anterior tooth. **B,** Posterior tooth.

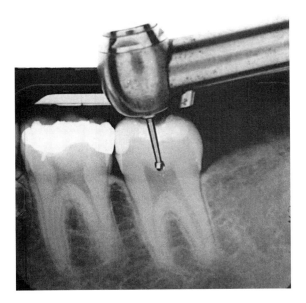

FIGURE 11-10
A technique for determining the distance from the occlusal surface to the roof of the pulp chamber. This is of obvious benefit during access preparation to prevent perforation.

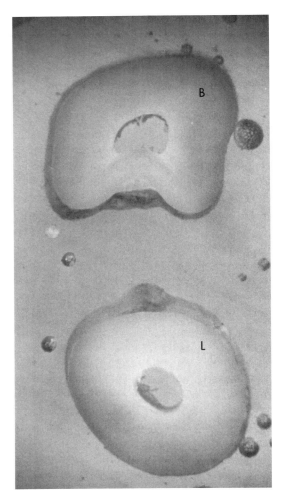

FIGURE 11-11
Maxillary first premolar roots. A common finding: cross section through buccal *(B)* and lingual *(L)* roots shows a concavity on the lingual surface and an irregular canal shape in the middle third of the buccal root. (Courtesy Dr. A. Tamse.)

PULP HORNS

Pulp horns represent what the dentist does not want to locate during restorative procedures but does want to locate during access preparation. Although they may vary in height and location, a single pulp horn tends to be associated with each cusp in a posterior tooth, and mesial and distal horns tend to be in incisors. Generally, the occlusal extent of the pulp horns corresponds to the height of contour in a younger tooth but lies closer to the cervical margin in an older tooth. Occasionally, an aberrant horn extends occlusally and is exposed as a result of caries or routine cavity preparation. Such abnormally high pulp horns may or may not be visible on radiographs.

During access preparation, the height and location of pulp horns may be more accurately determined by measuring from cusp tip to pulp horn or chamber roof using a bur and a handpiece (Figure 11-10).

PULP CHAMBER

The pulp chamber occupies the center of the crown and trunk of the root. Again, its shape, in both longitudinal and cross-sectional dimensions, depends on the shape of the crown and trunk; this configuration varies with tooth age and/or irritation.[11]

ROOT CANALS

Root canals extend the length of the root, beginning as a funneled orifice and exiting as the apical foramen. Significantly, most canals are curved, often in a facial-lingual direction. Therefore a curved canal is often undetectable on facial projection radiographs. As a result, the uninitiated or uninformed clinician may assume that a canal is straight and may overenlarge what is, in reality, a facial or lingual curvature, resulting in ledging or perforation. *The operator should always assume that a canal is curved.*

Canal shape varies with root shape and size, degree of curvature, and the age and condition of the tooth (see Figures 11-2 and 11-3). As a rule,

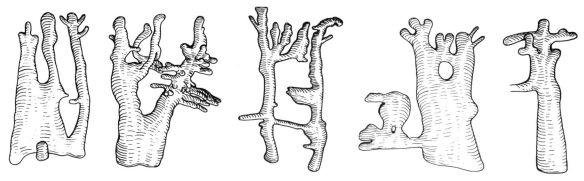

FIGURE 11-12
Three-dimensional reconstruction from histologic sections shows complex anatomic structure of apical pulp anatomy. (Adapted from Meyer W: *Dtsch Zahnaertzl Z* 25:1064, 1970.)

when two canals occur in a root, they tend to be more oval. In the deep facial-lingual root with mesial or distal (or both) concavities (hourglass- or kidney bean-shaped), a single canal may have a bowling pin, kidney-bean, hourglass, or ribbon shape. Regardless of the shape in the cervical third, in the apical curvature the root (and canal) tends to become more oval but may be somewhat flattened.[17]

The shape and number of canals in a root reflects the facial-lingual depth and shape of the root at each level (Figure 11-11); the deeper the root, the more likely that there are two separate, definitive canals. If the root tapers toward the apical third, there is a greater likelihood that the canals will converge to exit as a single canal.

Irregularities and aberrations are commonplace. This is particularly true in posterior teeth. Such aberrations include hills and valleys in canal walls, intercanal communications (isthmuses between two canals), cul-de-sacs, fins, and other variations (Figure 11-12). Again, these aberrations are usually not accessible to instruments or irrigants.

Remember that the chamber tends to occupy the center of the crown; a canal occupies the center of the root. When there are two canals in a root, each will often occupy the center of its own root "bulge."

ACCESSORY CANALS

Accessory (or lateral) canals are lateral branches of the main canal that form a communication between the pulp and periodontium. They contain connective tissue and vessels and may be located at any level from furcation[18,19] to apex, but tend to be more common in the apical third and in posterior teeth.[20] In other words, the more apical and the farther posterior the tooth, the more likely that accessory canals will be present. The relationship of accessory canals to pulp health and disease as well as to treatment is debatable.[21] They do not supply collateral circulation and therefore contribute little to pulp function and probably represent an anomaly that occurred during root formation.

These canals do form an exit for irritants from the pulp space to the lateral periodontium. They probably cannot be débrided during cleaning and shaping[1] but are occasionally filled with obturating materials during canal filling (Figure 11-13). The importance of obturating accessory canals is unknown.[22]

APICAL REGION

Development: The apex is the root terminus. It is relatively straight in the young mature tooth but tends to curve more distally with time. This curvature results from continued apical-distal apposition of cementum in response to continued mesial-occlusal eruption. Alterations in the apical region may also result from resorption and irregular cementum apposition. Thus apical anatomy tends to be nonuniform and unpredictable.[23]

Apical Foramen: The apical foramen varies in size and configuration with maturity. Before maturation, the apical foramen is open. With time and deposition of dentin and cementum, it becomes smaller and funneled. Significantly, the foramen usually does not exit at the true (anatomic) root apex[24,25] but is offset approximately 0.5 mm and seldom more than 1.0 mm from the true apex. The degree of deviation is unpredictable and may vary considerably from the average, particularly in the older tooth that has undergone cementum apposition (Figure 11-14). For this reason, root canal preparation and obturation end short of the anatomic root apex (Figure 11-15) as seen in the radiograph.[26] Usually, the

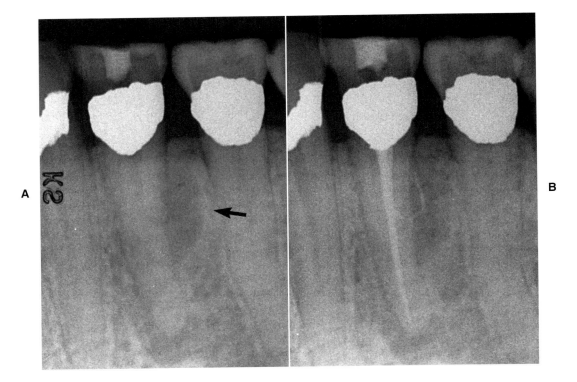

FIGURE 11-13
A, Resorptive bony lesion is visible *(arrow)*; this usually indicates an accessory canal (not visible) that is a pathway for irritants. **B,** The accessory canal is now obvious after obturation.

apical foramen is not visible radiographically. The clinician relies on averages or on electronic measuring devices to determine the extent of canal preparation and obturation.[23,24]

Variations in Anatomy: The only consistent aspect of the apex region is its inconsistency.[27,28] The canal may take twists and turns, divide into several canals to form a delta with ramifications on the apical root surface, or exhibit irregularities in the canal wall (Figure 11-16). Generally, these aberrations are neither detectable nor predictably negotiable and are neither well débrided nor obturated.

A common concept is that canals round out in this apical region. This is not always true. Canals are frequently a long oval or even ribbon-shaped apically.[29] These nonround canals cannot be enlarged to a round shape without perforating or weakening the roots.[29]

Apical Constriction: The presence of an apical constriction is unpredictable. It has been proposed that the cementodentinal junction forms the apical constriction; this is an incorrect concept. In fact, the junction is difficult to determine clinically with accuracy,[24] and the intracanal extent of cementum is variable. If an apical constriction is present, it is not visible on a radiograph and usually is not detectable by touch, even by the most skilled practitioner.

Variations of Root and Pulp Anatomy

Representative examples of the tooth groups are diagrammed in the Appendix, where both cross-sectional and longitudinal aspects are outlined. In addition, the pulp anatomy of each is shown in relation to the design of the access preparation.

Occasionally, teeth vary significantly in root or, more likely, in pulp anatomy. Such variations and abnormalities are most common in the maxillary lateral incisors, maxillary[30,31] and mandibular premolars,[32] and maxillary molars.[33,34] Unusual root morphology tends to be bilateral.[35]

DENS INVAGINATUS (DENS IN DENTE)

Dens invaginatus is most common in maxillary lateral incisors[36] that results from an infolding of the enamel organ during proliferation and is an error in morphodifferentiation (Figure 11-17). It often results in an early pulp-oral cavity communication requiring root canal treatment.[37] Dens invaginatus is most common in the maxillary lateral incisor and shows varying degrees of severity and complexity.[38,39] The more severe cases should be referred to a specialist because special treat-

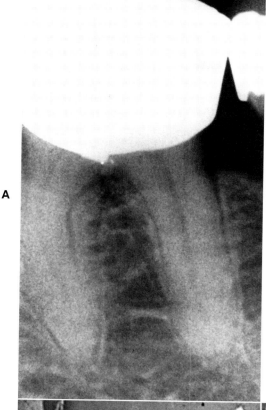

A

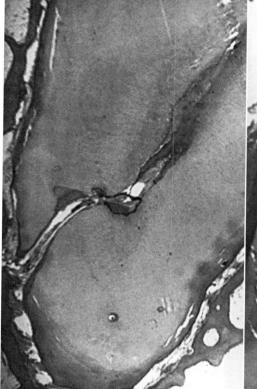

B

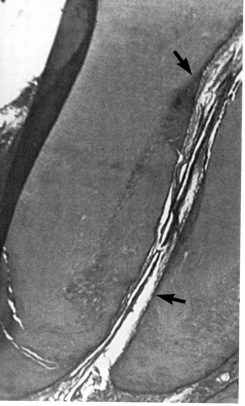

C

FIGURE 11-14

Variations in apical canal anatomy. **A,** The radiograph often does not demonstrate the size, shape, or curvature of canals apically. **B,** Mesial root apex showing abrupt curve and apical foramen exiting on the mesial well short of the anatomic apex. **C,** Distal root apex showing uniform canal with no constriction and variable levels *(arrows)* of cementodentinal junctions; these variabilities are common. (Cadaver specimen courtesy Dr. D. Holtzmann.)

FIGURE 11-15
A, Note that the apical foramina (*small arrows*) do not correspond to the true anatomic apex (*large arrows*). **B,** in most situations the apical terminus or seat of the preparation will vary from the apical foramen and radiographic apex. (**A** courtesy Dr. D. Melton.)

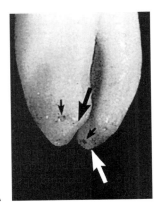

A

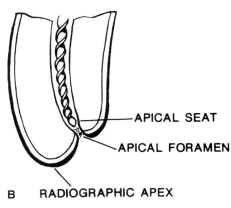

APICAL SEAT
APICAL FORAMEN
B RADIOGRAPHIC APEX

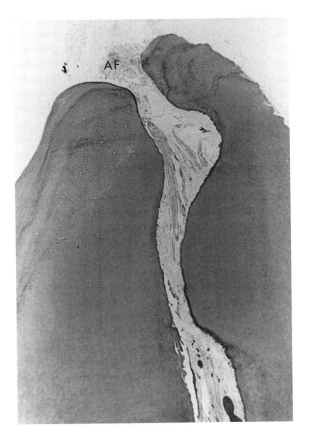

FIGURE 11-16
The apical region of the canal and apical foramen *(AF)* are often very irregular.

ment, such as surgery, is frequently required. The prognosis of any treatment often is questionable. The invagination is usually visible on radiographs; however, it is often small and obscure. The lingual pit on maxillary anterior teeth represents a minor form of dens invaginatus.

DENS EVAGINATUS

A variation of invaginatus,[40] dens evaginatus is most common in mandibular premolars and in individuals with Oriental ancestry (this includes Native Americans and Hispanics). Clinically, dens evaginatus initially appears as a small tubercle "bulge" on the occlusal surface, but it may not be obvious radiographically (Figure 11-18). These malformations often contain an extension of the pulp. When these fragile tubercles fracture off, the pulp is exposed and will become necrotic, requiring apexification. They are generally not difficult to treat, prophylactically, by removing the tubercle and capping, then restoring with amalgam.[41]

HIGH PULP HORNS

Occasionally, a pulp horn extends far into a cusp region, resulting in premature exposure by caries or accidental exposure during cavity preparation.

LINGUAL GROOVE

Usually found in maxillary lateral incisors, a lingual groove appears as a surface infolding of dentin oriented from the cervical toward the apical direction (Figure 11-19).[42] Frequently, this results in a deep narrow periodontal defect that occasionally communicates with the pulp, causing an endodontic/periodontal problem (Figure 11-20). Treatment is difficult and unpredictable; prognosis is poor.

DILACERATION

By definition, dilaceration is a severe or complex root curvature (see Figure 11-1). During root formation, structures such as the cortical bone of the maxillary sinus or mandibular canal or nasal fossa may deflect the epithelial diaphragm, resulting in a severe curvature. Many of these curvatures are

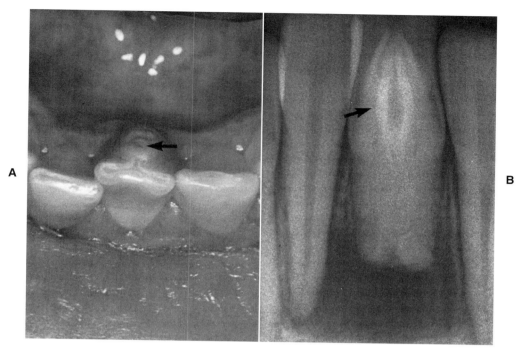

FIGURE 11-17

Dens invaginatus. **A,** The invagination is visible on the lingual surface (*arrow*) of this abnormally shaped incisor. **B,** The invagination is lined internally by enamel (*arrow*). By communicating with the pulp, the exposure resulted in pulp necrosis, apical pathosis, and arrested root development. These situations are difficult to treat.

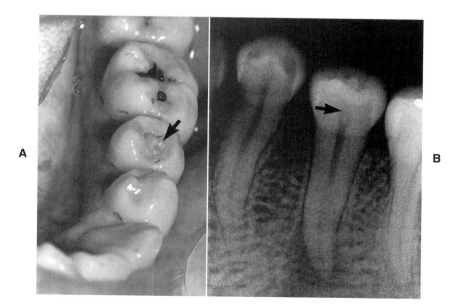

FIGURE 11-18

Dens evaginatus. The chamber extends to the occlusal surface. **A,** The defect is visible from the occlusal surface *(arrow)*. **B,** There is a communication through this to the pulp space *(arrow)*, with resultant necrosis and apical periodontitis. (Courtesy Dr. R. Johnson.)

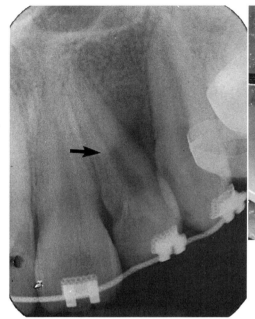

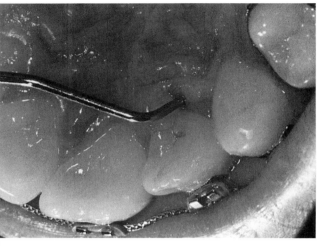

FIGURE 11-19
Lingual groove, which is an apparent infolding during root and crown formation. **A,** The groove is faintly visible on the periapical radiograph *(arrow)*. **B,** The groove is often detected on the surface with probing and is usually untreatable.

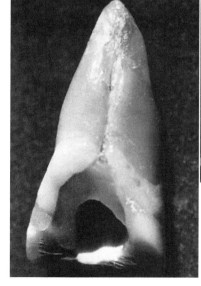

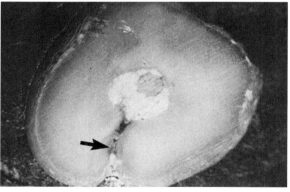

FIGURE 11-20
A, Lingual groove defect proved untreatable periodontally and endodontically. **B,** Cross section shows that the groove invagination (*arrow*) communicates with the pulp.

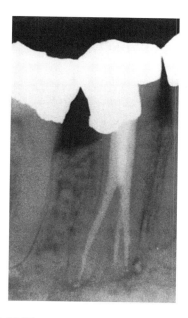

FIGURE 11-21
Premolar with three canals—a challenge to treat.

found in a facial-lingual plane and are not obvious on standard radiographic projections.

OTHER VARIATIONS

Many other pulp and root anomalies may occur.[43-47] Some occur in association with genetic disorders,[48] such as variations in the number of canals or roots (Figure 11-21), and teeth with unusual root canal configurations have an impact on treatment.[49,50] The astute clinician will be alert to these possibilities and will study radiographs and occlusal anatomy carefully. A not uncommon abnormality is the C-shaped canal (Figure 11-22). This usually occurs in mandibular molars. Because of the complex internal anatomy, prognosis of root canal treatment is questionable owing to difficulty in adequate débridement and obturation.[51] Additional treatment measures may be required, and patients with such canals should be considered for referral.

New technologies, using computer reconstruction of microtomography, are able to provide three-dimensional morphologic information on tooth and pulp anatomy.[12,52]

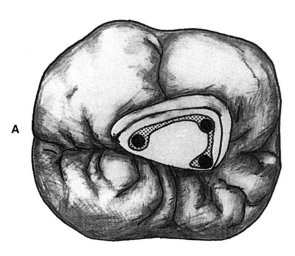

A

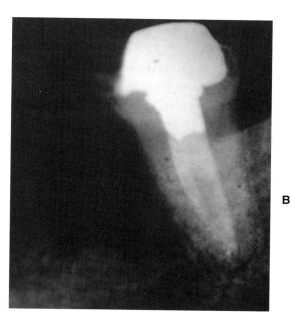

B

FIGURE 11-22
A, C-shaped pulp chamber. The C-shaped space may be continuous throughout the length of the root but is variable anatomically. More commonly, three separate canal orifices may be found within the groove. **B,** Obturated C-shaped molar with three canals joined by an interconnecting isthmus.

REFERENCES

1. Walton RE: Histologic comparison of different methods of pulp canal enlargement, *J Endod* 2:304, 1976.
2. Pineda F, Kuttler Y: Mesiodistal and buccolingual roentgenographic investigation of 7,275 root canals, *Oral Surg Oral Med Oral Pathol* 33:101, 1972.
3. Mueller AH: Anatomy of the root canals of the incisors, cuspids and bicuspids of the permanent teeth, *J Am Dent Assoc* 20:1361, 1933.
4. Vertucci F: Root canal anatomy of the human permanent teeth, *Oral Surg Oral Med Oral Pathol* 58:589, 1984.
5. Vertucci FJ: Root canal anatomy of the mandibular anterior teeth, *J Am Dent Assoc* 89:369, 1974.
6. Green D: Morphology of the pulp cavity of the permanent teeth, *Oral Surg Oral Med Oral Pathol* 8:743, 1955.
7. Kaffe I, Kaufman A, Littner MM, et al: Radiographic study of the root canal system of mandibular anterior teeth, *Int Endod J* 18:235, 1985.
8. Walton RE: Endodontic radiographic techniques, *Dent Radiog Photog* 46:51, 1973.
9. Skidmore A: The importance of pre-operative radiographs and determination of root canal configuration, *Quintessence Int* 10:55, 1979.
10. Johnson WT: Difficulties in locating the mesiobuccal canal in molars, *Quintessence Int* 16:169, 1985.
11. Stambaugh RV, Wittrock JW: The relationship of the pulp chamber to the external surface of the tooth, *J Prosthet Dent* 37:537, 1977.
12. Bjorndal L, Carlsen O, Thuesen G, et al: External and internal macromorphology in 3D-reconstructed maxillary molars using computerized X-ray microtomography, *Int Endod J* 32:3, 1999.
13. Bhaskar S: *Orban's oral histology,* ed 10, St Louis, 1986, Mosby.
14. Mauger M, Schindler W, Walker W III: An evaluation of canal morphology at different levels of root resection in mandibular incisors, *J Endod* 24:607, 1998.
15. Fogel H, Peikoff M, Christie W: Canal configuration in the mesiobuccal root of the maxillary first molar: a clinical study, *J Endod* 20:135, 1994.
16. Tamse A, Kaffe I, Littner MM, Shani R: Statistical evaluation of radiologic survey of pulp stones, *J Endod* 8:81, 1982.
17. Gani O, Visvisian C: Apical canal diameter in the first upper molar at various ages, *J Endod* 25:689, 1999.
18. Guttman J: Prevalence, location, and patency of accessory canals in the furcation of molars, *J Periodontol* 49:21, 1978.
19. Vertucci FJ, Anthony RL: A scanning electron microscopic investigation of accessory foramina in the furcation and pulp chamber floor of molar teeth, *Oral Surg Oral Med Oral Pathol* 62:319, 1986.
20. DeDeus WD: Frequency, location, and direction of the lateral, secondary, and accessory canals, *J Endod* 1:361, 1975.
21. Sinai IH, Soltanoff W: The transmission of pathologic changes between the pulp and the periodontal structures, *Oral Surg Oral Med Oral Pathol* 36:558, 1973.
22. Weine F: The enigma of the lateral canal, *Dent Clin North Am* 28:833, 1984.
23. Kuttler Y: Microscope investigation of root apexes, *J Am Dent Assoc* 50:544, 1955.
24. Dummer PM, McGinn JH, Rees DG: The position and topography of the apical canal constriction and apical foramen, *Int Endod J* 17:192, 1984.
25. Miyashita M, Kasahara E, Yasuda E, et al: Root canal system of the mandibular incisor, *J Endod* 23:479, 1997.
26. Wu M, Wesselink P, Walton R: Apical terminus location of root canal treatment procedures, *Oral Surg Oral Med Oral Pathol Oral Radiol Endod* 89:99, 2000.
27. Morfis A, Sylaras N, Georgopoulou M, et al: Study of the apices of human permanent teeth with the use of a scanning electron microscope, *Oral Surg Oral Med Oral Pathol Endod* 77:172, 1994.
28. Guttman J, Regan J: Historical and contemporary perspectives of the root apex, *Arab Dent J* 3:9, 1998.
29. Wu M, R'Oris A, Barkin D: Prevalence and extent of long oval canals in the apical third, *Oral Surg Oral Med Oral Pathol Oral Radiol Endod* 89:739, 2000.
30. Kartel N, Ozcelik B, Cimilli H: Root canal morphology of maxillary premolars, *J Endod* 24:417, 1998.
31. Tamse A, Katz A, Pilo R: Furcation groove of buccal root of maxillary first premolars—a morphometric study, *J Endod* 26:359, 2000.
32. Baisden MK, Kulild JC, Weller RN: Root canal configuration of the mandibular first premolar, *J Endod* 18:505, 1992.
33. Libfeld H, Rotstein I: Incidence of four-rooted maxillary second molars: literature review and radiographic survey of 1,200 teeth, *J Endod* 15:129, 1989.
34. Stropko J: Canal morphology of maxillary molars: clinical observations of canal configurations, *J Endod* 25: 446, 1999.
35. Sabala CL, Benenati FW, Neas BR: Bilateral root or root canal aberrations in a dental school patient population, *J Endod* 20:38, 1994.
36. Hulsmann M: Dens invaginatus. aetiology, classification, prevalence, diagnosis, and treatment considerations, *Int Endod J* 30:79, 1997.
37. Piatelli A, Trisi P: Dens invaginatus: a histological study of undemineralized material, *Endod Dent Traumatol* 9:191, 1993.
38. Oehlers F: Dens invaginatus. I. Variations of the invagination process and associated crown forms, *Oral Surg Oral Med Oral Pathol* 10:1204, 1957.
39. Gound TG: Dens invaginatus—a pathway to pulpal pathology: a literature review, *Pract Periodontics Aesthet Dent* 9:585, 1997.
40. Reichart PA, Methah D, Sukasem M: Morphologic findings in dens evaginatus, *Int J Oral Surg Oral Med Oral Pathol* 11:59, 1982.
41. McCulloch K, Mills C, Greenfield R, Coil J: Dens evaginatus: review of the literature and report of several clinical cases, *J Can Dent Assoc* 64:104, 1998.
42. Lara V, Consolaro A, Bruce R: Macroscopic and microscopic analysis of the palato-gingival groove, *J Endod* 26:345, 2000.
43. Beatty RG, Krell K: Mandibular molars with five canals. Report of two cases, *J Am Dent Assoc* 114:802, 1987.
44. Yang Z-P, Yang S-F, Lee G: The root and root canal anatomy of maxillary molars in a Chinese population, *Endod Dent Traumatol* 4:215, 1988.
45. Sieraski SM, Taylor GN, Kohn RA: Identification and endodontic management of three canalled maxillary premolars, *J Endod* 15:29, 1989.

46. Manning SA: Root canal anatomy of mandibular second molars, *Int Endod J* 23:34, 1990.

47. Melton DC, Krell KV, Fuller MW: Anatomical and histological features of C-shaped canals in mandibular second molars, *J Endod* 17:384, 1991.

48. Kelsen A, Love R, Kieser J, Herbison P: Root canal anatomy of anterior and premolar teeth in Down's syndrome, *Int Endod J* 32:211, 1999.

49. Sharma R, Pecora J, Lumley P, Walmsley A: The external and internal anatomy of human mandibular canine teeth with two roots, *Endod Dent Traumatol* 14:88, 1998.

50. Ferreira C, Gomes de Moraes I, Bernardineli N: Three-rooted maxillary second premolar, *J Endod* 26:105, 2000.

51. Fava L, Otani A, Otani I: The C-shaped root canal system and its endodontic implications: a clinical review, *Endod Pract* 2:18, 1999.

52. Mikrogeorgis G, Lyroudia K, Nikopoulos, et al: 3D computer-aided reconstruction of six teeth with morphological abnormalities, *Int Endod J* 32:88, 1999.

12

Richard E. Walton

Access Preparation and Length Determination

LEARNING OBJECTIVES

After reading this chapter, the student should be able to:

1 / Identify major objectives of access preparation in both anterior and posterior teeth.

2 / Describe why straight-line access is critical.

3 / Explain why removal of pulp horns in anterior teeth is important.

4 / Relate reasons and indications for removing caries or restorations during access preparation.

5 / Explain the reason and technique for removing the dentin shelf in anterior and posterior teeth.

6 / Describe the procedure, burs used, and sequence of operations to start and complete access preparations on various teeth.

7 / Identify common errors for specific teeth that may occur during access preparation.

8 / Recognize when these errors occur and know how to correct them (if they are correctable).

9 / Describe techniques for locating difficult-to-find chambers or canals.

10 / Account for conditions under which working length (distance from radiographic apex) varies.

11 / Demonstrate the step-by-step technique for obtaining estimated and final working lengths.

12 / Describe how to designate and maintain (and create, when necessary) a stable reference point.

13 / Describe electronic apex locators—how they function and when they are useful.

Refer to the Appendix:

14 / Diagram the portions of the tooth that must be removed to attain straight-line access to the canals. Illustrate this on sagittal sections of both anterior and posterior teeth.

15 / Diagram the outline form of the access preparation for all teeth.

16 / Show the location of each canal orifice relative to the occlusal or lingual surface.

| OUTLINE |

Access Preparation
Major Objectives
Access in Special Situations
Access Techniques
Errors
Working Length Determination
Reference Point
Technique for Determination
Alternative Techniques

T his chapter and the following two chapters (Chapters 13 and 14) cover the technical aspects of root canal treatment. Discussed are access and working length, cleaning and shaping, and obturation. These procedures occupy much of the clinician's effort; the steps involved are critical for success.

There are many ways to accomplish various tasks. A variety of techniques, instruments, and materials can be used to perform root canal treatment successfully. These three chapters represent basically one general approach. The recommended methods follow a sequence of procedures that have proved to be successful based on research and clinical usage. Other approaches or modifications may also result in success. There is not enough space here to describe all variations; these will be found in individual courses on endodontics or in other publications.

Access Preparation
MAJOR OBJECTIVES

Access preparation is the most important phase of the technical aspects of root canal treatment! Access is the key that opens the door to maximize cleaning, shaping, and obturation. These three procedures are difficult at best; without adequate access preparation, instruments and materials are difficult to control within the pulp system. Importantly, the time and effort devoted to access preparation pay dividends in the treatment steps that follow.

The three major objectives of access preparation are (1) attainment of *straight-line access*, (2) *conservation of tooth structure*, and (3) *unroofing of the chamber* to expose orifices and to remove pulp horns in anterior teeth. Of course, the approach and specific details for each of these vary in different teeth.

Straight-Line Access

As stated earlier, access preparation is very important; straight-line access is the most critical aspect. The ideal procedure would be to have instruments pass through the chamber without touching the walls and through the straight part of the canal undeflected. The initial curve of the instrument would then occur at the first bend of the canal, usually in the apical third of the root. This, of course, is not always possible because of crown-root relationships; however, this *straight-line access to the first canal curvature* is attempted (Figure 12-1).

Improved Instrument Control. Minimizing instrument curvature and deflection increases the

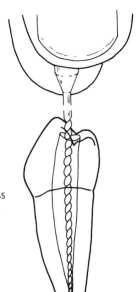

FIGURE 12-1
In the ideal straight-line access preparation, the instrument is not deflected until it reaches the first curve of the canal.

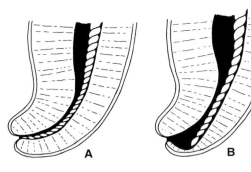

FIGURE 12-2
A, Small hand instruments (No. 20 or less) usually negotiate curves. **B,** Larger files overcome dentin resistance by straightening themselves and cutting raw dentin on the outside of the curve. Adequate straight-line access decreases this tendency for files to transport a curved canal.

operator's ability to manipulate files in as many areas of the canal as possible without grossly altering the internal canal anatomy.[1] Stainless steel files are relatively inflexible and resist deformation, particularly those of size 25 or above. Nickel-titanium files have more flexibility in larger sizes. In either case, any instrument in a curved canal always tries to straighten itself. A sharp stainless steel file larger than size 25 in a curved canal overcomes the resistance of confining dentin. It therefore cuts straight ahead and does most of its work removing raw dentin on the outside of the curve (Figure 12-2). This straight-ahead cutting is accentuated according to the severity of the curve and the size of the file. Therefore less curve in the coronal portion of the instrument makes the straightening effect toward the tip less pronounced. The end result is improved instrument control, resulting in better cleaning and shaping of the canal system with less chance of undesirable internal alterations such as *transportation, ledging,* and *"zipping."*[2,3]

Another advantage of straight-line access is the ease of introducing instruments into canals. Achieving straight-line access involves controlled funneling of canal orifices. These funnels guide the instrument tips into the canals, minimizing the frustration of repeated tap tap tapping of the file on the chamber floor while attempting to locate the canal orifice(s).

Improved Obturation. The same principles stated under instrument control apply to obturation. Straighter access to the apical portion (and the

greater the funneling of the canal orifice), makes the obturation easier and more effective. Because spreader or plugger depth is critical for a better seal throughout the length of the canal, it is important to introduce these instruments (with minimal curve) close to the apical preparation.[4]

Decreased Procedural Errors. The principle of improved instrument control through reduced curvature also applies to decreased procedural errors. The curved instrument straightens itself. Larger instruments have greater stiffness; therefore they more readily cut straight ahead (Figure 12-2). Straight-line access decreases canal curvature and provides better instrument control. There are three potential unfortunate accidents that may be result from inadequate straight-line access, which results in more transportation.

Ledge Formation.[5] The canal is straightened. Suddenly the file no longer negotiates the curve but bumps into a dead end. A radiograph made with the file in place shows the tip of the instrument now straight and pointing toward the outside of the curve.[6] It is now difficult (usually impossible) to renegotiate the original curve to complete débridement and obturation.

Apical Perforation. If the operator persists, the instrument will continue to straighten both itself and the canal; the eventual outcome will be a zipping perforation. Again, this possibility is reduced with straight-line access.

Furcal (Stripping) Perforation. Stripping results usually from over-rigorous planing and forcing in-

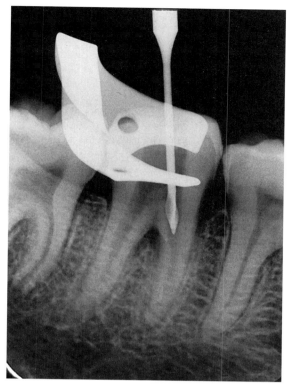

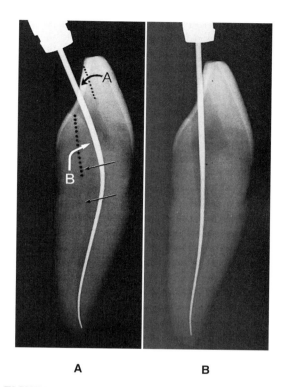

A   B

FIGURE 12-3
Using large rotary instruments such as this No. 5 Gates-Glidden bur against the furcation wall of a canal in molars is dangerous.

FIGURE 12-4
A, Totally inadequate access. The instrument tends to do all its work by cutting toward the facial aspect and will never reach into and débride portions of the canal toward the lingual aspect *(arrows)*. Straight-line access is achieved by removing the lingual dentin shelf *(B)* and the enamel triangle *(A)*. **B,** The result is straight access and improved instrument control.

struments or burs toward the furcation wall.[4] Stripping perforation of the furcation is usually devastating and is difficult to repair with predictable long-term success. Of course, stripping may also result from improper use of rotary instruments to achieve straight-line access (Figure 12-3). Files and burs should not be overused against the furcation portion of canal walls (the so-called *danger zone*) but directed toward the periphery (the *safety zone*).[7,8]

Tooth Structure Removal. Straight-line access consists of removal of dentin and enamel in selected regions (Figure 12-4). Dentin is removed internally at or just apical to the canal orifice (dentin or lingual shelf). Enamel is removed from the incisal surface of anterior teeth (enamel triangle) and toward the crown periphery (cusp tips) on posterior teeth.

The preferred site for removal and the most efficient in terms of improved instrument control and straight access is reduction of the dentin shelf. Not only does this

provide the desired decrease in instrument curvature, but it also "opens up" regions of the canal that would otherwise be sequestered. Such hidden areas tend to occur in roots that contain only a single canal. Because of canal constriction near the orifice, concavities will be found (usually toward the lingual aspect) in the midroot that are not otherwise accessible (Figure 12-4).

An axiom of canal preparation is that *instruments must physically contact and plane the walls to loosen the tissue and debris for removal.*[9] Unplaned areas often retain existing or potential irritants. Removal of a constriction or shelf during straight-line access permits files to reach more surface areas.

Conservation of Tooth Structure

Removal of excess enamel and dentin (in particular) weakens the tooth and increases the possibility of fracture or perforation. Generally, a preparation that allows adequate straight-line access need not require removal of much tooth structure. The key is to remove dentin and enamel in strategic areas, leaving other areas intact. A properly designed access preparation generally has little effect on decreasing cusp strength.[10]

Minimal Weakening of Tooth. Gouging out portions of the dentin wall invariably weakens the cusps and compromises the integrity of the marginal ridges, leading to diminished cuspal strength and an increased incidence of fracture.[11] In molars, the orifice location and access outlines show that it is generally unnecessary to extend the preparation into marginal ridges.[12] Marginal ridges with their underlying dentin are the basic facial-lingual strength of the tooth.[13] Unless they are already involved with caries or restorations, *marginal ridges should be left alone!*

Excessive removal of dentin apically beyond the orifice increases the chances of vertical root fracture. Extreme lateral forces may be created during condensation or placement of posts. Without doubt, the key factor affecting the strength of the crown and root is the amount of dentin remaining and not the so-called brittleness of dentin per se.[13,14]

The design and extent of permanent restorations are also affected by the amount of tooth structure removed during access preparation. Excessive removal may require a more complex restoration than would otherwise have been necessary. At times, a cusp that has adequate dentin

support and is bound by a strong, intact marginal ridge need not be covered.

Prevention of Accidents. Accidents mean perforations! Obviously, excessive removal of tooth structure in any region increases the likelihood of perforation. Except for vertical root fracture, perforation is the most devastating occurrence. Specific details on root perforations and their prognosis and repair are discussed in Chapter 18.

Unroofing of Chamber and Exposure of Pulp Horns

Unroofing of the chamber in all teeth is important to locate canals and permit adequate access to them. It also decreases the incidence of discoloration in anterior teeth. An attempt to economize on unroofing the chamber in an effort to preserve a small amount of dentin only increases the frustration level. However, unroofing the chamber does vary according to tooth groups, as follows.

Maximal Visibility. It is counterproductive to work through a "mousehole." Inadequate openings (Figure 12-5) through the occlusal surface or chamber roof do not permit adequate light to enter the chamber. In addition, clear visualization is compromised in all aspects of the chamber floor. Visibility is important in the posterior teeth. Molars, in particular, present difficulties in identifying canal orifices.

Location of Canals. Unroofing the chamber in molars is a prerequisite for locating canals, partic-

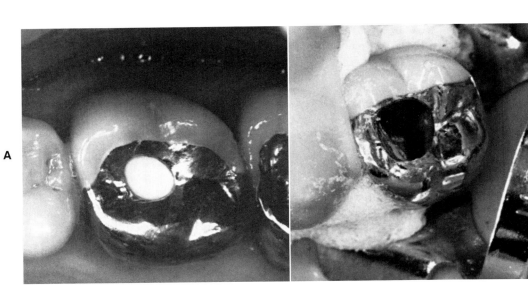

A

B

FIGURE 12-5
A, Inadequate opening would permit neither good visibility to locate canals nor adequate straight-line access.
B, Wide opening through occlusal surface of crown is correct. Note that the access does not extend to the porcelain to prevent its chipping.

ularly those that have displaced orifices. An example is the mesiobuccal (MB) canal in both maxillary and mandibular molars. These canals are the most difficult to locate because they lie farthest at the periphery and under the mesiobuccal cusp.

A particular challenge is the second (mesiolingual [ML]) canal in the MB root of maxillary molars.[15] This orifice is usually obscured by a shelf of dentin and requires special techniques of exposure.[16,17]

Improve Straight-Line Access. Areas of the roof of the chamber and dentin shelves that overlie canal orifices are particularly likely to impede straight-line access. They must be removed (Figure 12-6).

Exposure of Pulp Horns. Exposure of pulp horns in all teeth is critical, particularly in anterior teeth, because of future aesthetic considerations. Pulp horns contain debris and trap sealer remnants; both are liable to cause eventual discoloration, which may become manifest months or years after treatment. Pulp horns should be opened conservatively and with care. It is not necessary to remove excessive amounts of enamel or dentin to obtain access for removal of debris and sealer. The technique is described later in this chapter.

ACCESS IN SPECIAL SITUATIONS

Usually, access preparation is done under less than ideal conditions. Most teeth requiring root canal treatment have been affected by caries,

restorations, fractures, attrition, and so on. Frequently, these irritants have promoted deposition of dentin. This means that the preparation itself will not be "ideal" and must be altered to accommodate variations. *It is critical for the operator to recognize these variations and plan the access accordingly* (Figure 12-7) *before picking up the handpiece!*

Caries

Ordinarily, all caries are removed early in the access preparation phase. Ideally, caries are excavated before the chamber is entered to avoid contaminating the chamber and canals with later caries removal. The reason for not leaving caries is obvious; the pulp chamber will be heavily contaminated with bacteria, which may be introduced into the pulp system during canal preparation. Also, a temporary seal is not obtained unless the sealing material is in direct contact with clean and noncarious dentin.

There is one exception. When caries removal may lacerate the gingiva or compromise isolation, it is advisable to leave a very small remnant of caries temporarily. This thin band of caries at the gingival margin may remain until root canal treatment is complete (Figure 12-8). Then the carious remnants are removed before the postobturation temporary restoration is placed. However, to repeat, *all* caries internal to this region must be removed, preferably *before* the chamber is unroofed.

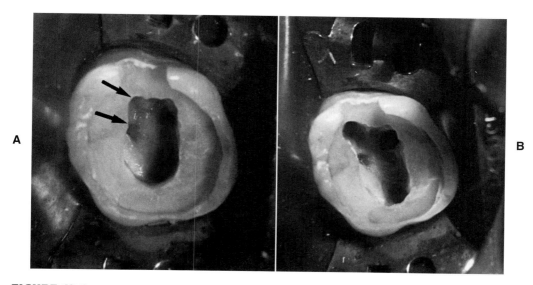

FIGURE 12-6

A, Inadequate access opening because dentin shelves obscure orifices, particularly the mesiobuccal and mesiolingual orifices *(arrows)*. **B,** Removal of these shelves gives good straight-line access to the canals in this maxillary molar.

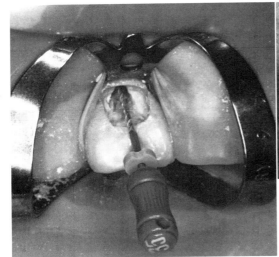

A

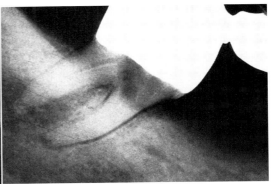

B

FIGURE 12-7
Unusual situations. **A,** Extensive caries permits access from the facial surface. **B,** The dentist did not recognize that the retainer was misoriented on the tooth; the bur was misaligned and perforated the mesial surface.

A hint: When caries under enamel are removed, a portion of enamel is left undermined. This undermining should be at the proximal edges, not under a cusp. These undercuts in the facial and lingual aid in retaining the temporary restoration.

Existing Permanent Restoration

There is a general idea that when a restoration is present, a textbook outline access preparation should be done through the restoration. This is not the case! A restoration generally provides more flexibility in designing the preparation because of the opportunity for a wider opening. Tooth structure is not being removed, only the restorative materials.

Ideal Situations. Removal of the entire restoration, whether a small occlusal amalgam or a full crown, is preferred. Total removal increases visibility and simplifies the search for and preparation of canals. However, total removal is often neither feasible nor desirable. Retaining the proximal component of an intact class II restoration that extends subgingivally will aid in isolation. A crown that is still serviceable and that will not be replaced ordinarily is retained because the casting may be destroyed on removal.

Extent of Opening. When the existing restoration will not be removed entirely, the opening should be expanded. This allows the operator to widen the access to attain better visibility and straighter access (see Figure 12-5). Obviously, a decision must be made early in treatment (preferably as a first consideration) whether to replace or repair the restoration (see Chapter 15). If it is to be repaired, the opening is minimized. An excep-

tion is a full gold crown, which permits a very wide access.

Porcelain Restorations. Access through these presents some special problems. Edge chipping and cracks are common; shattering or loss of segments of porcelain occasionally occurs.[18] To minimize these effects, preparations should be done slowly, with copious water spray.

Restoration Repair. Restoring the access opening through a crown with amalgam is permanent and maintains crown retention at original levels.[19] Therefore access usually does not ultimately compromise retention or strength.

Defective Restoration. Before access is begun and the rubber dam is placed, the margins of the restoration are checked carefully with an explorer. This is particularly important subgingivally. Open margins, recurrent caries, or other factors that may lead to communication with the pulp space after access preparation may jeopardize isolation during treatment and between appointments. If defective, the restoration must be removed entirely. It is very important not to discover a defective restoration *after* the access preparation is complete! This wastes time and compromises treatment. Such a determination is made before the rubber dam is placed and access is begun.

Existing Temporary Restoration

Frequently, a tooth requiring root canal treatment has been restored temporarily. The same basic principles apply as with the permanent restoration; that is, the entire temporary restoration is removed when feasible. When the entire temporary restoration will not be removed, the opening is overprepared at the expense of the material. Occasionally,

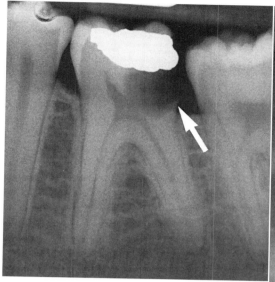

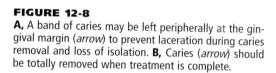

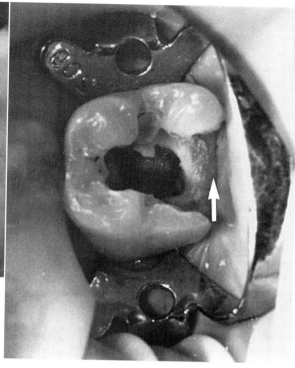

FIGURE 12-8
A, A band of caries may be left peripherally at the gingival margin (*arrow*) to prevent laceration during caries removal and loss of isolation. **B,** Caries (*arrow*) should be totally removed when treatment is complete.

a portion (usually proximal) of the temporary restoration may remain to improve isolation.

Temporary Crowns. Unless there are extenuating circumstances, temporary crowns are removed before isolation. This improves visibility, enhances access and canal preparation, and facilitates obturation. When left in place, temporary crowns frequently become loose and are displaced by the rubber dam clamp or leak during treatment and between appointments.

Bands. Ordinarily it is safer to remove bands because of their potential for leakage. However, if a band has been placed to help retain a temporary crown, it may aid in isolation. A well-fitting orthodontic band may remain and does not impinge on or hamper occlusal access. However, a rubber dam clamp may displace a band during the procedure. If the band is not removed, the clamp should be placed on an adjacent tooth.

Copper bands are notoriously poor for maintaining a seal (Figure 12-9). If they are already in place, the adequacy of adaptation should be determined. If in doubt, the band is removed and another isolation system is used (see Chapter 8).

Previous Partial Treatment

Root canal treatment started by another operator offers special challenges. The practitioner must make a periapical radiograph before instituting treatment (Figure 12-10). This is done for two reasons: first, to become aware of the situation and any previous mishaps (e.g., perforations, separated instruments, or misoriented access); and second, if such a mishap was caused by the first operator, the patient is made aware of the situation. Radiographs are made partly for protection; otherwise, responsibility for the mishap may be attributed to the second operator by the patient or by a jury.

Although some phases of treatment have been completed, it should not be assumed that treatment has been satisfactory to that point. For example, if access preparation and partial canal instrumentation have been done, the access may not have good straight-line preparation. The operator should be ready to correct another's faults or errors.

Timing and Reasons for Removal of a Restoration

Restoration removal, either total or partial, should be completed before the opening into the chamber is made. This saves time and also helps to prevent particles of the temporary or permanent restoration from precipitating into and blocking the canals. If it becomes necessary to

A

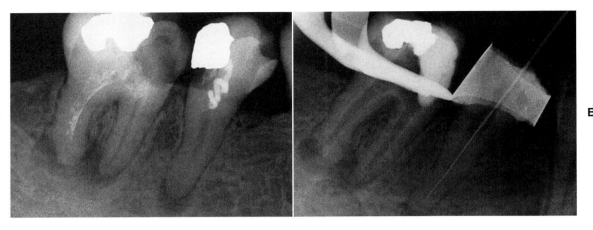

B

FIGURE 12-9
A, Two teeth requiring retreatment that will present isolation and access problems. **B,** Two methods of isolation for access are shown. The copper band on the premolar is poorly adapted and will irritate the gingiva and probably leak. The IRM on the molar is the preferred approach for temporary isolation.

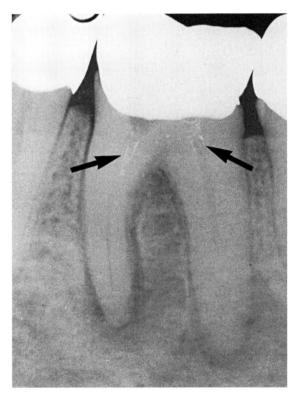

FIGURE 12-10
The reason for making preoperative radiographs is evident. A treatment attempt by an earlier operator left amalgam shaving *(arrows)* in the canals of the first molar. The shavings could easily be packed deeper and could block the canals. (Courtesy G. Obermayr.)

remove more restoration after unroofing the chamber, a cotton pellet is packed tightly onto the chamber floor to protect the orifices. This is only partially satisfactory; frequently the bur grabs and displaces the cotton pellet.

Altered Internal Anatomy

External irritants and age change the morphology of the pulp space. Anything that exposes dentin to the oral cavity often results in formation of additional layers of dentin in the chamber.

Dentin Formation. Generally, dentin that forms in response to surface irritants is irregular, thus giving rise to the term "irregular secondary (or tertiary) dentin". This dentin results from either the stimulation of existing odontoblasts or the destruction and replacement of odontoblasts by a unique cell that forms a hard tissue. Invariably, this irregular dentin forms at the base of tubules that communicate with the exposure or the irritation.

Areas of Altered Dentin. In most cases, the irritants responsible for dentin formation are obvious. These include things such as caries, restorations, areas of attrition or abrasion, and fractures. Each results in dentin exposure and irritation of the underlying pulp. A second means of identification is careful viewing of radiographs, directing particular attention to the pulp regions under areas of dentin irritation or exposure (Figure 12-11). Access should be designed accordingly.

Difficult-to-Locate Canals

Difficulty in locating canals is common; a canal or canals are certainly present in the root (as they always are) but cannot be located. Frequently, this difficulty can be anticipated. Isolation and radiographs assist in finding the canal.

Delay Isolation. Teeth may have extensive restorations or caries or may contain canals not visible on radiographs; these and other factors suggest difficulties in orientation and location of orifices. Occasionally, placement of a rubber dam may be delayed until the chamber or canals are located; this permits improved bur orientation to the long axis of the crown and root. Radiographs are studied to determine root direction, and the alveolus is examined to detect root prominence. The inclination of the root relative to the crown and to adjacent teeth is noted. A canal (if single) is located in the approximate center of the root. All these factors serve as a guide for the operator and the bur.

Although the best means of searching for and determining the location of a canal is to use a small file as an explorer, caution is needed because the airway is not protected unless a rubber dam is in place. A piece of floss is placed through the hole in the handle of the file or a gauze pack positioned at the back of the tongue for protection.

Once a canal is discovered or suspected, the rubber dam is placed immediately. A confirmatory radiograph with a file in place is recommended if there is a possibility that the "canal" might, in fact, be a perforation.

Exploratory Radiographs. Occasionally, as the bur search goes deeper into the root, radiographs are made to determine the position of the access preparation in the root. Two radiographs are made, one from the straight facial perspective and another from a mesial or a distal perspective. The canal is centered, and therefore the preparation should also be directed toward the center of the root. The facial projection gives a mesiodistal orientation; the angled radiograph provides a facial-lingual direction relative to where the canal should lie. Appropriate adjustments are made to direct the bur toward the center of the root. For specific details of this technique, refer to Chapter 9.

ACCESS TECHNIQUES

There is a basic approach to access preparation that applies in principle to all situations. Variations occur according to position, orientation, restoration, extent of caries, and other factors. Specific details for all situations are not discussed in this chapter. The operator must carefully ana-

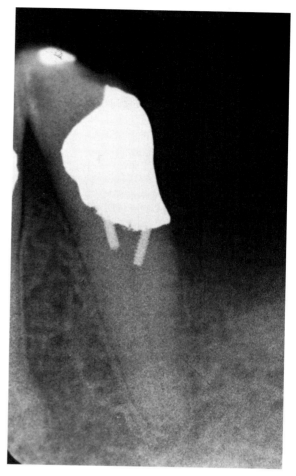

FIGURE 12-11
Caries, restorations, and pins on the premolar all alter the internal anatomy by stimulating formation of irregular secondary dentin. Thus, access is difficult and must be modified accordingly.

lyze each situation, formulate an approach, and then proceed with caution. If on initial assessment the case seems complex, the clinician should not attempt access preparation and thus create errors. The patient should initially be referred to an endodontist.

Burs

Although different designs and types of burs have been advocated, none has been demonstrated to be superior.[20] Special burs are manufactured primarily for access (Figure 12-12). These are effective but require practice. Conventional burs that function well include the straight and tapered fissure burs (Figure 12-13), occasionally supplemented by round burs.

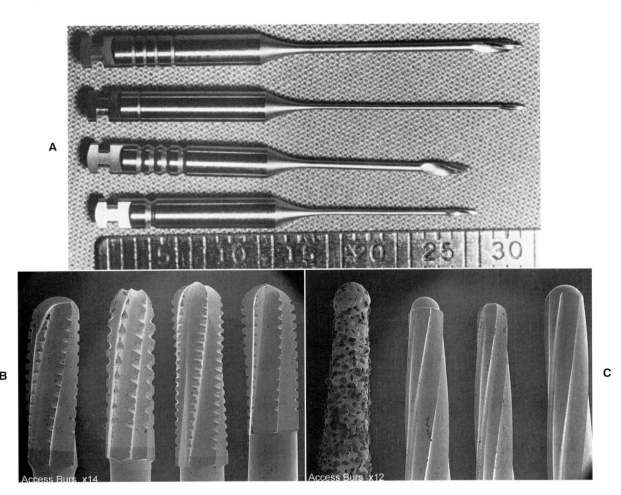

FIGURE 12-12
Access burs. **A,** Gates-Glidden drills; size is identified by the grooves on the shank. The drills also are available in two lengths. The shorter are useful in molars. **B,** These special end-cutting burs are good for opening through porcelain or metal. *Left to right:* Beaver by Dentsply Midwest, GW#2 by S S White, Transmetal by Dentsply Maillefer, H34L by Braessler. **C,** Non-end-cutting burs are for removing dentin shelves and finishing the outline. *Left to right:* Endo Access Bur, Endo Z, Multipurpose Bur—all three by Dentsply Maillefer; 269GK by Braessler. (**B** and **C** courtesy Dr. W. Johnson.)

Procedure

To repeat, there are three general objectives. (1) Expose and unroof the chamber for visibility. This includes removal of pulp horns in anterior teeth; removal of pulp horns is not always necessary in posterior teeth. (2) Conserve tooth structure by removing only the portions that must be removed. Restorations should be removed or at least opened widely. (3) Most important is to obtain straight-line access.

These objectives are accomplished as follows (Figure 12-13):

1. Rough out the access cavity well into the dentin, close to the chamber, with a high-speed handpiece (Figure 12-13, *A*).

2. Penetrate and unroof the chamber with a high-speed bur (Figure 12-13, *B*). It is prudent to measure on the radiograph the distance between the occlusal or incisal surface and the roof of the chamber. This marking is transferred onto the bur to serve as a landmark. It indicates the approximate bur depth to the chamber roof. When difficulty in locating the chamber is anticipated, a search should be made for the chamber region of greatest dimension (for example, over the lingual canal region in maxillary molars and over the distal canal in mandibular molars).

3. Locate canal orifices with the endodontic explorer. These are confirmed as canals by

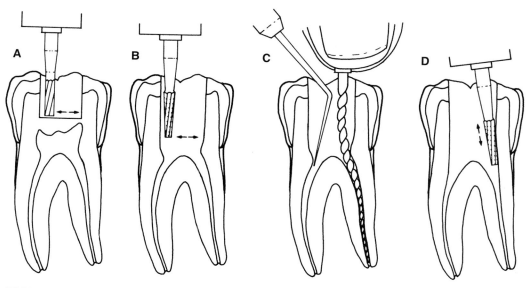

FIGURE 12-13

Basic steps in access preparation. **A,** The access cavity is outlined deep in the dentin and close to the chamber roof by the high-speed bur. **B,** Penetration and unroofing are achieved by low-speed latch-type burs or, as in this example, a tapered fissure high-speed bur. Other shaped burs are suitable also. **C,** Canal orifices are located with an endodontic explorer and are identified and negotiated to their estimated length with small files. **D,** The dentin shelves that overlie and obscure the orifices are removed.

penetrating them with small (No. 15 and 25) files (Figure 12-13, C). If there is doubt about which canal has been discovered, an angled radiograph is made with a file or files in place before proceeding. Frequently a canal that is thought to be of one type turns out to be another.

4. Remove dentin shelves that usually overlie and obscure canal orifices in molars with long-shank, small round, or small tapered fissure or diamond burs (Figure 12-13, D). Standard-length burs may be converted to surgical length by extension in the handpiece chuck. Gates-Glidden burs are not for removal of dentin from the chamber; these are for use at or beyond the orifice and in the canal.

5. Before obtaining straight-line access, canals are explored with small files to determine patency and whether the canal is large enough to accommodate Gates-Glidden burs. This evaluation is carried out as follows:
   a. A series of small files (No. 10 to 25) is set at the estimated working length for each canal.
   b. Each canal is explored starting with the smallest and progressing to the larger files at estimated length to establish patency.

6. Occasionally small instruments cannot be inserted to length; this may be caused by one of two problems:
   a. *Blockage.* The file passes easily but strikes a dead end, possibly owing to a small ledge or calcification deep in the canal. A small curve or bend is made at the tip of the file and an attempt is made to wiggle and tease the file tip past the blockage.
   b. *Constriction.* The instrument increasingly binds and then stops in the small canal. A lubricant (glycerin, liquid surgical soap, or topical anesthetic) is placed at the orifice with the tip of cotton pliers or with a small syringe. The lubricant is worked ahead of the file by pumping and spinning counterclockwise. This usually permits the file to slide several millimeters farther. Lubricant is also useful in initial enlargement and in placing larger files in the canal after the corrected working length is determined. Also, opening a canal coronally often facilitates passage to the apical end of the canal. More information on managing constrictions and blockages is found in Chapter 13.

7. Small canals must be sufficiently large and patent to permit passage of Gates-Glidden

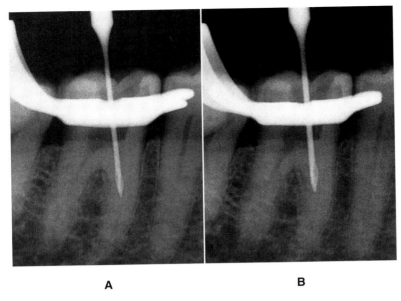

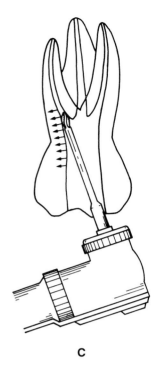

FIGURE 12-14
Gates-Glidden drill usage. **A,** No. 3 extends well past the orifice. **B,** No. 4 is used shorter than the No. 3 and can be used peripherally for straight-line preparation. **C,** These burs must be used only on peripheral walls and away from the furcation.

burs. In these smaller canals, this is best achieved by a "*passive step-back*" (preflaring) of the canals.[21] This provides nonforced enlargement and slight canal flaring; there is a reduction in procedural errors, which allows use of larger working length files, with more control.[22] The technique is as follows:

   a. The estimated working length (EWL) is determined (radiographic tooth length minus 3 mm).

   b. Irrigant (in larger canals) or a lubricant (in smaller canals) is worked apically.

   c. Small files that will pass without force to or close to EWL are then rotated (reamed) a few times to remove a small amount of dentin.

   d. Progressively larger files at successively shorter lengths are again rotated to remove small amounts of dentin. This is continued through several sized instruments.

8. After passive step-back preparation in small canals or in already larger canals, the coronal segment of the canal is ready for Gates-Glidden burs. These burs will now have a definite canal to follow and are less likely to bind or create a blind ending. Gates-Glidden burs (see Figure 12-12, *A*) for most situations are stainless steel in sizes 2, 3, and 4 (as indicated by the number of bands on the shank). No. 1 burs are too small to be effective, dull quickly, and break easily.[23] Sizes 5 and 6 are overly large and dangerous.

9. The No. 2 or 3 bur is run at medium speed and with light force several millimeters (the distance depends on canal size and curvature) into the canal, allowing the bur to make its own way, but away from the danger zone. The bur should be inserted in the same direction as the canal exits the chamber. It should not be forced laterally, and no attempt to gain straight-line access should be made with the No. 2 or 3 bur (Figure 12-14, *A*).

10. Use of the No. 4 bur follows almost to the depth of the No. 3 bur. To obtain straight-line access, the No. 4 bur is worked on the outstroke (Figure 12-14, *B*). This motion is directed toward the lingual aspect in anterior teeth and toward the periphery (or line angles) in posterior teeth, staying away from the danger zone (Figure 12-14, *C*).

   NOTE: *Gates-Glidden burs are always worked away* from the furcation in molars to avoid a stripping perforation. For example, to obtain straight-line access on the mesiobuccal canal of a maxillary molar, the No. 4 bur is worked toward a "standing up" position

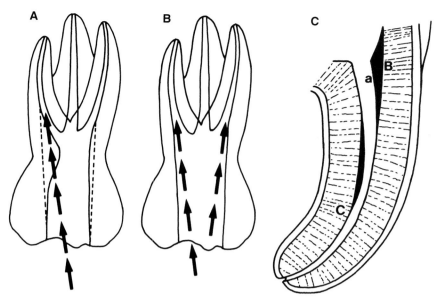

FIGURE 12-15
A, The *dashed lines* show where dentin must be removed to achieve straight-line access. **B,** The access so attained. **C,** The original canal *(a)* is modified by Gates-Glidden burs by removing tooth structure at *B* and *C.*

(safety zone region) on the mesiobuccal wall (Figure 12-15).

11. Straight-line access is checked with files, which should pass undeflected deep into the canals. Smaller (No. 3) Gates-Glidden burs carefully used in the canal close to the curve facilitate straight-line access (Figure 12-16).

Anterior Teeth

The procedure followed is basically that outlined in the preceding section, with the following special considerations.

Straight-Line Access. Access is evaluated with a file. When placed deep in the canal, the file should not be deflected from the incisal enamel. Ideally, the file should sit passively in the canal. If it does not, tooth structure may be removed from the incisal triangle[1] or, preferably, from the lingual shelf (see Figure 12-4). Usually lingual access extends deep under the cingulum. Also, a lingual canal in mandibular anterior teeth or premolars is often missed because of inadequate lingual extension and lack of straight-line access. In some cases (especially in mandibular anterior teeth), the preparation is extended close to the incisal edge to gain direct access.[24]

Pulp Horns Removed. Removal of pulp horns is evaluated with the small hooked end of an explorer (Figure 12-17). There should be no incisal

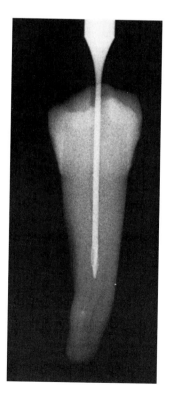

FIGURE 12-16
Gates-Glidden burs may be used deep in the canal or until resistance is felt at the curvature. The more these burs improve the access, the more efficient is the overall preparation of the canal.

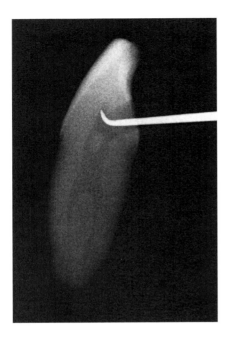

FIGURE 12-17
The hook end of an explorer detects unremoved pulp horns. This preparation requires opening and exposure of the horns and removal of the lingual shelf.

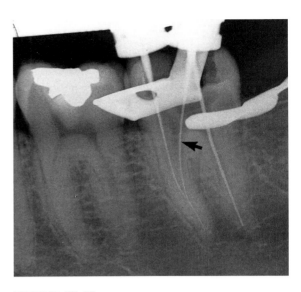

FIGURE 12-18
Mesial and distal files demonstrate good straight-line access. The middle file *(arrow)* is deflected by dentin shelves and offers poor straight-line access.

catch. The remaining pulp horns are opened and removed with small round burs.

Posterior Teeth

Straight-Line Access. Access is evaluated with files, which should not deflect off the enamel. In a single-canal premolar, the file should pass straight into the canal.[25] In a multicanaled tooth, the file handles ideally are parallel when all are placed in their respective canals simultaneously (Figure 12-18). This result is usually not totally feasible, but at least the file shaft should not deflect from the enamel on an opposite wall. A curvature on the thicker upper portion of the file imparts more straightening force on the apical portion of the file. Therefore a *straighter approach of the file in the curved canal decreases the probability of preparation error in the apical region.*

In other words, straight-line access to the canal in a curved root provides an opportunity to reach the apical region and to prepare the apical curvature more efficiently (by having to deal with only one curvature rather than two).

Pulp Horns Removed. It is not necessary to open the access excessively to remove pulp horns in molars and premolars.

Specific Preparations

In the diagrams of molar access (see the Appendix), the outline is centered mesiodistally. Canal orifices and chamber are centered and are not located mesially as commonly reported.[12] The Appendix illustrates pulp morphology and access preparations for each tooth group.

ERRORS

Unfortunately, mistakes occur. Most result from inadequate diagnosis and failure to recognize problems early. Others reflect a lack of knowledge either of internal anatomy or the desired end point of access preparation.

Misorientation

Internal Excess Removal. Excess removal of dentin constitutes needless destruction of dentin either in searching for the chamber or canals or in placing the access improperly.

Anterior Teeth. Usually the bur is directed too far labially or lingually and gouges the dentin internally (Figure 12-19).

Premolars. As with anterior teeth, the bur is directed too far labially or lingually as well as

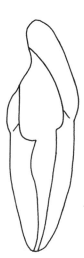

FIGURE 12-19
A common error encountered in achieving access on mandibular anterior teeth: gouging the facial or lingual surface internally.

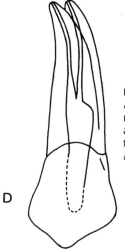

FIGURE 12-20
A common error encountered on maxillary premolars: misdirection and gouging internally toward the mesial concavity. *D,* Distal; *M,* mesial.

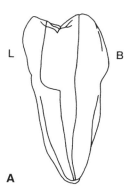
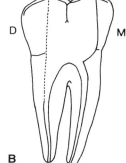
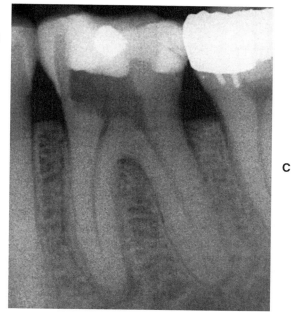

FIGURE 12-21
Common errors in access preparation of mandibular molars. **A,** Gouging toward the lingual surface because of the lingual inclination of the crown and lingual tipping of the tooth. *L,* lingual; *B,* buccal. **B,** Undermining of the marginal ridge and near-perforation on the mesial surface. The error was created by starting access too far mesially and directing the burs straight inferiorly. *D,* distal; *M,* mesial. **C,** Example of misdirected access preparations.

mesially or distally.[25] These teeth leave little room for error, particularly toward the mesial or distal aspect, which is narrow with cervical concavities (Figure 12-20).

Mandibular Molars. Two regions tend to be abused: the mesial aspect under the marginal ridge and the lingual surface beneath the lingual cusps. The teeth and the crowns tip mesially and lingually. A bur directed straight inferior will gouge these areas (Figure 12-21).

Maxillary Molars. As in mandibular molars, there is a tendency to remove dentin beneath the mesial marginal ridge (Figure 12-22).

Mistaken Canal. As stated earlier, it is common to become misoriented during molar access preparation and mistake one canal for another.

When in doubt, a file is placed and then an appropriate angled radiograph is made to identify the discovered canal.

Perforation

Perforation usually results from misorientation (Figure 12-23) or while searching for a canal. All perforations adversely affect prognosis; some doom the tooth to extraction.

Causes. The major cause for perforation is lack of knowledge of the internal tooth anatomy and failure to consider alterations. The second major cause is rushing to treat without careful evaluation. These considerations were described earlier in this chapter and are related to restorations, altered tooth position, or changes in internal anatomy caused by caries. When the practitioner is searching for canals in molars, most perforations occur into the furcation.

Treatment. Techniques for repairing perforations depend on their location, size, and other factors. Specific techniques are described in Chapter 18.

Prevention. Many errors can be prevented, minimized, or corrected before they become serious. One such preventive technique is to make a bitewing radiograph, which often identifies an impending problem (Figure 12-24).

Two tricks can be used to minimize misorientation by staying in the long axis of the root and crown during initial access: (1) A rubber dam is not placed until the canal is located; and (2) a pencil line is scribed on the crown, showing the long axis of the root (Figure 12-25).

Bur Separation

Using burs or drills improperly may result in breakage in the canal. Delicate tapered fissure burs should not be used deep into an orifice. Gates-Glidden drills should be worked into canals with continuous rotation; stopping probably will cause the drill to bind and then separate. These often lock in the canal and cannot be removed (Figure 12-26).

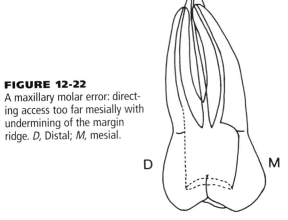

FIGURE 12-22
A maxillary molar error: directing access too far mesially with undermining of the margin ridge. *D,* Distal; *M,* mesial.

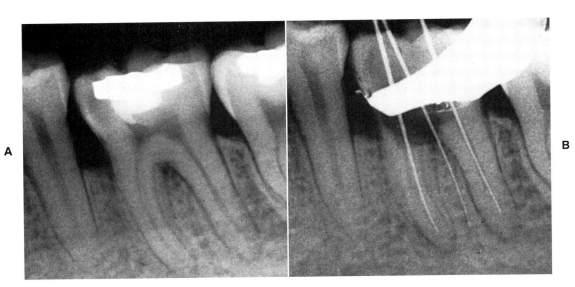

FIGURE 12-23
Misorientation resulting in perforation. **A,** Molar is inclined mesially and lingually. **B,** Incorrect access approach resulting in severe perforation on mesial and into furcation.

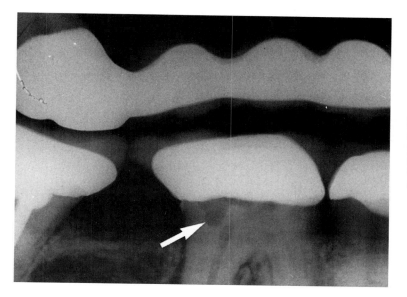

FIGURE 12-24
Misorientation of the access is obvious *(arrow)* on the bitewing radiograph. Identifying such an error early often prevents a serious consequence and permits correction. (Courtesy Dr. C. Koloffon.)

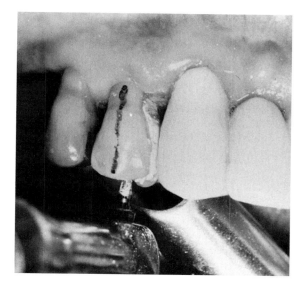

FIGURE 12-25
Techniques that help with difficult access. A line is scribed on the facial surface in the long axis of the tooth. Preparation is started without a rubber dam (until the canal is located); this aids in orientation.

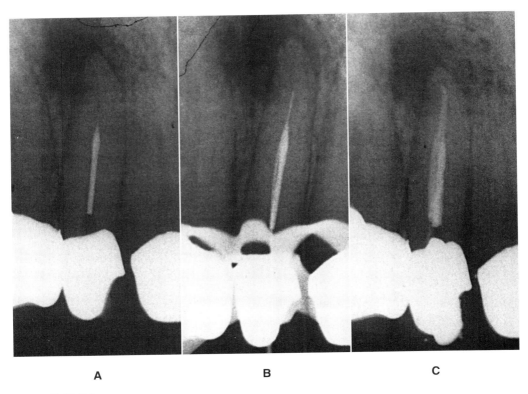

A   **B**   **C**

FIGURE 12-26
Gates-Glidden drill separation. **A,** Drill was stopped, causing binding and breakage up the shaft. **B,** The drill could not be removed, but was bypassed. **C,** The canal was prepared and obturated; the prognosis is good because canal is sealed apically and coronally.

Working Length Determination

The objective is to establish the length (distance from the apex) at which canal preparation and subsequent obturation are to be completed. Optimal length is 1 to 2 mm short of the apex, although this may vary slightly with different diagnoses.[26] Procedures may be terminated 0 to 2 mm from the apex if the pulp is necrotic and 0 to 3 mm if the pulp is vital.[27] Of course, lengths will vary according to many factors; these ideals are not always attainable. Apex location varies; these variations can be approximated but not usually determined using only a diagnostic radiograph.[28-30] Therefore this determination must be an estimate, using average measurements of distances from the apical foramen to the true apex and from the apical constriction (or within the canal) to the apical foramen.[31] Electronic apex locators are also helpful with length determination in many situations.

Prognosis and microbiologic studies as well as histologic experiments involving healing after obturation consistently show that it is preferable to confine instruments, chemicals, and obturating materials to the canal space.[32-37]

REFERENCE POINT

The reference point is the site on the occlusal or incisal surface from which measurements are made. This point is used throughout canal preparation and obturation.

Selection

A reference point is chosen that is stable and easily visualized during preparation. Usually this is the highest point on the incisal edge on anterior teeth and a buccal cusp tip on posterior teeth. The same reference point is best used for all canals in multirooted teeth. The mesiobuccal cusp tip is preferred in molars.

Stability

A reference point that will not change during or between appointments is selected. Examples of unstable reference points are undermined cusps or cements. If it is necessary to use an undermined cusp, it should be reduced considerably before access preparation. Areas other than cusp tips, such as marginal ridges or the floor of the chamber, are unreliable or difficult to visualize.

TECHNIQUE FOR DETERMINATION

After coronal access preparation and passive step-back, the working length is determined.[38]

Different techniques have been used, studied, and advocated for determining working length, including radiographic (conventional or digital), electronic, and tactile methods; none are totally accurate or infallible.[39] Electronic techniques are best used in certain situations, but must be confirmed radiographically; tactile methods are too unreliable. Radiographs are usually made to determine the working length. A workable technique is as follows.

Estimated Working Length

1. The diagnostic film, which is made using a paralleling technique, is measured from the reference point to the apex with a millimeter endodontic ruler.
2. From the radiographic tooth measurement, 3 mm is subtracted for the estimated working length. This takes into account the following:
   a. The relation of the radiographic apex to the actual apical foramen or constriction (approximately 1 mm).
   b. The magnification effect of the radiograph. Magnification of 2 mm (because of divergence of the central beam) is allowed for all teeth.
   c. This 3-mm decrease should generally leave the initial instrument placement slightly short of working length (a good "fudge" factor).
3. An instrument stop measured to the estimated working length is placed on each of a series of small files.
4. These files are used in successively larger sizes to explore the canal until a size is reached that binds (locks) at or slightly short of the estimated working length. If this is No. 25 or larger, a working length film is made with this file in place. If smaller than this, passive step-back is performed (described earlier). A radiograph is then made with a file binding tight. No. 8 or 10 files should *not be* used to take working length radiographs; small file tips fade out

and are usually not visible. On molar radiographs, No. 15 file tips are often obscure.
5. In a multicanaled tooth, files are usually placed in all canals.
6. If a root contains two canals (or may have an undiscovered canal), the cone should be positioned at a 20-to 30-degree horizontal deviation from the standard facial projection. (Exceptions are maxillary molars, for which at least a facial radiograph should be provided.)
7. A film is exposed with the instruments in place. Either conventional or digital radiography is suitable.[40,41] Usually one radiograph is sufficient; occasionally an additional film is necessary.

Corrected Working Length

The corrected working length is determined by measuring the discrepancy between the tip of the file and the radiographic apex. The file is then adjusted to 1 to 2 mm short of the radiographic apex.

Variations

The proper working length distance from the radiographic apex varies (Figure 12-27). A periradicular lesion resorbs bone and apical tooth structure.[42] The apical resorption may or may not be visible radiographically, but significantly alters apical anatomy (Figure 12-28). Working length distance from the apex is determined when the following are seen *radiographically*:[43]

1. No bone or root resorption: 1 mm from apex.
2. Bone but no root resorption: 1.5 mm from apex.
3. Bone and root resorption: 2 mm from apex.

The distance from the file to the apex is measured and then the file is adjusted to obtain the correct working length. An additional radiograph is not necessary for verification unless there is a discrepancy greater than 3 mm. If so, a confirmatory radiograph should be made.

ALTERNATIVE TECHNIQUES
Electronic Apex Locators

Electronic devices have been designed to determine canal length by "reading" when periodontal ligament has been reached by the file tip at the apical foramen. The electronic principle is relatively simple and is based on electrical resistance; when a circuit is complete (tissue is contacted by the tip of the file), resistance decreases markedly and current suddenly begins to flow (Figure 12-29).[44] According to the device, this event is signaled by a beep, a buzz, a flashing light, digital readouts, or a pointer on a dial.

The original electronic apex locators operated on the direct current principle. A problem with these devices was that conductive fluids such as hemorrhage, exudate, or irrigant in the canal would permit current flow and therefore a false reading. Newer devices (Figure 12-30) are impedance-based, using alternating current of two frequencies; these measure and compare two electrical impedances

that change as the file moves apically. The benefit is that these devices are much less affected by fluid conductive media in the canal.[45] The impedance-type apex locators have been demonstrated to be 80 to 95% accurate in identifying the apical foramen.[46,47] Therefore after obtaining a reading, 1 to 2 mm is subtracted as the corrected working length.

Although there are some variations with newer devices, most operate similarly. One electrode is attached to the patient (commonly a lip clip); the other electrode is clipped to the file. The patient

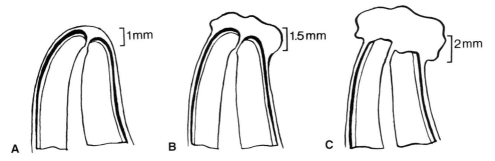

FIGURE 12-27
Determination of proper working length distance from apex. This distance varies according to radiographic findings: **A,** When there is no bone or root resorption: 1 mm from apex. **B,** Bone but no root resorption: 1.5 mm from apex. **C,** Both bone and root resorption: 2 mm from apex. (Courtesy Dr. A. Goerig.)

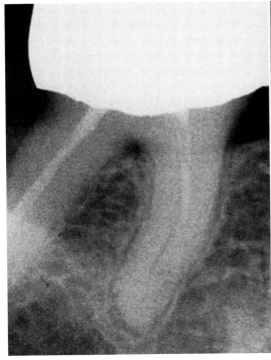

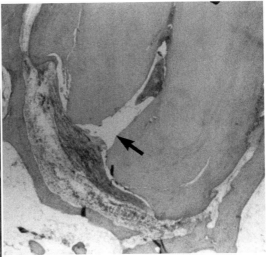

FIGURE 12-28
Apical resorption. **A,** Bone and root resorption at the apex. **B,** Viewing this histologically, the apex appears blunt and the canal has funneling resorption *(arrow).* The working length must be decreased to confine instruments to the canal. (Cadaver specimen, courtesy Dr. D. Holtzmann.)

therefore forms part of the circuit. When current flows, the operator is notified by one of the aforementioned signals. After the length adjustment is made, a confirmatory radiograph is made (angled when indicated) with an appropriate size file at this length.

These heavily marketed devices have engendered the interest and attention of clinicians and have been the subject of considerable research.[48] The apex locators are most useful for determining or confirming lengths on apices that are not clearly visible radiographically (Figure 12-31). They also are a good supplement to working radiographs and may improve length determination.[49] Importantly, this method does not replace radiographic techniques.[50] Radiographs not only determine working lengths, but angled working films also provide information regarding tooth and canal anatomy, curvatures, and relationships.

Electronic apex locators are also useful for identifying the presence and location of a perforation.[51] If a perforation is suspected, a file may be clipped to an apex locator. The file tip is then teased into the area of the suspected perforation. A positive reading would indicate contact with lateral periodontium.

Feeling the Apical Constriction

A popular belief is that a dentist with well-developed fingertip tactile sense can detect

when the file tip has reached the apical constriction. In most instances, this is unreliable.[22] Many apical regions do not in fact have a constriction; even those that do are at variable distances from the apical foramen.

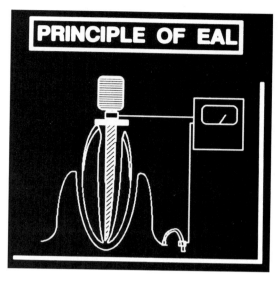

FIGURE 12-29
Electronic apex locators (EALs) operate on direct current, which is supplied by the unit on the upper right. One electrode is in contact with the metal shaft of the file; the other contacts soft tissue, usually by a lip clip. When the tip of the file touches tissue at the apical foramen, current begins to flow.

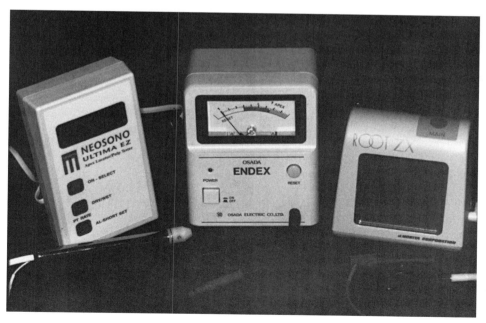

FIGURE 12-30
Examples of impedance-based electronic apex locators. These will function fairly accurately in either a wet or dry canal.

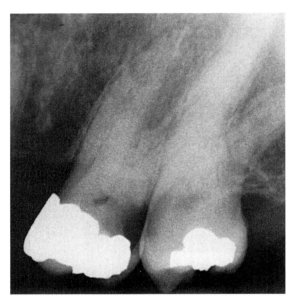

FIGURE 12-31
An apex locator would be very useful in determining the working length of this molar; all apices cannot be visualized radiographically because of superimposition over the other molar.

Patient Response

Another fallacious belief is that if the pulp is necrotic or if canal preparation is complete, an unanesthetized patient will detect the file tip when it reaches and contacts the vital tissue at the apical foramen. Supposedly, the patient then signals this event with an "eye blink" or other pain response. There are problems with this approach also. First, the procedure is painful for the patient. Second, a necrotic pulp frequently contains vital inflamed tissue that extends several millimeters into the canal.[34] This tissue may be very sensitive and respond to instrument contact short of the apex. Third, a patient feels pain after canal preparation is complete from hydraulic pressure even though instruments do not reach the apical region.

The opposite of pain with instruments *short* of length is lack of pain response when instruments are *beyond* the apex. This has been observed in some situations when, in an unanesthetized patient, an instrument has passed several millimeters out of the apex without being detected.

REFERENCES

1. LaTurno SA, Zillich RM: Straight-line endodontic access to anterior teeth, *Oral Surg Oral Med Oral Pathol* 59:418, 1985.
2. Leeb J: Canal orifice enlargement as related to biomechanical preparation, *J Endod* 9:463, 1983.
3. Abou-Rass M, Patoni FJ: The effects of decreasing surface tension on the flow of irrigating solutions in narrow root canals, *Oral Surg Oral Med Oral Pathol* 53:524, 1982.
4. Allison D, Michelich R, Walton R: The influence of method of canal preparation on the quality of apical and coronal obturation, *J Endod* 5:298, 1979.
5. Weine F, Kelly R, Lio P: The effect of preparation procedures on original canal shape and on apical foramen shape, *J Endod* 1:255, 1975.
6. Greene KJ, Krell KV: Clinical factors associated with ledged canals in maxillary and mandibular molars, *Oral Surg Oral Med Oral Pathol* 70:490, 1990.
7. Montgomery S: Root canal wall thickness of mandibular molars after biomechanical preparation, *J Endod* 11:257, 1985.
8. Abou-Rass M, Frank AL, Glick DH: Anticurvature filing method to prepare the root canal, *J Am Dent Assoc* 101:792, 1980.
9. Walton R: Histologic evaluation of different methods of enlarging the pulp canal space, *J Endod* 2:304, 1976.
10. Reeh E, Messer H, Douglas W: Reduction in tooth stiffness as a result of endodontic and restorative procedures, *J Endod* 15:512, 1989.
11. Panitvisai P, Messer H: Cuspal deflection in molars in relation to endodontic and restorative procedures, *J Endod* 21:57, 1995.
12. Wilcox L, Walton R, Case W: Molar access shape and outline according to orifice location, *J Endod* 15:315, 1989.
13. Sedgley C, Messer H: Are endodontically treated teeth more brittle? *J Endod* 18:332, 1992.
14. Wilcox L, Roskelley C, Sutton T: Relationship of root canal enlargement to finger-spreader induced vertical fracture, *J Endod* 23:533, 1997.
15. Stropko J: Canal morphology of maxillary molars: clinical observations of canal configurations, *J Endod* 25:447, 1999.
16. Weller R, Hartwell G: Impact of improved access and searching techniques on detection of the mesiolingual canal in maxillary molars, *J Endod* 15:2, 1989.
17. Ting P, Nga L: Clinical detection of the minor mesiobuccal canal of maxillary first molars, *Int Endod J* 25:304, 1992.
18. Haselton D, Lloyd P, Johnson W: A comparison of the effects of two burs on endodontic access in all-ceramic high Lucite crowns, *Oral Surg Oral Med Oral Pathol* 89:486, 2000.
19. McMullen A, Himel V, Sarkar N: An in vitro study of the effects endodontic access preparation and amalgam restoration have upon incisor crown retention, *J Endod* 16:269, 1990.
20. Stokes A, Tidmarsh B: Comparison of diamond and tungsten carbide burs for preparing endodontic access cavities through crowns, *J Endod* 14:550, 1988.
21. Torabinejad M: Passive step-back technique, *Oral Surg Oral Med Oral Pathol* 77:398, 1994.
22. Stabholz A, Rotstein I, Torabinejad M: Effect of preflaring on tactile detection of the apical constriction, *J Endod* 21:92, 1995.

23. Leubke N, Brantley W: Torsional and metallurgical properties of rotary endodontic instruments. II. Stainless steel Gates-Glidden drills, *J Endod* 17:319, 1991.

24. Mauger M, Waite R, Alexander J, Schindler W: Ideal endodontic access in mandibular incisors, *J Endod* 25:206, 1999.

25. Wilcox L, Walton R: The shape and location of mandibular premolar access openings, *Int Endodon J* 20:223, 1987.

26. Taintor J, Biesterfeld R, Valle G: Termination of the root canal filling, *Dent Surg* 3:54, 1979.

27. Wu M-K, Wesselink P, Walton R: Apical terminus location of root canal treatment procedures, *Oral Surg Oral Med Oral Pathol* 89:99, 2000.

28. Burch J, Hulen S: The relationship of the apical foramen to the anatomic apex of the tooth root, *Oral Surg Oral Med Oral Pathol* 34:262, 1972.

29. Mizutani T, Ohno N, Nakamura H: Anatomical study of the root apex in the maxillary anterior teeth, *J Endod* 18:344, 1992.

30. Olson AK, Goerig A, Cavataio R: The ability of the radiograph to determine the location of the apical foramen, *Int Endod J* 24:28, 1991.

31. Morfis A, Sylaras S, Georgopoulou M, et al: Study of apices of human permanent teeth with the use of a scanning electron microscope, *Oral Surg Oral Med Oral Pathol* 77:172, 1994.

32. Matsumoto T, Nagai T, Ida K: Factors affecting successful prognosis of root canal treatment, *J Endod* 13:239, 1987.

33. Debelian G, Olsen I, Tronstad L: Anaerobic bacteremia and fungemia in patients undergoing endodontic therapy: an overview, *Ann Periodontol* 3:281, 1998.

34. Ricucci D: Apical limit of root canal instrumentation and obturation. Part 1. Literature review, *Int Endod J* 31:384, 1998.

35. Ricucci D, Langeland K: Apical limit of root canal instrumentation and obturation, part 2. A histological study, *Int Endod J* 31:394, 1998.

36. Seltzer S, Soltanoff W, Sinai I, et al: Biologic aspects of endodontics. III. Periapical reactions to root canal instruments, *Oral Surg Oral Med Oral Pathol* 26:534, 1968.

37. Seltzer S, Solanoff W, Smith J: Biologic aspects of endodontics. V. Periapical tissue reactions to root canal instrumentation beyond the apex and root canal fillings short of and beyond the apex, *Oral Surg Oral Med Oral Pathol* 36:725, 1973.

38. Ibarrola J, Chapman B, Howard J, et al: Effect of preflaring on Root ZX apex locators, *J Endod* 25:625, 1999.

39. Katz A, et al: Tooth length determination: a review, *Oral Surg Oral Med Oral Pathol* 72:238, 1991.

40. Cederberg R, Tidwell E, Frederiksen N, Benson B: Endodontic working length assessment: comparison of storage phosphor digital imaging and radiographic film, *Oral Surg Oral Med Oral Pathol* 85:325, 1998.

41. Burger C, Mork T, Hutter J, Nicoll B: Direct digital radiography versus conventional radiography for estimation of canal length in curved canals, *J Endod* 25:260, 1999.

42. Malueg L, Wilcox L, Johnson W: Examination of external apical root resorption with scanning electron microscopy, *Oral Surg Oral Med Oral Pathol* 82:89, 1996.

43. Weine F: Endodontic therapy, ed 5, pp 395-405, St Louis, 1996, Mosby.

44. Sunada I: New method for measuring the length of the root canal, *J Dent Res* 41:375, 1962.

45. Lumley P: Impedance type electronic apex locators, *Endod Pract* 2:6, 1999.

46. Pagavino G, Pace R, Baccetti T: A SEM study of in vivo accuracy of the Root ZX electronic apex locator, *J Endod* 24:438, 1998.

47. Dunlap C, Remeikis N, BeGole E, Rauschenberger C: An in vivo evaluation of an electronic apex locator that uses the ratio method in vital and necrotic canals, *J Endod* 24:48, 1998.

48. Rivera E, Seraji M: Effect of recapitulation on accuracy of electronically determined canal length, *Oral Surg Oral Med Oral Pathol* 76:225, 1993.

49. Fouad A, Reid L: Effect of using electronic apex locators on selected endodontic treatment parameters, *J Endod* 26:364, 2000.

50. Fouad A, Krell K, McKendry D, et al: A clinical evaluation of five electronic root canal length measuring instruments, *J Endod* 16:446, 1990.

51. Fuss Z, Assooline L, Kaufman A: Determination of location of root perforations by electronic apex locators, *Oral Surg Oral Med Oral Radiol* 82:324, 1996.

13

Richard E. Walton and Eric M. Rivera

Cleaning and Shaping

LEARNING OBJECTIVES

After reading this chapter, the student should be able to:

1 / State reasons and describe situations for enlarging the cervical portion of the canal before performing straight-line access.

2 / Define how to determine the appropriate size of the master apical file.

3 / Describe objectives for both cleaning and shaping; explain how to determine when these have been achieved.

4 / Diagram "perfect" shapes of flared (step-back) and standardized preparations; draw these both in longitudinal and cross-sectional diagrams.

5 / Diagram probable actual shapes of flared (step-back) and standardized preparations in curved canals.

6 / Describe techniques for shaping canals that are irregular, such as round, oval, hourglass, bowling-pin, kidney-bean, or ribbon-shaped.

7 / Describe techniques, step-by-step, for standardized and flaring (step-back and/or crown-down) preparations.

8 / Distinguish between apical stop, apical seat, and open apex and discuss how to manage obturation in each.

9 / Describe the technique of pulp extirpation.

10 / Characterize the difficulties of preparation in the presence of anatomic aberrations that make complete débridement difficult.

11 / List properties of the "ideal" irrigant and identify which irrigant meets most of these criteria.

12 / Describe the needles and techniques that provide the maximal irrigant effect.

13 / Discuss the properties and role of chelating and decalcifying agents.

14 / Explain how to minimize preparation errors in small curved canals.

15 / Describe techniques for negotiating severely curved, "blocked," or constricted canals.

16 / Describe, in general, the principles of application of ultrasonic devices for cleaning and shaping.

17 / Evaluate, in general, alternative means of cleaning and shaping and list their advantages and disadvantages.

18 / Discuss nickel-titanium hand and rotary instruments and how the physical properties of this metal affect cleaning and shaping.

19 / Discuss the properties and role of intracanal, interappointment medicaments.

OUTLINE

Objectives
  Cleaning
  Shaping
  Master Apical File Determination
  Apical Preparation

Techniques of Pulp Extirpation and Cleaning and Shaping
  Pulp Extirpation
  Standardized Preparation
  Flaring Preparation
  Passive Step-Back
  Apical Clearing
  Anatomic Aberrations

Chemical Adjuncts
  Irrigation
  Dentin Softening
  Lubricants
  Desiccants

Avoidance of Preparation Errors
  Problems
  Prevention
  Other Errors

Review of Basic Principles of Instrumentation

Nickel-Titanium Instrumentation
  Hand
  Engine-Driven Rotary
  Combination of Passive Step-Back and Rotary Instrumentation

Alternative Techniques of Cleaning and Shaping
  Balanced Forces
  Energized Vibratory Systems
  Other Mechanized Techniques
  Lasers

Intracanal Medicaments
  Applications
  Limitations and Contraindications
  Calcium Hydroxide

Objectives

The end points of cleaning and shaping must be recognized. In other words, is canal preparation complete, and what criteria are used to make that determination? Schilder[1] defined the general objectives of canal preparation as follows: "Root canal systems must be cleaned and shaped: cleaned of their organic remnants and shaped to receive a three dimensional hermetic filling of the entire root canal space."

Cleaning and shaping are action words that identify precisely the two major goals of canal preparation. In fact, the goals are quite different, even though both are accomplished simultaneously and with the same instruments and agents. Therefore, criteria for each are considered separately. In addition to cleaning and shaping, apical preparation is also an important goal.

CLEANING
Débridement

By definition, débridement is the removal of existing or potential irritants from the root canal system. The goal is elimination; in actual practice, there is usually only a significant reduction. These irritants consist of the following, either singly or in combination: bacteria, bacterial byproducts, necrotic tissue, organic debris, vital tissue, salivary byproducts, hemorrhage, and other contaminants. The components in a necrotic pulp space represent a potent irritant.

Technique. The principle of débridement is simple. Ideally, instruments contact and plane all walls to loosen debris. The chemical action of irrigants further dissolves organic remnants and destroys microorganisms. Irrigants then flush the loosened and suspended debris from the canal space. This rids the canal space of irritants. However, experiments have shown clearly that with the canal preparation techniques currently available, such complete débridement is very difficult and in most cases nearly impossible.[2-4] Despite a practitioner's best efforts, remnants usually persist after the most careful chemomechanical preparation of the canal (Figure 13-1). So, realistically, the objectives are (1) to reduce these irritants to a subsignificant level and (2) to obturate so that the remnants are sequestered within the canal. Histologic and ultrastructural studies have demonstrated the presence of tissue elements and debris at all levels and in all areas of the canal, particularly in regions inaccessible to files (Figures 13-1 and 13-2).

Limitations. The root canal system is a very difficult environment in which to operate. To reemphasize an important concept, *files must contact and*

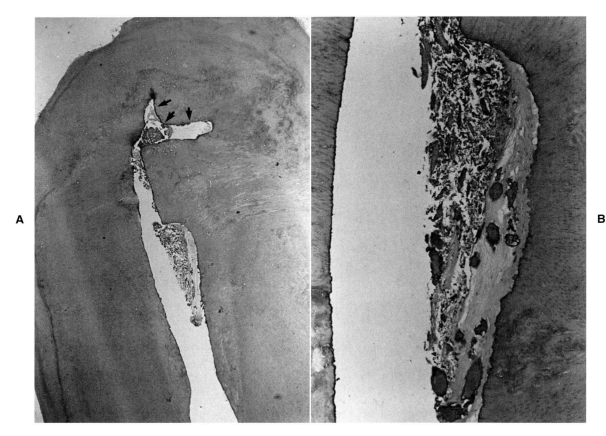

FIGURE 13-1
A, Remnants of tissue and debris are present in apical ramifications *(arrows)* and in a concavity in the canal wall.
B, Remnants in the concavity comprise a mixture of connective tissue, dentin chips, and other debris. This is a region in which the wall was not contacted by files during canal preparation.

plane the walls to débride effectively (see Figure 13-1). Such contact is often impossible owing to the design and physical properties of instruments and the irregularities of the pulp system.

Intracanal instruments were designed originally without consideration to the space in which they were to do their work. Reamers and files are best suited to enlarge a relatively straight, slightly tapered canal for post space. Their design and physical properties preclude effective débridement of actual canals. The interior of canals is bumpy with dips, concavities, intercanal communications, cul-de-sacs, inaccessible fins, apical ramifications, and other sequestered regions that these instruments have no chance of reaching. An additional complication is the usually curved canal that must be negotiated with relatively inflexible intracanal instruments.

It would seem that these débridement problems could be overcome by enlarging canals to greater sizes and by using irrigants or other chemicals that would break down tissue and bacterial remnants. However, increasing canal enlargement may not improve débridement and has other disadvantages, such as weakening the tooth.[5] Irrigating solutions also have limitations; these are discussed in detail later in this chapter.

Because of the difficulties with and inadequacies of instruments, irrigants, and techniques, the outcome is usually incomplete débridement of canals. There may be sufficient debris to compromise success; however, obturation may sequester these irritants, but this sequestration may not last indefinitely. With time, sealer may be washed out, or other communications may develop. Thus, the debris may now harbor and feed bacteria. Then irritants are produced that pass via the main or lateral canals to the periodontium. The result may be short-term treatment success but long-term failure. Thus, it is important to maximize canal débridement during cleaning and shaping.

Criteria. Unfortunately, there are no totally reliable, easily definable criteria for determining the end point of débridement. One suggestion has been to obtain clean shavings. However, shavings are difficult to see on files at all, whether clean or

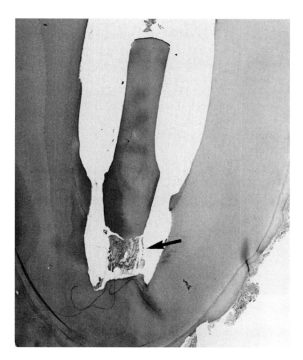

FIGURE 13-2
Facial-lingual section through the mesial root of a first molar. The intercommunicating isthmus *(arrow)* contains tissue after canal preparation. These regions are common and are inaccessible to instruments and irrigants.

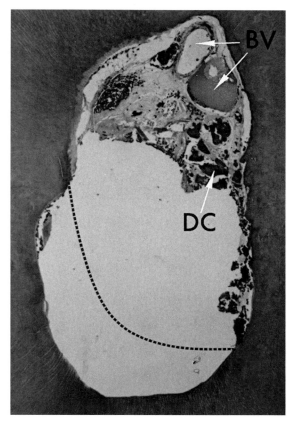

FIGURE 13-3
Canal cross section (after preparation) shows the ineffectiveness of débridement at times. The dashed line indicates the approximate dimension of the original canal. Residue includes intact tissue with blood vessels *(BV)* mixed with dentin chips *(DC)*. Note that instruments have done most of their work by stripping away the dentin outside the original canal and have left other areas untouched.

dirty. When this criterion has been used in studies evaluating canal débridement, there is little relationship between clean shavings and the quality of débridement.[4] Attainment of clean irrigating solution is another criterion. However, this is also inaccurate and serves only as a crude indictor.

Achievement of *glassy smooth* walls is the preferred result.[6] Smoothness is evaluated by firmly pushing the side of the tip of a small instrument along each wall on the outstroke. The walls should become and feel smooth in all dimensions. Although the best indicator to date, this criterion is not totally accurate either. Other and better determinants are yet to be identified.

SHAPING

Schilder[1] outlined the principles of shaping as follows: "To develop a continuously shaped conical form from apical to coronal. The apical preparation should be as small as is practical and in its original position spatially." In addition, removal of a uniform layer of dentin in all dimensions and all regions of the canal is also desirable. Is such uniform removal of dentin from all canal walls achievable? The answer is "seldom" for either straight or slightly curved canals and "almost never" for more curved canals. The same problem occurs in shaping as in cleaning. The nature of canal dimensions, shape, and curves as well as the physical properties of shaping instruments prevents the possibility of a uniform, tapered, flowing preparation.

Essentially all canals are curved, and most instruments are relatively inflexible. It has been suggested that instruments be precurved to fit the canal. However, the files will cut to the outside of the curvature ("transportation") regardless of whether files are precurved[7,8] and whether the files are stainless steel or nickel-titanium.[9] In curved canals, files do most of their work by stripping away layers of raw dentin from one or two walls in certain areas (Figure 13-3); they may not touch or may enlarge many other regions of the canal.[10] Recognizing these deficiencies, the dentist attempts to minimize this action by using certain techniques of preparation.

Enlargement

The eternal question is, how much should the canal be enlarged? The answer is simple (although implementation is difficult): enough to permit adequate débridement as well as manipulation and control of obturating materials and instruments, but not so much that the chances of making procedural errors and needlessly weakening the root are increased.

Taper

Generally, taper should be sufficient to permit deep penetration of spreaders or pluggers when obturating with gutta-percha. Excessive taper may result in unnecessary removal of dentin and weakening of the root.

Criteria

Adequate shaping basically reflects adequacy of preparation for obturation. That is, whether the technique is lateral or vertical condensation, the canal must be flared and enlarged to permit control and to achieve adequate depth for spreader or plugger insertion during obturation.[11]

To test adequacy, selected obturating instruments are "tried-in" during canal shaping. When taper is sufficient to permit spreader penetration deep into the canal (0 to 1 mm from the apical stop) with some space adjacent for gutta-percha, the flare is adequate (Figure 13-4).[12] With lateral condensation, the deeper the spreader penetrates during its initial insertion alongside the gutta-percha, the better the apical seal.[12] With vertical condensation, sufficient flare is required to allow placement of pluggers within 3 to 5 mm of working length.

MASTER APICAL FILE DETERMINATION

The *master apical file* (MAF) is by definition the largest file that binds *slightly* at the corrected working length. The MAF is determined by passively placing successively larger files at the correct working length until a size is reached that slightly binds at the tip. This determination is made after straight-line access (see Chapter 12). Straight-line access allows files to be introduced without binding through the chamber and into the canal until the first canal curve is reached, thus eliminating interference cervical to the apical constriction.[13] After MAF determination, the next procedure is step-back cleaning and shaping.

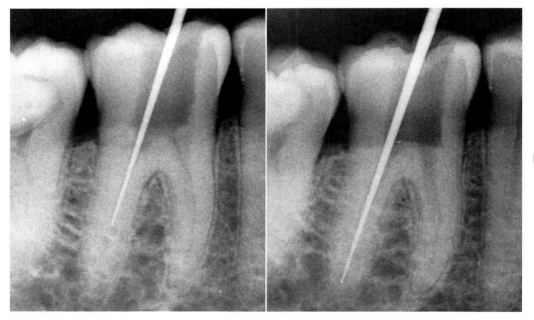

A　　　　　　　　　　　　　　　　　　　　　　　　　　　　　**B**

FIGURE 13-4
A, Canal preparation has inadequate flare, limiting spreader penetration. **B,** Canal preparation has greater taper to allow deep spreader penetration and better obturation.

APICAL PREPARATION

An additional objective is adequate preparation of the apical region. Length is important, but even more critical is the creation of an apical "matrix" or constriction. The apical matrix has two purposes: (1) to help confine instruments, materials, and chemicals to the canal space; and (2) to create (or retain) a barrier against which gutta-percha can be condensed. Depending on apical foramen configuration and canal shape and size, an apical stop, apical seat, or open apex will be created (Figure 13-5). Whichever of these three occurs, the result will influence the choice of the obturation technique and possibly affect the ultimate prognosis.[14]

The *apical patency* concept has been proposed as another means of managing the apex.[15] The technique is to perform apical "trephination," i.e., to pass small files through the apical foramen (without widening it) at times during canal preparation. The idea is that this will prevent hard or soft tissue blockage of the foramen, thereby improving débridement and reducing irritants. There is no experimental support for the apical patency approach. In fact, repeated use of files through the apex and extruded sealer will damage periradicular tissues and cause inflammation.

Variations

Apical Stop. A barrier at the preparation end is an apical stop.

Apical Seat. Lack of a complete barrier but the presence of a constriction represents an apical seat.

Open Apex. The apical preparation resembles an open cylinder (neither barrier nor constriction). Open apex is undesirable and will probably not confine materials to the canal space. In addition, there is no semblance of a matrix against which to condense gutta-percha; often, no apical seal will be created.

Criteria

An instrument one or two sizes smaller than that used for apical preparation (i.e., the MAP) is the instrument used for evaluation. If this smaller instrument is placed to length, tapped around, and hits a dead end in all areas, this is an *apical stop*. If the file meets some resistance but can be passed through the constriction, this is an *apical seat*. If the instrument passes unimpeded through the apical preparation, neither seat nor stop is present; this represents an *open apex*. Lack of a stop or seat is undesirable and is usually preventable.

A mnemonic that can be used to remember stop, seat, and open is as follows: Santa Claus attempts to go down the chimney. If the damper is closed, his feet strike that impediment and he proceeds no farther; that is a *stop*. If the damper is open but small, his feet and legs will pass through but not his *seat*. If a damper is not present, his feet, legs, seat, and torso pass through with ease (an open apex); the same thing tends to occur with gutta-percha and sealer during condensation.

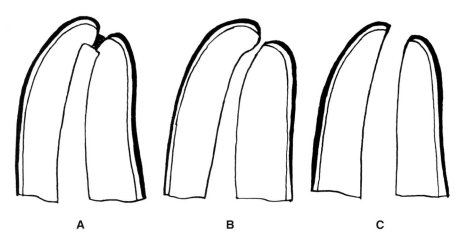

| A | B | C |

FIGURE 13-5
Apical preparations. **A,** Apical stop: Creation of a small ledge at working length. **B,** Apical seat: Permits passage of a small instrument through the apical foramen. **C,** Open apex: Preparation is wide open with no barrier or constriction. It is difficult to obtain a seal and to contain obturating materials. (Courtesy Dr. A. Goerig.)

Techniques of Pulp Extirpation and Cleaning and Shaping

Preparation includes removal of vital pulp (extirpation) as well as cleaning and shaping. Cleaning and shaping methods have historically varied according to the situation and the obturating material selected. However, at present, two basic approaches are used: the *standardized* taper and the *flaring* (stepback or crown-down) taper. There are several variations in methods used to achieve these.

PULP EXTIRPATION
Bulk Removal

Pulpotomy is removal of the coronal vital pulp.

Extirpation of the vital radicular pulp with a broach does not represent *pulpectomy*, which is total removal of pulp tissue. Rather, portions of pulp are dislodged and pulled out, leaving shredded remnants. This is a *partial pulpectomy*. Complete removal is not accomplished until working length is established and considerable canal preparation has been done.

Complete removal of necrotic and vital radicular pulp is referred to as débridement (cleaning and shaping). To perform a pulpotomy or pulpectomy, there must be vital pulp tissue present. There is no descriptive term for the removal of necrotic pulp tissue; however débridement of the canal space is necessary. The description "access with no vital pulp" or "débridement with no vital pulp" should be used instead of "pulpotomy" or "pulpectomy" to describe situations in which the pulp is necrotic.

The preferred time for pulp extirpation is during access. Completion of access preparation is difficult without good visibility, which is difficult with continuous hemorrhage into the chamber from a torn pulp stump. The best time to extirpate is when the chamber is unroofed and canals are discovered. Another indication for extirpation is persistent tissue sensitivity in a particular canal. The hyperreactive pulp is broached out quickly, facilitating canal preparation if the patient is comfortable.

Technique

A barbed broach should fit the canal dimensions approximately (according to radiographic size) but does not bind. The larger the instrument, the better it will "grab" tissue. However, a too-large instrument risks binding in dentin with possible breakage. Caution must be used with broaches because they are somewhat fragile instruments and are difficult to remove when separated.

The broach is measured at estimated length and teased into the canal short of working length. The handle is rotated a few times and then withdrawn. The broach is not reused if it is bent or has bound in the canal—a new instrument is selected. If tissue is not removed, a larger size is tried. A technique used in larger canals is the "broach wrap." Two smaller broaches are inserted, and then the handles are wrapped several times around each other; this often engages and dislodges the pulp.

STANDARDIZED PREPARATION

This is the classic technique initially described as the preferred method of cleaning and shaping.[16]

Objective

The desired end result is the creation of a preparation that has the same size, shape, and taper as a standardized instrument. The technique was an outgrowth of size standardization, which was introduced in the 1950s as a guide for endodontic instrument manufacturers.[17] At that time, an attempt was made to apply these standards as a guide to canal enlargement. In fact, creating a true standardized tapered preparation is difficult in ideal situations and impossible in curved canals.[10,18,19]

Standardized preparation is indicated for silver cone obturation but may also be used for guttapercha.[20] However, the operator must exercise care, particularly in curved canals. Preparation with large instruments around curves transports the preparation, which tends to create irregularities (ledges and zips) and subsequent problems.

Method

The technique is shown in Figure 13-6.

FLARING PREPARATION

This is a tapered preparation, using a step-back or crown-down technique or a combination of the two. The concept of the step-back (also known as flaring or serial preparation) technique is relatively recent. It was first described by Clem[21] in 1969 and became popular when a series of research reports[2,4] indicated its superiority over the standardized preparation techniques. In addition, the step-back technique creates a smoother flow and a more tapered preparation from apical to coronal direction. The step-back technique with stainless steel instruments is currently the most widely taught and used technique.[22] The crown-down (also known as step-down) technique is also

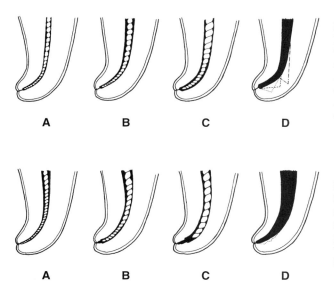

FIGURE 13-6
Standardized technique. **A** to **C,** The objective is to attempt to prepare the canal to uniform size using successively larger instruments to working length. **D,** In reality, instruments larger than No. 20 or 25 (depending on curvature) tend to cut straight ahead, resulting in apical "transportation," ledges, or creation of a new canal, as indicated by the *dotted* and *dashed lines*.

FIGURE 13-7
Step-back technique. **A,** Canals are prepared to a small size at the apical length. **B** and **C,** Larger files are used sequentially to decreasing lengths. **D,** The result is a preparation with small apical enlargement and a marked taper from apical to coronal. Small steps usually remain in the apical area.

relatively new and also creates a tapered preparation. Flaring techniques that use nickel-titanium hand or engine-driven rotary instruments are becoming increasingly popular. Also popular are techniques that use a combination of step-back and crown-down with hand and/or rotary instrumentation. These will be further discussed later in this chapter.

Objective

The objective is to keep the apical preparation as small as practical (but well débrided) with an increasing taper throughout the canal. Also, the final apical preparation should be at or close to the original canal position. It is desirable to remove a layer of dentin from all canal walls from apical to coronal. Such removal has been shown to be difficult but is more achievable with the flaring techniques.

Method

The basic method of canal preparation for any flaring technique is as follows:

1. Negotiate the canal space with small files to length.
2. Remove coronal dentin (enlarge the coronal canal) to facilitate placement of larger files in the middle and apical regions. This is performed with Gates-Glidden burs, orifice openers, or hand files.
3. Determine the size of the file that corresponds with the size of the most apical canal space. This is the "master apical file."

4. Enlarge the apical and middle canal spaces with a flaring preparation (step-back or crown-down) to clean and shape.

The description to follow is a hand preparation technique with stainless steel and/or nickel-titanium files. First, access preparation, passive step-back,[23] and working length are performed as detailed in Chapter 12.

Straight-line access is also completed and MAF size is determined. The step-back technique (Figure 13-7) is then executed as follows. Note that apical preparation has two phases, initial and final. The initial phase is small to minimize transportation. In the final phase the apical preparation is increased three to four sizes larger during apical clearing; this will improve débridement and obturation. The apical clearing technique is explained later in this chapter.

Apical Preparation. This is the next step after straight-line access is made and the MAF size is determined. To keep the canal small but débrided, the apical 1 to 2 mm of the canal is enlarged by reaming (cutting by rotation), generally to only one or two sizes larger than the MAF. *Care is required to not overprepare the apical region, particularly in the curved canal!*

As the curvature becomes greater, a smaller apical preparation is needed. If the canal is small and the curvature is more than slight, the MAF is usually no larger than a No. 20 file. A straight or slightly curved canal allows more latitude for a larger MAF.

If the apical portion of the curved canal is anatomically larger than a No. 25 file, to minimize transportation, *no attempt should be made to enlarge this region further than the size of the file that shows slight binding.* Again, whichever instrument binds slightly at length is used; this will be the MAF. Step-back is begun from this point.

Taper. After apical preparation, tapering of the remaining canal is created by shortening the working length of each successively larger instrument by 0.5 mm and by performing peripheral filing (Figure 13-8).[24] This creates the step-back.

Recapitulation. After each step-back file is used, recapitulation is performed by returning to length with the MAF (or smaller file) (Figure 13-9).[25] The instrument is rotated carefully to loosen debris but not enlarge the apical canal.

Irrigation. At least 2 ml of irrigant is used between each file size after recapitulation (Figure 13-9).

Size of Preparation. Step-back instrumentation up to *at least* a size 70 file is usually necessary. This should give adequate débridement of most of the canal as well as sufficient taper to permit deep spreader (or plugger) penetration. A larger step-back is indicated in larger canals.

Final Apical Enlargement. This will improve débridement of the apical portion of the canal. See the upcoming section on "Apical Clearing."

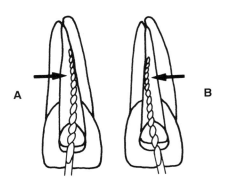

FIGURE 13-8
Peripheral filing. The end portions of the files are pressed successively against each of the four walls *(arrows)*. The action is similar to that used with a paintbrush. (Courtesy Dr. G. Scott.)

Crown-Down

The "crown-down pressureless" technique[26] and the step-down technique[27] are modifications of the step-back technique. Crown-down, step-down, and step-back procedures produce a similar outcome, resulting in a flaring preparation with small apical enlargement. Like the step-back, these techniques are particularly useful in fine curved canals of maxillary and mandibular molars (Figure 13-10). Advocates propose that the canals will be somewhat débrided before the instruments are placed in the apical region, thereby decreasing the chance of debris extrusion.

The crown-down is often suggested as a basic approach using nickel-titanium rotary instruments. Although there is some evidence that these techniques are effective and result in a desirable preparation shape,[26,27] there is no proof that they are superior clinically to step-back instrumentation with hand files. However, the logic of these approaches makes them good alternatives.

PASSIVE STEP-BACK

The passive step-back technique uses a combination of hand instruments (files) and rotary instruments (Gates-Glidden drills and Peeso reamers) to achieve adequate coronal flare before apical root canal preparation.

The passive step-back technique provides an unforceful and gradual enlargement of canals in an apical-coronal direction. In addition, it is applicable in every canal type, is easy to master, reduces procedural accidents, and is convenient for both operator and patient.

Instruments

No. 10 to 40 K-type files, No. 2 and 3 Gates-Glidden drills, and Peeso engine reamers as well as high-speed round and diamond burs will suffice for most situations.

Clinical Techniques and Rationale

Step One: Access Preparation. With the use of an appropriate sized bur in a high-speed handpiece,

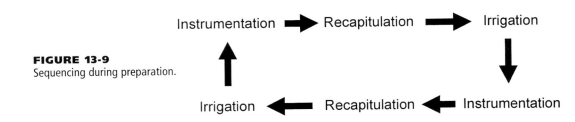

FIGURE 13-9
Sequencing during preparation.

the pulp chamber is penetrated and unroofed. After the canal orifice is located, the access cavity wall(s) are flared adjacent to the orifice with a thin, tapered diamond bur. With use of the diagnostic film, a No. 15 file is placed in the canal at the estimated working length of the root canal either as determined radiographically or with an electronic apex locator.

Step Two: Passive Step-Back Hand Instrumentation. After depositing sodium hypochlorite in the pulp chamber, a No. 10 or 15 K-type file is placed to the radiographic apex with a very light one eighth to one quarter turn and push-pull strokes to establish apical canal patency with little or no resistance. With the same motion, No. 20, 25, 30, 35, and 40 K-type files are carried into the canal as far as they can be inserted passively to remove small amounts of dentin. After passage of these files, the canal is irrigated with sodium hypochlorite solution.

Step Three: Passive Use of Gates-Glidden Drills. A No. 2 Gates-Glidden drill is inserted into the mildly flared canal to a point where it binds slightly. It is then pulled back about 1 to 1.5 mm and the slow-speed handpiece is activated. With an up-and-down motion and slight pressure, the desired canal wall(s) is planed and flared. A similar technique is used to plane and flare the coronal region with No. 3 Gates-Glidden drill. A No. 4 Gates-Glidden drill is used in large canals. The root canals should be irrigated with sodium hypochlorite solution between the engine-driven instrument.

Step Four: Passive Use of Peeso Reamers. A No. 2 Peeso reamer is placed into the canal to a point where it binds slightly. It is then pulled back about 1 to 1.5 mm and the slow-speed handpiece is activated. With a gentle up-and-down motion, the coronal portion of the canal is shaped and flared further. With the use of a similar technique, the coronal 2 to 3 mm can be flared with a No. 3 Peeso reamer.

Step Five: Confirmation of Working Length. Because flaring and removal of curvatures reduce the working length, it is essential to confirm the corrected working length before apical preparation. After placing a No. 15 (patency file) or No. 20 file in the canal, the working length should be confirmed either with a radiograph or an electronic apex locator.

Step Six: Apical Preparation. After the canal is flared and the corrected working length is determined, a No. 20 file should penetrate to the working length without any resistance. The canal is then prepared with sequential use of progressively larger instruments placed successively short of the working length. Narrow or curved root canals should not be enlarged beyond the size of No. 25 or 30 files.

Evaluation Criteria

There are basically three criteria for evaluation of canal preparation.

1. *Débridement.* After preparation, the MAF tip is pressed firmly against each wall on the outstroke. All walls should feel smooth.
2. *Taper.* The selected spreader passes easily to or within 1 mm of the working length with

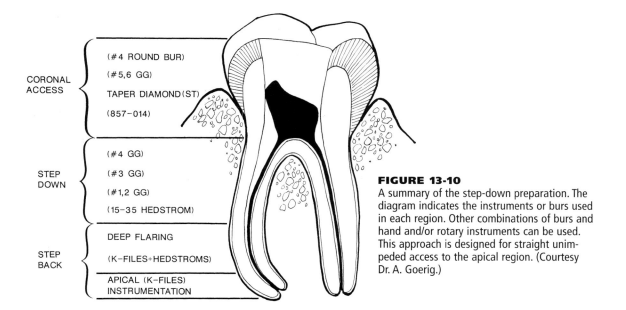

CORONAL ACCESS
- (#4 ROUND BUR)
- (#5,6 GG)
- TAPER DIAMOND(ST)
- (857−014)

STEP DOWN
- (#4 GG)
- (#3 GG)
- (#1,2 GG)
- (15−35 HEDSTROM)

STEP BACK
- DEEP FLARING
- (K−FILES+HEDSTROMS)
- APICAL (K−FILES) INSTRUMENTATION

FIGURE 13-10
A summary of the step-down preparation. The diagram indicates the instruments or burs used in each region. Other combinations of burs and hand and/or rotary instruments can be used. This approach is designed for straight unimpeded access to the apical region. (Courtesy Dr. A. Goerig.)

APICAL CLEARING

Final Apical Enlargement

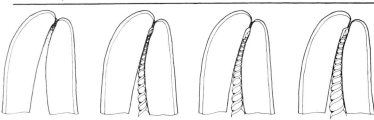

Dry Reaming

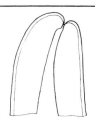

FIGURE 13-11
Apical clearing has two steps: final apical enlargement and dry reaming. Note removal of dentin chips apically and accentuation of the apical stop. The last instrument used is the final apical file *(upper right, lower center).*

space alongside for the master gutta-percha cone.

3. *Apical Preparation.* A seat or a stop or neither (open apex) is identified by using a file smaller than the MAF at the working length.

These three criteria were described earlier in this chapter.

APICAL CLEARING

Apical clearing results in (1) better débridement, (2) enhanced obturation, and (3) a more defined apical stop.[28] Performed in a prepared canal with an apical stop, apical clearing enlarges the apical region at the corrected working length (Figure 13-11). There are two steps: *final apical enlargement* and *dry reaming.*

Apical clearing is indicated *only* if there is an apical stop. Further apical enlargement in the presence of an apical seat or open apex configuration increases the chance of an overfill by removing dentin chips that are forming a partial plug or seal, or it may actually open the apex further.

Final Apical Enlargement. This step is performed after canal preparation is complete and has met the criteria of adequate cleaning and shaping. Instead of final recapitulation, instruments three to four sizes larger than the MAF are carefully spun (reamed) in a clockwise manner at the working length in the wet canal. Therefore, the final apical size in a smaller canal would be No. 35 or 40. Final irrigation with 2 to 3 ml of irrigant per canal is

followed by drying with paper points. This minimal, careful use of files in a tapered (flared) canal will better débride the apical few millimeters and will not cause transportation or ledging.[28]

Final apical enlargement is not done in canals greater than a size 40. If MAF size is already greater than 40 and there is an apical stop, dry reaming is done with the MAF only.

Dry Reaming. The files used will remove dentin chips that pack apically during drying (Figure 13-12). Dry reaming is done after final apical enlargement and irrigation and drying with paper points. The last size file used for final apical enlargement (or the MAF if larger than a size 40) is then spun carefully in a clockwise manner to length. This is the *final apical file.*

ANATOMIC ABERRATIONS

The root canal system, contrary to the usual diagrammatic representation, is irregular. Mother Nature does not form dentin internally with a uniform pattern; therefore, there are many regions containing tissue that lie outside the main canal. These relatively inaccessible areas must be considered during preparation and are recognized as potential causes of long-term failure.

Types

These aberrations are subclassified as intercanal isthmi, cul-de-sacs, lateral canals, apical ramifications, and concavities. Numbers and irregularities of anatomic aberrations increase in the posterior

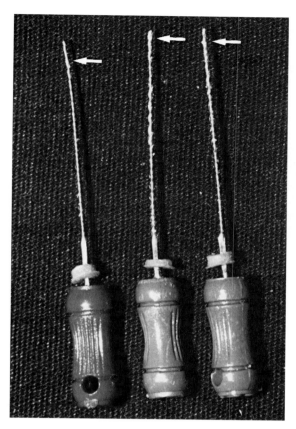

FIGURE 13-12
Apical clearing. Apical enlargement has been done with Nos. 25, 30, and 35 files *(left to right)*. Note the dentin shavings *(arrows)* on the apical regions of the files.

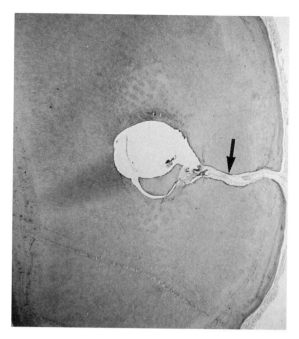

FIGURE 13-13
A lateral canal *(arrow)* in this cross section of a root in the apical third. Although the main canal has been well débrided, tissue remains intact in the lateral canal. This is a typical finding.

teeth,[29] reflecting the larger roots of molars and most premolars as well as their complex pattern of formation.

Significance

All these aberrations are relatively inaccessible to intracanal instruments.[30] Regardless of the technique or chemicals used, isthmi (see Figure 13-2), cul-de-sacs, lateral canals (Figure 13-13), and apical ramifications (Figures 13-1 and 13-14) are generally not débrided at all. Fins and concavities, if exposed to irrigants, may be partially cleaned, probably owing to the surface solvent or flushing action of the irrigant. Not only are all these aberrations largely undébrided, but also bits of tissue and dentin chips may actually be pushed into these areas after being loosened from the main canal.

NOTE: Maximal débridement will occur predictably only when the files contact and plane all walls. The ability to achieve maximum instrument contact is enhanced with good straight-line access (Figure 13-15).

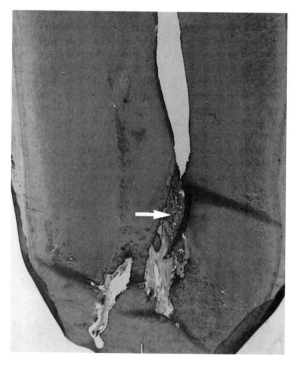

FIGURE 13-14
Apical ramifications. These are similar to the lateral canals in that they communicate pulp-to-periodontium. These regions also contain tissue and preparation debris *(arrow)* that is not removed by instruments and irrigants.

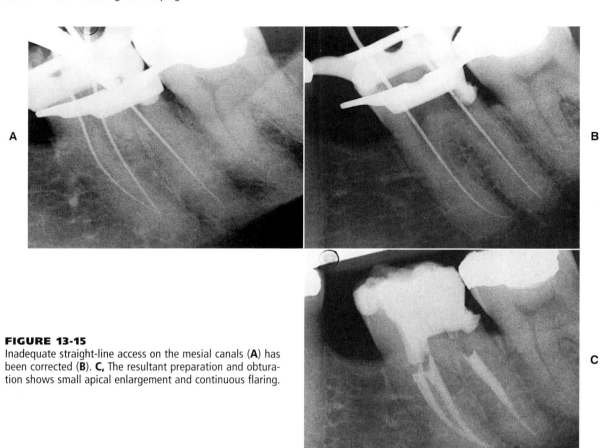

FIGURE 13-15
Inadequate straight-line access on the mesial canals (**A**) has been corrected (**B**). **C,** The resultant preparation and obturation shows small apical enlargement and continuous flaring.

The importance of minimizing the volume of tissue remnants in canals after preparation is obvious. If these irritants are sufficiently large and potent, have access to the periodontium, and are not otherwise "neutralized" by host defenses, disease and eventual failure will occur because of inflammation. This principle was discussed in detail earlier in this chapter. The bottom line is that there are regions that cannot be débrided and these may compromise treatment and, ultimately, success. Therefore, some factors that cause failure are beyond the capability of the dentist to manage.

Chemical Adjuncts

As man does not live by bread alone, the pulp system is not cleaned and shaped by instruments alone. Important adjuncts are *irrigants* and agents that aid in débridement and that may alter dentin to facilitate enlargement. All vary in relative effectiveness. Other adjuncts are *lubricants,* which facil-itate the negotiation of small canals, and *desiccants*, which aid in drying before obturation.

IRRIGATION

With filing, the other important process in canal débridement is irrigation. In theory, files loosen and disrupt materials within canals and remove dentin from the walls as shavings; the whole sludge is then flushed out with an irrigant. This process is more theoretical than actual. Irrigants and irrigation are only moderately effective. The most important factor is the delivery system of the irrigant and not the solution per se.

Irrigants

Many types of solutions have been used, such as distilled water, concentrated acids, and antimicrobials. Unfortunately, although numerous studies have been done in vitro (not in a clinical mode), the relative effectiveness of different irrigants has not been clearly demonstrated in clinical usage. Therefore, much information is theoretical.

Although the major function of an irrigant is to flush debris from the canal, the irrigant may have additional properties that aid in cleaning and shaping. Below are outlined the characteristics of an ideal irrigant.

Properties of Ideal Irrigant

- *Tissue or Debris Solvent.* In regions inaccessible to instruments, the irrigant could dissolve or disrupt soft tissue or hard tissue remnants to permit their removal.[31-33]
- *Toxicity.* The irrigant should be noninjurious to periradicular tissues.
- *Low Surface Tension.* This property promotes flow into tubules[34] and into inaccessible areas.[35] Alcohol added to an irrigant decreases surface tension and increases penetrability[36]; whether this enhances débridement is unknown.
- *Lubricant.* Lubrication helps instruments to slide down the canal. All liquids have this effect, some more than others.
- *Sterilization (or at Least Disinfection).*[37,38]
- *Removal of Smear Layer.* The smear layer is a layer of microcrystalline and organic particle debris spread on the walls after canal preparation. There are solutions that chelate and decalcify remove the smear layer.[39-41] At present it is not known whether the smear layer should be removed. One advantage is that the smear layer seems to inhibit bacterial colonization.[42]
- *Other Factors.* Other factors relate to irrigant utility and include availability, moderate cost, user friendliness, convenience, adequate shelf life, and ease of storage. An additional important requirement is that the chemical not be easily neutralized in the canal to retain effectiveness.

Solutions. Sodium hypochlorite, in various concentrations, is the most popular and most advocated irrigant. This inexpensive, readily available, easily used chemical usually rates the best in research. However, experimental evidence does not necessarily correspond directly to clinical effectiveness. Although in vitro studies[43] indicate that sodium hypochlorite dissolves tissues readily, experiments in extracted teeth and clinical usage in patients are less impressive. Most histologic and scanning electron microscope studies[44-46] do not show that the tissue dissolution or sterilization properties of sodium hypochlorite are consistently effective.

The difference between in vitro and in vivo studies may be that in the clinical situation, irrigating solutions have limited surface contact and are buffered (neutralized). In the canal, irrigants would not have extensive and intimate contact with all areas of tissue.[47] In addition, the irrigant has little access to sequestered areas and aberrations and, therefore, leaves regions undébrided.[46]

The same phenomenon of noncontact may limit the antibacterial action of irrigants. Although experiments have shown that sodium hypochlorite is very effective in vitro[48] and does reduce bacterial populations in canals and in tubules,[49] bacteria usually are not totally eliminated.[50-52] The same problem of limited contact in hidden areas compromises bactericidal action.

Another disadvantage of sodium hypochlorite is toxicity. It is capable of causing tissue damage and has access to periradicular tissue in small amounts.[53,54] However, the limited extrusion of sodium hypochlorite is unlikely to be significant because it is diluted and buffered by tissue fluids apically.

Chelators (calcium removers), such as ethylenediaminetetraacetic acid (EDTA) or citric acid, remove the smear layer. The combination of chelators alternating with sodium hypochlorite has potential as the ultimate clinical débriding agent to soften dentin[55] and to reduce the smear layer and organic debris.[40] As yet, this theory has been tested only in bench-top studies and not in clinical trials.

The use of *hydrogen peroxide* (H_2O_2), alone or alternating with sodium hypochlorite, is not beneficial. This once popular method was thought to have a nascent bubbling action to facilitate debris removal; however, improved débridement does not occur.[56,57]

Other sterilizing agents have been tested. A common antimicrobial solution used in dentistry is chlorhexidine. In both in vivo and in vitro experiments chlorhexidine has been shown to significantly reduce numbers of bacteria.[58] However, sodium hypochlorite is probably more effective[59] and offers the distinct advantages of ease of use, some tissue dissolution, and much lower cost.

Recommendation. A suggested concentration of sodium hypochlorite is common household bleach (5.25%) diluted with equal parts of water for a 2.6% solution. This is just as effective as full strength and is safer and more pleasant for both patient and dentist.

Technique

Needles. Different types of needles are available, but none has a demonstrated advantage. What is important is the gauge, which should be small. A 27- or 28-gauge needle is preferred. These needles have the potential to pass farther into the canal for better delivery and flushing. Smaller needles tend to clog; this tendency is minimized by aspirating air into the needle after each irrigation.

Usage. Needle penetration and volume of irrigant are the most important factors. The needle introduces irrigant to flush the canal *only coronal* to the extent of penetration.[57,60] Therefore, a smaller gauge needle, in conjunction with canal enlargement and copious and frequent irrigation, will produce better flushing (Figure 13-16).

An interesting recent innovation is the use of nickel-titanium needles. These are flexible and reportedly can be inserted deeply into small, curved canals. If this claim proves to be correct, they should provide improved flushing of canals.

Safety. To avoid forcing irrigant or debris out of the apex, the needle tip must not bind in the canal. Careful insertion and slight withdrawal after binding (or a slight pumping action during irrigation) minimizes this potentially serious occurrence that creates a "hypochlorite accident."[61] This free backflow is particularly important when there is no apical stop or when the apical foramen opens directly into the maxillary sinus.

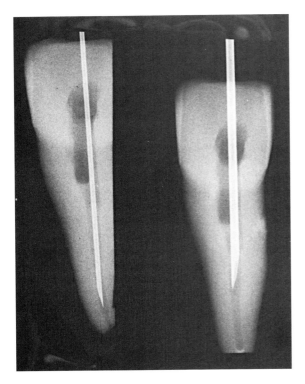

FIGURE 13-16
Depth of irrigating needle penetration is critical. A 27-gauge needle *(left)* is closer to length (preferred) than the 25-gauge needle *(right)*. No flushing occurs except coronal to the needle.

DENTIN SOFTENING

Dentin softeners can potentially facilitate instrument passage and canal enlargement by removing mineral components from the dentin walls or eliminating obstructions.[62,63] Whether dentin softeners are clinically advantageous is doubtful.

Chelators

By definition, the organic substances called chelators remove metallic ions (such as calcium) by binding them chemically. These agents have been promoted as commercial products, usually in combination with lubricating or bubbling agents (oxygen releasers).

Types. The two most common chelators are EDTA and dilute (10%) citric acid.[64]

Action. As dentin-softening agents, chelators have not provided impressive results in either in vitro or in vivo studies. EDTA works very slowly,[65] probably more slowly than the cutting action of the file. This is particularly true in the apical regions of small canals, where the amount of chelating agent that can be introduced is limited.[66] The combination of EDTA and bubbling agents also does not seem to increase the volume of tissue removed or aid in flushing. Limited information is available about citric acid.[64]

Effectiveness. A time and motion study[67] demonstrated that chelators alone or in combination with sodium hypochlorite did not reduce the time required for canal preparation. EDTA was ineffective; the combination of 10% citric acid used alternately with sodium hypochlorite slightly decreased the time needed for enlargement.

There is no proof that chelators soften or remove canal obstructions sufficiently to permit passage of instruments. In fact, softening agents for this purpose are contraindicated because they slightly alter the walls, thereby limiting the ability of instruments to be guided along hard dentin. If these softening chemicals are used, they should be placed in canals only after instruments have been used to length and the canal preparation has been started. As a further precaution, these chemicals should not remain in the canal for any period of time without instrumentation.

Decalcifiers

By definition, decalcifiers are chemicals that remove mineral salts in solution. Decalcifying agents are commonly used in histologic preparation of mineralized tissues, but they have not been demonstrated to be useful in canal enlargement.

Acids. Strong inorganic acids, such as hydrochloric and sulfuric acids, have been used as enlargement aids. Organic acids such as concentrated citric acid (30% to 50%) have also been proposed for irrigation and softening. These concentrated acids are too potent. Therefore, their toxicity is high and their decalcifying action too rapid to control. They are not recommended.

LUBRICANTS

Lubricants are helpful in passing of instruments to length during exploration and negotiation of small constricted canals. If small files bind progressively tighter and stop short of working length, this indicates a need for a lubricating substance. Lubricants may not be beneficial when the file stops abruptly, which indicates a ledge or obstruction that must be bypassed.

Types

Glycerin is a good lubricant. This mild alcohol is very slippery, self-sterilizing, inexpensive, and nontoxic. Also it is slightly soluble, permitting removal once it has completed its function. Soap (liquid or bar) or topical anesthetic may also be used. However, liquid soap (unless sterile) or bar soap may be contaminated with bacteria.

Commercial preparations of EDTA usually contain lubricants (wax or glycerin). These are suitable as lubricants but should be used with caution when one is negotiating a tight canal; EDTA may soften the walls slightly, thus permitting the file tips to gouge and ledge.

Usage

For glycerin or sterile liquid soap, a drop is placed at the orifice by picking up a small amount with cotton pliers, placing the tip at the orifice, and opening the pliers slightly. This introduces small, controlled amounts of the liquid (Figure 13-17). Another method is to introduce glycerin with a tuberculin (or other small) syringe.

The file is worked up and down through the glycerin and into the canal using a pumping action and counterclockwise spin. This carries the lubricant ahead of the file. Usually the file can then be worked (teased) closer to length. Lubricant may even be used to facilitate initial enlargement through two or three file sizes.

DESICCANTS

Concentrated solutions of 70% to 90% alcohol (methanol or ethanol) may be used as a final irrigant to dry the canal and remove traces of other chemicals. Whether this is beneficial has not been determined. The same irrigating syringe used in the same manner as that used for chemical irrigation is indicated for alcohol. Only a small amount of alcohol (1 to 2 ml per canal) is needed.

Avoidance of Preparation Errors

Preparation errors are most common in small, round, curved, long canals. As stated earlier, instruments are not designed to enlarge small curves; they attempt to straighten themselves[68] and cut the outside of the curve in the apical region.[7,69] Histologic sections of these curved canals after preparation are dramatic. The files have done most of their work by stripping away layers of raw dentin from certain areas but accomplishing nothing in other regions (see Figure 13-3).[70] Using increasingly larger instruments only aggravates the effect. The outcome will be largely undesirable. Careful instrument use is the key.[71] In addition, a flaring (step-back or crown-down) technique involves small instruments in the apical curvature and larger, less flexible instruments in the straighter portion of the canal. This preparation tends to create fewer problems. More informa-

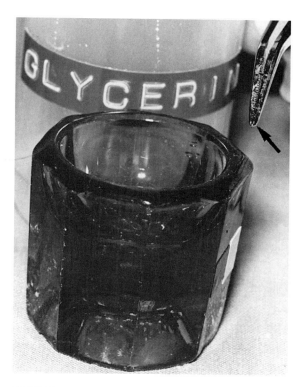

FIGURE 13-17
Glycerin is an excellent lubricant. A drop (arrow) is transported from a dappen dish to the canal orifice in the beaks of cotton pliers or may be introduced with a syringe.

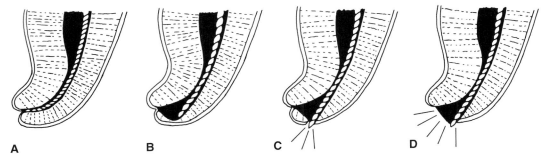

A   **B**   **C**   **D**

FIGURE 13-18
Hazards of overenlarging the apical curvature. **A,** Correct preparation is maintained when small flexible instruments, less than No. 25, are used to negotiate the curvature. **B,** Larger instruments increase stiffness and cutting efficiency and transport the apical preparation. **C,** Continued enlargement results in perforation. **D,** Apical region is zipped when large instruments are continually forced apically.

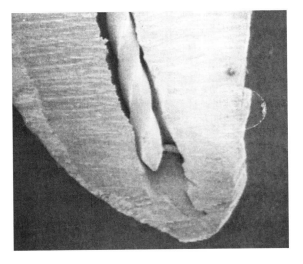

FIGURE 13-19
Transportation, creating a small ledge. The apical region of a curved canal shows too-large file overpreparation and straightening of the canal with creation of a small ledge outside the curvature. (Courtesy Dr. P. Ardines.)

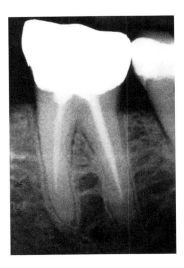

FIGURE 13-20
Both mesial and distal canals were straightened, ledged, and obturated short of working length. The preparation and the obturation are not centered in the root. The long-term prognosis is compromised; significant areas of canals remain undébrided and unobturated.

tion on preventing and managing canal preparation problems is found in Chapter 18.

PROBLEMS
Overinstrumentation

A major mistake is overenlargement of small, curved canals. The files cut to the outside of the curvature (a process called *transportation*) in an attempt to straighten themselves and cut to the inside of the curve in the cervical region. This results from using too-large instruments or overusing smaller instruments in the apical curved portion of the canal (Figure 13-18). The greater the curvature[72] and the longer and smaller the canal, the higher is the potential for the fol-

lowing unfortunate occurrences.[69,73] Each problem adversely affects short-term or long-term prognosis by compromising obturation[74] or by creating a frank perforation.

Ledge Formation

Degree of curvature is the problem: the greater the curve, the more likely is the formation of a ledge.[72] As the instrument straightens, the tip begins to gouge into raw dentin (Figure 13-19). It also tends to cut straight ahead; the operator may accentuate this action by boring deeper in dentin in an attempt to regain lost length. The file now has the sensation of banging into a dead end short of length; this is the feeling of a *ledge*. A radiograph

A   **B**

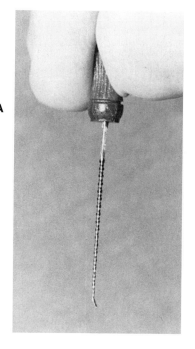

A

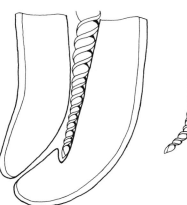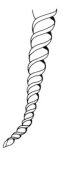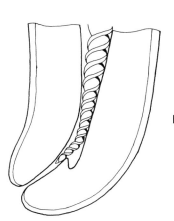

B

FIGURE 13-21
The consequences of ledging and "boring" a new canal. **A,** Not only did perforation occur, but also an area of the canal *(arrow)* remains undébrided and unobturated. **B,** At 2-year recall, the periradicular lesion remains, thus constituting a treatment failure.

FIGURE 13-22
Correcting a ledge. **A,** Ledges or obstructions are occasionally bypassed by placing a small bend at the instrument tip. **B,** To negotiate the file past blockages or ledges, the tip is teased along the canal wall to attempt to locate the original canal.

shows that the instrument or obturation no longer follows the original curve (Figure 13-20). Relocating and renegotiating the original canal is a problem; correcting the ledge is difficult, even if the original canal is renegotiated (Figure 13-21).

Trying to regain the original working length will result in boring straight ahead into raw dentin. Continued boring will create a perforation away from the apical foramen.

A technique (usually unsuccessful, but worth a try) that may aid in relocating the main canal is to place a bend in the apical 1 to 2 mm of a No. 15, 20, or 25 file (Figure 13-22). The tip is teased along the wall in the direction of the original

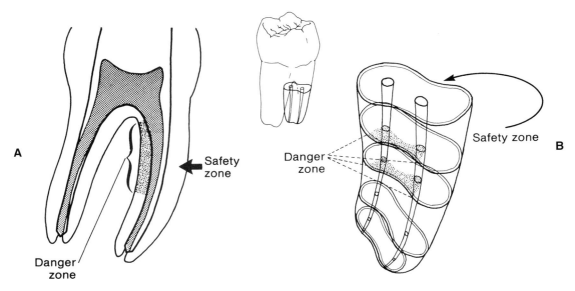

FIGURE 13-23
A and **B,** Safety zones and danger zones of molar roots. Rotary and hand instruments should be used in the canal toward the safety zone. (Adapted courtesy Dr. M. Abou-Rass.)

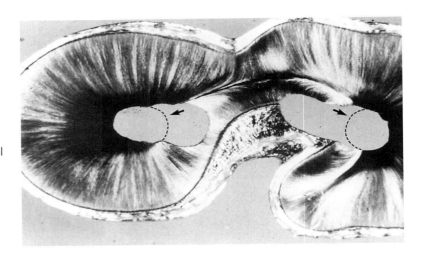

FIGURE 13-24
Inadequate access and overzealous enlargement in the danger zone are evident in this mesial root of a mandibular molar. Dashed lines *(arrows)* indicate approximate original canal dimensions. (Courtesy Dr. H. Rodriguez.)

canal. Also, this technique is helpful in bypassing created blockages.

Zipping of the Apical Canal

Transportation may create a reverse funnel of the apical preparation as the file straightens the curved canal. If the preparation is continued past the apex and is straightened, a long or "zipping" perforation results. It is then difficult to control obturating materials adequately to obtain a good seal[74] owing to the reverse funnel shape.

Stripping Perforation

Strip perforation is, in most cases, very damaging. The cervical portion of the instrument (file or Gates-Glidden bur) straightens the canal in multirooted teeth, leading eventually to communication with the furcation. The canal and dentin facing the furcation constitute a "danger" zone (Figure 13-23).

In the danger zone there is less tooth structure compared with the more peripheral portion (safety zone) of the root dentin.[75] There is a tendency, particularly in canals without straight-line access, to remove dentin from the danger zone (Figure 13-24).[76]

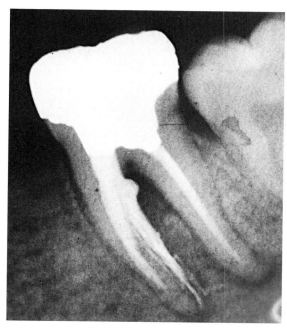

FIGURE 13-25
Stripping perforation. Overpreparation in the danger zone perforated the furcation. Obturating materials are forced interradicularly. Prognosis is very poor.

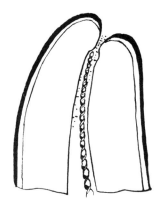

FIGURE 13-26
Recapitulation. Small files are used often to working length to loosen debris to permit removal by irrigation.

Recapitulation is another preventive technique (Figure 13-26).[25] This removal of debris with small files helps to avoid canal straightening. Also, frequent and copious *irrigation*, particularly after recapitulation, minimizes packing of dentin chips. This apical accumulation of chips promotes deflection and straightening of the instrument tip.

OTHER ERRORS

Mistakes such as separated instruments, canal blockages, overpreparation beyond the apex, and the preceding procedural errors are discussed in more detail in Chapter 18. Also discussed are prevention and management.

Review of Basic Principles of Instrumentation

Some principles apply regardless of the technique of instrumentation used.

A stripping perforation may also occur during straight-line access preparation by overusing Gates-Glidden burs into the danger zone.

A stripping perforation into the furcation generally results in failure[77] if obturating material extrudes into the periodontium (Figure 13-25). Prevention is the key; these types of perforations are very difficult to correct.

PREVENTION

These problems are easy to create; to prevent them is a challenge. The most important steps are passive step-back for preflaring, then good straight-line access, and then judicious use of instruments around curves to maintain a small apical preparation! Larger files used around curves accomplish relatively little débridement. **To repeat**, small canals with more than a slight curvature should usually undergo apical preparation with no larger than a size 20 MAF.

Another approach for more curved canals is a *repeat step-back technique*. This involves minimal dentin removal (about 1-mm increments) around the curve during the first step-back. Then more aggressive dentin removal is done at 0.5-mm increments during the second step-back.

1. Files are always worked in a canal filled with irrigant.
2. Copious irrigation is done between each file size.
3. Exploration is always done with smaller files to gauge canal size and configuration.
4. Passive step-back (preflaring) with hand instruments will facilitate placing larger working length files (either hand or rotary) and will reduce transportation.
5. Canal enlargement is gradual, using sequentially larger files from apical to coronal, regardless of flaring technique.
6. Debris is loosened and dentin is removed from all walls on the outstroke (circumfer-

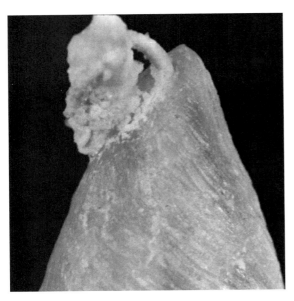

FIGURE 13-27
Extrusion of a "worm" of debris through the apical foramen. This represents an irritant that may be sufficient to initiate or exacerbate existing periapical inflammation.

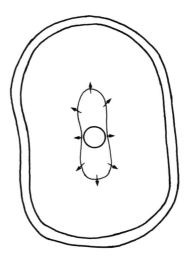

FIGURE 13-28
Files should be used peripherally in an attempt to remove a layer of dentin from all walls, recognizing that the canals are usually irregular in shape.

ential filing) or with a rotating (reaming) action at or close to working length.

7. Instrument binding or dentin removal on insertion should be avoided. Files are teased to length using a "twiddling" action. Twiddling is a back-and-forth rotating motion of the files (giving a quarter turn) between the thumb and forefinger, continually working apically. Careful file insertion (twiddling) followed by planing on the outstroke will help to avoid apical packing of debris and minimize extrusion of debris apically (Figure 13-27).

8. *Reaming* is accomplished by twiddling the instrument to length and then working it back and forth until it rotates freely and continuously in a clockwise direction. Reaming is accomplished using either reamers or K-type files.

9. *Filing* is a dentin stripping or planing motion accomplished on the pull stroke. The file is twiddled to length, rotated clockwise until it locks (the amount of rotation needed depends on the size of the canal and the instrument), and then withdrawn while the instrument tip is pushed alternately against all walls (Figure 13-28). The pushing motion is analogous to the action of a paintbrush. Overall, this is a *turn and pull* motion.

10. After each insertion and planing pull of the file, the file is removed and the flutes are cleaned of debris; the file is then reinserted into the canal to plane the next wall.

11. Debris is removed from the file by wiping it with an alcohol-soaked gauze or cotton roll.[78] An alternative but less effective technique is to spear the file up and down in the alcohol-soaked sponge or in other sponge systems used for instrument storage (Figure 13-29).

12. The canal is effectively cleaned *only* where the files actually contact and plane the walls. Inaccessible regions are poorly débrided.

13. Recapitulation is done to loosen debris by often returning to working length and rotating the MAF or a smaller size (see Figure 13-26). The walls should not be planed, nor should the canal be enlarged during recapitulation.

14. Small, long, curved, round canals are the most difficult and tedious to enlarge. They require extra caution during preparation, being the most prone to transportation.

15. Too-aggressive overenlargement of curved canals by files attempting to straighten themselves is likely to lead to procedural errors (Figure 13-30).

16. Overpreparation of canal walls toward the furcation leads into the danger zone; root dentin is thinner in this area.

A 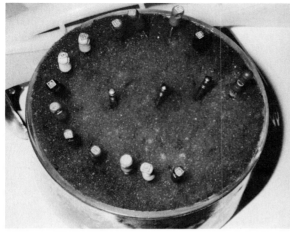 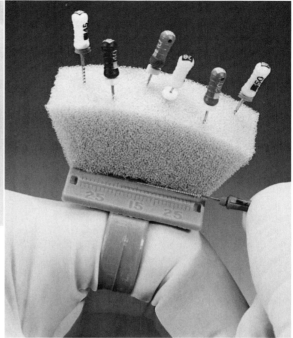 B

FIGURE 13-29
A, A sponge in a glass or plastic dish soaked with alcohol is ideal for organizing, cleaning, and storing files and Gates-Glidden burs during the appointment. **B**, A special storage and measuring device is conveniently fit on the index finger. (**B** courtesy Dr. G. Glickman.)

17. It is neither desirable nor necessary to try to remove created steps or other slight irregularities created during canal preparation.
18. Everything (instruments, irrigants, debris, and obturating materials) should be contained within the canal. These are all known physical or chemical irritants that will induce inflammation and may delay or compromise healing.
19. Creation of an apical stop may be impossible if the apical foramen is already very large. An apical taper (seat) is attempted, but with care. Overusing large files aggravates the problem by creating an even larger apical opening.
20. Forcing or continuing to rotate (either clockwise or counterclockwise) a file that binds is dangerous. This tends to untwist, wrap-up, weaken, and break the instrument.

Nickel-Titanium Instrumentation

The importance of nickel-titanium (NiTi) instruments has recently become significant.[79] This metal, when cut to the shape of a file, has desirable physical properties.[80] These relate to the flexibility of the instrument without memory (the instrument can be bent significantly, but returns to its original shape). In contrast to stainless steel

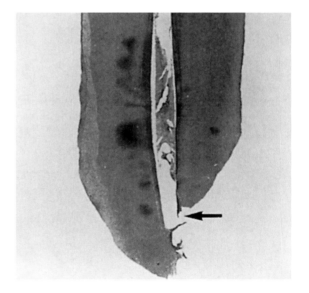

FIGURE 13-30
Overenlargement has resulted in perforation *(arrow)* and an open apex. The canal contains blood, a frequent finding after apical perforation.

(which is less flexible), NiTi may be used in a rotary, slow speed (150 to 300 rpm) handpiece. The physical properties of NiTi instruments (variable tapering cross-sectional flat radial land design, noncutting tips, and parallel core) are discussed in greater detail in Chapter 10. NiTi is used for both hand and engine-driven rotary instruments.[81]

HAND

NiTi hand files have advantages and disadvantages compared with more commonly used stainless steel files.[82] The major advantages are flexibility and superelastic behavior (memory) upon deformation. These are useful when a small, curved canal is prepared; there is evidence of less transportation.[83] Other claimed advantages include strength, anticorrosive properties, and no weakening after sterilization.

Disadvantages include cost (much more expensive), inability to precurve, lack of some stiffness (stiffness is desirable when trying to locate or negotiate a small canal), and a tendency for breakage if overused. NiTi hand instruments seem to be less efficient in removing dentin compared with stainless steel files because of their cross-sectional and flute designs.

NiTi hand files are used in a manner similar to that used for stainless steel files. These techniques are described earlier in this chapter.

ENGINE-DRIVEN ROTARY
Systems

A variety of NiTi rotary file systems have been developed by different manufacturers (each with its own instrumentation technique). General features will be described in this chapter; specific features and techniques are described in promotional materials, videotapes, and other publications for each system.

Many designs of NiTi instruments are available. Most resemble a basic file, with flutes along the length and a latching or attaching system to affix the file to a handpiece. Some are available in different tapers and with noncutting tips (Figure 13-31). Another unique design (Lightspeed) resembles a Gates-Glidden drill, with a small shaft and a short, flame-shaped cutting head; this instrument also has a latch to attach to a rotary handpiece (see Chapter 10, Figure 10-7). Both types can be used with either conventional or special low-torque, controlled speed motor systems, (Figure 13-32) including battery-operated handpieces.[84]

Techniques

After negotiating the canals and determining the corrected working length, NiTi rotary instruments are used to flare either with the step-back or the crown-down methods. Straight-line access to the canal space is established (usually with Gates-Glidden drills or with special orifice shapers). A small hand file (No. 10 stainless steel) is used to explore the canal to the corrected length. Hand instrumentation (reaming) is performed at the corrected length through two or three sizes with either stainless steel or NiTi files. This is followed by rotary instrumentation.

The rotary NiTi instruments are used in the apical portion of the canal at or short (usually

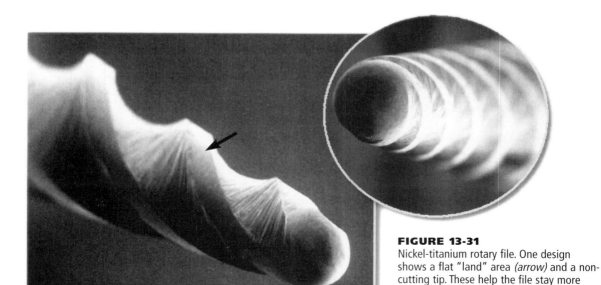

FIGURE 13-31
Nickel-titanium rotary file. One design shows a flat "land" area *(arrow)* and a noncutting tip. These help the file stay more centered in the canal during preparation. (Courtesy Tulsa Dentsply Dental.)

2 to 4 mm) of the corrected working length. The files are continuously rotated with the foot pedal of the electric or air turbine motor handpiece fully depressed for constant speed and torque. Very light pressure is used along with lubrication (irrigant) to place the NiTi rotary instrument into the canal until resistance is felt. The instrument is then immediately withdrawn in a smooth motion from the canal space, although recommendations of advancement of the instrument apically in an up-and-down "pecking" motion have also been made. Slow speed is preferred to minimize instrument distortion.[85,86] Light pressure (force is never used!) is applied; the instrument is withdrawn when resistance is felt to prevent breakage.[87] After each withdrawal, the flutes are cleaned with wet gauze or an alcohol sponge, and the file is examined for distortions and/or deformations (unwinding or wrapping-up of the flutes).

This process is repeated by using a sequence of larger instruments to the desired length, with recapitulation and irrigation between each instrument size. Patience and careful insertion with light pressure is necessary, allowing the system to do the work, particularly in canals with calcific metamorphosis. Instrumentation of the apical portion of the canal space is usually performed in a step-back manner with hand (stainless steel or NiTi) instruments to form an apical matrix.

The Lightspeed technique has a somewhat different approach, using only the "pecking" action to prepare the canal; this is also done in a crown-down mode.[88] Débridement effectiveness with these unique instruments seems similar to that with hand preparation.[89]

NiTi rotary instrumentation has advantages as well as disadvantages compared with stainless steel hand instrumentation. Because of their flexibility, the files have less tendency to transport curved canals. Finger fatigue is less because the handpiece is doing much of the work. Somewhat less time is required to prepare the canal. Preliminary evidence indicates that débridement effectiveness is comparable to that with hand instrumentation.[90] There are also disadvantages. Expense is greater if one of the special motor systems is purchased; in addition, the files are costly. Files are prone to breakage, without warning, particularly if overused.[91] Overall, no difference is seen with NiTi rotary instruments for either quality of débridement or prognosis; there are no substantive data on either.

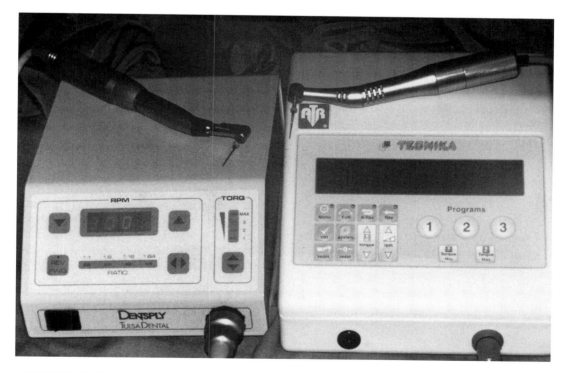

FIGURE 13-32
Two control units ("motors") for handpieces that drive nickel-titanium rotary files. The unit on the left allows control of speed and torque; that on the right is programmable for these two functions plus a variety of other functions.

COMBINATION OF PASSIVE STEP-BACK AND ROTARY INSTRUMENTATION

The crown down or step down technique with rotary instruments is advocated by the manufacturers for shaping of canals with rotary NiTi files. The main disadvantage of this recommendation is the possibility of instrument separation. To reduce the frequency of this procedural accident, coronal flaring as recommended for the passive step-back technique (as described earlier in this chapter) is used before rotary instruments are used to shape the apical portion of the canal. This flaring enhances irrigation of the apical third and removes irritants. In addition, the use of this technique before the use of rotary instruments creates straighter line access to the apical canal and less transportation during apical preparation with rotary instruments.[23] This procedure reduces the chances for instrument separation, packing debris, ledging, straightening the apical portion of the canal, and root perforation.

The steps are as follows:

1. After the pulp chamber is completely unroofed, an estimated working length is determined from a preoperative radiograph. After apical-canal patency is established with a No. 10 or 15 K-type file, the canal is passively (without binding) flared using No. 15 to 45 K-type files.
2. After filing, Gates-Glidden drills (Nos. 2 and 3 and in large canals No. 4) are used in an up-and-down motion without lateral pressure. To further enlarge and flare the coronal portion of the canal, Nos. 2 and 3 Peeso reamers are used passively.
3. After copious irrigation with sodium hypochlorite, a new working length with an apex locator is determined and confirmed radiographically.
4. With the use of rotary NiTi files (sizes 15 to 25) and a "pecking" motion, the apical portion of the canal is enlarged to the working length. With the use of larger rotary NiTi files (sizes 30 to 40), the coronal portion of the canal is flared progressively at successively shorter lengths (increments of 0.5 to 1mm).
5. The canal is irrigated with sodium hypochlorite, and the working length is confirmed by a radiograph or an apex locator before obturation.

Alternative Techniques of Cleaning and Shaping

Other approaches to canal preparation have been devised. Some of these have generated great interest and enthusiasm, whereas others have attracted little attention. Because conventional preparation with hand instruments is somewhat difficult and time-consuming, the search continues for something more effective and less involved. Interestingly, automated devices that create cavitation and hydrodynamic turbulence with continuous irrigant exchange are being tested.[92] These or other devices probably will evolve in the future to simplify treatment modalities.

Some unique approaches have been introduced, including ultrasonic and sonic devices as well as the newer engine-driven, slow-speed handpieces that make use of special nickel-titanium files; these techniques and devices have generated much interest. Other, older mechanical devices (handpieces) are also in use. These, including alternative hand techniques, are briefly reviewed here.

BALANCED FORCES

The balanced forces method is a somewhat different approach; the technique also uses an altered instrument design.[93] The files used have a modified tip that is noncutting. Canal preparation involves counterclockwise rotation combined with apical pressure. There is evidence that this method allows the instrument to stay more centered in the canal during preparation, causing less transportation.[94,95] However, it has not been demonstrated whether this ultimately results in better clinical success or whether there is a significant advantage in cleaning and shaping with this technique or instruments.[96]

ENERGIZED VIBRATORY SYSTEMS

Sonic and ultrasonic techniques were introduced in the 1980s. Some authors proposed that these techniques were the "wave of the future." They have not, however, proved to be panaceas. In addition, some questions remain unanswered and there has been insufficient clinical usage over time to allow endorsement with or without reservations. Ultrasonic and sonic techniques have been suggested to have a role when used in combination with hand instruments.[97]

These vibratory systems were developed in the hope of replacing or supplementing hand instrumentation. Nickel-titanium rotary instruments seem to be filling that role; the vibratory systems currently are little used for canal preparation.

Ultrasonic Instruments

Physics. Essentially, endosonic machines are an adaptation of the ultrasound apparatus used for scaling. The power source (either electromagnetic or piezoelectric) is transferred to a special insert that holds an instrument similar to a file. The file is energized as ultrasonic energy is transmitted through the insert. The file then vibrates at approximately 25,000 vibrations per second.

The energy from the file is transmitted to a fluid medium (irrigant) within the canal, which transfers the energy to the dentin walls. This energized solution shows *acoustic streaming*, which is the "rapid movement of particles of fluid in vortex-like motion about a vibrating object."[98] The swirls and whirlpools of moving fluid supposedly help loosen debris from the canal walls.

Application. The devices seem to be most effective for cleaning and shaping canals that are easier to prepare.[99] For more difficult situations, such as small curved canals, ultrasonic instruments are no more or less effective than standard hand instrument techniques.[100-103] In more uniform canals, where the instrument can be fully energized, ultrasonic devices may provide superior débriding qualities. However, if the instrument is curved or binds in the canal, it may not have the same vibratory activity and therefore is less energized (Figure 13-33).[104]

Effectiveness. Research and clinical usage have led to the following conclusions. *Débridement* may be quite good in the straighter canals but less so in small, curved canals. *Flushing* seems to be effective, with irrigant flowing to the tip of the file when it is energized properly.[105] Whether this technique is superior to conventional irrigation with a syringe has not been shown.

Endodontists have found ultrasonic instruments useful for removing posts, silver points, paste fills, and separated instruments.[103,106-108]

Sonic Instrumentation

Special handpieces have been developed that vibrate root canal instruments of various designs. The handpiece is run from the standard high-speed air line of the dental unit. When activated, the instruments whip in an oval, whirling motion at a frequency of approximately 1500 to 8000 vibrations per second (Figure 13-34). The file vibrates against and scrapes the canal walls. Irrigating solution (water) is delivered to and directed along the file into the canal. In limited tests, the sonic instrument appeared to enlarge and débride the canal safely and effectively.[109,110] In usage tests under rigorous conditions (in small curved canals), sonic handpieces did not perform as well as the step-back

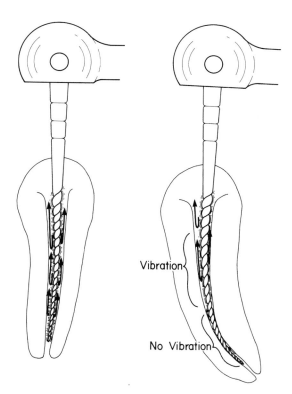

FIGURE 13-33
Theory of the difference in ultrasonic vibrations noted in a straight versus a curved canal. Instrument and irrigation patterns may be very active in the straight canal *(left)*. The curve dampens the energy of the file and reduces or eliminates its vibratory action *(right)*.

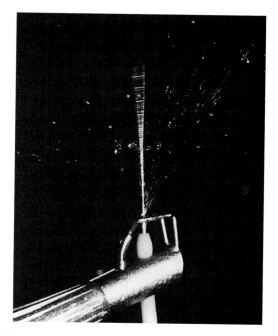

FIGURE 13-34
A sonic handpiece transmits a whipping vibration and an irrigant to a specially designed file.

preparation but results were approximately equal to those with ultrasonic devices.[100,101]

Sonic handpieces seem to have fallen into disuse because of their limitations.

OTHER MECHANIZED TECHNIQUES

Stainless Steel Rotary. It seems like a great idea to adapt conventional stainless steel instruments to standard handpieces that would mechanically clean and shape canals. This should be faster and less tedious than manipulating files with fingers. However, because of the relative inflexibility of stainless steel, these techniques are ineffective and fraught with danger, particularly in curved canals.

Many approaches, instruments, and special handpieces have been designed to perform canal preparation. Reamers have added latches for attachment to standard handpieces. Instruments similar to a broach are latched to fit into a special handpiece that vibrates alternately back and forth. Handpieces that rotate back and forth in a quarter circle and up and down a few millimeters are available; these also grasp the handles of certain files.

There are problems with these devices that use stainless steel instruments. First, they generally do not débride well.[76,111] Second, they tend to push debris in an apical direction, particularly the instruments using an up-and-down motion.[112] Third, they tend to markedly straighten and ledge curved canals without creating a taper.[76,111] These are not recommended.

LASERS

Lasers have been experimentally applied as aids in root canal treatment. As yet, there are no demonstrated useful applications in canal preparation.

Intracanal Medicaments

Intracanal medicaments have traditionally been integral to root canal treatment and have been considered important to success (Box 13-1). In fact, at one time, a common assumption that success, both short-term and long-term, depended on the chemical placed in the canal between appointments. It was also recognized that medicaments possess potentially harmful side effects; each is an active, toxic chemical or therapeutic agent. The question was and still is, Are the benefits worth the risks? The answer is mainly no.[113] There is no demonstrated usefulness for the traditional phenolic or fixative agents such as camphorated monochlorophenol (CMCP), formocresol, and Cresatin. Calcium hydroxide $(Ca(OH)_2)$ is of a different class and is promising as an antimicrobial agent.

Uses and actions of most of these agents are largely based on empiricism and opinion.[114] Clinicians and lecturers in the past applied these agents without investigation. Thus, popular intracanal medicaments were designed and proposed for (1) antimicrobial activity in the pulp and periapex, (2) neutralization of canal remnants to render them inert, and (3) control or prevention of post-treatment pain. Again, the phenolic and fixative agents have no beneficial effects when used as intracanal medicaments between appointments.

Habits, beliefs, and clinical impressions are potent influences. Pressured by the focus of infection theories of the early 1900s, practitioners adapted strong antimicrobial agents for root canal treatment. The goal was to render the canals and periradicular tissues sterile and to prevent supposed dissemination of dangerous bacteria throughout the body.

As the focal infection theory diminished in importance, the use as well as the significance of antimicrobial medicaments also diminished. Intracanal bacterial populations are best reduced or even eliminated by careful instrumentation and irrigation.[51,115] Thus, the use of traditional medicaments,

---

BOX 13-1

Groupings of Commonly Used Intracanal Medicaments

Phenolics
  Eugenol
  Camphorated monoparachlorophenol (CMCP)
  Parachlorophenol (PCP)
  Camphorated parachlorophenol (CPC)
  Metacresylacetate (Cresatin)
  Cresol
  Creosote (beechwood)
  Thymol
Aldehydes
  Formocresol
  Glutaraldehyde
Halides
  Sodium hypochlorite
  Iodine-potassium iodide
Steroids
Calcium hydroxide
Antibiotics
Combinations

From Walton R: Intracanal medicaments, *Dent Clin North Am* 28:783, 1984.

owing to lack of evidence of usefulness and toxicity, is in decline. In contrast, calcium hydroxide $(Ca(OH)_2)$ usage is increasing because of its demonstrated antimicrobial properties, coupled with some initial evidence of its aiding in reducing periapical inflammation.[116] However, the long-term outcome (success or failure) with the use $Ca(OH)_2$ as an intracanal medicament is uncertain.[117]

APPLICATIONS

Studies to test medicament effectiveness show that they either do not perform as expected or occasionally have the opposite effect. There are, however, exceptions, including steroids and calcium hydroxide.

Antibacterial Action. The most popular antimicrobials are calcium hydroxide, CMCP, and formocresol. These are potent microbe killers under ideal laboratory test conditions; their effectiveness in clinical use is doubtful,[118] although calcium hydroxide does inhibit intracanal bacterial growth[119] and alters the biologic properties of bacterial lipopolysaccharide.[120]

Pain Relief. Certain intracanal medicaments are claimed to reduce pain by anodyne, antimicrobial effect, or both. Reducing or preventing inflammation presumably decreases its byproduct, pain.

Clinical studies on phenolics, formocresol, and calcium hydroxide show that routine use as intracanal medicaments has no effect on prevention or control of pain.[121-124] However, steroids have been demonstrated to decrease post-treatment pain somewhat, but with mixed results. These drugs, whether applied topically (for example, through the canal)[125] or systemically, alter the inflammatory or vascular response sufficiently to affect lower levels of pain.[126] However, steroids do not reduce the incidence of flare-ups (severe pain).[124] In endodontic applications their action seems to be minor and affects only milder degrees of pain.

Canal Contents Rendered Inert. Chemicals used for this purpose are fixatives, or aldehyde derivatives. They fix fresh tissues for histologic study; however, aldehydes do not effectively fix necrotic or decomposed tissues. Fixed tissues are not inert.[127] In fact, when both necrotic and vital tissues are fixed with aldehydes, they become more toxic and antigenic.

LIMITATIONS AND CONTRAINDICATIONS

Intracanal Environment. The chemical or therapeutic action of medicaments depends on direct contact of the agent with microbes or tissue. This is a drawback to chemicals used in the pulp space; these substances probably do not reach all areas in the canal and into dentinal tubules where bacteria or tissues are hidden and their action is limited to the surface only.

Duration. To be effective, most agents should remain chemically active during the time between appointments. Phenolics dissipate and may lose their activity within 24 hours.[118] Calcium hydroxide retains antimicrobial activity for prolonged periods and can inhibit regrowth of bacteria. The duration of steroid activity is unknown.

Sustained-release delivery systems of various intracanal medicaments have been evaluated in vitro, but their clinical effectiveness has not been clearly demonstrated.[128-130]

Toxicity. Any chemical that kills bacteria will also kill host cells. Both in vitro (bench type) and in vivo (animal and clinical use) studies show that phenolics and aldehydes are generally potent cell killers.[131,132] Another potential adverse side effect is allergenicity. Some medicaments act as haptens and alter tissues to become foreign substances, which then elicit an immune response.[133] This action may be responsible for their localized adverse effects on pulp or periapical tissues.[134] Neither calcium hydroxide nor steroid compounds have significant toxicity.

Distribution. There is ample evidence that substances placed in the pulp, with or without tissue, have ready access to periradicular tissues and even to the systemic circulation.[135-137] Although the dangers of this distribution are unknown,[138] the use of potent chemicals that have no demonstrated beneficial effects is questionable.

Taste and Smell. The phenolics in particular possess a pungent odor and foul taste. These medicaments soak into and through the temporary restoration into the oral cavity. Patients report a disagreeable medicinal taste; many find this most objectionable. Some dentists believe that if a patient reports a bad taste, the temporary seal is defective and will leak saliva into the canal; there is no evidence to support this presumption.

CALCIUM HYDROXIDE

Properties. Calcium hydroxide is available in different forms, combinations, and proprietary compounds.[139] When sealed in the canal for either short- or long-term use, a number of actions have been attributed to it.[119,140] Most have not been clearly substantiated in clinical trials. Calcium hydroxide may be used as a canal dressing between appointments, particularly when pulp necrosis has been diagnosed.

Although the antibacterial properties of calcium hydroxide pastes are effective when evalu-

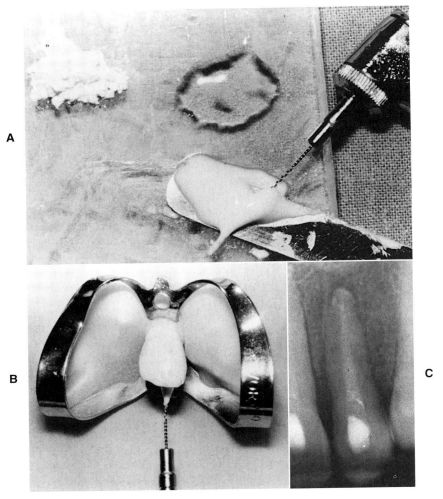

FIGURE 13-35
Calcium hydroxide placement. Powder is mixed with glycerin to toothpaste consistency (**A**) and placed with a lentulo spiral (**B**). Proper fill appears dense (**C**). Slight overfill is not a problem.

ated over short time periods,[119,140] little is known concerning their long-term antimicrobial efficacy. This is a clinically relevant concern, because high numbers of bacteria within the canal space and/ or tubules may represent a source of continual microbial challenge to originally placed calcium hydroxide.[119]

Calcium hydroxide also has some tissue-altering effects,[141-143] but it does not aid in débridement when placed in the canal space.[46]

Placement. Calcium hydroxide should ideally be placed deep and densely in the canal space so that its biological effect can be exerted in close proximity to the appropriate tissues. Techniques that deliver dry calcium hydroxide powder alone are diffi-

cult or impossible in smaller, more curved canals. In most cases, the calcium hydroxide must be mixed with a liquid such as anesthetic solution water, glycerin, other intracanal medicaments, or methyl cellulose to facilitate placement.[144] To use, calcium hydroxide is mixed with glycerin (water is less effective in terms of density to length) to a thick paste and placed in the canal with either a plugger or spun into a lentulo spiral (Figure 13-35) using a counter-clockwise motion.[145] The lentulo spiral (use with caution!) is most effective device for carrying calcium hydroxide paste to length in small, curved canals.[145,146] The powder alone may be placed with a Messing gun or pluggers in large, straight canals.[147]

REFERENCES

1. Schilder H: Cleaning and shaping the root canal, *Dent Clin North Am* 18:269, 1974.
2. Bolaños OR, Jensen JR: Scanning electron microscope comparison of the efficacy of various methods of root canal preparation, *J Endod* 6:815, 1980.
3. Turek T, Langeland K: A light microscopic study of the efficacy of the telescopic and Giromatic preparation of root canals, *J Endod* 8:437, 1982.
4. Walton RE: Histologic evaluation of different methods of enlarging the pulp space, *J Endod* 2:304, 1976.
5. Wilcox L, Roskelley, Sutton T: The relationship of root canal enlargement to finger-spreader induced vertical root fracture, *J Endod* 23:533, 1997.
6. Walton RE: Current concepts of canal preparation, *Dent Clin North Am* 36:309, 1992.
7. Weine FS, Kelly RF, Lio PJ: The effect of preparation procedures on the original canal shape and on apical foramen shape, *J Endod* 1:255, 1975.
8. Johnson WT: Instrumentation of the fine curved canals found in the mesial roots of maxillary and mandibular molars, *Quintessence Int* 17:309, 1986.
9. Kosa D, Marshall G, Baumgartner C: An analysis of canal centering using mechanical instrumentation techniques, *J Endod* 25:441, 1999.
10. Jungmann CL, Uchin RA, Bucher JF: Effect of instrumentation on the shape of the root canal, *J Endod* 1:66, 1975.
11. Kavanagh D, Lumley PJ: An in vitro evaluation of canal preparation using Profile .04 and .06 taper instruments, *Endod Dent Traumatol* 14:16, 1998.
12. Allison DA, Weber CR, Walton RE: The influence of the method of canal preparation on the quality of apical and coronal obturation, *J Endod* 5:298, 1979.
13. Leeb J: Canal orifice enlargement as related to biomechanical preparation, *J Endod* 9:463, 1983.
14. Wu M-K, Wesselink P, Walton R: Apical terminus of root canal treatment procedures, *Oral Surg Oral Med Oral Pathol* 89:99, 2000.
15. Mullaney T, Cailleteau J, Duell R: The case for patency in apical root canal enlargement, *Endod Pract* 1:3, 1998.
16. Ingle JI: A standardized endodontic technique using newly designed instruments and filling materials, *Oral Surg Oral Med Oral Pathol* 14:83, 1961.
17. Ingle JI: The need for endodontic instrument standardization, *Oral Surg Oral Med Oral Pathol* 8:1211, 1955.
18. Haga CS: Microscopic measurements of root canal preparations following instrumentation, *J Br Endod Soc* 2:41, 1969.
19. Schneider SW: A comparison of canal preparations in straight and curved canals, *Oral Surg Oral Med Oral Pathol* 32:271, 1971.
20. Kerekes K, Tronstad L: Long term results of endodontic treatment performed with a standardized technique, *J Endod* 5:83, 1979.
21. Clem WH: Endodontics in the adolescent patient, *Dent Clin North Am* 13:483, 1969.
22. Cailleteau J, Mullaney T: Prevalence of teaching apical patency and various instrumentation and obturation techniques in United States dental schools, *J Endod* 23:394, 1997.
23. Torabinejad M: Passive step-back technique, *Oral Surg Oral Med Oral Pathol* 77:398, 1994.
24. Alodeh MH, Dummer PMH: A comparison of the ability of K-files and Hedstrom files to shape simulated root canals in resin blocks, *Int Endod J* 22:226, 1989.
25. Rivera EM, Seraji M: Effect of canal patency on accuracy of electronically determined working length, *Oral Surg Oral Med Oral Pathol* 75:225, 1993.
26. Morgan LF, Montgomery S: An evaluation of the crown-down pressureless technique, *J Endod* 10:491, 1984.
27. Goerig A, Michelich R, Schultz H: Instrumentation of root canals in molars using the step-down technique, *J Endod* 8:550, 1982.
28. Parris J, Wilcox L, Walton RE: Effectiveness of apical clearing: histological and radiographical evaluation, *J Endod* 20:219, 1994.
29. Pineda F, Kuttler Y: Mesiodistal and buccolingual roentgenographic investigation of 7275 root canals, *Oral Surg Oral Med Oral Pathol* 33:101, 1972.
30. Siqueira J, Araujo M, Garcia P, et al: Histological evaluation of the effectiveness of five instrumentation techniques for cleaning the apical third of root canals, *J Endod* 23:499, 1997.
31. Rosenfeld EF, James GA, Burch BS: Vital pulp tissue response to sodium hypochlorite, *J Endod* 4:140, 1978.
32. The SD: The solvent action of sodium hypochlorite on fixed and unfixed necrotic tissue, *Oral Surg Oral Med Oral Pathol* 47:558, 1979.
33. Baumgartner JC, Cuenin PR: Efficacy of several concentrations of sodium hypochlorite for root canal irrigation, *J Endod* 18:605, 1992.
34. Berutti E, Marini R, Angeretti A: Penetration ability of different irrigants into dentinal tubules, *J Endod* 23:725, 1997.
35. Abou-Rass M, Patonai FJ: The effects of decreasing surface tension on the flow of irrigating solutions in narrow root canals, *Oral Surg Oral Med Oral Pathol* 53:524, 1982.
36. Cunningham WT, Cole JS, Balekjian A: Effect of alcohol on the spreading ability of sodium hypochlorite endodontic irrigant, *Oral Surg Oral Med Oral Pathol* 54:333, 1982.
37. D'Arcangelo C, Varvara G, DeFazio P: An evaluation of the action of different root canal irrigants on facultative aerobic-anaerobic, obligate anaerobic, and microaerophilic bacteria, *J Endod* 25:351, 1999.
38. Foley DB, Weine FS, Hagen JC, et al: Effectiveness of selected irrigants in the elimination of *Bacteroides melaninogenicus* from the root canal system: an in vitro study, *J Endod* 9:236, 1983.
39. McComb D, Smith DC: A preliminary electron microscopic study of root canals after endodontic procedures, *J Endod* 1:238, 1975.
40. Baumgartner JC, Mader C: A scanning electron microscopic evaluation of four root canal irrigation regimens, *J Endod* 13:147, 1987.
41. Takeda F, Harashima T, Kimura Y, Matsumoto K: A comparative study of the removal of smear layer by three endodontic irrigants and two types of laser, *Int Endod J* 32:32, 1999.

42. Drake DR, Wiemann AH, Rivera EM, et al: Bacterial retention in canal walls in vitro: effect of smear layer, *J Endod* 20:78, 1994.

43. Grossman L, Meiman B: Solution of pulp tissue by chemical agents, *J Am Dent Assoc* 28:223, 1941.

44. Moodnik RM, Dorn SO, Feldman MJ, et al: Efficiency of biomechanical instrumentation: an electron microscope study, *J Endod* 2:261, 1976.

45. Walker TL, del Rio CE: Histological evaluation of ultrasonic débridement comparing sodium hypochlorite and water, *J Endod* 17:66, 1991.

46. Yang S-F, Rivera EM, Walton RE, Baumgardner K: Solvent effect of calcium hydroxide and sodium hypochlorite in root canal spaces, *J Endod* 22:521, 1996.

47. Senia ES, Marshall FJ, Rosen S: The solvent action of sodium hypochlorite on pulp tissue of extracted teeth, *Oral Surg Oral Med Oral Pathol* 31:96, 1971.

48. Ayhan H, Sultan N, Cirak M, et al: Antimicrobial effects of various endodontic irrigants on selected microorganisms, *Int Endod J* 32:99, 1999.

49. Heling I, Chandler NP: Antimicrobial effect of irrigant combinations within dentinal tubules, *Int Endod J* 31:8, 1998.

50. Grahnen H, Krasse B: The effect of instrumentation and flushing of non-vital teeth in endodontic therapy, *Odontol Rev* 14:167, 1963.

51. Bystrom A, Sundqvist G: The antibacterial action of sodium hypochlorite and EDTA in 60 cases of endodontic therapy, *Int Endod J* 18:35, 1985.

52. Bystrom A, Sundqvist G: Bacteriologic evaluation of the efficacy of mechanical root canal instrumentation in endodontic therapy, *Scand J Dent Res* 89:321, 1981.

53. Hühlsmann M, Hahn W: Complications during root canal irrigation—literature review and case reports, *Int Endod J* 33:186, 2000.

54. Pashley EL, Birdsong NL, Bowman K, et al: Cytotoxic effects of NaOCl on vital tissue, *J Endod* 11:525, 1985.

55. Saleh A, Ettman W: Effect of endodontic irrigation solutions on microhardness of root canal dentin, *J Dent* 27:43, 1999.

56. Svec TA, Harrison JW: Chemomechanical removal of pulpal and dentinal debris with sodium hypochlorite and hydrogen peroxide vs normal saline solution, *J Endod* 3:49, 1977.

57. Abou-Rass M, Piccinino M: The effectiveness of four clinical irrigation methods on the removal of tooth canal debris, *Oral Surg Oral Med Oral Pathol* 54:323, 1982.

58. Leonardo M, Filho T, Silva L, et al: In vivo antimicrobial activity of 2% chlorhexidine used as a root canal irrigating solution, *J Endod* 25:167, 1999.

59. Siqueira J, Batista M, Fraga R, de Uzeda M: Antibacterial effects of endodontic irrigants on black-pigmented gram-negative anaerobes and facultative bacteria, *J Endod* 24:414, 1998.

60. Ram A: Effectiveness of root canal irrigation, *Oral Surg Oral Med Oral Pathol* 44:306, 1977.

61. Mehra P, Clancy C, Wu J: Case report: formation of a facial hematoma during endodontic therapy, *J Am Dent Assoc* 131:67, 2000.

62. Nygaard-Ostby L: Chelation in root canal therapy. *Odont Tidskr* 65:3, 1957.

63. Stewart G, Kapsimalis P, Rappaport H: EDTA and urea peroxide for root canal preparation, *J Am Dent Assoc* 78:335, 1969.

64. Wayman BE, Kopp WM, Pinero GJ: Citric and lactic acids as root canal irrigants in vitro, *J Endod* 5:258, 1979.

65. Goldberg F, Abramovich A: Analysis of the effect of EDTAC on the dentinal walls of the root canal, *J Endod* 3:101, 1977.

66. Verdelis K, Eliades G, Oviir T, Margelos J: Effect of chelating agents on the molecular composition and extent of decalcification at cervical, middle and apical root dentin locations, *Endod Dent Traumatol* 15:164, 1999.

67. Mykleby B, Krell K: Speed of canal preparation using different endodontic irrigants: a time-motion study (Abstract), *J Endod* 10:188, 1985.

68. Lentine FN: A study of torsional and angular deflection of endodontic files and reamers, *J Endod* 5:181, 1979.

69. Lim KC, Webber J: The effect of root canal preparation on the shape of the curved root canal, *Int Endod J* 18:233, 1985.

70. Wilcox LR, Swift ML: Endodontic retreatment in small and large curved canals, *J Endod* 17:313, 1991.

71. Torabinejad M: Endodontic mishaps: etiology, prevention, and management, *Alpha Omegan* 83:42, 1990.

72. Greene K, Krell K: Clinical factors associated with ledged canals in maxillary and mandibular molars, *Oral Surg Oral Med Oral Pathol* 70:490, 1990.

73. Kapalas A, Lambrianidis T: Factors associated with root canal ledging during instrumentation, *Endod Dent Traumatol* 16:229, 2000.

74. Wu M-K, Fan B, Wesselink P: Leakage along apical root fillings in curved root canals. Part I: effects of apical transportation on seal of root fillings, *J Endod* 26:210, 2000.

75. Lim S, Stock C: The risk of perforation in the curved canal: anticurvature filing compared with the stepback technique, *Int Endod J* 20:33, 1987.

76. Abou-Rass M, Jastrab RJ: The use of rotary instruments as auxiliary aids to root canal preparation of molars, *J Endod* 8:78, 1982.

77. Meister FJ, Lommel TJ, Gerstein H, et al: Endodontic perforations which resulted in alveolar bone loss. Report of five cases, *Oral Surg Oral Med Oral Pathol* 47:463, 1979.

78. Murgel CA, Walton RE, Rittman B, Pecora JD: A comparison of techniques for cleaning endodontic files after usage: a quantitative scanning electron microscopic study, *J Endod* 16:214, 1990.

79. Thompson SA: An overview of nickel-titanium alloys used in dentistry, *Int Endod J* 33:297, 2000.

80. Walia HM, Brantley W, Gerstein H: An initial investigation of the bending and torsional properties of Nitinol root canal files, *J Endod* 14:346, 1988.

81. Rhodes J, Pitt Ford T, Lynch J, et al: A comparison of two nickel-titanium instrumentation techniques in teeth using microcomputed tomography, *Int Endod J* 33:279, 2000.

82. Coleman C, Svec T: Analysis of Ni-Ti versus stainless steel instrumentation in resin simulated canals, *J Endod* 23:232, 1997.

83. Pettiette MT, Metzger Z, Phillips C, Trope M: Endodontic complications of root canal therapy performed by dental students with stainless-steel K-files and nickel-titanium hand files, *J Endod* 25:230, 1999.

84. Gambarini G: Rationale for the use of low-torque endodontic motors in root canal instrumentation, *Endod Dent Traumatol* 16:95, 2000.

85. Gabel WP, Hoen M, Steiman HR, et al: Effect of rotational speed on nickel-titanium file distortion, *J Endod* 25:752, 1999.

86. Dietz D, Di Fiore P, Bahcall J, Lautenschlager E: Effect of rotational speed on the breakage of nickel-titanium rotary files, *J Endod* 26:68, 2000.

87. Yared G, Bou Dagher F, Machtou P: Cyclic fatigue of profile rotary instruments after clinical use, *Int Endod J* 33:204, 2000.

88. Barbakow F, Lutz F: The 'Lightspeed' preparation technique evaluated by Swiss clinicians after attending continuing education courses, *Int Endod J* 30:46, 1997.

89. Bechelli C, Orlandini SZ, Colafranceschi M: Scanning electron microscope study on the efficacy of root canal wall debridement of hand versus Lightspeed instrumentation, *Int Endod J* 32:484, 1999.

90. Schafer E, Zapke K: A comparative scanning electron microscopic investigation of the efficacy of manual and automated instrumentation of root canals, *J Endod* 26:660, 2000.

91. Zuolo M, Walton R: Instrument deterioration with usage: nickel titanium versus stainless steel, *Quintessence Int* 28:397, 1997.

92. Lussi A, Portmann P, Nussbacher U, et al: Comparison of two devices for root canal cleansing by the noninstrumentation technology, *J Endod* 25:9, 1999.

93. Roane JB, Sabala CL, Duncanson MG: The "balanced force" concept for instrumentation of curved canals, *J Endod* 11:203, 1985.

94. Sepic AO, Pantera EA, Neaverth EJ, et al: A comparison of Flex-R and K-type files for enlargement of severely curved molar root canals, *J Endod* 15:240, 1989.

95. Charles T, Charles J: The 'balanced force' concept for instrumentation of curved canals revisited, *Int Endod J* 31:166, 1998.

96. Zuolo ML, Walton RE, Imura N: Histologic evaluation of three endodontic instrument/preparation techniques, *Endod Dent Traumatol* 8:125, 1992.

97. Torabinejad M: Passive step-back technique: a sequential use of ultrasonic and hand instruments, *Oral Surg Oral Med Oral Pathol* 77:402, 1994.

98. Ahmad M, Pitt-Ford T, Crum L: Ultrasonic débridement of root canals: an insight into the mechanisms involved, *J Endod* 13:93, 1987.

99. Cunningham WT, Martin H: A scanning electron microscope evaluation of root canal débridement with the endodontic ultrasonic synergistic system, *Oral Surg Oral Med Oral Pathol* 53:527, 1982.

100. Langeland K, Liao K, Pascon EA: Work-saving devices in endodontics: efficacy of sonic and ultrasonic techniques, *J Endod* 11:499, 1985.

101. Reynolds MA, Madison S, Walton RE, et al: An in vitro histological comparison of the step-back, sonic and ultrasonic instrumentation techniques in small curved root canals, *J Endod* 13:307, 1987.

102. Goldman M, White RR, Moser CR, et al: A comparison of three methods of cleaning and shaping the root canal in vitro, *J Endod* 14:7, 1988.

103. Heard F, Walton R: Scanning electron microscope study comparing four root canal preparation techniques in small curved canals, *Int Endod J* 30:323, 1997.

104. Lumley PJ, Walmsley AD, Walton RE, et al: Effect of precurving endosonic files on the amount of debris and smear layer remaining in curved root canals, *J Endod* 18:616, 1992.

105. Krell K, Johnson R: Irrigation patterns of ultrasonic diamond coated files, *J Endod* 12:129, 1986.

106. Krell KV, Neo J: The use of ultrasonic endodontic instrumentation in the re-treatment of a paste-filled endodontic tooth, *Oral Surg Oral Med Oral Pathol* 60:100, 1985.

107. Jordan RD, Krell KV, Aquilino SA, et al: Removal of acid-etched fixed partial dentures with modified ultrasonic scaler tips, *J Am Dent Assoc* 112:505, 1986.

108. Nagai O, Tani N, Kayaba Y, et al: Removal of broken instruments, *Int Endod J* 19:83, 1986.

109. Zakariasen KL, Zakariasen KA, McMinn MM: Today's sonics: using the combined hand/sonic endodontic technique, *J Am Dent Assoc* 123:67, 1992.

110. Tronstad L, Barnett F, Schwartzben L: Effectiveness and safety of a sonic vibratory endodontic instrument, *Endod Dent Traumatol* 1:69, 1985.

111. Weine F, Kelly R, Bray L: Effect of preparation with endodontic handpieces on original canal shape, *J Endod* 2:298, 1976.

112. O'Connell DT, Brayton SM: Evaluation with two automated endodontic handpieces, *Oral Surg Oral Med Oral Pathol* 39:298, 1975.

113. Doran MG, Radtke PK: A review of endodontic medicaments, *Gen Dent* 46:484, 1998.

114. Walton RE: Intracanal medicaments, *Dent Clin North Am* 28:783, 1984.

115. Ingle JI, Zeldow BJ: An evaluation of mechanical instrumentation and the negative culture in endodontic therapy, *J Am Dent Assoc* 57:471, 1958.

116. Katebzadeh N, Hupp J, Trope M: Histological periapical repair after obturation of infected root canals in dogs, *J Endod* 25:364, 1999.

117. Weiger R, Rosendahl R, Löst C: Influence of calcium hydroxide intracanal dressings on the prognosis of teeth with endodontically induced periapical lesions, *Int Endod J* 33:219, 2000.

118. Messer H, Shepard C, Chen R-S: The duration of effectiveness of root canal medicaments, *J Endod* 10:240, 1984.

119. Bystrom A, Claesson R, Sundqvist G: The antibacterial effect of camphorated paramonochlorophenol, camphorated phenol and calcium hydroxide in the treatment of infected root canals, *Endod Dent Traumatol* 1:170, 1985.

120. Safavi KE, Nichols FC: Alteration of biological properties of bacterial lipopolysaccharide by calcium hydroxide treatment, *J Endod* 20:127, 1994.

121. Maddox D, Walton RE, Davis C: Incidence of post-treatment endodontic pain related to medicaments and other factors, *J Endod* 3:447, 1977.

122. Kleir D, Mullaney T: Effects of formocresol on post-treatment pain of endodontic origin in vital molars, *J Endod* 6:566, 1980.

123. Torabinejad M, Kettering JD, Cummings RR, et al: Factors associated with endodontic interappointment emergencies of teeth with necrotic pulps, *J Endod* 14:261, 1988.

124. Trope M: Relationship of intracanal medicaments to endodontic flare-ups, *Endod Dent Traumatol* 6:226, 1990.

125. Moskow A, Morse DR, Krasner P, et al: Intracanal use of corticosteroidal solution as an endodontic anodyne, *Oral Surg Oral Med Oral Pathol* 58:600, 1984.

126. Marshall JG, Walton RE: The effect of intramuscular injection of steroid on post-treatment endodontic pain, *J Endod* 10:5, 1984.

127. Thoden van Velzen S, Van den Hooff R: The influence of dead and fixed dead tissue in the living organism. III. The tissue reaction to implantation of autologous dead tissue fixed with formaldehyde or glutaraldehyde, *Neth Dent J* 82:6, 1975.

128. Tronstad L, Barnett F, Londono A, et al: Clinical efficacy of an endodontic antiseptic in a controlled release delivery system, *Endod Dent Traumatol* 4:79, 1988.

129. Heling I, Steinberg D, Kenig S, et al: Efficacy of a sustained-release device containing chlorhexidine and $Co(OH)_2$ in preventing secondary infection of dentinal tubules, *Int Endod J* 25:20, 1992.

130. Gilad J, Teles R, Goodson M, et al: Development of a clindamycin-impregnated fiber as an intracanal medication in endodontic therapy, *J Endod* 25:722, 1999.

131. Spangberg L, Engstrom G, Langeland K: Biologic effects of dental materials. III. Toxicity and antimicrobial effect of endodontic antiseptics in vitro, *Oral Surg Oral Med Oral Pathol* 36:856, 1973.

132. Chang Y-C, Tai K-W, Chou L, Chou M-Y: Effects of camphorated parachlorophenol on human periodontal ligament cells in vitro, *J Endod* 25:779, 1999.

133. Thoden van Velzen S, Feltkamp-Vroom T: Immunologic consequences of formaldehyde fixation of autologous tissue implants, *J Endod* 3:179, 1977.

134. Wemes JC, Jansen HW, Purdell-Lewis D, et al: Histologic evaluation of the effect of formocresol and glutaraldehyde on the periapical tissues after endodontic treatment, *Oral Surg Oral Med Oral Pathol* 54:329, 1982.

135. Meyers DR, Shoaf HK, Dirksen TR, et al: Distribution of C-formaldehyde after pulpotomies with formocresol, *J Am Dent Assoc* 96:805, 1978.

136. Walton R, Langeland K: Migration of materials in the dental pulp of monkeys, *J Endod* 4:167, 1978.

137. Araki K, Isaka H, Ishii T, Suda H: Excretion of ^{14}C-formaldehyde distributed systemically through root canals following pulpectomy, *Endod Dent Traumatol* 9:196, 1993.

138. Fager FK, Messer HH: Systemic distribution of camphorated monochlorophenol from cotton pellets sealed in pulp chambers, *J Endod* 12:225, 1986.

139. Fava LRG, Saunders WP: Calcium hydroxide pastes: classification and clinical indications, *Int Endod J* 32:257, 1999.

140. Safavi KE, Nichols FC: Effect of calcium hydroxide on bacterial lipopolysaccharide, *J Endod* 19:76, 1993.

141. Hasselgren G, Olsson B, Cvek M: Effects of calcium hydroxide and sodium hypochlorite on the dissolution of necrotic porcine muscle tissue, *J Endod* 14:125, 1985.

142. Andersen M, Lund A, Andreasen JO, et al: In vitro solubility of human pulp tissue in calcium hydroxide and sodium hypochlorite, *Endod Dent Traumatol* 8:104, 1992.

143. Yang S-F, Rivera EM, Baumgardner KR, et al: Anaerobic tissue dissolving abilities of calcium hydroxide and sodium hypochlorite, *J Endod* 21: 613, 1995.

144. Özçelik B, Tasman T, Ogan C: A comparison of the surface tension of calcium hydroxide mixed with different vehicles, *J Endod* 26:500, 2000.

145. Rivera EM, Williams K: Placement of calcium hydroxide in simulated canals: comparison of glycerin versus water, *J Endod* 20:445, 1994.

146. Sigurdsson A, Stancill R, Madison S: Intracanal placement of $Ca(OH)_2$: a comparison of techniques, *J Endod* 18:367, 1992.

147. Krell KV, Madison S: The use of the Messing gun in placing calcium hydroxide powder, *J Endod* 11:233, 1985.

14

Obturation

LEARNING OBJECTIVES

After reading this chapter, the student should be able to:

1 / Recognize the clinical criteria that determine when to obturate.

2 / List the criteria for the ideal obturating material.

3 / Describe the purpose of obturation and the reasons why inadequate obturation may result in treatment failure.

4 / Identify the two core obturating materials most commonly used and list their constituents and physical properties.

5 / Describe the advantages and disadvantages of each core material.

6 / Discuss the indications and contraindications for obturating with each core material.

7 / Differentiate between "standardized" and "conventional" sizes of gutta-percha cones and discuss when each is indicated.

8 / Define and differentiate between lateral and vertical condensation and suggest where each is indicated.

9 / Describe the lateral condensation technique.

10 / Discuss the significance of depth of spreader penetration during condensation.

11 / Describe the vertical condensation technique.

12 / Describe briefly other techniques used for obturation, including thermoplasticization, thermocompaction, paste injection, gutta-percha carrier systems, and sectional obturation.

13 / Describe the custom cone (chloroform-softened) technique and discuss when it is indicated.

14 / Describe the preparation of the canal for obturation.

15 / Review the techniques for final drying and apical clearing.

16 / Discuss the technique for fitting the master cone.

17 / List criteria for the ideal sealer.

18 / Describe a technique for mixing and placing sealer.

19 / Discuss the technique for removing excess sealer and obturating material from the chamber and why this process is necessary.

20 / Discuss the clinical and radiographic criteria for evaluating the quality of obturation.

OUTLINE

Objectives of Obturation

Potential Causes of Failure
Apical Seal
Coronal Seal
Lateral Seal
Length of Obturation
Lateral Canals
Vertical Root Fractures

Timing of Obturation
Patient Symptoms
Pulp and Periradicular Status
Degree of Difficulty
Culture Results
Number of Appointments

Core Obturating Materials
Solid Materials
Pastes (Semisolids)

Sealers
Desirable Properties
Types
Mixing
Placement

Obturation Techniques with Gutta-Percha
Selection of Technique
Lateral Condensation
Solvent-Softened Custom Cones
Vertical Condensation
Alternative Techniques

Evaluation of Obturation
Symptoms
Radiographic Criteria

Objectives of Obturation

The obturation phase of root canal treatment receives a great deal of attention. Historically, obturation has been accorded the role of the most critical step and the cause of most treatment failures. An early and often quoted report[1] stated that most treatment failures could be attributed to inadequate obturation. Such retrospective surveys have major limitations. This study consisted of radiographic assessment of healing at various periods of time after root canal treatment.[1] The observed failures were correlated with apparently poorly obturated canals (as evaluated on radiographs). The fallacy in this reasoning is evident; just because two events are associated does not prove cause and effect.

In other words, although canals in these failed treatments may not have demonstrated dense fills, other factors may have caused irritation of the periradicular tissues and failure. These include (1) loss of the coronal seal, (2) inadequate débridement, (3) missed canals, (4) vertical root fractures, (5) significant periodontal disease, (6) coronal fractures, and (7) procedural errors such as loss of length, ledging, zipping, and perforations.

Significantly, a periradicular lesion may heal after débridement without obturation. Although this is not an acceptable treatment option (an unobturated canal would result in long-term treatment failure), it does demonstrate an important concept: *What is removed from the root canal system is more important than what is inserted in the system.* Obturation is important, but not the most significant factor for success.

The objective of obturation is to create a complete seal along the length of the root canal system from the coronal opening to the apical termination. The importance of establishing and maintaining a *coronal* seal has been overlooked; the coronal seal is probably more important than the apical seal in long-term success.[2]

Potential Causes of Failure

Most treatment failures related to deficiencies in obturation are long-term failures. A low volume of irritant or slow release of irritant into periradicular tissues produces damage that is not apparent in the short term. *Persistence or development of periradicular pathosis may not be evident for months or even years after treatment.* Therefore, recall evaluation to assess the response to treatment is important.

Obturation-related failures occur in different ways.

APICAL SEAL
Irritating Remnants in Canals

Bacteria, tissue debris, and other irritants are usually not totally removed during cleaning and shaping (refer to Chapter 13). These constitute a potential source of irritation that may lead to failure. It is likely, and there is evidence, that sealing in these irritants during obturation may prevent their escape into the surrounding tissues. Obviously, this seal must remain intact indefinitely because this reservoir of irritants persists forever. Interestingly, some bacteria sealed in the canal may lose viability, probably because of lack of substrate.[3] Possibly, other bacteria remain dormant, waiting for the introduction of substrate, to proliferate and create havoc. Even dead bacteria or their remnants can be irritating or antigenic and cause inflammation.

Percolation

By definition, percolation is movement of fluids into a small space, usually by capillary action. The potential for communication exists between the pulp space and the periapex.[1,4-7] Tissue fluids with plasma proteins may seep into this space and then degrade into irritating chemicals; these irritants may then diffuse back into the periapical tissues and induce inflammation. Another possibility is that periradicular tissue fluids supply substrate (growth medium) to bacteria remaining in the root canal space. With proliferation, bacteria and their toxins could then return to periapical tissues to cause inflammation.

A vicious cycle is established. Periapical inflammation produces exudation and transudation of fluid as well as an accumulation of cellular debris composed primarily of inflammatory and tissue cells. These irritants and inflammatory fluids then pass into the canal space, and the cycle is repeated.

CORONAL SEAL
Irritants from Oral Cavity

A coronal seal is important. If the myriad of irritants in the oral cavity gain access to periradicular tissues, they may cause inflammation and treatment failure. Irritants include substances in saliva such as microorganisms, food, chemicals, or other agents that pass through the mouth.

If coronal gutta-percha or sealer obturation is exposed to saliva, dissolution of sealer and leakage over a relatively short period of time may occur.[8-11] This results in leakage of bacteria, toxins, and chemicals into and around the gutta-percha.[12,13] The consequences of sealer loss are obvious; communication from the oral cavity to the periapex or periodontium will eventually be complete via a lateral canal or apical foramen.

It is not possible to determine clinically whether communication from the oral cavity to the periapex has been established. Therefore, it is unwise to restore a tooth with a canal that may contain saliva, bacteria, food debris, or other irritants. Coronal exposure of the obturating material for more than a short period of time through loss of restoration, recurrent caries, or open margins requires retreatment. The time of exposure requiring retreatment is undetermined, but probably depends on varied factors, such as quality of obturation, length of canal(s) and surface area of exposure.

Restoration

Both design and placement of the final restoration are critical. This aspect of treatment is an integral part of obturation. The restoration acts as a protector and is the primary coronal seal, whether temporary or final.[14] These factors are discussed in detail in Chapter 15.

LATERAL SEAL

Although not as critical as the apical and coronal seals, establishment of a seal in the inner middle aspect of the canal is also important. Lateral canals are occasionally found in these regions; they constitute a potential communication for irritants or, possibly, percolation from the canal interior to the lateral periodontium (Figure 14-1).

LENGTH OF OBTURATION

Extent of obturation relative to the apex is also important. Ideally, obturating materials should remain within the canal.

Overfill

Overfills are undesirable. Prognosis studies consistently show that failures increase with time when the primary obturating material has been extruded.[12-17] Histologic examination of periapical tissues after overfilling typically shows increased inflammation with delayed or impaired healing.[18,19] Patients probably experience more postobturation discomfort after overfills. Two

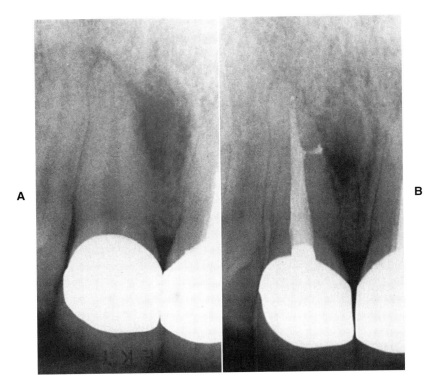

FIGURE 14-1
A, Pulp necrosis with apical and lateral radiolucent lesions. **B,** On obturation, a lateral canal was detected communicating with periodontium. This lesion should heal after removal of necrotic pulp tissue in the main canal and then obturation.

other problems with overfills are irritation from the material itself and lack of an apical seal.

Obturating Materials. Whether the obturating material is core or sealer, both are irritants to a greater or lesser degree.[20,21] Silver points and gutta-percha (slightly) as well as sealers (in particular) are toxic when they are in contact with tissues. Sealers invoke a foreign body response and inflammation.[21-23]

Lack of Apical Seal Secondary to Overfill. This may be even more important than irritation from the materials. Gutta-percha, like amalgam, requires a matrix to condense against. Imagine trying to condense and form amalgam into a class II preparation without a metal matrix! The same is true of gutta-percha and sealer. Absence of an apical matrix may prevent lateral spreading and sealing during condensation.

A tapered apical preparation with no core materials and a small amount of sealer passing out of the foramen is not a significant problem. The taper forms an adequate matrix for gutta-percha condensation; irritation from the sealer should resolve. However, when there is gross overfill of both primary obturating materials and sealer, per-

sistent inflammation[18] and failure often ensue (Figure 14-2).

Underfill

Underfill results when both preparation and obturation are short of the desired working length or when the obturation does not extend to the prepared length. Either instance may contribute to treatment failure, particularly long term (Figure 14-3).

The "ideal" preparation or obturation length is 1 to 2 mm short of the apex (Figure 14-4).[24] Preparation or obturation short of this length leaves existing or potential irritants in the apical canal. Periapical inflammation may develop over an extended period of time, depending on the volume of irritants or the balance established between irritants and the immune system.

Compared with overfill, underfill is less of a problem, as indicated by prognosis and histologic studies. Therefore, the axiom is, *if there is going to be an error, err on the short side;* try to confine everything to the canal space.

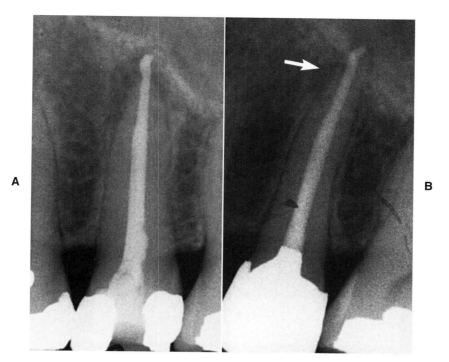

FIGURE 14-2
Gross overfill. **A,** The mass of gutta-percha has been extruded, indicating lack of an apical stop or seat. **B,** At 10-year recall, persistent pathosis *(arrow)* suggests a poor apical seal (lack of an apical matrix).

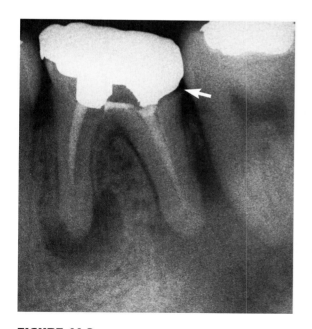

FIGURE 14-3
Failure caused by operator errors. The mesial canals are underprepared (inadequate debridement) and incompletely obturated; the distal *(arrow)* has a poorly adapted restoration (coronal leakage).

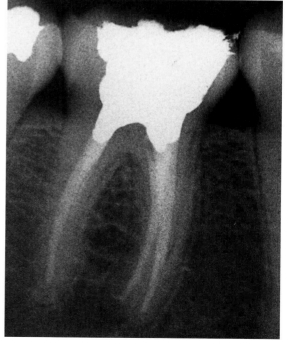

FIGURE 14-4
Desired lengths and preparations. The canals are prepared and obturated to a tapered shape approximately 2 mm from each apex.

LATERAL CANALS

The role of lateral (accessory) canals in root canal treatment has been a subject of debate.[25] These canals connect pulp space and periodontium. Irritants in the root canal system, such as bacteria and necrotic debris, may leak into the lateral periodontium and initiate inflammation (see Figure 14-1).

Histologic examination of roots after débridement shows that lateral canals are rarely if ever débrided.[26] There is no significant difference in the ability of various obturation techniques to fill the main canal. However, certain techniques tend to force materials into the lateral canals (Figure 14-5).[27]

When the main canal space is adequately débrided and obturated, lateral lesions adjacent to lateral canals heal as readily as periapical lesions. This occurs whether or not obturating material has been expressed into the lateral canal.

The conclusion is that obturation of lateral canals is inconsequential to the outcome of most root canal treatments despite proponents of certain techniques that claim to fill lateral canals.[28]

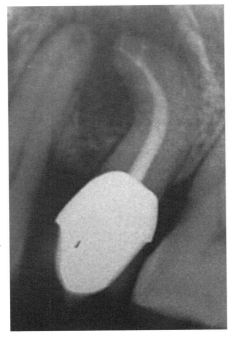

FIGURE 14-5
This premolar was obturated using a procedure (the diffusion technique) that involves dissolving the gutta-percha in chloroform. This tends to obturate the accessory and lateral canals but provides a poor apical seal.

VERTICAL ROOT FRACTURES

Vertical root fracture is a devastating occurrence that usually requires removal of the tooth or fractured root. Signs and symptoms as well as radiographic findings show that bone loss and soft tissue lesions are common.[29,30] Lateral forces exerted during obturation or postplacement are major etiologic factors owing to their wedging action.[31-37] The pathogenesis, findings, and prevention of vertical fractures are discussed further in Chapter 28.

Timing of Obturation

To answer the questions, When is treatment to be completed? Is it time to obturate?, the following factors are considered: signs and symptoms, pulp and periapical status, and difficulty of procedure. Combinations of these factors affect decisions made about number of appointments and timing of obturation.

PATIENT SYMPTOMS

In general, if the patient presents with severe symptoms and the diagnosis is acute apical periodontitis or abscess, obturation is contraindicated. These are emergency situations, and it is preferable to manage the immediate problem and delay definitive treatment. Even an acute apical abscess may be treated in a single appointment.[38] However, this is not good treatment; if the patient continues to have problems, management is more difficult if the canal is filled.

Painful irreversible pulpitis is a different situation. Because the inflamed pulp (which is the pain source) is to be removed, obturation may be completed at the same appointment. However, treatment of these problems requires caution because of difficulties in management of a patient in pain.

PULP AND PERIRADICULAR STATUS
Vital Pulp

Regardless of the inflammatory status of the pulp, and if time permits, the procedure may be completed in a single visit.

Necrotic Pulp

Without significant symptoms, obturation may be completed during the same appointment as canal preparation. Pulp necrosis with asymptomatic periradicular pathosis (that is, chronic apical periodontitis, suppurative apical periodontitis, or condensing osteitis) *alone* is not necessarily a contraindication to single-appointment treatment at least as related to postobturation symptoms.

There may be an advantage, however, to multiple appointments related to healing of apical pathosis. Recent studies indicate the benefits of treating these patients in two visits.[39-41] Placement of an intracanal antimicrobial dressing such as calcium hydroxide reduces bacteria and reduces inflammation somewhat. Calcium hydroxide in the canal for 7 days can effectively inhibit bacteria.[42] A recent prognosis study comparing single-visit versus two-visit with intracanal calcium hydroxide treatment did not demonstrate differences in long-term prognosis, however.[43] At present, there are no definitive conclusions about when single- or multiple-visit procedures are indicated.

One situation that contraindicates single-visit care is the presence and persistence of exudation in the canal during preparation. The potential for post-treatment exacerbation is increased if the periapical lesion is productive and generates continual suppuration. If the canal is sealed, pressure and corresponding tissue destruction may proceed rapidly. In these cases, canal preparation is completed, followed by calcium hydroxide placement. A dry cotton pellet is placed over the calcium hydroxide and the access is sealed with a temporary restoration. Generally, exudation will be diminished and controllable at a subsequent appointment; obturation may then be completed.

DEGREE OF DIFFICULTY

Complex cases are time consuming and are better managed in multiple appointments.

CULTURE RESULTS

Some practitioners rely on culturing canal contents to indicate timing of completion of treatment. Although the evidence is not clear about the value of cultures as an aid in increasing success in root canal treatment, culture results are an indicator of long-term prognosis.[42,44,45] Some practitioners believe that persistent positive cultures may indicate a poorly débrided canal, missed canals, or resistant strains of bacteria; these conclusions have not been proved and are debatable. However, proponents recommend that at least one negative culture be obtained before obturation, which requires more than one appointment. Currently, this approach is seldom used.

NUMBER OF APPOINTMENTS

The decision about the number of appointments needed usually occurs during initial treatment planning. The decision to schedule another appointment, when made *during* an appointment, reflects a change of circumstances such as the patient or dentist is tired or has lost patience.

Core Obturating Materials

Primary obturating materials are usually solid or semisolid (paste or softened form). They comprise the bulk of material that will fill the canal space and may or may not be used with a sealer. However, a sealer is essential with all core obturating materials.

These materials may be introduced into the canals in different forms and may be manipulated by different means once inside. Imaginations (and marketing) run rampant, resulting in a variety of materials and techniques. However, a small number of widely accepted and taught materials and techniques are used for obturation. These are discussed in some detail; alternatives are mentioned briefly.

SOLID MATERIALS

Solids have major advantages over semisolids (pastes). Although various materials have been tried, the only one universally accepted currently is gutta-percha as the primary material. This has withstood the test of time and research, and is by far the most commonly used material.[47-49] A major

---

Desirable Properties of Obturating Materials

Grossman suggested that the ideal obturant should[46]

- Be easily introduced into the canal.
- Seal the canal laterally as well as apically.
- Not shrink after being inserted.
- Be impervious to moisture.
- Be bactericidal or at least discourage bacterial growth.
- Be radiopaque.
- Not stain tooth structure.
- Not irritate periapical tissues or affect tooth structure.
- Be sterile or easily sterilized.
- Be easily removed from the root canal.

At this time, no material satisfies all these criteria. Gutta-percha with a suitable sealer is the closest match.

advantage of gutta-percha over semi-solid paste types is the ability to control length as well as the reasonable ability to adapt to irregularities and to create an adequate seal.

Gutta-Percha

Composition. The primary ingredient of a gutta-percha cone is zinc oxide (±75 percent). Gutta-percha accounts for approximately 20 percent and gives the cone its unique properties such as plasticity. The remaining ingredients are binders, opaquers, and coloring agents.

Shapes. Gutta-percha cones are available in two basic shapes: the "standardized" and the "conventional" (Figure 14-6). Standardized cones are designed to have the same size and taper as the corresponding endodontic instruments. That is, a No. 40 cone should correspond to a No. 40 file.

Interestingly, there is no uniformity in gutta-percha sizing. For example, the contents of a box or vial of No. 40 standardized gutta-percha cones vary in size from No. 35 to No. 45 and has inconsistent tips and shapes.[50] This lack of uniformity is not critical; canal shape after preparation is also variable.

Conventional cones use a different sizing system. The tip of the cone has one size and the body of the cone another. They are available in various combinations. For example, a fine tip end-medium body would be referred to as a fine-medium cone. Generally, conventional cones have a smaller tip with a relatively wider body compared with standardized cones.

Gutta-percha master cones tend to be selected according to the method of canal preparation or to match the master apical fill size. This is not universal, however; operator preferences vary considerably, indicating that size and shape of the cone are relatively unimportant.

Advantages. Gutta-percha has withstood the test of time, having been introduced as an obturating material more than 160 years ago. It is the standard to which other obturating materials are compared. First, because of plasticity, gutta-percha adapts with compaction to irregularities in prepared canals; second, it is relatively easy to manage and manipulate despite some complex obturation techniques; third, gutta-percha is easy to remove from the canal, either partially to allow post placement or totally for retreatment; and last, gutta-percha has relatively little toxicity, being nearly inert over time when in contact with connective tissue.[20,51] Another advantage of gutta-percha is that it tends to be self-sterilizing, as it will not support bacterial growth. If there is a possibility of cones being contaminated, they are predictably sterilized by immersion in 1% (or greater) sodium hypochloride for 1 minute.[52]

Sealability. Regardless of the technique used (condensation or plasticization), studies have consistently shown that gutta-percha without sealer will not seal.[4,53-55] Disadvantages of gutta-percha are a lack of adhesion to dentin and a slight elasticity, which causes a rebound and pulling away from the canal walls. Warmed gutta-percha shrinks during cooling. Gutta-percha mixed with solvents such as chloroform or eucalyptol shrinks with evaporation of the solvent.[56] Therefore, a sealer must be used to fill and seal the spaces between the gutta-percha cones and between the gutta-percha and the canal wall. Also gutta-percha should be added to the canal in increments.

Methods of Placement. As stated earlier, placement methods are varied and imaginative. Most popular is lateral condensation, followed by vertical condensation. Other techniques involve either

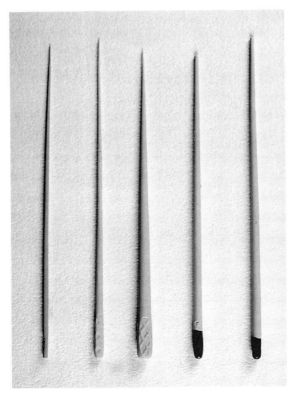

FIGURE 14-6
Comparison of conventional with standardized cones. The three conventional cones (from *left to right:* fine fine, medium fine, and fine) have a heavier body and a finer tip and are easier to manipulate than the small, standardized, color-coded cones (sizes 35 and 40) on the right. (Courtesy Dr. W. Johnson.)

chemical or physical alteration of the gutta-percha in an attempt to render the material more plastic or more adaptable.

Another variation is a system that includes a solid core (carrier) surrounded by a cone of gutta-percha. The carrier may be stainless steel, titanium, plastic, or a segment of a file. After preparation, the carrier and gutta-percha are warmed and placed in the canal as a unit.

Other devices have been introduced that involve warming to plasticize and inject gutta-percha. These will be discussed in more detail later in this chapter.

Indications. Gutta-percha is the material of choice in most situations. Some exceptions are severely curved, inaccessible canals in which gutta-percha or obturating instruments would be difficult or impossible to manage. However, if curvatures of canals are that severe, the patient should be referred to an endodontist.

Silver Points

Silver points were designed to correspond to the last file size used in preparation, to presumably fill the canal precisely in all dimensions. Because of the complexity of shape of the root canals, this is fallacious; it is impossible to predictably prepare canals to a uniform size and shape.[57]

Although the short term sealability success of silver points seemed comparable to that of gutta-percha, silver points are a poor long-term choice as a routine obturating material.[55,56,58,59] Their major problems relate to nonadaptability (Figure 14-7) and toxicity from corrosion.[60] Also, because of their tight frictional fit and hardness, silver cones are difficult to remove totally (retreatment) or partially (post space preparation).[61] Also, if silver cones are contacted with a bur, their seal may be broken.

In summary, *silver cones are contraindicated* as an obturating material.

Files as Core Materials

Files used as core materials are an interesting concept. Because preparation is accomplished with files, why not fill the canal with sealer, force or "screw" a file into place at the correct working length, and then cut it at the canal orifice? This technique has not gained popular acceptance, although there have been advocates.

A major disadvantage is that, because of their design and the complexity of root canals, files do not provide a complete seal.[59] Their fluting precludes a close fit, and sealer will not occupy the rest of the space. In addition, retrieval is difficult if retreatment or a post space is needed. Files as a primary core material are contraindicated.

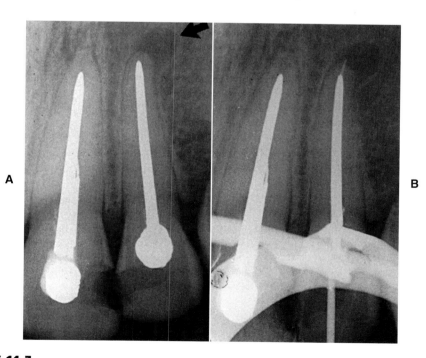

FIGURE 14-7
A, Apparent good obturation, but a persistent lesion *(arrow)* is seen on the lateral incisor, indicating treatment failure. **B,** The reason for the failure is poor adaptation; a No. 25 file readily passes lingual to the silver point.

PASTES (SEMISOLIDS)

Why not develop a paste or cement that can be mixed in a liquid or putty form, inject the material to length, fill the entire canal, and then allow the material to set? This would be fast, the paste would fill the entire canal space, and obturation would be much simpler. In addition, this method would permit use of a material that would adhere to dentin and create an absolute seal.

Although the concept is appealing, there are significant practical difficulties. However, it certainly has been attempted, and work on developing such a material continues. The major disadvantages of paste materials are lack of length control, unpredictability, and shrinkage.

Types

Zinc Oxide and Eugenol. Zinc oxide and eugenol may be mixed pure (no additives) to intermediate thickness. Other formulations combine zinc oxide-eugenol (ZnOE) with various additives. The types known as N2 or RC2B are most common. These are derivations of Sargenti's formula and contain opaquers, metallic oxides (lead) or chlorides (mercuric), steroids (at times), plasticizers, paraformaldehyde, and various other ingredients. Claims of antimicrobial properties, biologic therapeutic activity, and superiority are made for these paste formulations; no proof exists that they contribute any beneficial aspects to obturation. In fact, most of these additives are quite toxic.[62]

Plastics. It has been suggested that a resin-based sealer such as AH26 and Diaket be used as the sole obturating material. These sealers have the same disadvantages as pastes and, therefore, have not attained popular use.

Techniques of Placement

Various approaches and instruments have been devised or modified for insertion of pastes or sealers. Two popular methods are injection and placement with a lentulo spiral.

Injection is accomplished using a syringe-type device with a barrel and special needles.[63] The paste is mixed and placed in the barrel, a screw handle is inserted and twisted, and the paste is extruded through the special needle-like tips. The needles are placed deep in the canal, and the paste is expressed as the needles are slowly backed out of the canal. Advocates claim that this method completely fills the canal from the apical portion to the canal orifice.

Instrument placement is done with lentulo spiral drills. The paste is mixed, the drill is coated, and then it is placed and spun deep in the canal. As with the syringe device, the canal is supposedly filled with paste as the drill is slowly withdrawn.

Both techniques are more attractive in theory than in fact. Neither technique has demonstrated an ability to seal effectively or to fill the root canal system. Because of lack of control, both injection and placement by lentulo spiral drill have major deficiencies and are contraindicated.

Advantages and Disadvantages of Pastes

The *advantages* are obvious: paste techniques are fast and relativity easy to use and involve the use of a single material. The equipment needed, at least with the lentulo spiral technique, is relatively simple, comprising only a limited assortment of special drills.

The *disadvantages* outweigh the advantages by far. First, the universal problem with any non-solid core material is length control. It is difficult to avoid overfills (Figure 14-8) or underfills (Figure 14-9). Theoretically, radiographs should be made many times during obturation to assess length and density as the material is being injected or placed. Obviously, this is time consuming and subjects the patient to needless radiation.

Another major disadvantage is sealability. These techniques seal inconsistently: sometimes well, other times poorly.[64,65] This unpredictability may be related to three factors: (1) large voids or discrepancies within the material or adjacent to the walls; (2) shrinkage of ZnOE on setting, which leaves a space for microleakage; and (3) solubility of pastes in tissue or oral fluids. In addition, injection devices are difficult to clean and maintain.

Sealers

A basic concept is that sealer is more important than the core obturating material. Sealer accomplishes the objective of providing a fluid-tight seal; the core occupies space, serving as a vehicle for the sealer.[66] Sealer must be used in conjunction with the obturating material regardless of the technique or material used. This makes the physical properties and placement of the sealer important.

DESIRABLE PROPERTIES

Grossman outlined the criteria for an ideal sealer.[66] None of the currently available sealers possesses all these ideal properties, but some have more than others. His criteria are as follows.

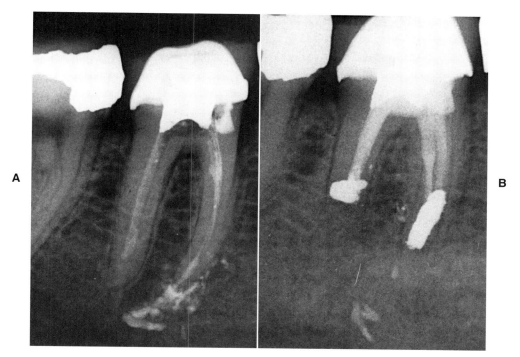

FIGURE 14-8
Mandibular paresthesia after treatment. **A,** Using an injection technique, unset paste was forced out the apex into the mandibular canal causing chemical damage to the inferior alveolar nerve. **B,** Periradicular surgery corrected the endodontic problem, but failed to resolve the paresthesia.

Tissue Tolerance

The sealer and its components should cause neither tissue destruction nor cell death. All commonly used sealers show a degree of toxicity.[21] This toxicity is greatest when the sealer is unset but tends to diminish after setting and with time.[67,68]

No Shrinkage with Setting

Sealer should remain dimensionally stable or even expand slightly on setting.

Slow Setting Time

Sealer should provide adequate working time for placement and manipulation of obturating material, then set reasonably soon after obturation is complete. It is desirable to have sealer unset if post space is made immediately.

Adhesiveness

Adhesiveness is a most desirable property. A truly adhesive material would form an absolute bond

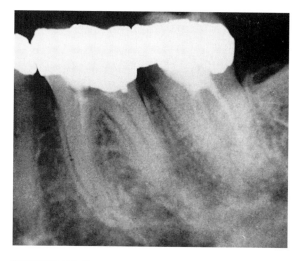

FIGURE 14-9
Frequent problems with inadequate preparation combined with paste fills: gross underfill and numerous voids, leading to long-term failure.

between the core material and dentin, closing off any spaces. ZnOE-based sealers have no adhesion; plastics have some.

Radiopacity

Sealer should be readily visible on radiographs. However, the more radiopaque the sealer, the more it obscures voids in the obturation. Some clinicians prefer a highly radiopaque sealer to mask discrepancies.

Absence of Staining

Remnants should not cause future staining of the crown. Currently, all tested sealers, particularly ZnOE-based sealers or those containing heavy metals, stain dentin.[69,70]

Solubility in Solvent

Occasionally post space or retreatment may be necessary days, months, or years after obturation. The sealer should be soluble in a solvent. Different sealers have different degrees of solubility in different solvents and with varying mechanical techniques.[71,72]

Insolubility to Oral and Tissue Fluids

Sealer should not disintegrate when in contact with tissue fluids. Sealers are somewhat soluble, particularly when in contact with oral fluids.[9,73]

Bacteriostatic Properties

Although a bactericidal sealer would seem to be desirable, a substance that kills bacteria will also be toxic to host tissues. At a minimum, the sealer should not encourage bacterial growth.[74]

Creation of a Seal

This is an obviously important physical property. The material must create and maintain a seal apically, laterally, and coronally.

TYPES

Generally, there are four major types of sealers: ZnOE-based, plastics, glass ionomer, and those containing calcium hydroxide. Other variations and compounds have been proposed or are marketed as sealers; these should be considered experimental.

Certainly, the standard sealer with which all others are compared is the Grossman formula-

tion. This has withstood the test of time and usage, although some of plastics (resins) also now are widely used and have many desirable properties. Calcium hydroxide and glass ionomer types are newer and have interesting properties but also significant drawbacks.

Zinc Oxide-Eugenol-Based

The major advantage of ZnOE-based sealer types is their long history of successful usage. Obviously, their positive qualities outweigh their negative aspects (staining, very slow setting time, non-adhesion, and solubility).

Grossman's Formulation. The formula is as follows:

> *Powder:* zinc oxide (body), 42 parts; stabellite resin (setting time and consistency), 27 parts; bismuth subcarbonate, 15 parts; barium sulfate (radiopacity), 15 parts; sodium borate, 1 part
> *Liquid:* eugenol

Most ZnOE sealers in use and available today are variations of this original formula. A problem with this formulation is the very slow setting time, more than 2 months, as studied in a usage test.[75]

Other Types. ZnOE forms the base for other sealers, some of which have been used more commonly than others. These will not be discussed further here.

Plastics

Plastics are much less commonly used and accepted, at least in the United States. Some have very desirable properties, however.

Epoxy. Epoxy is available in a powder-liquid formula (AH26). Its properties include antimicrobial action, adhesion, long working time, ease of mixing, and very good sealability.[76,77] Its disadvantages are staining, relative insolubility in solvents, some toxicity when unset, and some solubility to oral fluids. A recently introduced variation (AH-Plus) has similar physical properties, but better biocompatibility because it releases less formaldehyde and a supposed decrease in dentin staining by elimination of silver from the formula.[78]

Other Plastics. These are primarily of the methyl methacrylate type and are not commonly used.

Calcium Hydroxide

Calcium hydroxide sealers have been introduced in which the calcium hydroxide is incorporated in a ZnOE or plastic base. These sealers supposedly have biologic properties that stimulate a calcific barrier at the apex; however, these properties have not been conclusively demonstrated in clinical or experimental use. Calcium hydroxide sealers show antimicrobial properties[79] and adequate short-term sealability.[80] Questions have been raised about their long-term stability (greater solubility) and tissue toxicity.[81] Until further experimental and clinical data are available, these sealers have no demonstrated advantages and are not recommended.

Glass Ionomer

Endodontic formulations of glass ionomer[82] have been introduced recently. This material has the advantage of bonding to dentin, seems to provide an adequate apical and coronal seal, and is biocompatible.[83-86] However, its hardness and insolubility make retreatment and post space preparation more difficult.[87]

Others

Various luting agents and basing and restorative materials have been tried and tested as endodontic sealers.[88,89] Examples are zinc phosphate cement, composite, and polycarboxylate cement. These materials have not proved satisfactory.

MIXING

The common sealer types should be mixed carefully to a thick consistency. They should string approximately 2 to 3 inches. The thicker the mix, the better are the properties of the sealer, particularly in regard to stability, superiority of seal, and diminished toxicity.[90]

PLACEMENT

Various techniques have been advocated for placement of sealer, which is done before insertion of the core material. The sealer may be placed with paper points, with files, with ultrasonic activation of files, with special drills (lentulo), as a coating on the primary cone, or by injecting with special syringes. Although different methods have shown varying degrees of effectiveness in sealer application, no technique has proved superior.[91-94] In fact, sealers may not completely cover the interface between gutta-percha and canal wall after obturation.[95]

A simple and effective technique is to coat the walls by picking up sealer on the final apical file or a one-size smaller file (Figure 14-10). The file is teased to length and spun counterclockwise,

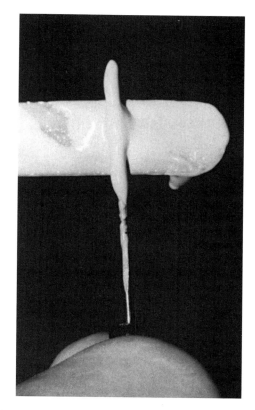

FIGURE 14-10
An easy, effective method of sealer application. The file covered with sealer will be inserted and spun counterclockwise to coat the canal walls.

which has the effect of carrying the sealer apically and coating the walls. Flooding the canal with sealer is neither necessary nor desirable.

Sealer is not placed in all canals at once unless it gives a long working time. Removing sealer that has set is difficult. The Grossman formulations and epoxy resins are slow setting and may be placed in all canals.[75]

Obturation Techniques with Gutta-Percha

Different approaches are available, depending on the size of the prepared canal, the final shape of the preparation, and irregularities within the canal. The overriding factor is operator preference.[96]

SELECTION OF TECHNIQUE

The two traditional techniques are lateral and vertical condensation; sealability is similar in both.[97,98] Again, the choice is dictated primarily by preference and custom, although there may be special situations indicating a particular use of each technique. Both must be used with a sealer.

More recent approaches have been introduced that depend upon warming and softening formulations of gutta-percha with special devices and instruments and then placing the gutta-percha incrementally. Some of these techniques and devices are heavily promoted and will be discussed later in the chapter.

Other methods are also used; most involve alteration of the entire gutta-percha cone with a solvent such as chloroform or eucalyptol. These are technique sensitive and therefore are not widely used or taught in the United States. They are not discussed in this textbook; details are found in other published sources.

A variation of lateral condensation is the solvent-softened (or custom-fitted tip) technique, which is outlined later in this chapter.

LATERAL CONDENSATION

Lateral condensation is the most popular technique of obturation, both in practice and as taught in most institutions.[99] Therefore, this technique will be described in detail.

Indications

Lateral condensation of gutta-percha may be used in most situations. Exceptions are severely curved or abnormally shaped canals or those with gross irregularities such as internal resorption. However, lateral condensation may be combined with other obturation approaches. In general, if the situation is not amenable to lateral (or vertical, if that is the usual approach) condensation, it is too difficult for the general practitioner and the patient should be referred to an endodontist.

Advantages

Lateral condensation is relatively uncomplicated, requires a simple armamentarium, and seals and obturates as well as any other technique in conventional situations.[100,101] A major advantage it has over most other techniques is length control.[98] With an apical stop and with careful use of the spreader, the length of the gutta-percha filling is managed well. Additional advantages include ease of retreatment, adaptation to the canal walls, positive dimensional stability, and the ability to prepare post space.[100,101]

Disadvantages

There are no major disadvantages to lateral condensation other than difficulties in obturating severely curved canals, an open apex, and canals with internal resorptive defects.

Technique

Although there are variations, a workable and acceptable technique is presented here. Variations of lateral condensation are described in other textbooks and manuals.

Spreader or Plugger Selection. Selection and try-in should be performed during the cleaning and shaping of the canal. Finger spreaders or pluggers are preferred over standard (long-handled) spreaders because of better tactile sensations, improved apical seal, better instrument control (Figure 14-11), and reduced dentin stress during obturation.[34,102] Use of these finger instruments

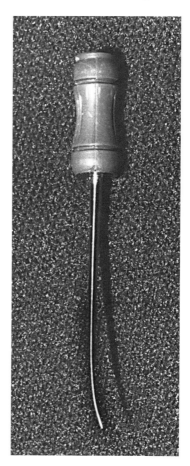

FIGURE 14-11
Hand spreaders may be precurved to improve manipulation into curved canals.

likely decreases the incidence of vertical root fractures during obturation. Finger spreaders/ pluggers also can be inserted more deeply than standard hand spreaders (Figure 14-12).

Nickel-titanium finger spreaders have been introduced recently. Because of their flexibility, these spreaders seem to produce less wedging force while penetrating deeper.[103,104] Their advantage may be less tendency to produce vertical root fractures. These spreaders do behave differently because of their flexibility and require practice for efficient use.

Master Cone Selection. Either a standardized or a conventionally shaped, fine gutta-percha cone may be adapted as a master cone. Apical preparations that are very irregular in shape, are larger than a No. 50 file, have no apical stop, or have an apical seat greater than a No. 40 file should have the custom solvent-softened cone (described later).

Large standardized cones (No. 50 and above) are used in the custom cone technique in canals larger than a No. 50 file. Conventional cones are cut and adapted to canals less than a No. 50 file.

Fitting the Master Cone. Apical clearing (when indicated) is important before the master cone is fitted (see Chapter 13). After apical clearing is completed, the steps are as follows:

1. Because the master cone fits only in the apical portion of the apically cleared, flared canal, the amount of resistance shown to removal is slight (Figure 14-13). A slight frictional fit is acceptable; the so-called tugback is unnecessary.[105] However, there should be a definite stop when the cone fits into place. The cone is fitted to within 1 mm of working length.

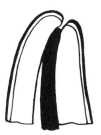

FIGURE 14-13
The master cone needs only a slight frictional fit in the very apical region. This permits deep spreader penetration between the gutta-percha and the canal wall.

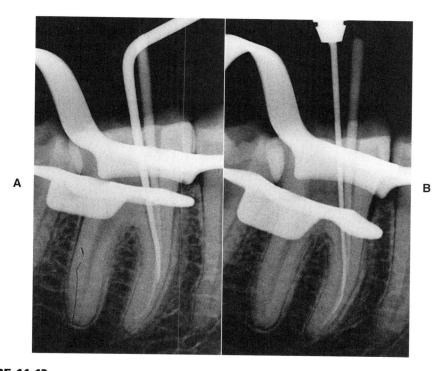

FIGURE 14-12
Comparison of hand spreader with finger pluggers or spreaders. **A,** The stiff, more tapered hand spreader will not negotiate the curve. **B,** The smaller, more flexible finger spreader permits deeper penetration and produces a superior apical seal.

2. A cone may be too small as indicated by a buckling in the apical few millimeters (Figure 14-14, *A*). A larger sized apical end is made by cutting 1-mm segments off the master cone until the slight fit is obtained (Figure 14-14, *B*). Frequently, the cone cannot be inserted quite to working length. This is acceptable only if (a) the apical area has been cleared of debris and (b) the spreader pene-

trates to within 1 mm of the prepared length. A cleared apical area and deep spreader penetration will usually push the gutta-percha and sealer apically to fill the remaining 1 mm (Figure 14-15).[106]

3. The master cone is removed by grasping it at the reference point, and the length is verified by measuring it on a ruler, then corrected if necessary.

4. Master cone length (not lateral fit) is evaluated radiographically. Again, the cone should be no more than 1 mm short of the prepared length. The traditional close radiographic fit of the master cone in the apical third is unrelated to the quality of the final seal.[105]

5. If the master cone length is not within 1 mm of the prepared canal length, either (a) dry reaming is repeated to be certain there is no debris, or (b) another, smaller cone is adapted.

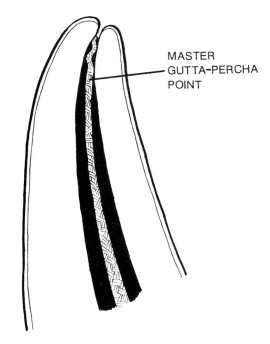

MASTER GUTTA-PERCHA POINT

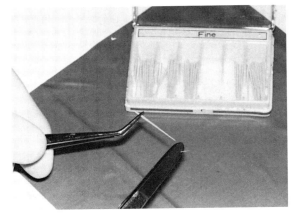

FIGURE 14-14
A, A cone that appears buckled on the radiograph or on removal is much too small. **B,** A larger cone should be selected or clipped to form a larger size at the tip.

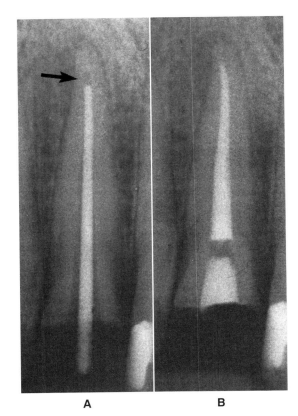

FIGURE 14-15
A, The master cone need not extend along the entire length if the preparation *(arrow)* has been apically cleared. **B,** Deep spreader penetration then often pushes the gutta-percha and sealer apically to fill the prepared space. (Courtesy Dr. J. Parsons.)

6. A gutta-percha cone that extends beyond the apical foramen shows the lack of an apical stop. This requires a custom solvent-softened cone or selection and modification of a shorter, larger cone.

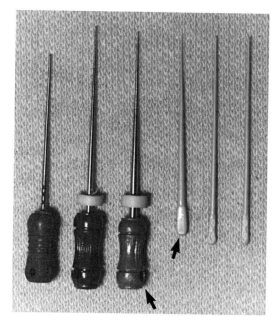

FIGURE 14-16
An assortment of obturation instruments and gutta-percha cones. From *left to right:* A 21-mm fine plugger with measurement markings on the shaft; a 25-mm medium fine plugger; a 25-mm fine plugger; a conventional fine gutta-percha point; and No. 35 and No. 40 standardized gutta-percha cones. A good combination for most situations is the fine gutta-percha point *(right arrow)* and the fine finger plugger *(left arrow).*

Steps in Obturation. Although there are many combinations of obturating instruments and different types of gutta-percha, a suggested combination for routine situations is a fine finger plugger and fine accessory cone (Figure 14-16). There is no precise correlation between size of accessory point and size of finger spreader.[107] Specific steps are as follows (Figure 14-17):

1. Sealer is mixed and applied to canal walls.
2. The master cone (without sealer coating) is inserted slowly to allow air and excess cement to escape.
3. Before the spreader is inserted and removed, an accessory cone is picked up with locking pliers at the measured length, ready to be inserted.
4. The measured spreader is inserted between the master cone and the canal wall using firm (apical only) pressure (5 to 7 pounds as for amalgam condensation) to within 1 to 2 mm from working length. Spreader taper is the mechanical force that laterally compresses and spreads gutta-percha, creating a space for an additional accessory cone.
5. The spreader is freed for removal by back-and-forth rotation around its axis. The spreader is removed and the measured accessory (fine) gutta-percha cone is immediately inserted into the space created.
6. (Optional) A radiograph may be made after one or two cones are placed. If there are length problems, the cones are retrieved. A new master cone is fit at a connected length.
7. This procedure is repeated until the spreader can no longer be pressed beyond

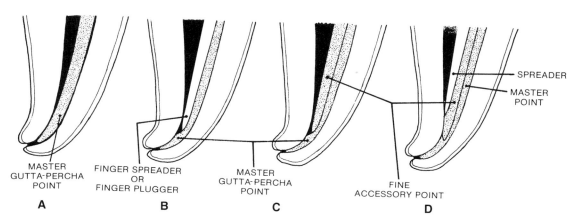

FIGURE 14-17
The steps of lateral condensation. **A,** The master cone is fitted. **B,** A finger spreader or plugger is inserted, ideally to 1 to 2 mm of the prepared length. **C,** The spreader is rotated and removed, and an accessory cone is placed in the space created. **D,** The process is repeated.

the apical third of the canal (approximately three to seven accessory cones). The last insertion is an accessory cone, not the spreader! The spreader need not be stepped all the way out of the canal, adding accessory cones. Obturation may be evaluated with a radiograph at this time.

8. Excess gutta-percha is seared off with a hot instrument (Glick No. 1, a heated plugger, or a battery-controlled heating device (Figure 14-18). This is done approximately 1 mm apical to the gingival margin in anterior teeth and 1 mm apical to the canal orifice in posterior teeth.

9. The cervical portion of the warm gutta-percha is vertically condensed firmly using the Glick No. 1 or a No. 5-7 heater-plugger.[108]

Ultrasonic Condensation. A variation is lateral condensation with ultrasonic activation of the spreader. With this technique the spreader is placed next to the master cone and activated without a water coolant. Apical pressure is exerted, and the spreader is inserted to a predetermined length. Advantages are that the ultrasonic action may spread the sealer, the friction of the spreader may thermoplasticize the gutta-percha, and the force required to place the spreader may be less.[109,110]

> **Suggestion:** If two or more canals are obturated, condensation is performed separately in each. Each canal is completed and the excess removed before the next is begun.

Finishing Touches

The procedure is completed as follows:

1. The chamber is cleaned thoroughly with cotton pellets soaked in alcohol or chloroform; unset sealers are soluble in these solutions. Remnants of gutta-percha or sealer (in particular) may cause future discoloration (Figure 14-19).

2. A temporary or permanent restoration is placed. Appropriate temporization or restoration (semipermanent or permanent) is discussed in Chapter 15.

3. A radiograph is made with the restoration in place and the clamp removed.

Correcting Obturation Problems

Occasionally, voids or length problems will be apparent on the radiograph taken during or after obturation. These should be corrected *now*, before the sealer sets!

For voids, gutta-percha is removed with hot pluggers until the spreader can be reinserted just beyond the void or discrepancy. Then, a fresh mix of sealer is prepared. Lateral condensation is performed as described previously; sealer is added back to the canal by coating each accessory cone.

An advantage of making an obturation verification radiograph before the excess gutta-percha is seared off is that the entire mass can usually be removed by grasping the cones with the fingers.

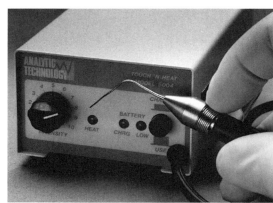
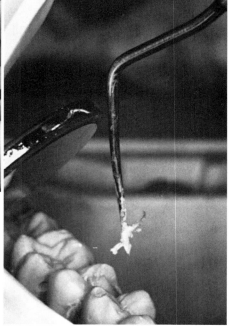

A

B

FIGURE 14-18
A, A convenient battery-controlled heating device holds an assortment of tips. **B,** The tip is rapidly heated for removal of excess gutta-percha from the chamber, or from the canal when creating a post space.

Fitting a new master cone and reobturation is then possible.

If the excess gutta-percha has been seared off, an overfill can sometimes be corrected before the sealer sets by removing all gutta-percha with files or broaches. When extruded beyond the apex, the overfilled gutta-percha is difficult to recover through the canal, particularly after the sealer sets. Extruded sealer can only be retrieved surgically.

Obturating materials extruded beyond the apex are irritants and affect healing, but generally they do not completely prevent resolution (Figure 14-20) unless there is gross overfill of core material. ZnOE-based sealers often resorb from periapical tissues over time.[111] These situations should not be treated surgically unless failure to heal is evident on recall examination.

SOLVENT-SOFTENED CUSTOM CONES

Different solvents have been proposed and tested. The two that have been proven to be useful clinically and that are used most often are chloroform and halothane; however, concerns about toxicity have been expressed. Some concerns about chloroform are unfounded; recent evaluations show that, if used judiciously, chloroform is safe for retreatment and for the formation of custom cones.[112,113] Described here is a technique using chloroform; halothane is used in a similar manner.

An impression of the apical 3 or 4 mm of the canal is made in the gutta-percha master cone. It is basically a "cone within a cone," as only the cone surface is softened and then shaped. The objective is to fit the cone closely into the apical portion to try to create a better seal but primarily to prevent extrusion of gutta-percha beyond the apex. In fact, solvent softening does not result ultimately in a better apical seal.[114-116]

Indications

Basically there are two indications: (1) an apical stop is lacking or (2) a stop is present but the apical portion of the canal is very large or irregular.

Technique

The steps are as follows:

1. The master cone selected is usually a larger standardized cone that, when inserted, stops 2 to 4 mm short of the working length.
2. The master cone tip (apical 3 to 4 mm) is softened by dipping it in chloroform for 1 to 2 seconds (Figure 14-21). Halothane dipping is done for 3 to 4 seconds.
3. The cone is tamped apically in the canal several times. Then, the cone is grasped at the reference point, removed, and measured. Softening and tamping are repeated until the cone goes to working length. The cone is

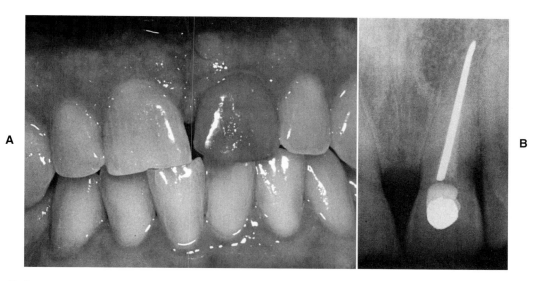

FIGURE 14-19
Often discoloration is caused by improper technique and is preventable. **A,** A too-frequent unfortunate occurrence: gradual discoloration after root canal treatment. **B,** Causes include sealer remnants and a silver point extending into the chamber and amalgam restoring the lingual access. This tooth will be difficult to bleach because the stains are from metallic ions.

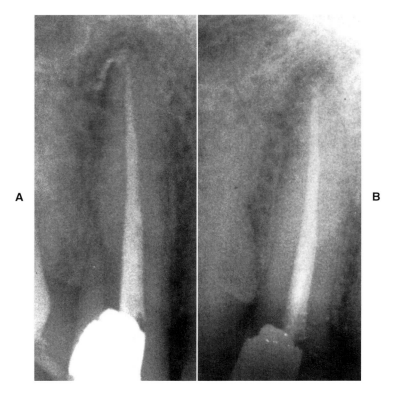

FIGURE 14-20
A, This is not a serious overfill. The core obturating material is confined to the canal. **B,** Recall examination shows healing and resorption of sealer.

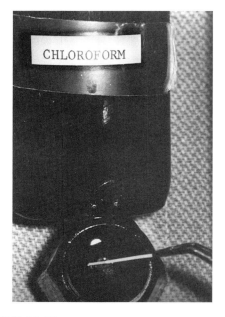

FIGURE 14-21
The softened custom cone technique. The apical portion (3 to 4 mm) is dipped in chloroform for 1 to 2 seconds and then tamped in the canal.

marked or bent for orientation; it must be replaced exactly in the same position during obturation.

4. The cone is removed, and the solvent is allowed to evaporate. The cone should not be left in the canal for any length of time while soft; the softening will continue and the tip may separate when the master cone is removed. The cone tip should show an impression of the apical preparation (Figure 14-22).

5. The cone is replaced and a confirmatory radiograph is made. The cone need not extend to working length but may be slightly shorter, up to 1 mm.

6. Sealer is mixed thick. The canal walls are not coated, only the apical third of the master cone. The cone is carefully inserted to length without wiping off all the sealer on the walls.

7. The standard lateral condensation procedure follows with spreader insertion, rotation, removal, accessory cone placement, and so on. More sealer is added by coating each accessory cone before placement.

8. A radiograph may be made to evaluate the obturation before the excess is seared off.

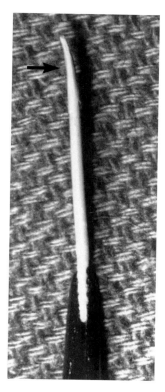

FIGURE 14-22
After the softened cone has been tamped into the canal and removed, it should show an impression of the apical region *(arrow)*.

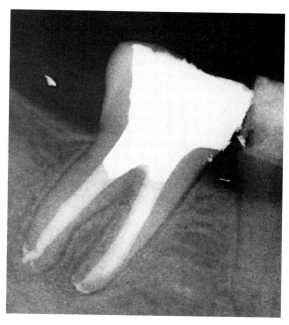

FIGURE 14-23
Warm vertical condensation. Larger canal preparations are indicated to accommodate obturating instruments (heater-pluggers). Also, this technique tends to apically extrude sealer and softened gutta-percha.

The mass can be pulled out and reobturation done if necessary.

VERTICAL CONDENSATION

Vertical condensation is also an effective technique; studies show its sealability is comparable to that of lateral condensation. Although vertical condensation is not widely taught in dental schools, the technique is becoming more popular. With the introduction of new devices and techniques, the warm vertical compaction technique is somewhat more user friendly and is less time consuming.

Indications

In general, vertical condensation can be used in the same situations as lateral condensation. It is preferred in a few circumstances, such as with internal resorption and with root end induction.

Advantages and Disadvantages

Its principal advantage over lateral condensation is the ability to adapt the warmed and softened

gutta-percha to the irregular root canal system.[117,118] Disadvantages include difficulty of length control, a more complicated procedure, and a larger assortment of required instruments. Also, a somewhat larger canal preparation is necessary to allow manipulation of the instruments (Figure 14-23).

Technique

The warm vertical compaction technique requires a heat source and various sized pluggers for compaction of the thermoplasticized gutta-percha. Schilder pluggers begin at 0.4 mm in diameter and increase by 0.1 mm for each of the successive instruments with 1.1 mm being the largest instrument. Pluggers are also available in ISO standardized sizes.

The technique consists of fitting a gutta-percha cone with a taper similar to the canal, short of the apex and applying heat using a flame-heated carrier. The gutta-percha is softened by the heat and becomes plastic. Pluggers are then placed in the canal with apical pressure to produce a hydraulic force that moves the gutta-percha apically, against the canal walls, and into canal irregularities such as accessory canals. Gutta-percha is then added in small increments; each increment of gutta-percha is heated and softened and packed vertically until the entire canal is filled. Detailed descriptions of the technique appear elsewhere.[119]

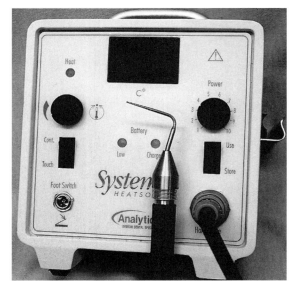

FIGURE 14-24
Device for heating gutta-percha. A controlled current causes rapid heating of the plugger, which then softens a prefit gutta-percha cone in the canal.

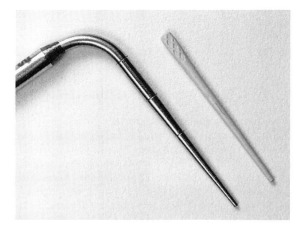

FIGURE 14-25
"Continuous wave of condensation" plugger is designed to size-match the rotary file used to prepare the canal. Pluggers are also approximately matched to nonstandardized gutta-percha in an attempt to obturate the apical portion of a canal with a single cone.

Other Warm Vertical Approaches

A recent modification of the warm vertical compaction technique is termed the "continuous wave of condensation." Prerequisites for this technique are a tapering canal preparation, a constricted apical preparation, and an accurate cone fit. The technique is often used after preparation with nickel-titanium rotary files of greater taper. The heat source is an electric device that supplies heat to a plugger on demand (Figure 14-24). Pluggers are available in nonstandardized sizes that match the nonstandardized gutta-percha cones or in standardized sizes that match files of greater taper (Figure 14-25). In addition, two hand pluggers of differing diameters are used to sustain and condense the gutta-percha apically.

Heat is applied at a prescribed temperature (200° C) for a short period of time as determined by the operator. By applying a constant source of heat to a prefitted gutta-percha cone, hydraulic pressure can be applied in one continuous motion. As the plugger moves apically, the fit becomes more precise and the hydraulic pressure is increased, forcing the gutta-percha into canal irregularities. Details of the continuous wave of condensation technique are available in other publications.[120]

There are inherent risks. When thermoplasticization or any technique that physically alters gutta-percha is used, there is the potential for extrusion into the periradicular tissues as well as possible damage to the periodontal ligament and supporting alveolar bone from heat. An increase of 10° C above body temperature appears to be a critical threshold for damaging osseous tissues.[96,121] Flame-heated carriers reach high temperatures and pose the greatest threat of damage to the periodontal structures.[122-125] When used properly, the injectable gutta-percha technique and the continuous wave condensation technique appear to produce temperature changes that are below the critical threshold.[125-127]

Sectional Obturation

A recent innovation, this technique involves a two-phased sectional approach. A small apical segment of gutta-percha is placed ("downpacked"), followed by a backfilling of gutta-percha. This technique seems relatively fast and may prove useful, but requires more investigation.[128] Details of the technique appear elsewhere.[129]

Thermoplasticized Injection

With this technique, specially formulated gutta-percha is warmed and then injected into the prepared canal with a device (Figure 14-26) that works like a caulking gun.[130] When used in conjunction with a sealer, thermoplasticized injection provides an adequate seal.[131] This technique is useful in special situations (Figure 14-27). However, lack of length control and shrinkage upon cooling are disadvantages.

Solvent Techniques

Solvent techniques involve the total or partial dissolution of gutta-percha in solvents, primarily chloroform or eucalyptol (see Figure 14-5). These have names such as chloropercha, eucapercha, diffusion technique, or chloroform resin. Often,

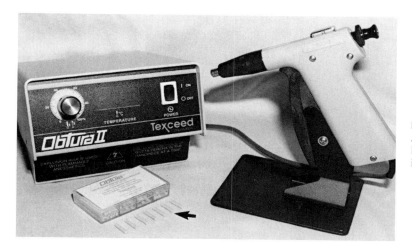

FIGURE 14-26
A thermoplasticizing device. A high-heat gun softens gutta-percha *(arrow)* into an injectable plastic mass.

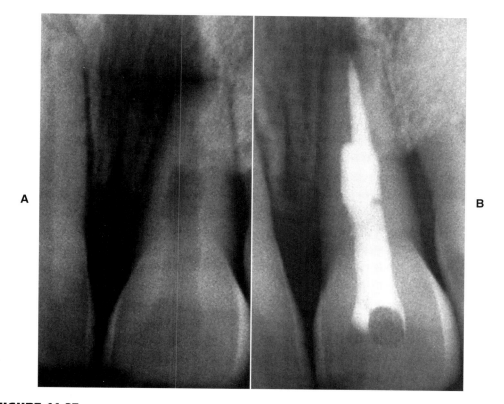

FIGURE 14-27
A, Internal resorptive defect is a good indication for **B,** obturation with a thermoplasticized gutta-percha technique. (Courtesy Dr. M Gomez.)

these techniques are not used in conjunction with a standard sealer but depend on softened gutta-percha to adapt closely. The problem is that gutta-percha shrinks away from the walls as the solvents evaporate. Extensive leakage is generally seen with these techniques,[56] and some have a poorer long-term prognosis.[132]

Gutta-Percha Carrier Systems

These systems use a central carrier (stainless steel, titanium, or plastic) coated with gutta-percha. The carrier is flexible yet it provides rigidity for the overlying gutta-percha. The obturators are standardized, so the carriers correspond to the size of instruments. After canal preparation, the canal is dried and lightly coated with sealer. The appropriate size obturator is heated in a special oven and firmly placed to working length. The carrier is then sectioned 1 to 2 mm above the orifice to the canal. These carrier/gutta-percha systems are equivalent to conventional gutta-percha obturation with apical sealing, but do not consistently create a coronal seal.[133,134]

Advantages of the technique include ease of placement and the potential for the plasticized gutta-percha to flow into canal irregularities. Disadvantages include a tendency for extrusion of material periapically, an inability to control the density of fill in irregularly shaped canals, difficulties in removing carrier and gutta-percha during retreatment, and variable adaptation of components in the canal.[134,135] Overall, there are no demonstrated advantages to routine use of these systems.

ALTERNATIVE TECHNIQUES

Other techniques involve primarily mixing and placement of unset material into the canal. Either chemical or physical changes cause the material to set into a semisolid or solid form. Many materials have been tried; clinical validation research on them usually is sparse or absent. None have yet proved feasible for various reasons related to either the material or the techniques of insertion. Again, length control and obturation voids are major difficulties.[136] Included with some of these techniques are materials as such amalgam, glass ionomer, composites, silicone pastes, semisoft acrylics N2 or RC2B paste ("Sargenti" technique), and ZnOE paste with various additives.

In addition to problems with physical properties, generally there are many biologic disadvantages as well.[137] In particular, the pastes with formaldehyde or heavy metal additives (e.g., Sargenti formulations) show more short-term and long-term toxicity than the standard accepted materials.[138-140] Although there are advocates for the so-called Sargenti technique, which continues to be practiced, experimental and clinical evidence weighs heavily against this approach. In addition, there are warnings and, in some countries and states, bans against it. There is also a federal ban on importation and interstate sales of the N2 or RC2B paste. Perhaps for these and other reasons, malpractice lawsuits and out-of-court settlements have consistently been decided for the plaintiff and against the dentist employing the Sargenti technique and the paste.

However, on the horizon are some interesting and radical approaches to preparation and obturation using hydrodynamics and vacuum techniques.[141] These are still experimental, lacking clinical verification, but show promise.

Evaluation of Obturation

Surprisingly, evaluation of obturation is difficult. The only means of immediate assessment is radiographic, which is imprecise at best. However, radiographic evaluation has been the standard and at least provides some criteria with which to judge obturation quality.

SYMPTOMS

The presence of symptoms for a few days after obturation is common and probably is unrelated to an inadequate seal. This reflects a different phenomenon.

RADIOGRAPHIC CRITERIA

Good obturation (fluid-tight seal) cannot be seen on a radiograph. Only fairly gross discrepancies are visible; these voids or deficiencies may or may not relate to lack of seal and may result in long-term failure.[142] The evaluative criteria as determined by studying the obturation radiograph (Figure 14-28) are as follows.

Radiolucencies

Voids within the body or at the interface of obturating material and dentin wall represent incomplete obturation.

Density

Material should be of uniform density from coronal to apical aspects. The coronal region (and large canals) are more radiopaque than the

FIGURE 14-28
Evaluation of obturation: an example showing several deficiencies and correction. **A,** Length: apical portion shows slight overfill; shape: there is not consistent taper (the fill is narrower in the cervical region); density: voids are present throughout; coronal removal: material remains in the chamber. **B,** Improved access, cleaning and shaping, correct obturation, and restoration. Healing is evident. (Courtesy Dr. A. Stabholz.)

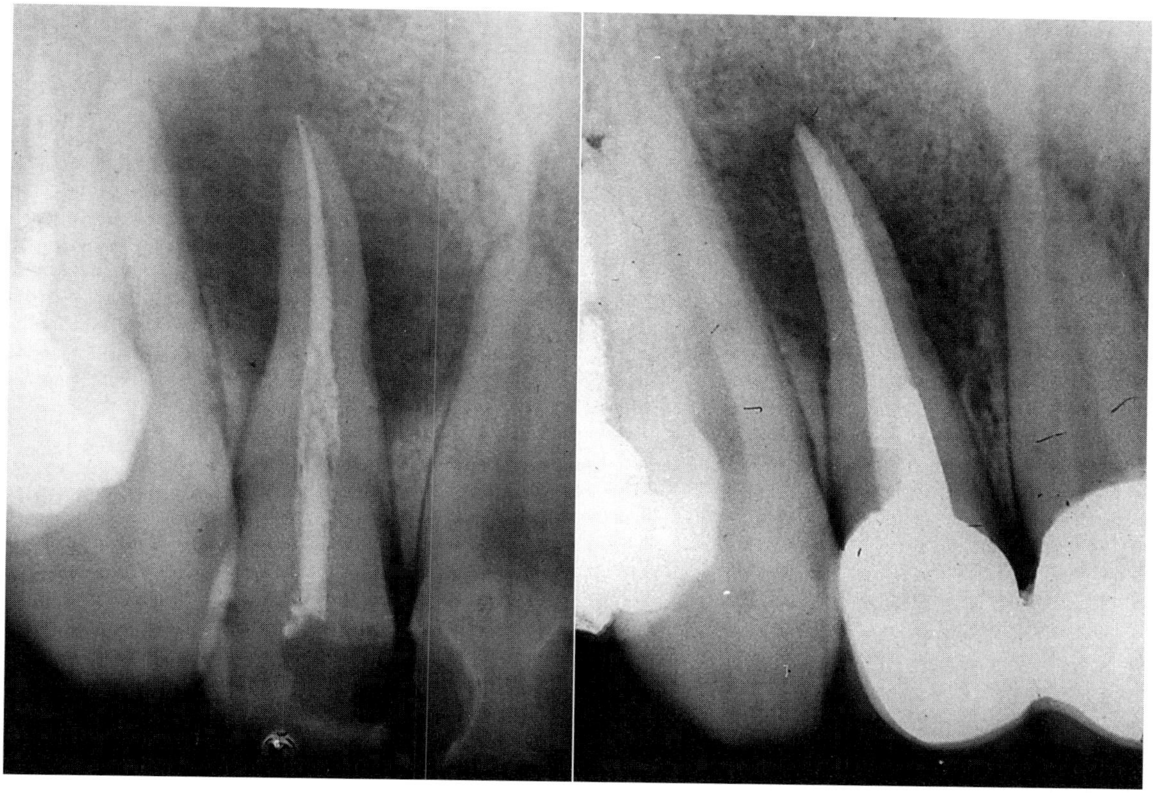

apical region because of differences in mass of material. The margins of gutta-percha should be sharp and distinct with no fuzziness, indicating close adaptation.

Length

The material should extend to the prepared length and be removed apical to the gingival margin (anterior teeth) and orifices (posterior teeth).

Taper

The gutta-percha should reflect the canal shape; that is, it should be tapered from coronal to apical regions. Taper need not be uniform but should be consistent. Ideally, the apical region should taper nearly to a point unless the canal in this region was not small before preparation.

Restoration

Whether permanent or temporary, the restoration should be contacting enough dentin surface to ensure a coronal seal.

REFERENCES

1. Ingle JL, Beveridge E, Glick D, Welchman J: The Washington study. In Ingle JI, Bakland LK, editors: *Endodontics,* ed 4, Baltimore, 1994, Williams & Wilkins.
2. Ray H, Trope M, Buxt P, Switzer S: Influence of various factors on the periapical status of endodontically treated teeth, *Int Endod J* 28:12, 1995.
3. Delivanis PD, Mattison GD, Mendel RW: The survivability of F43 strain of *Streptococcus sanguis* in root canals filled with gutta-percha and Procosol cement, *J Endod* 9:407, 1983.

4. Marshall FJ, Massler M: Sealing of pulpless teeth evaluated with radioisotopes, *J Dent Med* 16:172, 1961.

5. Kapsimalis P, Evans R: Sealing properties of endodontic filling materials using polar and nonpolar isotopes. *Oral Surg Oral Med Oral Pathol* 22:386, 1966.

6. Delivanis PD, Chapman KA: Comparison and reliability of techniques for measuring leakage and marginal penetration, *Oral Surg Oral Med Oral Pathol* 53:410, 1982.

7. Wu MK, Wesselink PR: Endodontic leakage studies reconsidered. Part I. Methodology, application and relevance, *Int Endod J* 2:37, 1993.

8. Swanson KS, Madison S: An evaluation of coronal microleakage in endodontically treated teeth. Part I. Time periods, *J Endod* 13:56, 1987.

9. Madison S, Swanson K, Chiles S: An evaluation of coronal microleakage in endodontically treated teeth. Part II. Sealer types, *J Endod* 13:109, 1987.

10. Khayat A, Lee SJ, Torabinejad M: Human saliva penetration of coronally unsealed obturated root canals, *J Endod* 19:458, 1993.

11. Magura ME, Kafrawy AH, Brown CE Jr, Newton CW: Human saliva coronal microleakage in obturated root canals: an in vitro study, *J Endod* 17:324, 1991.

12. Barrieshi K, Walton R, Johnson W, Drake D: Coronal leakage of mixed anaerobic bacteria after obturation and post space preparation, *Oral Surg Oral Med Oral Pathol Oral Radiol Endod* 84:310, 1997.

13. Barthel C, Moshonov J, Shuuping G, Ørstavik D: Bacterial leakage versus dye leakage in obturated root canals, *Int Endod J* 32:370, 1999.

14. Pisano D, DiFiore P, McClanahan S, et al: Intraorifice sealing of gutta-percha obturated root canals to prevent coronal microleakage, *J Endod* 24:659, 1998.

15. Strindberg LZ: The difference in the results of pulp therapy on certain factors, *Acta Odontol Scand Suppl* 14:21, 1956.

16. Odesjo B, Hellden L, Salonen L, Langeland K: Prevalence of previous endodontic treatment, technical standard and occurrence of periapical lesions in a randomly selected adult, general population, *Endod Dent Traumatol* 6:265, 1990.

17. Smith C, Setchell D, Harty F: Factors influencing the success of conventional root canal therapy—a five-year retrospective study, *Int Endod J* 26:321, 1993.

18. Seltzer S, Soltanoff W, Smith J: Periapical tissue reactions to root canal instrumentation beyond the apex and root canal fillings short of and beyond the apex, *Oral Surg Oral Med Oral Pathol* 36:725, 1973.

19. Smith RG, Patterson SS, El-Kafrawy AH: Histologic study of the effects of hydrocortisone on the apical periodontium of dogs, *J Endod* 2:376, 1976.

20. Feldman G, Nyborg H: Tissue reactions of root canal filling materials. 1. Comparison between gutta-percha and silver amalgam implanted in rabbits, *Odontol Rev* 13:1, 1962.

21. Rappaport HM, Lilly GE, Kapsimalis P: Toxicity of endodontic filling materials, *Oral Surg Oral Med Oral Pathol* 18:785, 1964.

22. Olsson B, Sliwkowski A, Langeland K: Subcutaneous implantation for the biologic evaluation of endodontic materials, *J Endod* 7:355, 1981.

23. Wenger JS, Tsaknis PJ, del Rio CE, Ayer WA: The effects of partially filled polyethylene tube intraosseous implants in rats, *Oral Surg Oral Med Oral Pathol* 46:88, 1978.

24. Wu M, Wesselink P, Walton R: Apical terminus location of root canal treatment procedures, *Oral Surg Oral Med Oral Pathol* 89:99, 2000.

25. Weine F, Buchanan L: Controversies in clinical endodontics: Part 1. The significance and filling of lateral canals, *Compend Contin Educ Dent* 17:1028, 1996.

26. Walton R: Histologic evaluation and comparison of different methods of pulp canal enlargement, *J Endod* 2:304, 1976.

27. Reader CM, Himel VT, Germain LP, Hoen MM: Effect of three obturation techniques on the filling of lateral canals and the main canal, *J Endod* 19:404, 1993.

28. Weine F: The enigma of the lateral canal, *Dent Clin North Am* 28:833, 1984.

29. Walton RE, Michelich RJ, Smith GN: The histopathogenesis of vertical root fractures, *J Endod* 10:48, 1984.

30. Meister F Jr, Lommel TJ, Gerstein H: Diagnosis and possible causes of vertical root fractures, *Oral Surg Oral Med Oral Pathol* 49:243, 1980.

31. Silver-Thorne M, Joyce T: Finite element analysis of anterior tooth root stresses developed during endodontic treatment, *J Biomech Eng* 121:108, 1999.

32. Pints DL, Matheny HE, Nicholls J: An in vitro study of spreader loads required to cause vertical root fracture during lateral condensation, *J Endod* 9:544, 1983.

33. Holcomb J, Pitts D, Nicholls J: Further investigation of spreader loads required to cause vertical root fracture during lateral condensation, *J Endod* 13:277, 1987.

34. Dang DA, Walton RE: Vertical root fracture and root distortion: effect of spreader design, *J Endod* 15:294, 1989.

35. Murgel CA, Walton RE: Vertical root fracture and dentin deformation in curved roots: The influence of spreader design, *Endod Dent Traumatol* 6:273, 1990.

36. Obermayr G, Walton RE, Leary JM, Krell KV: Vertical root fracture and relative deformation during obturation and post cementation, *J Prosthet Dent* 66:181, 1991.

37. Lertchirakarn V, Palamara J, Messer H: Load and strain during lateral condensation and vertical root fracture, *J Endod* 25:99, 1999.

38. Southard D, Rooney T: Effective one-visit therapy for the acute apical abscess, *J Endod* 10:580, 1984.

39. Sjogren U, Figdor, Persson S, Sundqvist G: Influence of infection at the time of root filling on the outcome of endodontic treatment of teeth with apical periodontitis, *Int Endod J* 30:297, 1997.

40. Katebzadeh N, Hupp J, Trope M: Histological periapical repair after obturation of infected root canals in dogs, *J Endod* 25:364, 1999.

41. Trope M, Delano E, Ørstavik D: Endodontic treatment of teeth with apical periodontitis: single vs. multivisit treatment, *J Endod* 25:345, 1999.

42. Sjögren U, Figdor D, Spangberg L, Sundqvist G: The antimicrobial effect of calcium hydroxide as a short-term intracanal dressing, *Int Endod J* 4:119, 1991.

43. Weiger R, Rosendahl R, Lost C: Influence of calcium hydroxide intracanal dressings on the prognosis of

teeth with endodontically induced periapical lesions, *Int Endod J* 33:219, 2000.

44. Zeldow BJ, Ingle JI: Correlation of the positive culture to the prognosis of endodontically treated teeth: a clinical study, *J Am Dent Assoc* 66:23, 1963.

45. Engstrom B, Segerstad L, Ramstrom G, Frostell G: Correlation of positive cultures with the prognosis for root canal treatment, *Odontol Rev* 15:257, 1964.

46. Grossman L: *Endodontic practice*, ed 11, p 242, Philadelphia, 1988, Lea & Febiger.

47. Marlin J, Schilder H: Physical measurements of gutta-percha, *Oral Surg Oral Med Oral Pathol* 32:260, 1971.

48. Friedman CE, Sandrik JL, Heuer MA, Rapp GW: Composition and physical properties of gutta-percha endodontic filling materials, *J Endod* 3:304, 1977.

49. Johansson BI: A methodological study of the mechanical properties of endodontic gutta-percha, *J Endod* 6:781, 1980.

50. Goldberg F, Grufinkel J, Spielberg C: Microscopic study of standardized gutta-percha points, *Oral Surg Oral Med Oral Pathol* 47:275, 1979.

51. Wolfson E, Seltzer S: Reaction of rat connective tissue to some gutta-percha formulations, *J Endod* 1:395, 1975.

52. Cardoso C, Kotaka C, Redmerski R, et al: Rapid decontamination of gutta-percha cones with sodium hypochlorite, *J Endod* 25:498, 1999.

53. Curson I, Kirk E: An assessment of root canal-sealing properties of root canal sealing cements, *Oral Surg Oral Med Oral Pathol* 26:229, 1968.

54. Skinner RL, Himel VT: The sealing ability of injection-molded thermoplasticized gutta-percha with and without the use of sealers, *J Endod* 13:315, 1987.

55. Miletic I, Anic I, Pezelj-Ribaric S, Jukic S: Leakage of five root canal sealers, *Int Endod J* 32:415, 1999.

56. Zakariasen KL, Stadem PS: Microleakage associated with modified eucapercha and chlorapercha root-canal-filling techniques, *Int Endod J* 15:67, 1982.

57. Schneider S: A comparison of canal preparation in straight and curved canals, *Oral Surg Oral Med Oral Pathol* 32:271, 1971.

58. Johnson WT, Zakariasen KL: Spectrophotometric analysis of micro-leakage in the fine curved canals found in the mesial roots of mandibular molars, *Oral Surg Oral Med Oral Pathol* 56:305, 1983.

59. Timpawat S, Jensen J, Feigal RJ, Messer HH: An in vitro study of the comparative effectiveness of obturating curved root canals with gutta-percha cones, silver cones, and stainless steel files, *Oral Surg Oral Med Oral Pathol* 55:180, 1983.

60. Zielke DR, Brady JM, del Rio CE: Corrosion of silver cones in bone: A scanning electron microprobe analysis, *J Endod* 1:11, 1975.

61. Krell K, Fuller M, Scott G: The conservative retrieval of silver cones in difficult cases, *J Endod* 10:269, 1984.

62. Serper A, Ucer O, Onur R, Etikan I: Comparative neurotoxic effects of root canal filling materials on rat sciatic nerve, *J Endod* 24:592, 1998.

63. Krakow A, Berk H: Efficient endodontic procedures with the use of the pressure syringe, *Dent Clin North Am* 9:387, 1965.

64. Fogel B: A comparative study of five materials for use in filling root canal spaces, *Oral Surg Oral Med Oral Pathol* 43:284, 1977.

65. Beatty R, Vertucci F, Zakariasen K: Apical sealing efficacy of endodontic obturation techniques, *Int Endod J* 19:237, 1986.

66. Grossman L: *Endodontic practice*, ed 11, p 255, Philadelphia, 1988, Lea & Febiger.

67. Kettering KD, Torabinejad M: Cytotoxicity of root canal sealer: a study using HeLa cell and fibroblast, *Int Endod J* 2:60, 1984.

68. Hashieh I, Pommel L, Camps J: Concentration of eugenol apically released from zinc oxide-eugenol-based sealers, *J Endod* 25:713, 1999.

69. van der Burgt T, Mullaney TP: Tooth discoloration induced by endodontic sealers, *Oral Surg Oral Med Oral Pathol* 61:84, 1986.

70. Parsons J, Walton R: Coronal discoloration from sealers: a longitudinal analysis, *J Endod* (in press).

71. Wilcox LR, Krell KV, Madison S, Rittman B: Endodontic retreatment: evaluation of gutta-percha and sealer removal and canal reinstrumentation, *J Endod* 13:453, 1987.

72. Grossman LI: Solubility of root canal cements, *J Dent Res* 57:927, 1978.

73. Higginbotham TL: A comparative study of the physical properties of five commonly used root canal sealers, *Oral Surg Oral Med Oral Pathol* 24:89, 1967.

74. Ørstavik D: Antibacterial properties of root canal sealers, cements and pastes, *Int Endod J* 14:27, 1981.

75. Allan N, Walton R, Schaffer M: Setting times for endodontic sealers under clinical usage and in vitro conditions, *J Endod* 27:421, 2000.

76. Heling I, Chandler N: The antimicrobial effect within dentinal tubules of four root canal sealers, *J Endod* 22:257, 1996.

77. Limkangwalmongkol S, Abbott PV, Sandler AB: Apical dye penetration with four root canal sealers and gutta-percha using longitudinal sectioning, *J Endod* 18:535, 1992.

78. Leonardo M, Bezerra da Silva L, Filho M, et al: Release of formaldehyde by 4 endodontic sealers, *Oral Surg Oral Med Oral Pathol Oral Radiol Endod* 88:221, 1999.

79. Fuss Z, Weiss E, Shalhav M: Antibacterial activity of calcium hydroxide-containing endodontic sealers on *enterococcus faecalis* in vitro, *Int Endod J* 30:397, 1997.

80. Barnett F, Trope M, Rooney J, Tronstad L: In vivo sealing ability of calcium hydroxide-containing root canal sealers, *Endod Dent Traumatol* 5:23, 1989.

81. Zmener O, Guglielmotti MB, Cabrini RL: Biocompatibility of two calcium hydroxide-based endodontic sealers: A quantitative study in the subcutaneous connective issue of the rat, *J Endod* 14:229, 1988.

82. Saunders WP, Saunders EM, Herd D, Stephens E: The use of glass ionomer as a root canal sealer: a pilot study, *Int Endod J* 25:238, 1992.

83. Lalh M, Titley K, Torneck C, Friedman: The shear bond strength of glass ionomer cement sealers to bovine dentin conditioned with common endodontic irrigants, *Int Endod J* 32:430, 1999.

84. Almeida W, Leonardo M, Filho T, Silva L: Evaluation of apical sealing of three endodontic sealers, *Int Endod J* 33:25, 2000.

85. Friedman S, Komorowski R, Maillet W, et al: In vivo resistance of coronally induced bacterial ingress by an experimental glass ionomer cement root canal sealer, *J Endod* 28:1, 2000.

86. Leonardo M, Almeida W, Bezerra da Silva L, Utrilla L: Histological evaluation of the response of apical tissues to glass ionomer and zinc oxide-eugenol based sealers in dog teeth after root canal treatment, *Endod Dent Traumatol* 14:257, 1998.

87. Moshonov J, Trope M, Friedman S: Retreatment efficacy 3 months after obturation using glass ionomer cement, zinc oxide-eugenol, and epoxy resin sealers, *J Endod* 20:90, 1994.

88. Barry GN, Fried IL: Sealing quality of two polycarboxylate cements used as root canal sealers, *J Endod* 1:107, 1975.

89. Zidan O, El Deeb ME: Use of a dentin bonding agent as a root canal sealer, *J Endod* 11:176, 1985.

90. Benatti O, Stolf WL, Ruhnke LA: Verification of the consistency, setting time, and dimensional changes of root canal filling materials, *Oral Surg Oral Med Oral Pathol* 46:107, 1978.

91. Stamos D, Gutmann J, Gettleman B: In vivo evaluation of root canal sealer distribution, *J Endod* 21:177, 1995.

92. Kahn F, Rosenberg P, Schertzer L, et al: An *in-vitro* evaluation of sealer placement methods, *Int Endod J* 30:181, 1997.

93. Wiemann AH, Wilcox LR: In vitro evaluation of four methods of sealer placement, *J Endod* 17:444, 1991.

94. Aguirre A, El Deeb M, Aguirre R: The effect of ultrasonics on sealer distribution and sealing of root canals, *J Endod* 23:759, 1997.

95. Hall M, Clement D, Dove S, Walker W: A comparison of sealer placement techniques in curved canals, *J Endod* 22:638, 1996.

96. Greene HA, Wong M, Ingram TA: Comparison of the sealing ability of four obturation techniques, *J Endod* 16:423, 1990.

97. Director RC, Rabinowitz JL, Miline RS: The short-term sealing properties of lateral condensation, vertical condensation and Hydron using ^{14}C human serum albumin, *J Endod* 8:149, 1982.

98. Rhome BH, Solomon EA, Rabinowitz JL: Isotopic evaluation of the sealing properties of lateral condensation, vertical condensation, and Hydron, *J Endod* 7:458, 1981.

99. Cailleteau J, Mullaney T: Prevalence of teaching apical patency and various instrumentation and obturation techniques in United States dental schools, *J Endod* 23:394, 1997.

100. Sakkal S, Weine FS, Lemian L: Lateral condensation: inside view, *Compendium* 12:796, 1991.

101. Amditis C, Blackler SM, Bryant RW, Hewitt GH: The adaptation achieved by four root canal filling techniques as assessed by three methods, *Aust Dent J* 37:439, 1992.

102. Simons J, Ibanez B, Friedman S, Trope M: Leakage after lateral condensation with finger spreaders and D-11-T spreaders, *J Endod* 17:101, 1991.

103. Joyce A, Loushine R, West L, et al: Photoelastic comparison of stress induced by using stainless-steel versus nickel-titanium spreaders in vitro, *J Endod* 24:714, 1998.

104. Schmidt K, Walker T, Johnson J, Nicoll B: Comparison of nickel-titanium and stainless-steel spreader penetration and accessory cone fit in curved canals, *J Endod* 26:42, 2000.

105. Allison DA, Michelich RJ, Walton RE: The influence of master cone adaptation on the quality of the apical seal, *J Endod* 11:166, 1981.

106. Yared GM, Bou Dagher FE: Elongation and movement of the gutta-percha master cone during initial lateral condensation, *J Endod* 19:395, 1993.

107. Hartwell GR, Barbieri SJ, Gerard SE, Gunsolley JC: Evaluation of size variation between endodontic finger spreaders and accessory gutta-percha cones, *J Endod* 17:8, 1991.

108. Yared G, Bou Dagher F, Machtou P: Influence of the removal of coronal gutta-percha on the seal of root canal obturation, *J Endod* 23:146, 1997.

109. Baumgardner K, Krell K: Ultrasonic condensation of gutta-percha: an in vitro dye penetration and scanning electron microscopic study, *J Endod* 16:253, 1990.

110. Zmener O, Banegas G: Clinical experience of root canal filling by ultrasonic condensation of gutta-percha, *Endod Dent Traumatol* 15:57, 1999.

111. Augsberger RA, Peters DD: Radiographic evaluation of extruded obturation materials, *J Endod* 16:492, 1990.

112. McDonald MN, Vire DE: Chloroform in the endodontic operatory, *J Endod* 18:301, 1992.

113. Allard U, Andersson L: Exposure of dental personnel to chloroform in root-filling procedures, *Endod Dent Traumatol* 8:155, 1992.

114. Keane KM, Harrington GW: The use of chloroform softened gutta-percha master cone and its effects on the apical seal, *J Endod* 10:57, 1984.

115. Smith JJ, Montgomery S: A comparison of apical seal: chloroform versus halothane-dipped gutta-percha cones, *J Endod* 18:156, 1992.

116. Yancich PP, Hartwell GR, Portell FR: A comparison of apical seal: chloroform versus eucalyptol-dipped gutta-percha obturation, *J Endod* 15:257, 1989.

117. Wolcott J, Himel V, Powell W: Effect of two obturation techniques on the filling of lateral canals and the main canal, *J Endod* 23:632, 1997.

118. DuLac K, Nielsen C, Tomazic T, et al: Comparison of the obturation of lateral canals by six techniques, *J Endod* 25:376, 1999.

119. Schilder H: Vertical compaction of warm gutta-percha. In Gerstein H, editor, *Techniques in clinical endodontics,* Philadelphia, 1983, WB Saunders.

120. Buchanan S: Continuous wave of condensation technique, *Endod Pract* 2:7, 1998.

121. Eriksson A, Albbrektsson T: Temperature threshold levels for heat-induced bone tissue injury; a vital microscopic study in the rabbit, *J Prosthet Dent* 50:101,1983.

122. Hand R, Hugel E, Tsaknis P: Effects of a warm gutta percha technique on the lateral periodontium, *Oral Surg Oral Med Oral Pathol* 36:872, 1973.

123. Marciano J, Michailesco P: Dental gutta percha; chemical composition, x-ray identification, enthalpic studies and clinical implications, *J Endod* 15:149,1989.

124. Lee F, VanCura J, BeGole E: A comparison of root surface temperatures using different obturation heat sources, *J Endod* 24:617, 1998.

125. Silver G, Love R, Purton D: Comparison of two vertical condensation obturation techniques: Touch 'n Heat modified and System B, *Int Endod J* 32:287, 1999.

126. Weller RN, Koch K: In vitro radicular temperatures produced by injectable thermoplasticized gutta-percha, *Int Endod J* 25:593, 1999.

127. Floren J, Weller RN, Pashly D, Kimbrough W: Changes in root surface temperatures with in vitro use of the System B HeatSource, *J Endod* 25:593, 1999.

128. Santos M, Walker W, Carnes D: Evaluation of apical seal in straight canals after obturation using the Lightspeed sectional method, *J Endod* 25:609, 1999.

129. Senia S: Canal diameter: the forgotten dimension, *Endod Pract* 3:34, 2000.

130. Marlin J, Krakow A, Desilets R, Gron P: Clinical use of injection-molded thermoplasticized gutta-percha for obturation of the root canal systems: a preliminary report, *J Endod* 7:277, 1981.

131. Evans JT, Simon JHS: Evaluation of the apical seal produced by injected thermoplasticized gutta-percha in the absence of smear layer and root canal sealer, *J Endod* 12:101, 1986.

132. Ørstavik D, Kerekes K, Eriksen HM: Clinical performance of three endodontic sealers, *Endod Dent Traumatol* 3:178, 1987.

133. Dummer PM, Kelly T, Meghji A, et al: An in vitro study of the quality of root fillings in teeth obturated by lateral condensation of gutta-percha or Thermafil obturators, *Int Endod J* 26:99, 1993.

134. Baumgardner K, Taylor J, Walton R: Canal adaptation and coronal leakage: lateral condensation compared to Thermafil, *J Am Dent Assoc* 126:351, 1995.

135. Juhlin J, Walton RE, Dovgan JS: Adaptation of Thermafil components to canal walls, *J Endod* 19:130, 1993.

136. Kothari P, Hanson N, Cannell H: Bilateral mandibular nerve damage following root canal therapy, *Br Dent J* 180:189, 1996.

137. Langeland K, Walton R: Sargenti (N2) technique. In Clark J, editor. *Clinical dentistry,* Philadelphia, 1982, Harper & Row.

138. Newton CW, Patterson SS, Kafrawy AH: Studies of Sargenti's technique of endodontic treatment: six-month and one year responses, *J Endod* 6:509, 1980.

139. West NM, England MC, Safavi K, Green DB: Level of lead in blood of dogs with RC-2B root canal fillings, *J Endod* 6:598, 1980.

140. Pitt Ford T: Tissue reactions to two root canal sealers containing formaldehyde, *Oral Surg Oral Med Oral Pathol* 60:661, 1985.

141. Lussi A, Imwinkelried S, Stich H: Obturation of root canals with different sealers using non-instrumentation technology, *Int Endod J* 32:17, 1999.

142. Youngson C, Nattress B, Manogue M, Speirs A: In vitro radiographic representation of the extent of voids within obturated root canals, *Int Endod J* 28:77, 1995.

15

Harold H. Messer and Peter R. Wilson

Preparation for Restoration and Temporization

LEARNING OBJECTIVES

After reading this chapter, the student should be able to:

1 / Describe the role of the restoration in longevity of endodontically treated teeth.

2 / Explain the importance of coronal seal in successful root canal treatment.

3 / Summarize factors contributing to loss of tooth strength, and describe the structural importance of remaining tooth tissue.

4 / Describe requirements of an adequate restoration and how it protects and seals coronally.

5 / Outline postoperative risks to the unrestored tooth.

6 / Discuss the rationale for immediate restoration and list indications for delaying final restoration.

7 / Identify restorative options before commencing root canal treatment.

8 / Discuss advantages and disadvantages of direct and indirect restorations.

9 / Outline indications for post placement in anterior and posterior teeth.

10 / Describe common post systems and advantages and disadvantages of each.

11 / Describe core materials and their placement.

12 / Describe techniques for restoring an access opening through an existing restoration.

13 / List the principal temporary filling materials and describe techniques for their placement and removal.

14 / Describe temporization of extensively damaged teeth.

15 / Outline techniques and materials used for long-term temporization.

OUTLINE

Longevity of Endodontically Treated Teeth

Coronal Seal

Structural and Biomechanical Considerations
Structural Changes in Dentin
Loss of Tooth Structure
Biomechanical Considerations

Requirements for an Adequate Restoration

Restoration Timing
The Ideal: Immediate Restoration
Indications for Delaying Final Restoration
Semipermanent Temporary Restoration

Restoration Design
Principles and Concepts
Planning the Definitive Restoration

Preparation of Canal Space and Tooth
Post Selection
Post Space Preparation

Retention and Core Systems
Anterior Teeth
Posterior Teeth
Pins

Restoring Access Through an Existing Restoration

Temporary Restorations
Objectives of Temporization
Routine Access Cavities
Extensive Coronal Breakdown
Temporary Post Crowns
Long-Term Temporary Restorations

T he need for careful restoration is reflected in the fact that more endodontically treated teeth are lost because of restorative factors than because of failure of the root canal treatment itself.[1,2] Options for restoration are considered before root canal treatment is begun, although the final decision on the most appropriate restoration is often made only as treatment progresses. The profusion of restorative techniques and materials makes planning appear complex; however, in most cases restoration is usually straightforward.

This chapter considers principles of restoration rather than detailed techniques, which are beyond the scope of this textbook. Conservation of tooth structure is emphasized, though not at the expense of preserving the treated tooth as a functional unit.

Longevity of Endodontically Treated Teeth

The effort and expense of root canal treatment and restoration require that the tooth function effectively for a prolonged period. Surprisingly few clinical studies have addressed the question of how long endodontically treated teeth survive. The numerous studies evaluating treatment success and failure have focused on endodontic aspects (development or persistence of a periapical lesion, with accompanying signs and symptoms), which are generally amenable to further management.[3] Few retrospective clinical studies have evaluated rates and causes of tooth loss; these have consistently demonstrated the importance of the restoration.

An 8- to 9-year follow-up study reported that 11% of root canal treated teeth were extracted, most for restorative or periodontal reasons.[2] Survival rates in excess of 90% after 10 years have been reported.[4,5] Many restorative variables influence the success rate achieved in clinical practice, and much lower survival rates can be expected with inadequate restoration.[6,7] Many endodontically treated teeth require extraction because of crown fracture from inadequate restoration, but inappropriate use of posts also leads to an unacceptably high rate of clinical failure.[1] Under ideal conditions, a loss rate from restorative failures of 1% to 2% per year may be achievable.

Coronal Seal

Root canal treatment will ultimately fail if the obturating materials become exposed to oral fluids. Coronal leakage is a major cause of failure.[8,9] Even a well-obturated canal with appropriate use of sealer cement does not provide an enduring barrier to bacterial penetration; the restoration (both temporary and permanent) provides the coronal seal.[10] Exposure of obturating materials to oral fluids through a lost restoration, marginal discrepancy, or recurrent caries leads eventually to sealer disintegration and bacterial contamination of the canal system.[8] The restoration must provide the coronal seal either as a separate step (for example, placing a barrier over canal orifices) or more commonly as an integral part of the restoration by virtue of its marginal sealing ability.[9,11] Posts (particularly prefabricated posts) and cores do not create a seal until the crown is placed. [12,13]

Lack of an intact sealing restoration is an important factor in assessing the cause of a persistent or developing periapical lesion. Fortunately, this is usually correctable by endodontic and restorative retreatment. Another concern is an inadequate temporary seal, both during treatment and after treatment is complete but before final restoration. There is not sufficient information to know how much exposure time to oral fluids mandates retreatment, although 3 months maximum exposure has been suggested as a general guideline.[10]

Structural and Biomechanical Considerations

Restorative failures commonly include cusp fractures or some form of crown-root fracture (split tooth)[1] (Figure 15-1). It is important to understand the basis for this fracture susceptibility when designing restorations. Access preparation superimposed on an extensively carious or restored tooth leads to further loss of tooth structure. Unsupported cusps (particularly those without an adjacent intact marginal ridge) associated with a large access opening are more prone to fracture. Excessive preparation of the canal space for a post further weakens the root and introduces significant stress areas.[14,15]

STRUCTURAL CHANGES IN DENTIN

A deeply entrenched clinical perception persists that root canal treated teeth become brittle, supposedly losing resilience as the moisture content of dentin declines after pulp loss. This perception is unsupported experimentally. Few studies have compared physical properties of endodontically treated versus nontreated human teeth with vital pulps. The moisture content of endodontically treated teeth was not reduced, even after 10 years.[16] Also, a comparison of these two groups revealed no significant differences in strength, toughness,

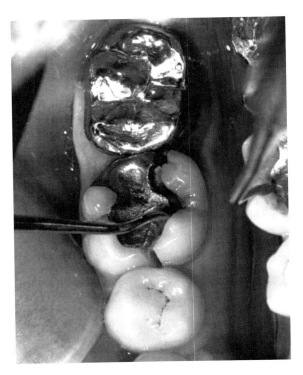

FIGURE 15-1
Crown-root fracture (split tooth) of a root canal treated tooth restored with amalgam but lacking cusp protection. (Courtesy Dr. H. Colman.)

and hardness of dentin.[17,18] Thus, susceptibility to fracture cannot be reliably attributed to structural changes in dentin after loss of pulp vitality or after root canal treatment.

LOSS OF TOOTH STRUCTURE

Teeth are measurably weakened even by occlusal cavity preparation; greater loss of tooth structure further compromises strength. Loss of one or both marginal ridges is a major contributor to reduced cuspal stiffness (strength), which predisposes teeth to fracture.[19,20] Access has only a minor effect on decreasing cuspal strength when the access cavity is surrounded by solid walls of dentin. In a tooth already seriously compromised by caries, trauma, or large restorations, the access cavity is more significant, particularly if the adjacent marginal ridge has been lost.[21] Excessive coronal flaring results in greater susceptibility to cusp fractures.[22]

BIOMECHANICAL CONSIDERATIONS

Cuspal flexure (movement under loading) will weaken premolars and molars over time.[20,21] As cavity preparations become larger and deeper, unsupported cusps become weaker and show more deflection under occlusal loads. Greater cuspal flexure leads to cyclic opening of margins between the tooth and the restorative material. Fatigue is also a factor; cusps become progressively weaker with repetitive flexing. Hence, the restoration must be designed to minimize cuspal flexure to protect against fracture and marginal leakage.

Requirements for an Adequate Restoration

The permanent restoration must (1) provide a coronal seal, (2) protect the remaining tooth structure, (3) minimize cuspal flexure, and (4) satisfy function and esthetics.

Restoration Timing

The unrestored, temporized tooth without a permanent restoration is a candidate for problems! Unless there are specific reasons for delay, final restoration is completed as soon as practical after root canal treatment.[8,23] In teeth requiring restoration of only the access (for example, minimally restored anterior teeth), the final restoration is best placed immediately after obturation. It may be necessary to defer restoration, but the delay should be minimal rather than to wait until after recall examination.

THE IDEAL: IMMEDIATE RESTORATION

The tooth is at its weakest after access and remains so until it is appropriately restored. The temporary restoration will not provide complete protection against occlusal forces even when the tooth is out of occlusion or splinted with an orthodontic band. Fracture during or soon after treatment is all too common (Figure 15-2) and is usually preventable.

Most temporary restorative materials have low wear and fracture resistance; substantial occlusal wear or material fracture may occur within weeks. Immediate restoration is preferred. It is unnecessary to wait for radiographic evidence of healing before the final restoration is placed. Even for many teeth having a guarded prognosis, prompt permanent restoration may improve the prognosis because of the better protection. In the event of failure, retreatment is usually possible through the restoration. Surgical management will not disturb the permanent restoration either.

INDICATIONS FOR DELAYING FINAL RESTORATION

Almost the only reason to delay the permanent restoration is a questionable prognosis where fail-

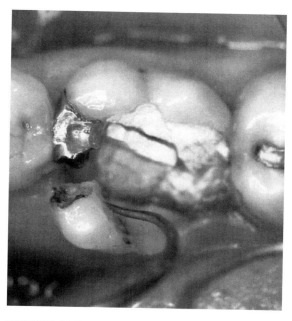

FIGURE 15-2
Interappointment fracture of a weakened tooth associated with incomplete removal of the previous restoration. Cusp protection and/or cusp reduction usually will prevent this occurrence.

ure would lead to extraction. A compromised prognosis may exist because of procedural difficulties or for nonendodontic reasons. These include canals that are not negotiable or incompletely obturated and procedural problems (for example, a broken instrument or perforation). The proposed use of the tooth as a bridge abutment may demand evidence of healing before an expensive prosthesis is placed. However, few indications justify delaying restoration.

With a guarded prognosis, the rationale for postponing final restoration is based on the nature of further management if failure occurs. Decision-making for managing failure is covered in Chapter 20. If failure is likely to result in extraction, the expense of a final restoration may dictate delay until the outcome is more certain. If correction requires surgery, there is no reason to delay restoration.

SEMIPERMANENT TEMPORARY RESTORATION

If final restoration is delayed, the temporary restoration must last as long as necessary (up to a year). It must protect, seal, and meet functional and esthetic demands. A good semipermanent posterior temporary restoration is an amalcore that onlays weakened cusps, thus providing functional and sealing protection. If a crown is to be placed later, the final crown preparation can be completed without

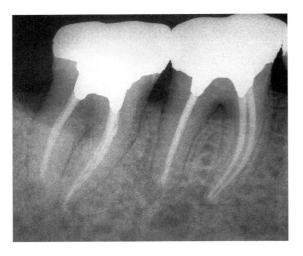

FIGURE 15-3
Chamber and canal orifices retain an amalgam core, taking advantage of natural undercuts. The teeth can be prepared for crowns without removing the amalcore, or the amalgams may be the permanent restoration if the cusps are adequately protected. (Courtesy Dr. P. Parashos.)

removing the core (Figure 15-3). Comparable anterior restorations are more challenging owing to esthetic factors and difficulties with coronal seal. A temporary post crown will not provide an adequate seal.[13] It is preferable to place a cast post and core immediately (which provides a better coronal seal) when a temporary crown is indicated.[12,13]

Restoration Design
PRINCIPLES AND CONCEPTS

Three practical principles for function and durability are the following:

1. *Conservation of tooth structure.* Most teeth requiring treatment are already compromised structurally; further dentin removal should be minimized.[22,24] On the other hand, cuspal reduction and capping may be necessary. Routinely decoronating and rebuilding an endodontically treated tooth is an outdated measure.
2. *Retention.* The coronal restoration is retained by the core and remaining dentin. If the core requires retention, then the canal system is used, with provision of a post. The post weakens and may perforate the root and should be placed only to retain the core.[14,24]
3. *Protection of remaining tooth structure.* In posterior teeth, this applies to protecting unsupported cusps to minimize flexure and fracture. The restoration is designed to transmit functional loads through the tooth to the suspensory apparatus.

PLANNING THE DEFINITIVE RESTORATION

Restoration planning begins before root canal treatment is started. The plan may be modified after the restoration and/or after caries is removed and the access is prepared and as treatment progresses. Visualizing the restorative preparation in advance ensures that structural requirements of the core will be preserved.

For anterior teeth, the choice of final restoration is somewhat limited. Wherever possible, restoration of the access (e.g., acid-etch composite) is used; this is sufficient for teeth that are otherwise largely intact. For more extensively damaged teeth (trauma, large proximal restorations), full coronal coverage supported by a post/core is indicated. The choices for premolars and molars are more varied.[25]

Direct Restoration

Restorations inserted directly into the prepared cavity (amalgam or composite) may be conservative, but a requirement is that the restoration protects against coronal fracture. Indications include the following:

1. Minimal tooth structure has been lost before and during root canal treatment. A conventional access cavity in a tooth with intact marginal ridges is restored without further preparation.
2. Prognosis is uncertain, requiring a durable semipermanent restoration.
3. Ease of placement and cost.

Many posterior teeth may be restored with amalgam if unsupported cusps are adequately protected.[26] A conventional class II amalgam will not achieve this, and ordinarily should not be used.[6,27] As a general guideline, cusps adjacent to a lost marginal ridge should be onlaid, with sufficient thickness of amalgam (at least 3 to 4 mm) to resist occlusal forces. This is a significant reduction. Premolars are more vulnerable to fracture than molars and should have both cusps onlaid when a marginal ridge is involved.[6] In molars, coverage only of cusps adjacent to a lost marginal ridge will generally be adequate if the remaining cusps and marginal ridge are not undermined. The amalgam should extend into the pulp chamber and canal orifices to aid retention.

Advantages of amalgam as a permanent restoration include significantly less cost and fewer appointments; the longevity of extensive amalgam restorations is similar to that of cast

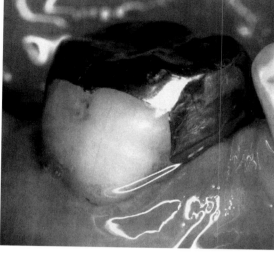

FIGURE 15-4
Cast gold onlay incorporates a reverse bevel for additional protection against cuspal flexure.

restorations.[28] The amalgam may subsequently serve as a core for indirect cast restoration if indicated (see Figure 15-3).

Composite resins have a limited role in direct restoration of posterior teeth.[29] With an occlusal access surrounded by enamel, acid-etch composites may prove sufficient. Bonded restorations (amalgam and composite) will probably be more widely used in the future, as bonding materials and techniques continue to improve.[29,30] However, at present amalgam bonding has few documented benefits in long-term clinical usage, and bond failure is likely to be catastrophic for otherwise unsupported cusps.[31,32]

Indirect restorations

Cast restorations (onlays, ¾ and full crowns) provide the greatest occlusal protection and are optimal if there is extensive loss of tooth structure. The attractiveness of onlays is that the cavity design usually requires little additional tooth tissue removal other than for the cusp onlays (Figure 15-4). The access cavity should be sealed with an amalcore or glass ionomer, which forms a base for the casting. The strength of gold allows conservative tooth reduction and a reverse bevel for greater cusp reinforcement.

A full crown is a reliable, strong restoration that protects against crown-root fracture.[4,24,33] Tooth reduction often removes most remaining coronal tooth structure; for retention, a core must be placed (and occasionally a post) to retain the core. To plan the core shape, there must be

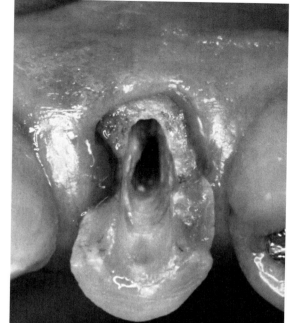

A

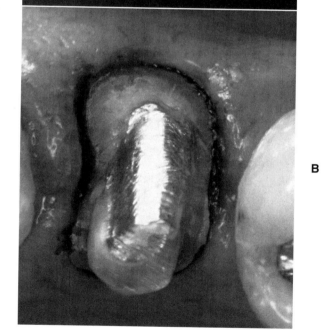

B

FIGURE 15-5
A, The gingival margin of the premolar is obscured by gingival overgrowth. **B**, The margins have been exposed by electrosurgery, and the core has been fabricated and cemented.

complete exposure of the margins. Gingival retraction cord and electrosurgery are useful for exposure, and prevent undersized cores being made because of incomplete viewing of the margins (Figure 15-5).

Full crowns should be used only when there is insufficient coronal tooth structure present for a more conservative restoration or if functional or parafunctional stresses require the splinting effect of full coronal coverage. Full crowns have been overused based on the mistaken concept that the treated tooth is weak and requires maximal protection.

Preparation of Canal Space and Tooth

POST SELECTION

A post retains the core; the need for a post is dictated by the amount of remaining coronal tooth structure. A major disadvantage is that posts do not reinforce the tooth, but further weaken it by additional removal of dentin and by creating stresses that predispose to root fracture.[7,14,24]

A post system should be selected that fits the requirements of the tooth and restoration. The tooth and restoration should not be prepared and adapted to the post system; rather, the post system and preparation design should be selected as appropriate to the situation.

There is much debate on how the post should interact with the tooth under load. Should the post material be similar in stiffness to root dentin (carbon fiber), somewhat stiffer (titanium and gold), or much stiffer (stainless steel and cobalt-chromium alloys)?[34] Stiffer posts may lead to tooth fracture, whereas the more flexible posts deform with the tooth, and tend to fail without fracturing the tooth.[35] Bonding between the post and the tooth may allow the restored tooth to deform more with loading, compared with the conventional approach of the indirect restoration being much more rigid than the tooth. Long-term clinical trials will determine how posts should interact with teeth, and what degree of stiffness functions best.

A further consideration is that of radiopacity; titanium posts have a radiopacity similar to that of gutta-percha, which can create clinical uncertainty.[36] All post designs are predisposed to leakage, particularly temporary post/core/crown systems.[13]

POST SPACE PREPARATION

Both chamber and canal may retain the restoration, and, in many instances, are essential. When a post is required for core retention, the minimum post space (length, diameter, and taper) should be prepared consistent with that need. Preparation consists of removing gutta-percha to the required

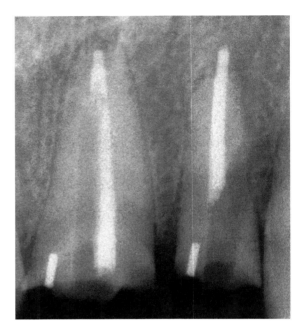

FIGURE 15-6
Post space preparation has led to a perforation in one incisor and unnecessary weakening of the other as a result of divergence from the canal space during gutta-percha removal by rotary instruments.

length, followed by enlargement and shaping to receive the post. Caution is required; removing excess gutta-percha results in a defective apical seal.[37,38] Also, excessive dentin removal seriously weakens the root, which may predispose to root fracture.[39] A perforation may occur if the cutting instrument deviates from the canal or if the preparation is too large or extends beyond the straight portion of the canal (Figure 15-6). Radiographs may be deceptive as a guide to root curvature and diameter by disguising root concavities and faciolingual curves.[40] As a general rule, post diameter should be minimal, particularly apically, and not more than one third of the root diameter.[41] Tapered post preparation prevents a step at the apical post space, which predisposes to wedging and root fracture.

Removal of Gutta-Percha

Whenever possible, gutta-percha is removed immediately after obturation to ensure the most predictable apical seal.[42] At this stage the dentist is most familiar with the canal features, including shape, length, size, and curvature. Depending on the obturation technique, the canal may be filled only to the desired length, or gutta-percha may be removed to length using a hot instrument. The re-

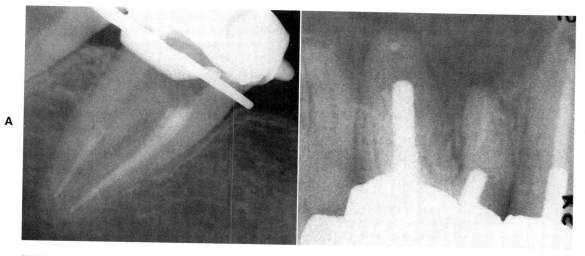

FIGURE 15-7
Gutta-percha removal. **A,** Enough remains in the distal canal to preserve the apical seal. **B,** Excessive removal from the palatal canal. This probably eliminated the apical seal and left a space between the post and gutta-percha. A radiograph taken before post placement would have allowed correction.

maining gutta-percha is then vertically condensed in the apical canal before the sealer has set. The obturation radiograph will confirm that sufficient gutta-percha remains (4 to 5 mm).

Gutta-percha removal at a subsequent appointment is satisfactory. Again, the safest procedure is use of a heated instrument. Gutta-percha is removed in increments to the desired length, using a heat carrier or plugger. Any instrument that penetrates to the desired depth can be used, so long as it has sufficient heat capacity. An alternative means of removal include solvents and mechanical. Problems with solvents such as chloroform, xylene, or eucalyptol include messiness and unpredictable depth of penetration. Use of rotary instruments, especially Peeso reamers, requires caution because of their tendency to diverge and perforate or at least seriously damage the root. They may also "grab" and displace the apical gutta-percha. Specially designed rotary nickel-titanium instruments rotating at low speeds may be more effective.

Whatever technique of removal is used, sufficient gutta-percha must remain to preserve the seal. At least 4 mm of gutta-percha is recommended (Figure 15-7), and this should be confirmed radiographically before the post is cemented.[37,38]

Finishing the Post Space

The post space is then further refined. If gutta-percha has been adequately removed, use of rotary instruments for final canal shaping should not be a problem. The bulk of the canal preparation has been achieved by the endodontic treatment, requiring only small refinements. Parallel sided drills generate significant temperature increase; final shaping should be by hand manipulation of the cutting instrument, since only small amounts of tooth need be removed.[43]

Retention and Core Systems

ANTERIOR TEETH

These teeth must withstand lateral forces from mandibular excursive movements, which if transmitted via a post, tend to split the root. Consideration should be given to the occlusal scheme. Where possible, the excursive load should be limited, with more force being borne by adjacent, more structurally sound teeth.

The optimal design is a cast metal post and core, prepared as a single unit. The post portion provides unit strength and retention, and the core cannot separate from the post. Custom fitting of the post and core permits minimal dentin removal both from canal space and coronally, plus maximum ferrule effect without crown lengthening (Figure 15-8).[44] Importantly, core shape should conform to the remaining coronal tooth structure, rather than machining the tooth for a standard core or technique. The small cross-sectional area of posts for mandibular incisors may result in casting porosities; it is possible to use a wrought gold alloy post as a basis for the addition of a cast core.

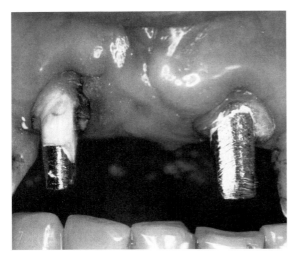

FIGURE 15-8
Cast post/cores in maxillary incisors. The preparation on the left shows extensive coronal dentin providing maximal ferrule effect; the preparation on the right illustrates minimal coronal dentin and little ferrule effect.

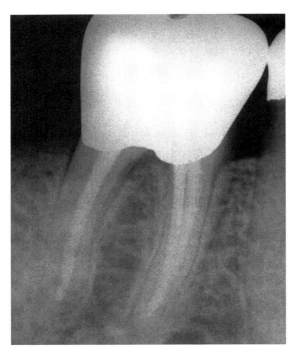

FIGURE 15-9
Molar correctly restored without a post and with a full crown. The decision to use a post depends on remaining coronal tooth structure and the retention provided by the chamber.

Use of a prefabricated post with direct core buildup is a last resort for an anterior tooth and is generally contraindicated. If used, a preformed post should be passive to minimize wedging forces. Also, passive fit facilitates removing the post for retreatment. Screw-retained posts are contraindicated—they predispose to vertical root fracture and are difficult to remove.

POSTERIOR TEETH

Premolars with substantial loss of coronal structure are also generally best restored with a cast post and core. Narrow mesiodistal root width does not permit adequate core thickness in association with a prefabricated post. Minimal enlargement during post space preparation is essential to preserve sufficient dentin thickness.[41] In maxillary premolars with two roots, only the palatal canal should be used for the post; the buccal furcation groove and narrow root preclude use of the buccal root.[41,45] A small, short (2 to 3 mm) post in the buccal canal provides some retention and antirotation.

Molars, which have larger pulp chambers, permit direct core options; the volume of the core is greater and the chamber shape provides retention. Most molars are restored with the direct core only, without a post (Figure 15-9). However, with minimal remaining coronal tooth structure and a small pulp chamber, a post may be placed in one canal for additional retention. Cast post/core systems are rarely necessary and should be considered only when essentially no coronal tooth structure remains.

The longest and straightest canal is preferred for the post, usually the palatal canal of maxillary molars and the distal canal of mandibular molars.[40] Other canals are narrower and more curved and are in weaker roots with surface concavities. These should be used only (and cautiously) if other factors preclude placement in the larger canals. Core retention is supplemented by extending the core material 2 to 3 mm into the remaining canal orifices.

A wide variety of passively seated prefabricated posts is available. Parallel-sided posts provide greater retention than tapered posts and do not wedge. They require more post space preparation; matching post size to canal size is important to minimize dentin removal. The post need not contact dentin throughout its length to achieve adequate retention (this is important in distal canals of mandibular molars, which are often broad cervically). Threaded screw posts should not be used.

Molar core design is simple and placement of the core requires little removal of tooth structure. A coronoradicular core of amalgam (amalcore) condensed into the chamber and slightly into canal orifices is preferred and provides a passive, strong core; an amalgam bonding agent may also be used.[45,46] With fast-setting amalgam, the crown may be prepared at the same visit, although preparation is easier when the material is fully set. An alternative is resin composite, which does not have the strength or long-term sealability of amalgam. However, composite resin has the advantage of allowing immediate crown preparation[47] (Figure 15-10). Glass ionomer cements do not have sufficient shear strength.

PINS

There is no need for retentive pins. The stresses and microfractures generated in dentin and the risk of perforation by pins outweigh any potential gain in retention of the restoration. Pins have been suggested for antirotation of the post/core; this is best achieved by other means such as a slightly out-of-round preparation.

Restoring Access Through an Existing Restoration

Occasionally, pulps undergo irreversible pulpitis or necrosis after placement of a crown, requiring root canal treatment (Figure 15-11).[33] Access through the restoration, with subsequent permanent repair of the opening is often preferred.

For the restoration to remain functional, three conditions must be met: (1) the interface between the restoration and the repair material must provide a good coronal seal; (2) retention of the restoration must not be compromised; and (3) the final core structure must support the restoration against functional or minor traumatic stresses. Access, particularly if overextended, may leave only a thin shell of dentin, especially in anterior teeth and premolars. Retention then depends almost entirely on the repair material. Fortunately, the chamber and canal are available to create a core that provides adequate retention and support in most instances. Placement of a dowel or post through an access or through an existing restoration adds no support and little retention and is rarely indicated.

The repair material should have high compressive and shear strength. In most situations, amalgam is preferred. It improves retention, maintains and even improves its seal with time, and is easily condensed into the entire chamber and access cavity as a single unit.[48] Composite resins, glass ionomer cements, and glass cermets do not have the requisite shear strength. Amalgam also functions well in anterior teeth with porcelain-fused-to-metal restorations. If esthetics is a problem, a new restoration is the first choice. A layer of composite can be placed over the amalgam core but serves only as a short-term repair. Inlays or gold foil to restore access openings through gold castings offer no advantage and do not merit the effort and cost.

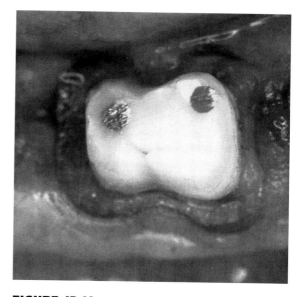

FIGURE 15-10
Restoration of a decoronated mandibular molar. Cemented parallel-sided posts retain a composite core. Inability to condense amalgam dictated the use of composite resin, placed and cured in many increments.

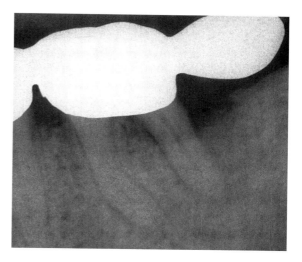

FIGURE 15-11
Pulp necrosis several years after preparation and placement of a cantilever bridge. Root canal treatment is required through the crown, with attendant risks of perforation and/or loss of retention.

Temporary Restorations

Many endodontic procedures involve multiple visits. Also, unless the final restoration is limited to a routine access cavity, root canal treatment and final restoration are usually not completed in the same appointment. A temporary restoration is

The temporary restoration must do the following:

1. Seal coronally, preventing ingress of oral fluids and bacteria and egress of intracanal medicaments.
2. Enhance isolation during treatment procedures.
3. Protect tooth structure until the final restoration is placed.
4. Allow ease of placement and removal.
5. Satisfy esthetics, but this is always as a secondary consideration to providing a seal.

Cotton Pellet

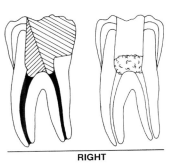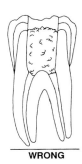

RIGHT   WRONG

FIGURE 15-12
Techniques for temporization. Shown on the left are the correct techniques; either minimal space is occupied by cotton or no cotton pellet is used, particularly if the proximal surface is to be restored. It is wrong to nearly fill the chamber with cotton, which leaves inadequate space and strength for the temporary restorative material (3 to 4 mm are required). (Courtesy Dr. L. Wilcox.)

thus required. The temporary restoration is normally in place for 1 to 4 weeks. In special situations such as apexification or delayed permanent restoration, the temporary restoration must last several months.

OBJECTIVES OF TEMPORIZATION

Objectives depend on the intended duration of use. Thus different materials are required, depending on time, occlusal load and wear, complexity of access, and loss of tooth structure.

ROUTINE ACCESS CAVITIES

Most access cavities involve only one surface and are surrounded by dentin walls or by porcelain or metal (if the restoration is retained). The temporary restoration must last from several days to several weeks. Numerous types are available, including premixed cements that set on contact with moisture (Cavit), intermediate restorative materials (IRM), glass ionomer cements, and specially formulated light-cured composite materials such as temporary endodontic restorative material (TERM).[49-51] Ease of use and good sealing ability make Cavit a good routine material, but low strength and rapid occlusal wear limit its use to short-term sealing of simple access cavities. Intermediate restorative materials provide improved wear resistance. TERM undergoes polymerization shrinkage followed by expansion resulting from water sorption. Its seal is comparable to that of Cavit, with superior strength and wear limits. More durable restorative materials (composites and glass ionomer cements) tend to provide the best seal.[51] It is not known whether experimental leakage differences based on bacterial leakage or dye penetration are significant clinically. Most critical are the thickness and placement of the material.

Techniques of Placement

The quality of the coronal seal depends on the thickness of the material, how it is compacted into the cavity, and the extent of contact with sound tooth structure or restoration. A minimum depth of 3 to 4 mm is required around the periphery and preferably 4 mm or more to allow for wear. In anterior teeth, the access is oblique to the tooth surface; care must be taken to ensure that the material is at least 3 mm thick in the cingulum area.

IRM and Cavit (or a similar material) are placed as follows. The chamber and cavity walls should be dry, with a thin layer of cotton (except in a class II situation) over the canal orifices to prevent canal blockage (Figure 15-12). Cavit is packed into the access opening with a plastic instrument in increments from the bottom up and pressed against the cavity walls and into undercuts (Figure 15-13). The excess is removed, and the surface is smoothed with moist cotton. The patient should avoid chewing on the tooth for at least 1 hour. TERM is prepackaged by the manufacturer in compules, ready for injection into the access. The material is inserted, packed with a plastic instrument, adjusted occlusally, and then light-cured.

EXTENSIVE CORONAL BREAKDOWN

Teeth without marginal ridges or with undermined cusps may require a stronger filling material (high-strength glass ionomer cement), with care being taken to ensure adequate thickness and good marginal adaptation proximally. Reducing the height of undermined cusps reduces

Blob Technique

Incremental Technique

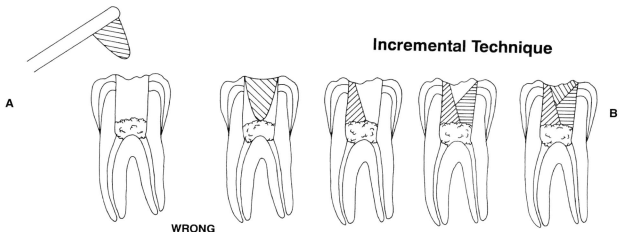

A

B

WRONG

FIGURE 15-13
Techniques for placing temporary restoration material. **A,** The "blob" technique is wrong because it does not seal the walls. **B,** The incremental technique, which adds successive layers, pressing each against the chamber walls, is correct. (Courtesy Dr. L. Wilcox.)

the risk of fracture. For severely broken-down teeth, a cusp-onlay amalgam or occasionally a well-fitting orthodontic band cemented onto the tooth (restored with glass ionomer cement) provides a durable temporary restoration. At the next appointment, access is cut through the restoration.

TEMPORARY POST CROWNS

Interappointment temporary crowns are generally contraindicated. In most situations if a crown is in place, it must be removed during the root canal procedure and then recemented after temporization of the access.

Esthetic restoration of anterior teeth is challenging if little coronal structure remains. A temporary crown retained with a post (preformed aluminum post, paper clip, or a sectioned large endodontic file) has inherent problems. Using the canal space for a temporary post precludes use of an intracanal medicament, and the coronal seal depends entirely on the temporary cement. The coronal seal is generally inadequate with a loosely fitting and mobile temporary post and crown.[13] If a temporary crown is placed, fabrication should preferably be done under rubber dam, with adjacent teeth also isolated to assist in preparing contacts.

The temporary post should fit the canal snugly (not binding) and extend apically 4 to 5 mm short of working length and coronally to within 2 to 3 mm of the incisal edge. A polycarbonate shell is

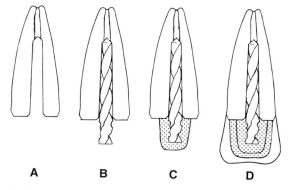

A   **B**   **C**   **D**

FIGURE 15-14
Technique sequence for anterior temporary post-core-crown fabrication. **A,** Post space is prepared. **B,** A temporary post of the proper size is fitted. **C,** A polycarbonate crown is adapted, filled with resin, and seated over the post. Excess resin is trimmed from the margins after the resin has set. **D,** The post/crown is cemented using a temporary cement such as Temp Bond.

trimmed to a good fit; self-curing material then is added to the inside of the shell to mold to the root face and attach to the post. The temporary luting cement (Temp Bond or similar cement) is placed on the coronal 3 to 4 mm of the post and root face, and the unit is cemented into place (Figure 15-14). A provisional removable partial overdenture is a useful alternative; access remains excellent, and there is little chance of disturbing the coronal seal between appointments.

LONG-TERM TEMPORARY RESTORATIONS

Restorations for procedures such as apexification may last for months, up to 2 years. For routine access openings, a durable restoration such as amalgam, glass ionomer cement, or acid-etch composite should be used, allowing sufficient thickness to ensure strength and a long-term seal. If the permanent restoration is delayed, these semipermanent temporary restorations are generally sufficient.

REFERENCES

1. Vire DE: Failure of endodontically treated teeth: classification and evaluation, *J Endod* 17:338, 1991.
2. Sjögren U, Hägglund B, Sundqvist G, Wing K: Factors affecting the long-term results of endodontic treatment, *J Endod* 16:498, 1990.
3. Friedman S: Treatment outcome and prognosis of endodontic therapy. In Orstavik D, Pitt Ford TR, editors, *Essential endodontology,* Oxford, 1998, Blackwell Science, p. 368.
4. Sorensen JA, Martinoff JT: Intracoronal reinforcement and coronal coverage: a study of endodontically treated teeth, *J Prosthet Dent* 51:780, 1984.
5. Weine FS, Wax AH, Wenckus CS: Retrospective study of tapered, smooth post systems in place for 10 years or more, *J Endod* 17:293, 1991.
6. Hansen EK, Asmussen E, Christiansen NC: In vivo fractures of endodontically treated posterior teeth restored with amalgam, *Endod Dent Traumatol* 6:49, 1990.
7. Goodacre CJ, Spolnik KJ: The prosthodontic management of endodontically treated teeth: a literature review. Part I. Success and failure data, treatment concepts, *J Prosthodont* 3:243, 1994.
8. Saunders WP, Saunders EM: Coronal leakage as a cause of failure in root-canal therapy: a review, *Endod Dent Traumatol* 10:105, 1994.
9. Ray H, Trope M: Periapical status of endodontically treated teeth in relation to the technical quality of the root filling and the coronal restoration, *Int Endod J* 28:12, 1995.
10. Magura ME, Kafrawy AH, Brown CE Jr, Newton CW: Human saliva coronal microleakage in obturated root canals: an in vitro study, *J Endod* 17:324, 1991.
11. Wolcott JF, Hicks ML, Himel VT: Evaluation of pigmented intraorifice barriers in endodontically treated teeth, *J Endod* 25:589, 1999.
12. Fogel HM: Microleakage of posts used to restore endodontically treated teeth, *J Endod* 21:376, 1995.
13. Fox K, Gutteridge DL: An in vitro study of coronal microleakage in root-canal-treated teeth restored by the post and core technique, *Int Endod J* 30:361, 1997.
14. Gutmann JL: The dentin—root complex: anatomic and biologic considerations in restoring endodontically treated teeth, *J Prosthet Dent* 67:458, 1992.
15. Sorensen JA, Engelman MJ: Effect of post adaptation on fracture resistance of endodontically treated teeth, *J Prosthet Dent* 64:419, 1990.
16. Papa J, Cain C, Messer HH: Moisture content of endodontically treated vs vital teeth, *Endod Dent Traumatol* 10:91, 1994.
17. Huang T–J, Schilder H, Nathanson D: Effects of moisture content and endodontic treatment on some mechanical properties of human dentin, *J Endod* 18:209, 1992.
18. Sedgley CM, Messer HH: Are endodontically treated teeth more brittle? *J Endod* 18:332, 1992.
19. Reeh ES, Messer HH, Douglas WH: Reduction in tooth stiffness as a result of endodontic and restorative procedures, *J Endod* 15:512, 1989.
20. Hood JAA: Biomechanics of the intact, prepared and restored tooth: some clinical implications, *Int Dent J* 41:25, 1991.
21. Panitvisai P, Messer HH: Cuspal deflection in molars in relation to endodontic and restorative procedures, *J Endod* 21:57, 1995.
22. Hansen EK, Asmussen E: Cusp fracture of endodontically treated posterior teeth restored with amalgam. Teeth restored in Denmark before 1975 versus after 1979, *Acta Odont Scand* 51:73, 1993.
23. Safavi KE, Dowden WE, Langeland K: Influence of delayed coronal permanent restoration on endodontic prognosis, *Endod Dent Traumatol* 3:187, 1987.
24. Assif D, Gorfil C: Biomechanical considerations in restoring endodontically treated teeth, *J Prosthet Dent* 71:565, 1994.
25. Morgano SM, Brackett SE: Foundation restorations in fixed prosthodontics: current knowledge and future needs, *J Prosthet Dent* 82:643, 1999.
26. Plasmans PJJM, Creugers NHJ, Mulder J: Long-term survival of extensive amalgam restorations, *J Dent Res* 77:453, 1998.
27. Linn J, Messer HH: Effect of restorative procedures on the strength of endodontically treated molars, *J Endod* 20:479, 1994.
28. Martin JA, Bader JD: Five year treatment outcomes for teeth with large amalgams and crowns, *Oper Dent* 22:72, 1997.
29. Steele A, Johnson BR: In vitro fracture strength of endodontically premolars, *J Endod* 25:6, 1999.
30. Roulet J-F: Benefits and disadvantages of tooth-coloured alternatives to amalgam, *J Dent* 25:459, 1997.
31. Mahler DB, Engle JH: Clinical evaluation of amalgam bonding in class I and II restorations, *J Am Dent Assoc* 131:43, 2000.
32. Davis R, Overton JD: Efficacy of bonded and non-bonded amalgam in the treatment of teeth with incomplete fractures, *J Am Dent Assoc* 131:469, 2000.
33. Valderhaug J, Jokstad A, Ambjornsen E, Norheim PW: Assessment of the periapical and clinical status of crowned teeth over 25 years, *J Dent* 25:97, 1997.
34. Asmussen E, Peutzfeld A, Heitmann T: Stiffness, elastic limit, and strength of newer types of endodontic posts, *J Dent* 27:275, 1999.
35. Martinez-Insua A, da Silva L, Santana U: Comparison of the fracture resistances of pulpless teeth restored with a cast post and core or carbon-fiber post with a composite core, *J Prosthet Dent* 80:527, 1998.

36. Kleier D, Shibilski K, Averbach RE: Radiographic appearance of titanium posts in endodontically treated teeth, *J Endod* 25:128, 1999.

37. Gish SP, Drake DR, Walton RE, Wilcox L: Coronal leakage: bacterial penetration through obturated canals following post preparation, *J Am Dent Assoc* 125:1369, 1994.

38. Kvist T, Rydin E, Reit C: The relative frequency of periapical lesions in teeth with root canal-retained posts, *J Endod* 12:578, 1989.

39. Wilcox LR, Roskelley C, Sutton T: The relationship of root canal enlargement to finger-spreader induced vertical root fracture, *J Endod* 23:533, 1997.

40. Perez E, Zillich R, Yaman P: Root curvature localizations as indicators of post length in various tooth groups, *Endod Dent Traumatol* 2:58, 1986.

41. Raiden G, Costa L, Koss S, Hernandez JL: Residual thickness of root in first maxillary premolars with post space preparation, *J Endod* 25; 502, 1999.

42. Fan B, Wu M-K, Wesselink PR: Coronal leakage along apical root fillings after immediate and delayed post space preparation, *Endod Dent Traumatol* 15:124, 1999.

43. Hussey DL, Biagioni PA, McCullagh JJP, Lamey P-J: Thermographic assessment of heat generated on the root surface during post space preparation, *Int Endod J* 30:187, 1997.

44. Sorensen JA. Engelman MJ: Ferrule design and fracture resistance of endodontically treated teeth, *J Prosthet Dent* 63:529, 1990.

45. Tamse A, Katz A, Pilo R: Furcation groove of buccal root of maxillary first premolars—a morphometric study, *J Endod* 26:359, 2000.

46. Nayyar A, Walton RE, Leonard LA: An amalgam coronal-radicular dowel and core technique for endodontically treated posterior teeth, *J Prosthet Dent* 43:511, 1980.

47. Davalou S, Gutmann JL, Nunn MH: Assessment of apical and coronal root canal seals using contemporary endodontic obturation and restorative materials and techniques, *Int Endod J* 32:388, 1999.

48. Mulvay PG, Abbott PV: The effect of endodontic access cavity preparation and subsequent restorative procedures on molar crown retention, *Aust Dent J* 41:134, 1996.

49. Deveaux E, Hildelbert P, Neut C, Romond C: Bacterial microleakage of Cavit, IRM, TERM, and Fermit: a 21-day in vitro study, *J Endod* 25:653, 1999.

50. Barthel CR, Strobach A, Briedigkeit H, et al: Leakage in roots coronally sealed with different temporary fillings, *J Endod* 25:731, 1999.

51. Uranga A, Blum J-Y, Esber S, et al: A comparative study of four coronal obturation materials in endodontic treatment, *J Endod* 25:178, 1999.

16

J. Craig Baumgartner

Endodontic Microbiology

LEARNING OBJECTIVES

After reading this chapter, the student should be able to:

1 / Define terms associated with endodontic microbiology.

2 / Describe portals of entry of microorganisms to the pulp and periradicular tissues.

3 / Understand the significance of bacteria in pulpal and periradicular diseases.

4 / Describe the predominant bacteria and discuss microbial virulence factors and the microbial ecosystem associated with endodontic infections.

5 / Describe the reaction of pulp and periradicular tissues to bacteria.

6 / Understand infection control as applied to endodontic practice.

7 / Discuss the rationale for débridement of the root canal system.

8 / Understand the importance of drainage in treating acute apical infections (abscess).

9 / Describe the indications and methods for microbial sampling of endodontic infections.

OUTLINE

Bacteria Associated with Endodontic Infections
Terminology
Portals of Entry to the Pulp
Caries and Pulpal Disease
Reaction of Pulp to Bacteria
Polymicrobial Infections
Microbial Ecosystem in the Root Canal

Association of Bacteria with Periradicular Disease
Virulence Factors
Correlations with Pathoses and Treatment

Infection Control

Treatment of Endodontic Infections
Débridement of the Root Canal System
Intracanal Medication
Drainage
When and How to Culture

Most pathoses of the dental pulp and periradicular tissues are either directly or indirectly related to microorganisms. Knowledge of the bacteria associated with endodontic pathoses is important in understanding the disease process and in developing a sound rationale for treatment. This chapter discusses microorganisms associated with pulpal and periradicular diseases, infection control, and the principles of treatment of endodontic infections.

Bacteria Associated with Endodontic Infections

TERMINOLOGY

Colonization is the establishment of bacteria or other microorganisms in a living host. Colonization occurs if appropriate biochemical and physical conditions are available for growth and inhibitory factors are inadequate to destroy the organisms. *Permanent colonization* in a symbiotic relationship with the host results in establishment of normal oral flora. These organisms participate in many beneficial relationships but are considered *opportunistic pathogens* if they gain access to a normally sterile area of the body and produce disease.

Infectious disease (infection) results if microorganisms damage the host and produce clinical signs and symptoms. Pulpal and periradicular pathoses (diseases) result from opportunistic pathogens infecting the pulp cavity and, at times, periradicular tissues.

Pathogenicity is the capacity of organisms to produce disease within a particular host. *Virulence* expresses the degree of pathogenicity in a host under defined circumstances. Stages in development of an endodontic infection include microbial invasion, colonization, multiplication, and pathogenic activity.

PORTALS OF ENTRY TO THE PULP

Microbes may take several routes to invade and infect the pulp. If enamel or cementum is missing, microorganisms may invade the pulp through exposed dentinal tubules. Caries are the most common source of bacterial penetration through the tubules. Bacteria can invade and multiply within permeable tubules. Importantly, bacterial penetration into dentinal tubules has been shown to be greater in teeth with necrotic pulps than in teeth with vital pulps.[1] Tubule permeability is reduced by the presence of various components of the dentinal fluid, the living odontoblastic processes, and the formation of peritubular dentin or tertiary dentin. Bacteria are preceded through the tubules by their byproducts and breakdown products, which may be pulp irritants. An example of this is the positive correlation between the presence of bacteria under restorations with pulpal inflammation.

Microorganisms may reach the pulp after direct pulpal exposure associated with caries, restorative procedures, or a traumatic injury that fractures, cracks, or displaces the tooth.[2] Pulp status is an important factor in susceptibility to microbial invasion. Vital pulp is very resistant to microbial invasion. Penetration of the surface of a healthy pulp by oral flora is relatively slow or may be blocked entirely. For example, if the pulp is exposed to the oral cavity following tooth fracture, the resulting inflammation, necrosis, and bacterial penetration extend no more than 2 mm into the pulp after 2 weeks. In contrast, a necrotic pulp is rapidly invaded and colonized by bacteria.[3]

There is also an intimate relationship between the pulp and periodontium via tubules, lateral or accessory canals, furcation canals, and the apical foramen. Pulpal necrosis and the egress of irritants by these routes may affect the periodontal ligament and surrounding attachment apparatus. The reverse seems less likely. It is debatable whether periodontal pathoses directly cause significant pulpal disease.[4,5] However, if periodontal disease involves the apex of a tooth, the pulp may become necrotic.[6] Presumably, pulpal inflammation results if bacteria can penetrate the lateral canals, furcation canals, or denuded dentin after periodontal treatment. The removal of cementum during periodontal therapy exposes dentinal tubules to oral flora. A study in humans after root planing demonstrated the presence of pulpitis, bacterial penetration into exposed dentinal tubules, and thermal sensitivity.[7]

Anachoresis is a process by which microorganisms are transported in the blood to an area of inflammation where they establish an infection. Investigators using animals have demonstrated the localization of blood-borne bacteria in inflamed pulp but not in instrumented unfilled canals.[8,9] How often (or whether) anachoresis contributes to pulpal or periradicular infections in humans has not been determined.

CARIES AND PULPAL DISEASE

The most common source of bacteria to the pulp is from caries. Bacteria associated with caries are not motile but apparently advance through the dentinal tubules by dividing (binary fission) and by dentinal fluid movement. In humans, mutans streptococci (mainly *Streptococcus mutans* and *Strep-*

tococcus sobrinus) have been associated with smooth surface and pit-fissure caries, whereas *Actinomyces* spp. have been associated with root caries. Although mutans streptococci are important in initiating caries, they may not be as important in the progression of deep caries. Bacteria in the deepest layers of caries are predominantly strict anaerobes.[10] After exposure of the dental pulp by caries, numerous species of opportunistic oral flora may invade and colonize necrotic tissue. This allows microbial selection by the ecosystem associated with infections of endodontic origin.[11,12]

REACTION OF PULP TO BACTERIA

Like other connective tissues, pulp responds to irritants with (1) nonspecific inflammation and (2) specific immunologic reactions. Pulpal inflammation from caries begins as an insidious chronic cellular response characterized by the presence of lymphocytes, plasma cells, and macrophages. The response to caries by the pulp-dentin complex includes the formation of peritubular dentin, decreased permeability of dentinal tubules, and often, production of tertiary dentin.[13,14] This irregular tertiary dentin is less tubular and presumably acts as a barrier to the invading caries. Generally, the pulp is not severely (not irreversibly) inflamed when caries do not penetrate to the pulp.

After pulp exposure by caries, numerous species of opportunistic oral flora may colonize the exposed tissue. Polymorphonuclear (PMN) leukocytes characteristic of acute inflammation are chemotactically attracted to the area. An accumulation of PMN leukocytes results in abscess formation. The pulp may remain inflamed for a long time or may undergo rapid necrosis. The dynamics of the pulpal reaction is related to the virulence of the bacteria, host response, amount of pulpal circulation, and degree of drainage. Because it is surrounded by hard tissue, the inflamed pulp is located in a unique low-compliance environment.[15] This low compliance causes increased intrapulpal pressure when extravascular inflammatory cells and fluids accumulate. The increased pressure further interferes with normal circulation and cell function, making the cells more susceptible to injury or death.

POLYMICROBIAL INFECTIONS

The intimate association between microorganisms and endodontic pathoses was demonstrated in rats by Kakehashi and associates.[16] After exposure of the dental pulp to the oral cavity, abscesses, pulpal necrosis, and periradicular inflammatory lesions developed in rats with normal microbial flora but not in germ-free rats. In the germ-free animals, pulpal inflammation resulting from exposure was minimal.[16] In humans, when bacteria reach the pulp, it may become inflamed but stay vital for some time, or quickly become necrotic. Microorganisms invade the necrotic pulp, multiply, and infect the root canal system, including the dentinal tubules (Figure 16-1). Once the pulp becomes necrotic, it becomes a reservoir for microorganisms, microbial byproducts, and microbial breakdown products. Endodontic infections include infections of both the pulp cavity and the periradicular diseased tissues.

Of about 500 species of bacteria recognized as normal oral flora, only a relatively small group are commonly isolated from infected pulp cavities. Strict anaerobic bacteria predominate, with some facultative anaerobes and, rarely, aerobes. Many bacteria (especially strict anaerobes) are difficult to cultivate. Differences in frequency of isolation from one study to another may be related to a number of variables including sampling technique, transport medium, culture medium, type of incubation, and method of identification.

Modern culturing techniques have demonstrated the association of polymicrobial opportunistic oral bacteria with pulpal and periradicular diseases. Sophisticated anaerobic technology provides an environment conducive to the growth of strict anaerobes. For example, in one study ex-

amining intact teeth with infected root canals, more than 90% of the bacteria were strict anaerobes (Table 16-1).[11] Another study isolated and identified bacteria from the apical 5 mm of infected root canals in teeth with carious pulpal exposures and associated periradicular lesions.[17] It was found that most (68%) of the isolates were strict anaerobes. The predominance of strict anaerobes suggests a selective process favoring the

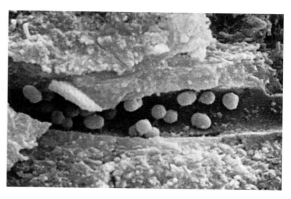

FIGURE 16-1
Cocci observed with scanning election microscopy in a tubule from a fractured root through a canal containing necrotic debris. Bacteria such as these, deep in tubules, may not be removed or killed during canal preparation or by intracanal medicaments.

TABLE 16-1		

Predominant Isolates from the Root Canals of 65 Teeth with Periapical Lesions

BACTERIAL SPECIES	NO. STRAINS ISOLATED	CHARACTERISTICS
Eubacterium spp.	59	Gram-positive rod, nonmotile
Peptostreptococcus spp.	54	Gram-positive cocci, nonmotile
Fusobacterium spp.	50	Gram-negative fusiform, nonmotile
Porphyromonas spp. (black-pigmented)	32	Gram-negative rod, nonmotile
Prevotella spp. (black-pigmented)	30	Gram-negative rod, nonmotile
Streptococcus spp.	28	Gram-positive cocci, nonmotile
Lactobacillus spp.*	24	Gram-positive rod, nonmotile
Wolinella spp.	18	Gram-negative rod, motile
Prevotella spp. (nonpigmented)	15	Gram-negative rod, nonmotile
Actinomyces spp.	14	Gram-positive rod, nonmotile
Propionibacterium spp.	7	Gram-positive rod, nonmotile
Capnocytophaga ochracea	7	Gram-negative fusiform, motile
Veillonella parvula	6	Gram-negative cocci, nonmotile
Selenomonas sputigena	6	Gram-negative rod, motile
Other spp.*	3	
Total number of strains isolated	353 (average 5.3 strains per root canal)	

Adapted from Sundqvist G: *Oral Microbiol Immunol* 7:257, 1992.
*Species isolated in low number or not identified to species level.

growth of anaerobes.[17] Importantly, the relative proportion of strict anaerobic bacteria to facultative bacteria increases with time, as does the total number of bacteria.[18]

The anaerobic genus *Bacteroides* has undergone major taxonomic revision, which has changed the nomenclature for the black-pigmented bacteria (BPB) associated with endodontic infections. Species of BPB were previously located in the genus *Bacteroides*. These species are nonmotile, non-spore-forming, Gram-negative rods. Three asaccharolytic species of BPB have been reclassified into a separate genus named *Porphyromonas* (Box 16-1).[19] Species of saccharolytic BPB have been reclassified into a separate genus named *Prevotella* (Box 16-1).[20] Several nonpigmented oral species of bacteria previously classified as *Bacteroides* have also been placed in the genus *Prevotella* (Box 16-1). The current nomenclature is used in this chapter.

Although no absolute correlation has been made between any species of bacteria and the clinical signs or symptoms of endodontic pathosis, BPB have been the most often implicated.[21-26] Other studies have found that *Porphyromonas gingivalis* and *Porphyromonas endodontalis* were isolated only from acute infections, whereas *Prevotella intermedia* was found with both symptomatic and asymptomatic infections.[27] Recently, with DNA methods, *Prevotella nigrescens* has been characterized as a species separate from *P. intermedia*.[28] Studies confirmed that *P. nigrescens* is the BPB most commonly cultivated from endodontic infections.[28-30]

Molecular methods have also been used to detect and identify the presence of another BPB, *Prevotella tannerae*, in endodontic infections. When the polymerase chain reaction was used to evaluate 118 microbial samples from endodontic infections, 60% of the samples tested positive for the presence of *P. tannerae*, although only 5 strains were cultivable.[31] Molecular methods will probably detect numerous other presently uncultivable microorganisms.

Other bacteria often associated with clinical signs and symptoms include *Prevotella buccae* and species of *Peptococcus*, *Peptostreptococcus*, *Eubacterium*, *Actinomyces*, and *Fusobacterium*.[24,26,32,33] Animal studies have demonstrated that purulent lesions may be induced with specific combinations of bacteria, especially strains of BPB.[18,34-36] However, no absolute causative relationship between specific microorganisms and endodontic disease have been defined.

Actinomyces and *Propionibacterium* species are able to persist in periradicular tissues in the presence of chronic inflammatory tissue.[37-39] Most of these infections apparently respond to conventional root canal treatment; however, surgery or antibiotics may be needed to resolve these infections.[37-39]

Recent studies have found a high incidence of the facultative anaerobe, *Streptococcus faecalis*, in root canals of teeth requiring retreatment of previous root canal therapy because of persistent inflammation.[40-42] A recent study found healing in 94% of the cases after a negative culture at the obturation appointment but only a 68% rate of healing if the cultures were positive at the time of obturation.[40] These studies support previous investigations that demonstrated absence of healing when canals are obturated in the presence of microbes in the root canal.[43]

Yeasts and viruses are also found in the pulp cavity. Fungi have been identified in root canals and in teeth refractory to endodontic treatment.[42-47] Viruses, including the human immunodeficiency virus (HIV), are present in the pulp and may be associated with endodontic disease.[48,49] The significance of intrapulpal viruses is unknown. A case report recently associated a herpes zoster infection with periodontal and endodontic disease.[50]

In summary, the microbial population in various endodontic pathoses and conditions has been

---

BOX 16-1

Recent Taxonomic Changes for Previous Bacteroides Species

Porphyromonas, black-pigmented (asaccharolytic *Bacteroides* species)
Porphyromonas asaccharolytica (usually nonoral)
*Porphyromonas gingivalis**
*Porphyromonas endodontalis**
Prevotella, black-pigmented (asaccharolytic *Bacteroides* species)
Prevotella melaninogenica
Prevotella denticola
Prevotella loescheii
Prevotella intermedia
Prevotella nigrescens†
Prevotella corporis
Prevotella tannerae
Prevotella, nonpigmented (saccharolytic *Bacteroides* species)
*Prevotella buccae**
Prevotella bivia
Prevotella oralis
Prevotella oris
Prevotella oulorum
Prevotella ruminicola

Studies have associated species with clinical signs and symptoms.
†Most commonly isolated black-pigmented bacteria from endodontic infections.

identified as being important, but is not yet thoroughly understood. This includes both the types of microorganisms and their significance. Future research should continue to clarify these issues.

MICROBIAL ECOSYSTEM IN THE ROOT CANAL

When a necrotic pulp is sampled, a mix of bacterial species are recovered. Because of the lack of circulation within a necrotic pulp, normal host defense mechanisms (inflammation and immunity) are absent or compromised. The pulp cavity supplies substrate and becomes a reservoir for invading microbes. The root canal system also is a special environment where selection results in a restricted group of bacteria. Tissue fluid and disintegrated cells from necrotic tissue form a substrate of nutrients (especially polypeptides and amino acids) essential for microorganisms. These nutrients, low oxygen tension, and bacterial interactions are the key ecologic determinants of which bacteria will predominate. Conditions favor the growth of anaerobes able to metabolize peptides and amino acids rather than carbohydrates. The growth of one bacterial species may depend on another commensal species, which supplies an essential nutrient as a metabolic byproduct. Figure 16-2 shows some of the possible complex nutritional relationships among bacteria in an infected root canal.[12]

Likewise, antagonistic relationships may develop among bacteria. Some by-products (e.g., ammonia) may be either a nutrient or a toxin, depending on the species of bacteria and the concentration of its by-products in the ecosystem. *Bacteriocins* are antibiotic-like proteins produced by one species of bacteria that inhibit the growth of other species.

Root canal treatment uses chemomechanical methods of débridement to disrupt, destroy, and remove the microbial ecosystem. This is accomplished through the cleaning and shaping process and the adjunctive use of antimicrobials within the pulp system. Effective obturation of the root canal space and coronal restoration prevents apical and coronal leakage and eliminates the pulp cavity as a reservoir of infection.

Association of Bacteria with Periradicular Disease

As stated earlier, the contents of infected root canals are potent irritants. The importance of bacteria and the development of apical periodontitis have been demonstrated.[16] Periradicular lesions

(disease) develop when the canal contains bacteria.[18,22,36,51] Evidence indicates that bacteria and bacterial by-products emanating from the root canal are the major irritants associated with periradicular inflammation. Bacterial by-products alone are capable of causing periradicular pathosis.[52]

VIRULENCE FACTORS

Bacterial virulence factors include fimbriae (pili), capsules, extracellular vesicles, lipopolysaccharides (LPSs), enzymes, short-chain fatty acids, polyamines, and low-molecular-weight products such as ammonia and hydrogen sulfide. Bacterial fimbriae are important for attachment to surfaces and to other bacteria. Fimbriae may be important in synergistic relationships between bacteria. Capsules are a significant resistance factor for bacteria, enabling them to avoid phagocytosis. BPB associated with endodontic infections may have such capsules.

Lipopolysaccharides

LPSs are found on the surface of Gram-negative bacteria and have numerous biologic effects that induce periradicular pathosis. LPSs have nonspecific antigens that are not well neutralized by antibodies. LPS antigens activate the complement cascade through both the classic and alternative pathways. When released from the cell wall, LPSs are known as endotoxins. A relationship has been established between the presence of endotoxins and the extent of periradicular inflammation.[52,53] Endotoxin is capable of diffusing across dentin. The content of LPSs in canals of symptomatic teeth with radiographically evident lesions and exudate is higher than that of asymptomatic teeth.[53-55]

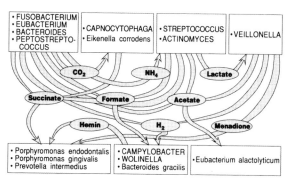

FIGURE 16-2
Possible nutritional relationships between bacteria in an infected root canal. A mixed microbial flora is necessary. Then, the dynamic interrelationships between the bacteria and host determine the degree of pathosis. (From Sundqvist G: *J Endod* 18:428, 1992.)

Enzymes

Bacteria produce enzymes (proteases) that neutralize immunoglobulins and complement components.[56-58] Recently the gene for collagenase, a metalloprotease associated with the spread of cellulitis, was detected in strains of *Porphyromonas gingivalis* isolated from endodontic infections.[59-61] In addition, hydrolytic enzymes released from PMN leukocytes in purulent infections have an adverse effect on surrounding tissues.

Extracellular Vesicles

Another type of irritant produced by Gram-negative bacteria is extracellular vesicles. These may be free endotoxin, blebs, and outer membrane fragments.[62] They have a trilaminar structure similar to that of the outer membrane of a Gram-negative bacterium (Figure 16-3). The vesicles contain enzymes or other products that affect host cells. These vesicles may be involved in hemagglutination, hemolysis, bacterial adhesion, and proteolytic activities.[62,63] They have the same antigenic determinants on their surface as their parent bacteria. They may protect the bacteria by neutralizing specific antibodies.

Fatty Acids

Anaerobic bacteria produce short-chain fatty acids such as propionic, butyric, and isobutyric acids. These acids are active virulence factors that affect neutrophil chemotaxis, degranulation, chemiluminescence, phagocytosis, and other intracellular changes. Research has shown that butyric acid offers greater inhibition of T-cell blastogenesis than does propionate or isobutyrate.[64] Butyric acid has been shown to stimulate production of interleukin-1, which is associated with bone resorption and periradicular pathosis.[64]

Polyamines

Biologically active polyamines have been found in infected canals.[65] Host cells and most bacteria, especially Gram-negative bacteria, contain large amounts of polyamines. Polyamines such as putrescine, cadaverine, spermidine, and spermine are involved in the regulation of cell growth, regeneration of tissues, and modulation of inflammation. Amounts of putrescine and total polyamines are higher in the necrotic pulps of teeth that are painful to percussion or those that have spontaneous pain. Teeth with a sinus tract have a significantly greater amount of cadaverine in the pulp space.[65] Although correlations such as these have been demonstrated, cause and effect relationships have not been proved for all virulence factors.

CORRELATIONS WITH PATHOSES AND TREATMENT

The association of specific species of bacteria with pulpal and periapical pathoses as well as with clinical signs and symptoms is not absolute. Endodontic infections are polymicrobial, with each species of bacteria having variable virulence factors. No single microorganism or group of bacteria has been proven to be more pathogenic than another. From a treatment point of view, all endodontic infections are considered polymicrobial and are treated accordingly. Root canal treatment of a necrotic pulp will disrupt the microbial ecosystem by removing bacteria, bacterial byproducts, and substrate from the root canal system.

In contrast to the necrotic debris and microbes sequestered in a pulp cavity, periradicular tissues have an excellent collateral blood supply, lymphatic drainage, and a large pool of undifferentiated cells. Eventually, periradicular pathoses develop primarily in response to microorganisms, microbial byproducts, and microbial breakdown products. The extent of the periradicular inflammatory reaction will depend on the severity of the irritation, its duration, and the host response. Mediators of both nonspecific inflammatory reactions and specific immunologic reactions participate in the formation and perpetuation of periradicular lesions (see Chapter 3).

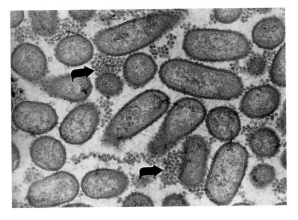

FIGURE 16-3
Extracellular vesicles *(arrows)* from the budding outer membrane of a strain of black-pigmented *Prevotella intermedia*, a suspected pathogen. The trilaminar structure is similar to that of the outer membrane of Gram-negative bacteria including lipopolysaccharides. These vesicles may be involved in hemagglutination, hemolysis, bacterial adhesion, and proteolytic activities (original magnification ×20,000).

Acute apical periodontitis (AAP) is the initial response that results from extension of pulpal inflammation to the periradicular tissues. Bacteria and their byproducts are usually involved in the process. Other factors that may be involved in AAP include inflammatory mediators from pulp, instrument trauma, and chemicals used during root canal treatment.

Microbiologic, histologic, and immunologic methods have been used to determine whether bacteria persist in the inflammatory tissue of asymptomatic chronic apical periodontitis (CAP). Whether bacteria can invade, colonize, and multiply in CAP is controversial. Different opinions result from different investigative techniques and interpretation of results. One prob-

lem with microbial sampling of periradicular lesions at the time of either periradicular surgery or tooth extraction is contamination of the sample by oral flora or by bacteria in the infected root canal. Results of culturing studies have been controversial and inconclusive.[66-69] Histologic evaluation of periradicular samples diagnosed as CAP rarely demonstrates bacteria in the tissue.[38,68,70,71] A scanning electron microscopic study demonstrated bacterial plaque on surgically resected root tips of teeth that were refractory to root canal treatment.[66] Other studies have shown a barrier of neutrophils or epithelium or an amorphous (necrotic) tissue between the bacteria in the canal and the periradicular inflammatory tissue (Figure 16-4).[38,70]

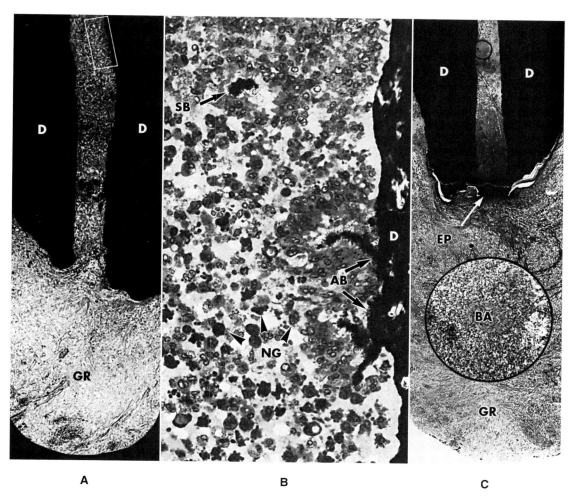

A   **B**   **C**

FIGURE 16-4

A, Resected apical third *(D)* of a human tooth with pulp necrosis and chronic apical periodontitis *(GR)*. **B,** The bacteria appear to be blocked by a wall of neutrophils *(NG)* or by **(C)** an epithelial plug *(EP)* in the apical foramen. Note dense aggregates of bacteria *(AB* in **B)** adherent to the dentin wall. Bacteria may clump *(SB* in **B)** or form loose collections *(BA* in *inset* in **C)** in the root canal. The infected canal becomes a sequestered reservoir for substrate and bacteria. (From Nair R: *J Endod* 13:31, 1987.)

Immunocytochemical methods have provided a means of identifying bacteria present in chronic periradicular lesions through the use of specific antisera to identify bacteria in the histologic sections. Only *Actinomyces israelii, Actinomyces naeslundii, Propionibacterium (Arachnia) propionica,* and *P. intermedia* have been identified using immunocytochemical methods in sections of periradicular lesions.[37,72,73] Any study that disturbs the periradicular tissues may allow their contamination with oral (or possibly intracanal) flora; also, the presence of a species of bacteria does not prove an etiologic relationship (cause and effect) with the periradicular pathosis.

Acute apical abscesses (AAAs), acute exacerbation of CAP (so-called "phoenix" abscesses), and suppurative apical periodontitis are characterized by large numbers of PMN leukocytes, necrotic tissue, and bacteria. Under certain circumstances (related to host resistance and virulence of bacteria) periradicular tissues are invaded and become involved in progressive infections (abscesses and cellulitis). The bacteria are polymicrobial and are similar to those isolated from infected root canals.[74-76] The number of strains of bacteria isolated from periradicular abscesses are on average more than five per sample, with most being strict anaerobes.[11,75,77] Thus, in both root canal infections and periradicular abscesses, a predominance of mixed strict anaerobes contributes to the disease.

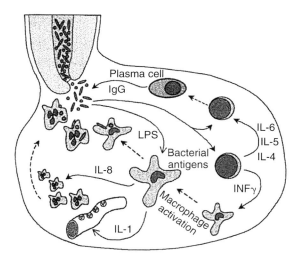

FIGURE 16-5
Protective role of activated macrophages and T-lymphocytes in periapical inflammatory granulomas. T-lymphocyte activation leads to antigen-specific B-lymphocyte activation and local production of specific antibodies. Healing will not occur until the bacteria are removed. (From Metzger ZV: *Endod Dent Traumatol* 16:3, 2000. © Munksgaard.)

Infection Control

Today's practice of dentistry, including endodontic procedures, requires universal precautions. All patients must be treated as if they have a transmissible disease. Precautions include preventing cross contamination between patients and health care providers. Not all exposures to microorganisms result in disease. Whether a disease is transmitted depends on the dose of the infective agent, the virulence of the microorganism, and the host resistance.

An effective way to reduce the dose of microorganisms is the use of physical barriers, which include the rubber dam, safety glasses or face shields, masks, gowns, and gloves. Once a rubber dam that seals against salivary contamination has been positioned, the tooth surface and surrounding rubber dam should be disinfected using sodium hypochlorite (NaOCl) or other accepted disinfectant. Irrigation of canals with sodium hypochlorite provides an additional chemical barrier against microorganisms for health care providers.

Endodontic procedures pose a risk for accidental percutaneous exposure to body fluids for both patient and dentist by burs, files, contaminated needles, instruments, spreaders and pluggers, Gates-Glidden drills, and so on. Techniques must be used to avoid accidental exposure to these sharp instruments. Disposable items are available to minimize the chances of contamination.

Treatment of Endodontic Infections

The microbial ecosystem of an infected root canal system and the subsequent inflammatory response of the periradicular tissue will persist until the source of irritation is removed (Figure 16-5). Treatment should establish an environment favorable for the host to resolve the disease. The key to successful treatment of periradicular disease is removal of the reservoir of infection (necrotic tissue, bacteria, and bacterial by-products) by thorough débridement.

DÉBRIDEMENT OF THE ROOT CANAL SYSTEM

Root canal débridement, as a part of the cleaning and shaping process, is the removal of substrates that support microorganisms. Because the root canal system is irregular, instruments do not reach all the fins, cul-de-sacs, indentations, and areas between the main canals. Irrigants flush out loose debris, provide lubrication, exert antimicrobial action, and dissolve some debris in the canal.

Sodium hypochlorite (NaOCl) (0.5% to 5.25%) is considered the irrigant of choice. NaOCl will dissolve some organic debris in areas not reached by instruments and is an excellent antimicrobial agent against those bacteria reached by the chemical.[78-86] The chemical activity of NaOCl should be maintained by frequent irrigation of the canals being instrumented.[78,84] A root canal system with necrotic pulpal debris may harbor bacteria in fins and other uninstrumented areas. Instrumentation combined with NaOCl irrigation accounts for tissue removal in the main canal but remains relatively ineffective in isthmi and fins.[87] Irrigants must reach the debris in these areas to be effective. Straight-line access and proper flaring of the root canal will enhance débridement and allow more efficient irrigation (see Chapter 13).

Instruments have been shown to produce an amorphous smear layer of burnished dentin and other debris about 1 to 4 μm thick on the root canal surface with plugs of the material extending up to 40 μm into the dentinal tubules.[88] The presence of a smear layer has been shown to affect the permeability of the dentin and to inhibit bacterial colonization; however, smear layer could harbor bacteria and decrease the effectiveness of intracanal antimicrobials.[79,89,90]

INTRACANAL MEDICATION

The antimicrobial function of intracanal medication between appointments is an important consideration. Microorganisms not removed from the canal will multiply.[85,91,92] Placement of a sterile dry cotton pellet may allow growth of bacteria.[86] Historically, intracanal medicaments were usually phenolics such as formocresol, camphorated parachlorophenol, eugenol, metacresylacetate, and halides (iodine-potassium iodide). These medicaments (particularly phenolics) are not recommended, being antigenic and cytotoxic, and function as antimicrobials for only a short time.[93-95] Clindamycin was recently tested as an intracanal medicament with questionable results.[96] There is concern that antibiotics that are normally used systemically may produce allergies or select for resistant organisms when used as intracanal medicaments.

Use of calcium hydroxide is recommended in canals with necrotic pulps after instrumentation. This chemical has a greater antimicrobial effect between appointments than the agents just listed.[97,98] Calcium hydroxide has some ability to dissolve pulp tissue in vitro but not in vivo.[87,99,100] However, intracanal use of calcium hydroxide may increase the effectiveness of sodium hypochlorite at the subsequent appointment, which should also enhance the effectiveness of antimicrobial agents.[101]

Calcium hydroxide powder should be mixed with water or glycerin to form a thick paste. This paste or a commercial preparation is placed in the pulp chamber with a plastic instrument, amalgam carrier, or syringe and carried down each canal by means of a lentulo spiral, a plugger, or counterclockwise rotation of files.[102] The paste is covered with a sterile cotton pellet and the access is sealed with a temporary restoration at least 3 mm thick to prevent coronal leakage of microbes or microbial by-products.[103-109]

DRAINAGE

Severe infections require a multifaceted approach including débridement, drainage, and pharmacotherapeutics. Débridement of the pulp space to remove the source of the infection is key along with drainage in managing an abscess or cellulitis. An abscess, which itself is a potent irritant, also has elevated osmotic pressure. This attracts more tissue fluid, thereby contributing to more edema and pain. Drainage from the canal or soft tissue decreases discomfort caused by inflammatory mediators and particularly the pressure of a fluctuant swelling containing purulent material. Incision of an indurated swelling is also effective because it releases blood and serous fluids that contain bacteria, bacterial byproducts, and inflammatory mediators. Good drainage also improves circulation to the area and improves delivery of antibiotics so a minimum inhibitory concentration may be reached. These procedures are discussed in detail in Chapter 17.

Antibiotics (antimicrobials) should be considered adjunctive treatment of more severe infections and are not a substitute for proper local treatment. The indications and recommendations for the use of antibiotics are discussed in Chapter 30.

WHEN AND HOW TO CULTURE

Because of the wide range of bacteria found in endodontic infections, the empirical administration of antibiotics may not be effective. Although culturing is rarely required, at times it may provide valuable information for better antibiotic selection. Great care must be taken to avoid contamination of the sample. In addition, the proper transport media must be obtained from the laboratory to ensure that the bacteria remain viable for culturing.

To prevent contamination by oral flora, a submucosal swelling should be sampled by needle aspiration. After anesthesia, the mucosal surface is dried and disinfected with Betadine or chlorhexidine. A 16- to 20-gauge needle is used to aspirate the exudate. The aspirate should be immediately injected into a container with prereduced transport media. Good communication with the laboratory technicians is important.

Gram staining should be performed on the sample to demonstrate which types of microorganisms predominate. The culture results should identify the predominant isolated microorganisms, which should not be identified merely as "normal oral flora."

Antibiotics are chosen to treat anaerobic infections based on the identification of the prominent microorganisms in the culture. A factor complicating the culture of anaerobes is that the identification may not be made for days or even weeks. In the future, once specific bacteria or combinations of bacteria are determined to be associated with endodontic pathoses, selective media, precise biochemical tests, immunofluorescence, and molecular methods may provide more rapid identification of pathogens.

REFERENCES

1. Nagaoka S, Youichi M, Hong L, et al: Bacterial invasion into dentinal tubules of human vital and nonvital teeth, *J Endod* 21:70, 1995.
2. Bergenholtz G: Inflammatory response of the dental pulp to bacterial irritation, *J Endod* 7:100, 1981.
3. Cvek M: A clinical report on partial pulpotomy and capping with calcium hydroxide in permanent incisors with complicated crown fractures, *J Endod* 4:232, 1978.
4. Torabinejad M, Kiger RD: Histological evaluation of a patient with periodontal disease, *Oral Surg* 59:198, 1985.
5. Bergenholtz G, Lindhe J: Effect of experimentally induced marginal periodontitis and periodontal scaling on the dental pulp, *J Clin Periodontol* 5:59, 1978.
6. Langeland K, Rodrigues H, Dowden W: Periodontal disease, bacteria, and pulpal histopathology, *Oral Surg* 37:257, 1974.
7. Wong R, Hirsch RS, Clarke NG: Endodontic effects of root planing in humans, *Endod Dent Traumatol* 5:193, 1989.
8. Allard U, Nord CE, Sjoberg L, Stromberg T: Experimental infections with *Staphylococcus aureus, Streptococcus sanguis, Pseudomonas aeruginosa,* and *Bacteroides fragilis* in the jaws of dogs, *Oral Surg* 48:454, 1979.
9. Delivanis PD, Fan VSC: The localization of bloodborne bacteria in instrumented unfilled and overinstrumented canals, *J Endod* 10:521, 1984.
10. Ando N, Hoshino E: Predominant obligate anaerobes invading the deep layers of root canal dentine, *Int Endod J* 23:20, 1990.
11. Sundqvist G: Associations between microbial species in dental root canal infections, *Oral Microbiol Immunol* 7:257, 1992.
12. Sundqvist G: Ecology of the root canal flora, *J Endod* 18:427, 1992.
13. Weber DF: Human dentine sclerosis: a microradiographic study, *Arch Oral Biol* 19:163, 1974.
14. Miller WA, Massler M: Permeability and staining of active and arrested lesions in dentine, *Br Dent J* 112:187, 1962.
15. Van Hassel HJ: Physiology of the human dental pulp, *Oral Surg* 32:126, 1971.
16. Kakehashi S, Stanley HR, Fitzgerald RJ: The effects of surgical exposures of dental pulps in germ-free and conventional laboratory rats, *Oral Surg* 20:340, 1965.
17. Baumgartner JC, Falkler WA, Jr.: Bacteria in the apical 5 mm of infected root canals, *J Endod* 17:380, 1991.
18. Fabricius L, Dahlén G, Öhman AE, Möller ÅJR: Predominant indigenous oral bacteria isolated from infected root canals after varied times of closure, *Scand J Dent Res* 90:134, 1982.
19. Shah HN, Collins MD: Proposal for reclassification of *Bacteroides asaccharolyticus, Bacteroides gingivalis,* and *Bacteroides endodontalis* in a new genus, *Porphyromonas, Int J Syst Bacteriol* 38:128, 1988.
20. Shah HN, Collins DM: *Prevotella,* a new genus to include *Bacteroides melaninogenicus* and related species formerly classified in the genus *Bacteroides, Int J Syst Bacteriol* 40:205, 1990.
21. Sundqvist GK: *Bacteriological studies of necrotic dental pulps* (thesis), Umea, Sweden, 1976, University of Umea.
22. Sundqvist G, Johansson E, Sjögren U: Prevalence of black-pigmented *Bacteroides* species in root canal infections, *J Endod* 15:13, 1989.
23. Griffee MB, Patterson SS, Miller CH, et al: The relationship of *Bacteroides melaninogenicus* to symptoms associated with pulpal necrosis, *Oral Surg* 50:457, 1980.
24. Yoshida M, Fukushima H, Yamamoto K, et al: Correlation between clinical symptoms and microorganisms isolated from root canals of teeth with periapical pathosis, *J Endod* 13:24, 1987.
25. Haapasalo M, Ranta H, Rantah K, Shah H: Black-pigmented *Bacteroides* spp. in human apical periodontitis, *Infect Immunol* 53:149, 1986.
26. Hashioka K, Yamasaki M, Nakane A, et al: The relationship between clinical symptoms and anaerobic bacteria from infected root canals, *J Endod* 18:558, 1992.
27. Haapasalo M, Ranta H, Ranta K, Shah H: Black-pigmented *Bacteroides* spp. in human apical periodontitis, *Infect Immunol* 53:149, 1986.
28. Gharbia S, Haapasalo M, Shah H, et al: Characterization of *Prevotella intermedia* and *Prevotella nigrescens* isolates from periodontic and endodontic infections, *J Periodontol* 65:56, 1994.
29. Bae K, Baumgartner J, Xia T, et al: SDS-PAGE and PCR for differentation of *Prevotella intermedia* and *P. nigrescens, J Endod* 25:324, 1997.
30. Dougherty W, Bae K, Watkins B, Baumgartner J: Black-pigmented bacteria in coronal and apical segments of infected root canals, *J Endod* 24:356, 1998.
31. Xia T, Baumgartner JC, David LL: Isolation and identification of *Prevotella tannerae* from endodontic infections, *Oral Microbiol Immunol* 15:273, 2000.
32. Heimdahl A, Von Konow L, Satoh T, Nord CE: Clinical appearance of orofacial infections of odontogenic origin in relation to microbiological findings, *J Clin Microbiol* 22:299, 1985.

33. Haapasalo M: *Bacteroides buccae* and related taxa in necrotic root canal infections, *J Clin Microbiol* 24:940, 1986.

34. Sundqvist GK, Eckerbom MI, Larsson ÅP, Sjögren UT: Capacity of anaerobic bacteria from necrotic dental pulps to induce purulent infections, *Infect Immunol* 25:685, 1979.

35. Baumgartner JC, Falkler WA Jr, Beckerman T: Experimentally induced infection by oral anaerobic microorganisms in a mouse model, *Oral Microbiol Immunol* 7:253, 1992.

36. Fabricius L, Dahlén G, Holm SE, Möller ÅJR: Influence of combinations of oral bacteria on periapical tissues of monkeys, *Scand J Dent Res* 90:200, 1982.

37. Happonen RP: Periapical actinomycosis: a follow-up study of 16 surgically treated cases, *Endod Dent Traumatol* 2:205, 1986.

38. Nair PNR: Light and electron microscopic studies of root canal flora and periapical lesions, *J Endod* 13:29, 1987.

39. O'Grady JF, Reade PC: Periapical actinomycosis involving *Actinomyces israelii*, *J Endod* 14:147, 1988.

40. Sjögren U, Figdor D, Persson S, Sundqvist G: Influence of infection at the time of root filling on the outcome of endodontic treatment of teeth with apical periodontitis, *Int Endod J* 30:297, 1997.

41. Molander A, Reit C, Dahlen G, Kvist T: Microbiological status of root-filled teeth with apical periodontitis, *Int Endod J* 31:1, 1998.

42. Sundqvist G, Figdor D, Persson S, Sjögren U: Microbiologic analysis of teeth with failed endodontic treatment and the outcome of conservative re-treatment, *Oral Surg* 85:86, 1998.

43. Nair PNR, Sjogren U, Krey G, et al: Intraradicular bacteria and fungi in root-filled, asymptomatic human teeth with therapy-resistant periapical lesions: a long-term light and electron microscopic follow-up study, *J Endod* 16:580, 1990.

44. Sen B, Safavi K, Spangberg L: Growth patterns of *Candida albicans* in relation to radicular dentin, *Oral Surg* 84:68, 1997.

45. Waltimo TMT, Sirén EK, Torkko HLK, et al: Fungi in therapy-resistant apical periodontitis, *Int Endod J* 30:96, 1997.

46. Waltimo T, Siren E, Orstavik D, Haapasalo M: Susceptibility of oral Candida species to calcium hydroxide in vitro, *Int Endod J* 32:94, 1999.

47. Baumgartner JC, Watts CM, Xia T: Occurrence of *Candida albicans* infections of endodontic origin, *J Endod* (in press).

48. Glick M, Trope M, Pliskin M: Detection of HIV in the dental pulp of a patient with AIDS, *J Am Dent Assoc* 119:649, 1989.

49. Glick M, Trope M, Pliskin E: Human immunodeficiency virus infection of fibroblasts of dental pulp in seropositive patients, *Oral Surg* 71:733, 1991.

50. Rauckhorst AJ, Baumgartner JC: Zebra. XIX. Herpes zoster, *J Endod* 26:469, 2000.

51. Möller AJR: Influence on periapical tissues of indigenous oral bacteria and necrotic pulp tissue in monkeys, *Scand J Dent Res* 89:475, 1981.

52. Dwyer TG, Torabinejad M: Radiographic and histologic evaluation of the effect of endotoxin on the periapical tissues of the cat, *J Endod* 7:31, 1981.

53. Horiba N, Maekawa Y, Abe Y, et al: Correlations between endotoxin and clinical symptoms or radiolucent areas in infected root canals, *Oral Surg* 71:492, 1991.

54. Horiba N, Maekawa Y, Matsumoto T, Nakamura H: A study of the distribution of endotoxin in the dentinal wall of infected root canals, *J Endod* 16:331, 1990.

55. Nissan R, Segal H, Pashley D, et al: Ability of bacterial endotoxin to diffuse through human dentin, *J Endod* 21:62, 1995.

56. Hashioka K, Suzuki K, Yoshida T, et al: Relationship between clinical symptoms and enzyme-producing bacteria isolated from infected root canal, *J Endod* 20:75, 1994.

57. Sundqvist GK, Carlsson J, Herrmann BF, et al: Degradation in vivo of the C3 protein of guinea-pig complement by a pathogenic strain of *Bacteroides gingivalis*, *Scand J Dent Res* 92:14, 1984.

58. Sundqvist G, Carlsson J, Herrmann B, Tärnvik A: Degradation of human immunoglobulins G and M and complement factors C3 and C5 by black-pigmented *Bacteroides*, *J Med Microbiol* 19:85, 1985.

59. Tamura M, Nagaoka S, Kawagoe M: Interleukin-1 stimulates interstitial collagenase gene expression in human dental pulp fibroblast, *J Endod* 22:240, 1996.

60. Barkhordar RA: Determining the presence and origin of collagenase in human periapical lesions, *J Endod* 13:228, 1987.

61. Odell L, Baumgartner J, Xia T, David L: Survey of collagenase gene *prtC* in *porphyromonas gingivalis* and *Porphyromonas endodontalis* isolated from endodontic infections, *J Endod* 25:555, 1999.

62. Shah HH: *Biology of the species Porphyromonas gingivalis*, Ann Arbor, Mich, 1993, CRC Press.

63. Kinder SA, Holt SC: Characterization of coaggregation between *Bacteroides gingivalis* T22 and *Fusobacterium nucleatum* T18, *Infect Immunol* 57:3425, 1989.

64. Eftimiadi C, Stashenko P, Tonetti M, et al: Divergent effect of the anaerobic bacteria by-product butyric acid on the immune response: suppression of T-lymphocyte proliferation and stimulation of interleukin-1 beta production, *Oral Microbiol Immunol* 6:17, 1991.

65. Maita E, Horiuchi H: Polyamine analysis of infected root canal contents related to clinical symptoms, *Endod Dent Traumatol* 6:213, 1990.

66. Tronstad L, Barnett F, Cervone F: Periapical bacterial plaque in teeth refractory to endodontic treatment, *Endod Dent Traumatol* 6:73, 1990.

67. Iwu C, MacFarlane TW, MacKenzie D, Stenhouse D: The microbiology of periapical granulomas, *Oral Surg* 69:502, 1990.

68. Wayman BE, Murata SM, Almeida RJ, Fowler CB: A bacteriological and histological evaluation of 58 periapical lesions, *J Endod* 18:152, 1992.

69. Sunde PT, Olsen I, Lind PO, Tronstad L: Extraradicular infection: a methodological study, *Endod Dent Traumatol* 16:84, 2000.

70. Walton RE, Ardjmand K: Histological evaluation of the presence of bacteria in induced periapical lesions in monkeys, *J Endod* 18:216, 1992.

71. Block RM, Bushell A, Rodrigues H, Langeland K: A histopathologic, histobacteriologic, and radiographic study of periapical endodontic surgical specimens, *Oral Surg* 42:656, 1976.

72. Nair PNR, Schroeder HE: Periapical actinomycosis, *J Endod* 10:567, 1984.

73. Barnett F, Stevens R, Tronstad L: Demonstration of *Bacteroides intermedius* in periapical tissue using indirect immunofluorescence microscopy, *Endod Dent Traumatol* 6:153, 1990.

74. Oguntebi B, Slee AM, Tanzer JM, Langeland K: Predominant microflora associated with human dental periapical abscesses, *J Clin Microbiol* 15:964, 1982.

75. Van Winkelhoff AJ, Carlee AW, de Graaff J: *Bacteroides endodontalis* and other black-pigmented *Bacteroides* species in odontogenic abscesses, *Infect Immunol* 49:494, 1985.

76. Brook I, Frazier EH, Gher ME: Aerobic and anaerobic microbiology of periapical abscess, *Oral Microbiol Immunol* 6:123, 1991.

77. Baumgartner JC, Watkins JB, Bae KS, Xia T: Association of black-pigmented bacteria with endodontic infections, *J Endod* 25:413, 1999.

78. Baumgartner JC, Ibay AC: The chemical reactions of irrigants used for root canal debridement, *J Endod* 13:47, 1987.

79. Baumgartner JC, Mader CL: A scanning electron microscopic evaluation of four root canal irrigation regimens, *J Endod* 13:147, 1987.

80. Harrison JW, Hand RE: The effect of dilution and organic matter on the antimicrobial property of 5.25% sodium hypochlorite, *J Endod* 7:128, 1981.

81. Hand RE, Smith ML, Harrison JW: Analysis of the effect of dilution on the necrotic tissue dissolution property of sodium hypochlorite, *J Endod* 4:60, 1978.

82. Senia ES, Marshall FJ, Rosen S: The solvent action of sodium hypochlorite on pulp tissue of extracted teeth, *Oral Surg* 1971:96, 1971.

83. Shih M, Marshall FJ, Rosen S: The bactericidal efficiency of sodium hypochlorite as an endodontic irrigant, *Oral Surg* 29:613, 1970.

84. Baumgartner JC, Cuenin PR: Efficacy of several concentrations of sodium hypochlorite for root canal irrigation, *J Endod* 18:605, 1992.

85. Byström A, Sundqvist G: The antibacterial action of sodium hypochlorite and EDTA in 60 cases of endodontic therapy, *Int Endod J* 18:35, 1985.

86. Byström A, Sundqvist G: Bacteriologic evaluation of the efficacy of mechanical root canal instrumentation in endodontic therapy, *Scand J Dent Res* 89:321, 1981.

87. Yang S, Rivera E, Walton R, Baumgardner K: Canal debridement: effectiveness of sodium hypochlorite and calcium hydroxide as medicaments, *J Endod* 22:521, 1996.

88. Mader CL, Baumgartner JC, Peters DD: Scanning electron microscopic investigation of the smeared layer on root canal walls, *J Endod* 10:477, 1984.

89. Drake DR, Wiemann AH, Rivera EM, Walton RE: Bacterial retention in canal walls in vitro: effect of smear layer, *J Endod* 20:78, 1994.

90. Galvan DA, Ciarlone AE, Pashley DH, et al: Effect of smear layer removal on the diffusion permeability of human roots, *J Endod* 20:83, 1994.

91. Sjögren U, Sundqvist G: Bacteriologic evaluation of ultrasonic root canal instrumentation, *Oral Surg* 63:366, 1987.

92. Byström A, Sundqvist G: Bacteriologic evaluation of the efficacy of mechanical root canal instrumentation in endodontic therapy, *Scand J Dent Res* 89:321, 1981.

93. Thoden van Velzen S, Feltkamp-Vroom T: Immunologic consequences of formaldehyde fixation of autologous tissue implants, *J Endod* 3:179, 1977.

94. Spangberg L, Engstrom B, Langeland K: Biologic effects of dental materials. 3. Toxicity and antimicrobial effect of endodontic antiseptics in vitro, *Oral Surg* 36:856, 1973.

95. Walton R: Intracanal medicaments, *Dent Clin North Am* 28:783, 1984.

96. Gilad JZ, Teles R, Goodson M, et al: Development of a clindamycin-impregnated fiber as an intracanal medication in endodontic therapy, *J Endod* 25:722, 1999.

97. Stuart KG, Miller CH, Brown CE, Newton CW: The comparative antimicrobial effect of calcium hydroxide, *Oral Surg* 72:101, 1991.

98. Bystrom A, Sundqvist G: The antibacterial action of sodium hypochlorite and EDTA in 60 cases of endodontic therapy, *Int Endod J* 1:35, 1985.

99. Metzler RS, Montgomery S: The effectiveness of ultrasonics and calcium hydroxide for the debridement of human mandibular molars, *J Endod* 15:373, 1989.

100. Andersen M, Lund A, Andreasen JO, Andreasen FM: *In vitro* solubility of human pulp tissue in calcium hydroxide and sodium hypochlorite, *Endod Dent Traumatol* 8:104, 1992.

101. Hasselgren G, Olsson B, Cvek M: Effects of calcium hydroxide and sodium hypochlorite on the dissolution of necrotic porcine muscle tissue, *J Endod* 14:125, 1988.

102. Sigurdsson A, Stancill R, Madison S: Intracanal placement of Ca(OH)$_2$: a comparison of techniques, *J Endod* 18:367, 1992.

103. Deveaux E, Hildelbert P, Neut C, et al: Bacterial microleakage of Cavit, IRM, and TERM, *Oral Surg* 74:634, 1992.

104. Gish SP, Drake DR, Walton RE, Wilcox LR: Coronal leakage: bacterial penetration through obturated canals following post preparation, *J Am Dent Assoc* 125:1369, 1994.

105. Madison S, Swanson K, Chiles SA: An evaluation of coronal microleakage in endodontically treated teeth. Part II. Sealer types, *J Endod* 13:109, 1987.

106. Torabinejad M, Ung B, Kettering JD: In vitro bacterial penetration of coronally unsealed endodontically treated teeth, *J Endod* 16:566, 1990.

107. Khayat A, Lee SJ, Torabinejad M: Human saliva penetration of coronally unsealed obturated root canals, *J Endod* 19:458, 1993.

108. Barrieshi K, Walton R, Johnson W, Drake D: Coronal leakage of mixed anaerobic bacteria after obturation and post space preparation, *Oral Surg* 84:310, 1997.

109. Alves J, Walton R, Drake D: Coronal leakage: endotoxin penetration from mixed bacterial communities through obturated, post-prepared canals, *J Endod* 24:587, 1998.

Endodontic Emergencies

LEARNING OBJECTIVES

After reading this chapter, the student should be able to:

1 / Identify causes of emergencies as they occur before treatment, between appointments, and after obturation.

2 / Recognize what constitutes a true emergency as opposed to urgency.

3 / Describe the emotional status of the emergency patient and explain how this complicates diagnosis and treatment.

4 / Describe the psychologic and physiologic factors that affect pain perception and pain reaction and how these are managed.

5 / List the factors that relate to greater frequency of interappointment or postobturation flare-ups.

6 / Describe and outline a sequential approach to endodontic emergencies:
   a. Determine the source of pain (pulpal or periradicular)
   b. Establish a pulpal and periradicular diagnosis
   c. Identify the etiologic factor of the pathosis
   d. Design an emergency (short-term) treatment plan
   e. Design a long-term treatment plan

7 / Outline a system of subjective and objective examinations and radiographic findings to identify the source of pain and the pulpal or periradicular diagnosis.

8 / Describe when pretreatment emergencies might occur and how to manage these emergencies.

9 / Outline the steps involved in treatment of painful irreversible pulpitis.

10 / Describe the steps involved in treatment of necrotic pulp with acute apical periodontitis.

11 / Describe treatment of acute apical abscess; include the indications and procedure for incision and drainage.

12 / Describe treatment of acute apical periodontitis after cleaning and shaping (interappointment) or after obturation (post-treatment).

13 / Detail the pharmacologic supportive therapy (analgesics, antibiotics, and anti-inflammatory agents) used in emergencies and their role in controlling inflammation or infection.

OUTLINE

Definition

Categories
  Pretreatment Emergency
  Interappointment and Postobturation
      Emergency

The Challenge
  Differentiation of Emergency and Urgency
  Development of a System

Pain Perception and Pain Reaction

Physical Condition

System of Diagnosis
  Medical and Dental Histories
  Subjective Examination
  Objective Examination
  Periodontal Examination
  Radiographic Examination
  Diagnostic Outcome

Treatment Planning

Pretreatment Emergencies
  Patient Management
  Profound Anesthesia
  Management of Painful Irreversible Pulpitis
  Management of Pulp Necrosis with Apical
      Pathosis
  Postoperative Instructions

Interappointment Emergencies
  Incidence
  Causative Factors
  Prevention
  Diagnosis
  Treatment of Flare-ups
  Medications

Postobturation Emergencies
  Causative Factors
  Treatment

E ndodontic emergencies are a challenge for both diagnosis and management. Knowledge and skill in several aspects of endodontics are required; failure to apply these will result in serious consequences for the patient. Incorrect diagnosis or incorrect treatment will fail to relieve pain and, in fact, may aggravate the situation. The clinician must have knowledge of pain mechanisms, patient management, diagnosis, anesthesia, therapeutics, and appropriate treatment measures for both hard and soft tissues.

This chapter discusses approaches to the diagnosis and treatment of various categories of emergencies. It includes a review of etiologic factors and details of a systematic approach to identifying and diagnosing the offending cause; then appropriate treatment is described.

These emergencies are a matter of concern to patients, dentists, and staff. Varying (but not uncommon) frequencies of pain or swelling occur in patients before, during, and after root canal treatment.[1-4] Causes of such emergencies are a combination of irritants that induce severe inflammation in the pulp and/or periradicular tissues.

Investigations into the role of host factors (age, gender, tooth type, and so on) contributing to the occurrence of endodontic emergencies have been inconclusive; clear cause-and-effect relationships have not been established. Most studies of interappointment pain have shown little or no direct relationship between emergencies and the factors (intracanal medication, occlusal reduction, and so on) that can be controlled by the operator.[1,5] Associated factors are those presented by the patient, such as the pulp or periapical diagnosis and the presenting levels of pain.[1-6]

Among major elements, the role of bacteria and their by-products in dental emergencies is well established. Bacteria are important causative agents of pathosis of the pulpal and periradicular tissues.[7,8] A mixed flora, including Gram-negative anaerobic bacteria, is related to clinical signs and symptoms of periradicular pathosis.[9,10] Bacterial by-products (including collagenase, chondroitinase, and hyaluronidase) isolated from root canals have also been related to clinical symptoms.[11]

Irritation of periradicular tissues results in inflammation and the release of a group of chemical mediators that initiate inflammation. The concentrations of some of these substances in the pulp and periradicular tissues are significantly higher in symptomatic than in asymptomatic lesions.[12] Pain results from two factors related to inflammation: (1) *chemical mediators* and (2) *pressure.* Chemical mediators cause pain either directly by lowering the response threshold of the sensory nerve fibers or indirectly by increasing vascular permeability and producing edema. Edema results in increased fluid pressure, which directly stimulates pain receptors. Of the two causes of pain, *pressure* is the more important.

Definition

By definition, endodontic emergencies are usually associated with pain and/or swelling and require immediate diagnosis and treatment. These emergencies are caused by pathoses in the pulp or periradicular tissues. They also include severe traumatic injuries that result in luxation, avulsion, or fractures of the hard tissues. Management of emergencies related to trauma will not be included in this chapter (see Chapter 25).

Categories

PRETREATMENT EMERGENCY

These are situations in which the patient is seen initially with severe pain and/or swelling. Problems occur with both diagnosis and treatment.

INTERAPPOINTMENT AND POSTOBTURATION EMERGENCY

Also referred to as the "flare-up," this problem occurs after an endodontic appointment. Although an upsetting event, this is easier to manage because the offending tooth has already been identified and a diagnosis has been previously established. Also, the clinician has knowledge of the prior procedure and will be better able to correct the problem.

The Challenge

It is satisfying and rewarding to successfully manage a distraught patient who has an emergency (Figure 17-1). In contrast, how distressing it is to have a patient with a flare-up after root canal treatment in a previously asymptomatic tooth! The aim is to increase occurrences in the first category and decrease those in the second.

DIFFERENTIATION OF EMERGENCY AND URGENCY

Whether a pretreatment, interappointment, or postobturation problem, it is important to differentiate between a *true emergency* and the less critical *urgency*. A *true emergency* is a condition requiring an

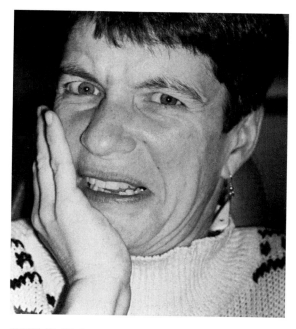

FIGURE 17-1
Patient is distraught from severe pulpal pain. This patient will be a challenge to diagnose and treat.

unscheduled office visit with diagnosis and treatment now! The visit cannot be rescheduled because of the severity of the problem. *Urgency* indicates a less severe problem; a visit may be scheduled for mutual convenience of the patient and the dentist. Key questions (that may be asked by telephone) to determine severity include the following:

1. Does the problem disturb your sleeping, eating, working, concentrating, or other daily activities? (A true emergency disrupts the patient's activities or quality of life.)
2. How long has this problem been bothering you? (A true emergency has rarely been severe for more than a few hours to 2 days.)
3. Have you taken any pain medication? Was the medication ineffective? (Analgesics do not relieve the pain of a true emergency.)

An affirmative answer to these questions requires an immediate office visit for management and constitutes a true emergency. Obviously, the patient's emotional and mental status must also be determined. To some patients, even a minor problem has major proportions and is disruptive.

DEVELOPMENT OF A SYSTEM

Because a misdiagnosis will probably result in improper treatment and an exacerbation of the problem, a systematic approach is mandatory!

The emotional status of the patient, pressures of time, and stress on dentist and staff should not affect such an orderly approach.

Pain Perception and Pain Reaction

Pain is a complex physiologic and psychologic phenomenon. Pain perception levels are not constant; pain thresholds as well as reactions to pain change significantly under various circumstances.[13] Psychologic components of pain perception and pain reaction comprise cognitive, emotional, and symbolic factors. The pain reaction threshold is significantly altered by past experiences and by present anxiety levels and emotional status. (Refer to Chapter 29 for more details on pain perception and reaction and pain threshold.)

To reduce anxiety and consequently obtain reliable information about the chief complaint and to receive cooperation during treatment, the clinician should (1) establish and maintain control of the situation, (2) gain the confidence of the patient, (3) provide attention and sympathy, and (4) treat the patient as an important individual.[13] By managing these pain components, pain perception and reaction thresholds are raised signifi-

cantly, greatly facilitating the procedure. Psychologic management of the patient is the most important factor in emergency treatment!

Physical Condition

In addition to the emotional factors that complicate the diagnosis of endodontic emergencies, physical conditions induced as a result of these situations also contribute to the problems. Pain or swelling may limit mouth opening, thereby hampering diagnostic procedures as well as treatment (Figure 17-2). In addition, hypersensitivity to thermal stimuli or pressure influences diagnosis and treatment.

System of Diagnosis

Patients in pain often provide information and responses that are exaggerated and inaccurate. They tend to be confused as well as apprehensive. It is easy (and tempting) to rush through the diagnosis to institute treatment for a suffering patient. After pertinent information regarding the medical and dental histories is obtained, both subjective questioning and an objective examination are performed carefully and completely.[14]

A rule of the true emergency is *one tooth is the offender*, i.e., the source of pain. In the excitement of the moment, the patient might believe that the severe pain is emanating from more than a single tooth. The clinician may become convinced also, leading to overtreatment.

MEDICAL AND DENTAL HISTORIES

Medical and dental histories should be reviewed first. If the patient is the dentist's own, the med-

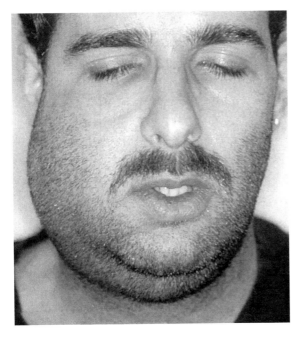

FIGURE 17-2
Severe submandibular swelling. The patient has limited mouth opening resulting from trismus.

> ### Diagnosis Sequence
>
> 1. Obtain pertinent information about the patient's medical and dental histories.
> 2. Ask pointed subjective questions about the patient's pain: history, location, severity, duration, character, and eliciting stimuli.
> 3. Perform an extraoral examination.
> 4. Perform an intraoral examination.
> 5. Perform pulp testing as appropriate.
> 6. Use palpation and percussion sensitivity tests to determine periapical status.
> 7. Interpret appropriate radiographs.

ical history is briefly reviewed and updated. If the patient is new, a standard, complete history is taken. An important medical complication may be easily overlooked in an emergency situation. Either a short or a complete dental history is taken. This includes recalling of dental procedures, a chronology of symptoms, or an earlier relevant comment by a dentist.

SUBJECTIVE EXAMINATION

When the patient is in pain, the subjective examination comprises careful questioning and is the most important aspect of diagnosis. Questions relate to the history, location, severity, duration, character, and eliciting stimuli of pain. Questions relating to the cause or stimulus that elicits or relieves the pain help select appropriate objective tests to arrive at a final diagnosis.

Pain that is elicited by thermal stimuli and/or is referred is likely to originate from the pulp. Pain that occurs on mastication or tooth contact and is well localized is probably periradicular.

The three important factors constituting the quality and quantity of pain are its spontaneity, intensity, and duration (see Chapter 4). If the patient reports any of these symptoms (and assuming that the patient is not exaggerating), significant pathosis is likely to be present. Careful questioning provides important information about the source of the pain and whether it is pulpal or periradicular. In fact, a perceptive, clever clinician should be able to arrive at a tentative diagnosis by means of a thorough subjective examination; objective tests and radiographic findings are then used for confirmation. For example, a reported complaint of severe, continuous (lingering) pain when the patient drinks cold beverages and marked tenderness on mastication indicates irreversible pulpitis and acute apical periodontitis. These stimuli are then repeated on an objective examination to confirm the patient's response.

OBJECTIVE EXAMINATION

Again, it is important in identifying the offending tooth to repeat tests that mimic what the patient reports subjectively. In other words, the best test is to repeat the stimulus that reportedly causes the pain. As in the previous example, applying cold and pressure should reproduce pain of basically the same type and magnitude as related by the patient. If similar subjective symptoms are not reproduced, this may not be a true emergency; the patient may be "over-reporting" (exaggerating the problem).

In addition, objective tests include extraoral and intraoral examination. Included are observation for swelling as well as mirror and explorer examination to note the presence of defective restorations, discolored crowns, recurrent caries, and fractures.

Periradicular tests include (1) palpation over the apex, (2) digital pressure on or wiggling of teeth (preferred if the patient reports severe pain on mastication), (3) light percussion with the end of the mirror handle, and (4) selective biting on an object such as a cotton swab or Tooth Slooth.

Pulp vitality tests are most useful to reproduce reported pain. Cold, heat, electricity, and direct dentin stimulation, however, usually indicate the pulp status (vital or necrotic).

PERIODONTAL EXAMINATION

A periodontal examination is always necessary. Probing helps in differentiating endodontic from periodontal disease. For example, a periodontal abscess can simulate an acute apical abscess (Figure 17-3). However, with a localized periodontal abscess, the pulp is usually vital (see Chapter 26). In contrast, an acute apical abscess is related to an unresponsive (necrotic) pulp. These abscesses occasionally communicate with the sulcus and have a deep probing defect. In addition to these tests, when the differential diagnosis is difficult, a test cavity may identify the pulp status and isolate the offending tooth.

RADIOGRAPHIC EXAMINATION

Radiographs are helpful, but have limitations. There is a tendency to over-rely on radiographs, often with unfortunate consequences. Periapical and bitewing radiography may detect the presence of interproximal and recurrent caries, possible pulpal exposure, internal or external resorption, and periradicular pathosis, among other entities.

DIAGNOSTIC OUTCOME

After carefully working through the sequence just described, the clinician should have identified the offending tooth and the tissue (pulpal or periradicular) that is the source of pain and should have recorded a pulpal or periradicular diagnosis. For many reasons, all or none of these conclusions may be clear. This may not be a true emergency, or the problem may be beyond the capability of the generalist and the patient should be referred (Figure 17-4). If the diagnosis is clear, however, treatment planning follows.

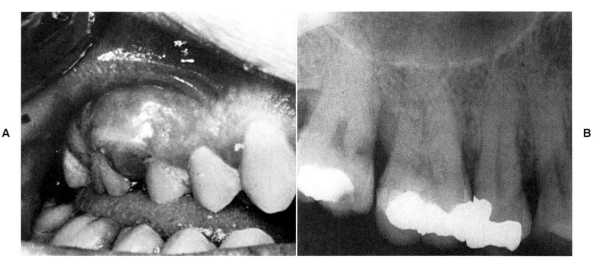

FIGURE 17-3
A, Periodontal abscess, **B,** Radiographic appearance. Positive responses to pulp testing differentiates this condition from an acute apical abscess.

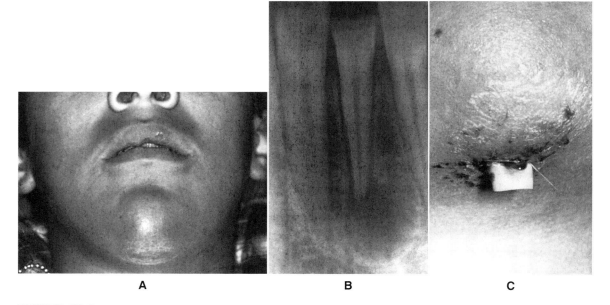

FIGURE 17-4
This patient has a complex problem and should be considered for referral. **A** and **B,** Submental space swelling resulting from trauma followed by acute apical abscess. **C,** Removal of the necrotic tissue was followed by extraoral incision and placement of a drain. (Courtesy Dr. V. Jones.)

Treatment Planning

As previously discussed, inflammation and its consequences, that is, increased tissue pressure and release of chemical mediators in the pulp or periradicular tissues, are the major causes of painful dental emergencies.[15,16] Therefore, reducing the irritant, or reduction of pressure or removal of the inflamed pulp or periradicular tissue should be the

immediate goal; this usually results in pain relief. Of the two, pressure release is the most effective.

Pretreatment Emergencies

These emergencies require a diagnosis and treatment sequencing. Each step is important: (1) categorizing the problem, (2) taking a medical history, (3) identifying the source, (4) making the diagnosis, (5) planning the treatment, and (6) treating the patient.

PATIENT MANAGEMENT

Patient management is always the most critical factor. The frightened patient in pain must have confidence that his or her problem is being properly managed.

PROFOUND ANESTHESIA

Obtaining profound anesthesia of inflamed painful tissue is a challenge. Adequate anesthesia, however, will instill confidence and cooperation and influence the patient's desire to save the offending tooth. Maxillary anesthesia is usually obtained by infiltration or block injections in the buccal and palatal regions. With mandibular teeth, in addition to an inferior alveolar and lingual nerve block, a long buccal injection may be helpful. Often (particularly with mandibular molars), although all "classic" signs of profound anesthesia are present, access into the dentin or pulp is painful. Periodontal, intrapulpal, or intraosseous injection controls the remaining sensitivity in most cases.[17] These supplemental injections are often given prophylactically, particularly with painful irreversible pulpitis.[18] Other conditions (for example, acute apical abscess) require other approaches. Chapter 7 contains details.

MANAGEMENT OF PAINFUL IRREVERSIBLE PULPITIS

Because the pain is the result of inflammation, primarily in the coronal pulp, removal of the inflamed tissue will usually reduce the pain.

Without Acute Apical Periodontitis

Complete cleaning and shaping of the root canals is the preferred treatment if time permits. With limited time, most pulpal tissue is extirpated with a broach (partial pulpectomy) in single-rooted teeth. In molars, a partial pulpectomy is performed on the largest canals (palatal or distal root). Pulpotomy (Figure 17-5) is usually effective in molars when minimal time is available.[19,20]

An old but still popular idea is that chemical medicaments sealed in chambers help control or prevent additional pain; this is not true. A dry cotton pellet alone is as effective in relieving pain as a pellet moistened with camphorated monochlorophenol (CMCP), formocresol, Cresatin, eugenol, or saline.[19] Therefore, after irrigation of the chamber or canals with sodium hypochlorite,

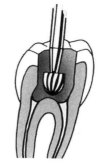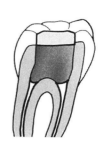

FIGURE 17-5
Removal of coronal pulp. Pulpotomy and placement of a dry cotton pellet and a temporary filling result in relief of pain from irreversible pulpitis.

a dry cotton pellet is placed and the access is sealed temporarily. A mild analgesic may be prescribed for patients with irreversible pulpitis. Antibiotics, however, are definitely not indicated.

With Acute Apical Periodontitis

In patients with extreme tenderness on percussion, a partial or total pulpectomy (as described above) is appropriate. Reducing the occlusion to eliminate contact has been shown to aid in relief of symptoms.[21] Trephination (artificial fistulation) by creating an opening through mucosa and bone is not useful and is contraindicated.[22,23]

MANAGEMENT OF PULP NECROSIS WITH APICAL PATHOSIS

The pain is related to periradicular inflammation, which results from potent irritants in the necrotic tissue in the pulp space. Treatment now is biphasic: (1) remove or reduce the pulp irritants and (2) relieve the apical fluid pressure (when possible). The diagnosis may be acute apical periodontitis (no significant periradicular resorption) or acute apical abscess with or without swelling.

Therefore, with pain and pulp necrosis there may be (1) no swelling, (2) localized swelling, or (3) diffuse, more extensive swelling. Each is managed differently. Of these three conditions, diffuse swelling is the least common.

Pulp Necrosis Without Swelling

These teeth may contain vital inflamed tissues in the apical canal and have inflamed painful periradicular tissues (acute apical periodontitis). Profound local anesthesia may be a problem, requiring a supplemental injection.

Alternatively, the lesion may have expanded and formed an abscess that is confined to bone.

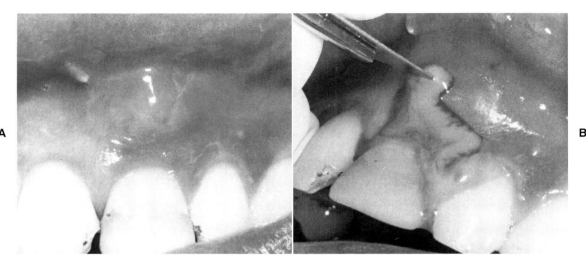

A

B

FIGURE 17-6
A, Localized swelling. **B,** Incision for drainage after cleaning and shaping of offending incisor. (Courtesy Dr. E. Rivera.)

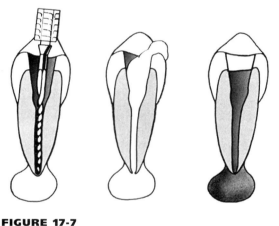

FIGURE 17-7
After opening into a root canal and establishment of drainage, instrumentation should be confined to the root canal system. Release of purulence removes a potent irritant (pus) and relieves pressure.

These are often painful, primarily because of fluid pressure in a noncompliant environment. The aim is to reduce the canal irritants and to try to encourage some drainage through the tooth.

Complete canal débridement, after determining the corrected working length, is the treatment of choice. If time is limited, partial débridement at the estimated working length is performed with light instrumentation with a passive stepback or crown-down technique to remove irritating debris. Canals are not enlarged without knowledge of the working length. During cleaning, canals are flooded and flushed with copious amounts of sodium hypochlorite. Finally, canals

are irrigated with the same solution, dried with paper points, filled with calcium hydroxide paste (if the preparation is large enough), and sealed with a dry cotton pellet and a temporary filling.

Some clinicians empirically place a cotton pellet lightly dampened with intracanal chemical medication in the pulp chamber before placing a temporary filling. There is no value to these medicaments. Administering a long-acting anesthetic, reassuring the patient, removing (or reducing) the irritant, and prescribing an analgesic will usually reduce postoperative pain significantly. Antibiotics are not indicated.[24] The patient is told that there will still be some pain (the inflamed, sensitive tissues are still present), but should subside during the next 2 or 3 days, as the inflammation decreases.

Pulp Necrosis with Localized Swelling

The abscess has now invaded regional soft tissues and at times, there is purulence in the canal. Radiographic findings range from no periapical change (rarely) to a large radiolucency.

Again, treatment is biphasic. First and most important is débridement (complete cleaning and shaping if time permits) of the canal or canals, and second in urgency is drainage (see Color Figure 17-1 immediately following page 308). Localized swelling (whether fluctuant or nonfluctuant) should be incised (Figure 17-6). Drainage accomplishes two things: (1) relief of pressure and pain and (2) removal of a very potent irritant—purulence.

In teeth that drain readily after opening, instrumentation should be confined to the root canal system (Figure 17-7). In patients with a periradicu-

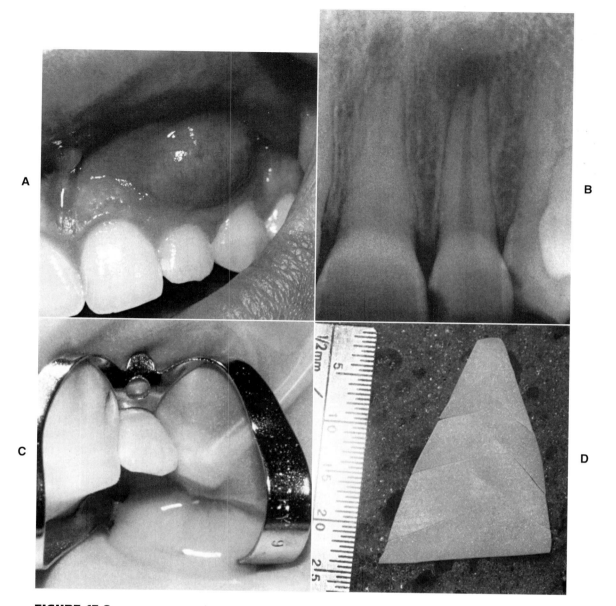

FIGURE 17-8
A, Localized fluctuant abscess as a result of periradicular pathosis after trauma. **B,** Radiographic appearance. **C,** Drainage was spontaneous when the tooth was opened. **D,** Christmas tree–shaped rubber drain placed after soft tissue incision. Antibiotics are unnecessary, but analgesics are indicated.

lar abscess but no drainage through the canal, penetration of the apical foramen with small files (up to 25) may initiate drainage and release of pressure. This release often does not occur because the abscess cavity does not communicate directly with the apical foramen. Occasionally there may be more than one abscess (Figure 17-8). One communicates with the apex while another, separate abscess is found in the vestibule. Because they do

not communicate, drainage must occur through both the tooth and a mucosal incision. Often, a drain is placed to permit continued drainage for 1 or 2 days or until débridement is complete. Several designs of drain are used (Figure 17-9).

Copious irrigation with sodium hypochlorite is performed throughout. The canals are then dried with paper points and filled with calcium hydroxide paste. After placement of a dry cotton

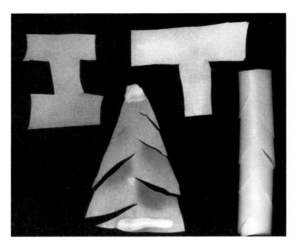

FIGURE 17-9
Different shapes of rubber drains. From left to right: I drain; Christmas tree drain; T drain; Penrose drain with oblique cuts. These designs are self-retentive and do not require suturing to the incision margins.

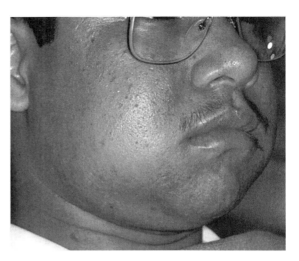

FIGURE 17-10
Progressively spreading swelling resulting from pulpal necrosis and acute apical abscess. The abscess moved rapidly into the buccal space. This patient has systemic signs of infection (elevated temperature). Localized treatment (extraction or pulp space debridement, incision for drainage) and antibiotics are indicated.

pellet, the access is sealed temporarily. These teeth should not be left open to drain, although leaving teeth open has been a common procedure. A canal exposed to the oral cavity is a potential home for introduced bacteria, food debris, and even viruses.[24] Occasionally, purulence will continue to fill the canal during the preparation (the so-called "weeping" canal). If this occurs, the patient should sit for a time. Usually, the flow will cease and the access may be closed.

These patients seldom have elevated temperatures or other systemic signs. Therefore, in acute apical abscess with localized swelling, the use of systemic antibiotics is not necessary, having been shown to be of no benefit.[25-27]

Pulp Necrosis with Diffuse Swelling

These rapidly progressive and spreading swellings are not localized and may have dissected into the fascial spaces (Figure 17-10). These patients occasionally have elevated temperature or other systemic signs and usually should be referred to a specialist.

Most important is removal of the irritant by canal débridement (cleaning and shaping is completed, if possible) or by extraction. The apical foramen may then be gently penetrated with a file to hopefully permit a flow of exudate (see Figure 17-8), although drainage often does not occur. Also at this time, swelling may be incised and a rubber drain inserted for 1 or 2 days. Occasionally the abscess localizes extraorally and subcuta-

neously, requiring extraoral incision for drainage (Figure 17-11).

Speed of recovery (whether the swelling is localized or diffuse) depends primarily on canal débridement and drainage. Because edema (fluid) has spread through the tissues, diffuse swelling decreases slowly, over a period of perhaps 3 to 4 days. As with patients undergoing removal of impacted third molars, pretreatment with nonsteroidal anti-inflammatory drugs may reduce the frequency and amount of postoperative discomfort.[14]

After placing calcium hydroxide paste and a dry pellet, the access is closed with a temporary filling. Systemic antibiotics are indicated for the diffuse, rapidly spreading swelling. The preferred and first (albeit empirical) choice is penicillin; the causative microorganisms are likely to be streptococci.[28,29] An alternative for penicillin-allergic patients is clindamycin.[29] Systemic steroids, advocated by some, are probably of no benefit. Analgesics for moderate to severe pain should be prescribed. Specific details on therapeutics are found in Chapter 30.

POSTOPERATIVE INSTRUCTIONS

Patients must be informed of their responsibilities and of what to expect. The pain and swelling will take time to resolve, proper nutrition and adequate intake of fluids are important, and medications must be taken as prescribed. The problem may recur or worsen (flare-up), requiring another emergency visit.[1] Communication after the visit is very important; calling the patient the

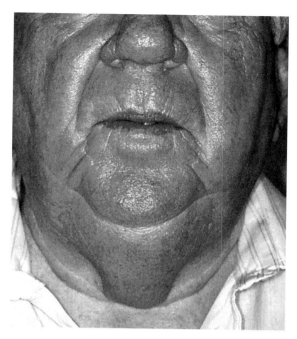

FIGURE 17-11
An acute apical abscess from a mandibular molar has rapidly spread to bilateral submandibular and cervical spaces. Also involved is the space of Burns. The result is a Ludwig's angina that requires immediate hospitalization. This patient is at risk for airway compromise and requires special procedures, including antibiotics, extraoral drainage, and airway management.

day after the appointment has been shown to reduce pain perception and analgesic needs[30] and allows the clinician the opportunity of monitoring the progress of the patient.

Interappointment Emergencies

The interappointment flare-up is a true emergency and is so severe that an unscheduled patient visit and treatment are required. Despite judicious and careful treatment procedures, complications such as pain, swelling, or both may occur. Regional temporary paresthesia has even been reported.[31] As with emergencies occurring before root canal therapy, these interappointment emergencies are undesirable and disruptive events and should be resolved quickly. Occasionally flare-ups are unexpected, although they can often be better predicted according to certain patient presenting factors.

INCIDENCE

Studies report varying incidences (1.4% to 25%) of flare-ups.[1,2,6,32-34] These variations may be due to the fact that different factors, conditions, and cri-

teria were examined. The problems with most of these studies are that they are retrospective, lack controls, have relatively small numbers of patients, or have undefined variables.[1] Prospective studies, which are better controlled, report an overall incidence of flare-ups of 1.4% to 3%.[1,33] Therefore, overall the occurrence is low, but it varies in certain situations. Most postoperative discomfort is in the mild range.[35]

CAUSATIVE FACTORS

The causative factors associated with flare-ups have also been examined. These factors generally can be categorized as related to the patient, to pulpal or periapical diagnosis, or to treatment procedures. Although many factors have been examined, a history of preoperative pain or swelling is the best predictor of interappointment emergencies.[1,5,6]

In other words, a patient who has a painful acute apical abscess that requires emergency treatment is much more likely to experience a flare-up. A tooth with a vital pulp, on the other hand, is unlikely to demonstrate severe interappointment symptoms while under treatment.

PREVENTION
Procedures

Use of long-acting anesthetic solutions, complete cleaning and shaping of the root canal system (possibly), analgesics, and psychologic preparation of patients (particularly those with preoperative pain) will decrease interappointment symptoms in the mild to moderate levels.[36] There are, however, no demonstrated treatment or therapeutic measures that will reduce the number of interappointment flare-ups. In other words, no particular relationship of flare-ups to actual treatment procedures has been shown.[1,5]

Verbal Instructions

Most important is the preparation of patients for what to expect after the appointment. They should be told that discomfort is likely; the discomfort should subside within a day or two. An increase in pain, noticeable swelling, or other adverse signs necessitate a call and sometimes a visit. This explanation reduces the number of calls from unnecessarily concerned patients.

Therapeutic Prophylaxis

A popular preventive approach has been the prescribing of antibiotics to minimize postoperative symptoms. This has been demonstrated to be not useful and needlessly exposes the patient to expensive, potentially dangerous drugs.[37,38] In contrast, certain analgesics and anti-inflammatory agents will reduce post-treatment symptoms. More information on therapeutics is included in Chapter 30.

DIAGNOSIS

The same basic procedure is followed as outlined earlier in this chapter for pretreatment emergencies, although with modifications. The problem has already been diagnosed initially; the operator has an advantage. However, a step-by-step approach to diagnose the existing condition reduces confusion and error; most important, it calms a patient who has been shaken by the episode of pain or swelling. After the underlying complications are identified, treatment is initiated.

TREATMENT OF FLARE-UPS

Reassurance (the "Big R") *is the most important aspect of treatment.* The patient is generally frightened and upset and may even assume that extraction is necessary. The explanation is that the flare-up is neither unusual nor irrevocable and will be managed. Next in importance is restoring the patient's comfort and breaking the pain cycle. For extended anesthesia or analgesia, administration of ropivacaine, etidocaine, or bupivacaine hydrochloride is recommended.

Interappointment emergencies are divided into patients with an initial diagnosis of a vital or a necrotic pulp and with or without swelling.

Previously Vital Pulps with Complete Débridement

Because this situation is unlikely to be a true flare-up, patient reassurance and the prescription of a mild to moderate analgesic often will suffice. Generally, nothing is to be gained by opening these teeth; the pain will usually regress spontaneously. Placing corticosteroids in the canal or giving an intraoral or intramuscular injection of these medications after cleaning and shaping reduces inflammation and somewhat lowers the level of moderate pain.[39-43] Flare-ups, however, have not been shown to be prevented by steroids, whether administered intracanal or systemically.[44]

Previously Vital Pulps with Incomplete Débridement

It is likely that tissue remnants have become inflamed and are now a major irritant. The working length should be rechecked, and the canal(s) should be carefully cleaned with copious irrigation of sodium hypochlorite. A dry cotton pellet is

then placed followed by a temporary filling, and a mild to moderate analgesic is prescribed.

Occasionally, a previously vital pulp (with or without complete débridement) will develop into an acute apical abscess. This will occur some time after the appointment and indicates that pulpal remnants have become necrotic and are invaded by bacteria.

Previously Necrotic Pulps with No Swelling

Occasionally these teeth develop an acute apical abscess (flare-up) after the appointment.[1] The abscess is confined to bone and can be very painful.

The tooth is opened and the canal is gently recleaned and irrigated with sodium hypochlorite. Drainage should be established if possible (see Figure 17-7). If there is active drainage from the tooth after opening, the canal should be recleaned (or débridement completed) and irrigated with sodium hypochlorite. The rubber dam is left in place after the tooth is opened; the patient is allowed to rest pain-free for at least 30 minutes or until drainage stops. Then, the canals are dried, calcium hydroxide paste is placed, and the access is sealed. The tooth should not be left open! If there is no drainage, the tooth should also be lightly instrumented and gently irrigated, medicated with calcium hydroxide paste, and then closed. The symptoms usually subside, but do so more slowly than if drainage was present. Again, patient education and reassurance are critical. A long-acting anesthetic and a strong analgesic are helpful; antibiotics are not indicated.[25,26]

Previously Necrotic Pulps with Swelling

These cases are best managed with incision and drainage (see Figure 17-6). In addition, it is most important that the canals have been débrided. If not, they should be opened and débrided, medicated with calcium hydroxide paste, and closed. Then incision and drainage with placement of a drain are completed.

Follow-up Care

With flare-ups, the patient should be contacted daily until the symptoms abate. Communication may be made by telephone; patients with more serious problems or those that are not resolving (many do not and require additional measures) should return to the dentist for treatment as described above, depending on findings. When symptoms recur or cannot be controlled, these patients should be considered for referral. Ultimate treatment by a specialist may include extra measures, such as apical surgery, or even hospitalization.

MEDICATIONS
Intracanal

Both local and systemic medications are part of the treatment regimen used for flare-ups. Phenolic intracanal medications include formocresol, CMCP, Cresatin, and eugenol. Other medications used in canals are steroid combinations and calcium hydroxide. None of these has been shown to prevent flare-ups; none helps in relieving flare-up symptoms.[44]

Systemic

Systemic drugs are usually limited to analgesics and antibiotics. Nonsteroidal anti-inflammatory agents are indicated if an analgesic effect is desired. Narcotics are useful to provide analgesia and sedation. Combinations of an opioid (codeine, oxycodone, pentazocine, and so on) and a non-steroidal agent are most effective for more severe pain. Antibiotics are indicated only if there is a diffuse, rapidly spreading cellulitis into the fascial spaces. Localized swelling does not indicate a need for antibiotic administration; surgical or canal drainage and complete canal débridement are necessary.[25,26] See Chapter 30 for more information on therapeutics.

Occasionally, but rarely, a flare-up or a presenting acute apical abscess may be serious or even life-threatening (Figure 17-12). These situations may require hospitalization and aggressive therapy with the cooperation of an oral surgeon.

Postobturation Emergencies

True emergencies postobturation are infrequent although pain at the mild level is common. There-

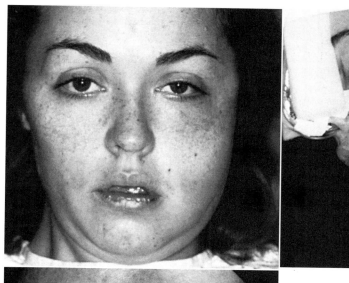
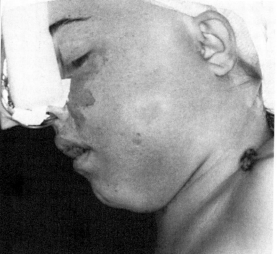
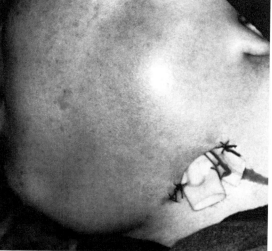

FIGURE 17-12

Progressively spreading swelling from a flare-up resulting in an acute apical abscess from a mandibular second molar. **A,** The swelling has extended to the temporal, submandibular, pharyngeal, and sublingual spaces. This condition compromised the patient's airway, requiring hospitalization for aggressive therapy including nasal intubation (**B**) and placement of extraoral drains (**C**). These severe infections are best managed by an oral surgeon.

fore, active intervention is seldom necessary; usually symptoms will resolve spontaneously.

CAUSATIVE FACTORS

Little is known about the etiologic factors involved in postoperative pain after obturation. Approximately one-third of endodontic patients experience some pain after obturation.[45] There is a correlation between the level of obturation and pain incidence, with overextension associated with the highest incidence of discomfort.[46] Postobturation pain also relates to preobturation pain; levels of pain reported after obturation tend to correlate to levels of pain before the appointment.[46,47]

TREATMENT

Information about possible discomfort for the first few days, reassurance about the availability of emergency services, and administration of mild analgesics significantly control the patient's anxiety and prevent overreaction. This in turn decreases the incidence of postobturation frantic telephone calls or "emergency" visits. Some patients, however, do develop serious complications and require follow-up treatment.

Retreatment is indicated when prior treatment obviously has been inadequate. Apical surgery is often required when an acute apical abscess develops, and there is uncorrectable, inadequate root canal treatment. If root canal treatment was acceptable, excision and drainage of swelling after obturation (an occasional occurrence) should be performed; usually the swelling resolves without further treatment. At times the patient reports severe pain, but there is no evidence of acute apical abscess, and the root canal treatment has been well done. These patients are treated with reassurance and analgesics; again, the symptoms usually subside spontaneously.

Patients with postobturation emergencies that do not respond to therapy should be referred to an endodontist for other treatment modalities, such as surgery.

REFERENCES

1. Walton R, Fouad A: Endodontic interappointment flare-ups: a prospective study of incidence and related factors, *J Endod* 18:172, 1992.
2. Mor C, Rotstein I, Friedman S: Incidence of interappointment emergency associated with endodontic therapy, *J Endod* 28:509, 1992.
3. Marshall JG, Liesinger AW: Factors associated with endodontic posttreatment pain, *J Endod* 19:573, 1993.
4. Albashaireh Z, Alnegrish A: Postobturation pain after single- and multiple-visit endodontic therapy. A prospective study, *J Dent* 26:227, 1998.
5. Torabinejad M, Kettering JD, McGraw C, et al: Factors associated with endodontic interappointment emergencies of teeth with necrotic pulps, *J Endod* 14:261, 1988.
6. Imura N, Zuolo ML: Factors associated with endodontic flare-ups: a prospective study, *Int Endod J* 28:261, 1995.
7. Kakehashi S, Stanley H, Fitzgerald R: The effect of surgical exposure of dental pulps in germ-free and conventional laboratory rats, *Oral Surg Oral Med Oral Pathol* 20:340, 1965.
8. Möller AJ, Fabricius L, Dahlen G, et al: Influence on periapical tissues of indigenous oral bacteria and necrotic pulp tissue in monkeys, *Scand J Dent Res* 89:475, 1981.
9. Griffee MG, Patterson SS, Miller CH, et al: The relationship of bacteroides melaninogenicus to symptoms associated with pulpal necrosis, *Oral Surg Oral Med Oral Pathol* 50:457, 1986.
10. Van Winkelhoff AJ, Carlee AW, Graaff DE: *Bacteroides endodontalis* and other black-pigmented bacteroides species in odontogenic abscesses, *Infect Immunol* 49:494, 1985.
11. Hashioka K, Suzuki K, Yoshida T, et al: Relationship between clinical symptoms and enzyme-producing bacteria isolated from infected root canals, *J Endod* 20:75, 1994.
12. Torabinejad M, Cotti E, Jung T: Concentrations of leukotriene B_4 in symptomatic and asymptomatic periapical lesions, *J Endod* 18:205, 1992.
13. Weyman BJ: Psychological components of pain perception, *Dent Clin North Am* 22:101, 1978.
14. Torabinejad M, Walton RE: Managing endodontic emergencies, *J Am Dent Assoc* 122:102, 1991.
15. Torabinejad M, Eby WC, Naidorf IJ: Inflammatory and immunological aspects of the pathogenesis of human periapical lesions, *J Endod* 11:479, 1985.
16. Torabinejad M: Mediators of acute and chronic periradicular lesions, *Oral Surg Oral Med Oral Pathol* 78:511, 1994.
17. Walton RE: The periodontal ligament injection as a primary technique, *J Endod* 16:62, 1990.
18. Nusstein J, Reader A, Nist R, et al: Anesthetic efficacy of the supplemental intraosseous injection of 2% lidocaine with 1:100,000 epinephrine in irreversible pulpitis, *J Endod* 24:487, 1998.
19. Hasselgren G, Reit C: Emergency pulpotomy: pain relieving effect with and without the use of sedative dressings, *J Endod* 15:254, 1989.
20. Oguntebi B, De Schepper E, Taylor T, et al: Postoperative pain incidence related to the type of emergency treatment of symptomatic pulpitis, *Oral Surg Oral Med Oral Pathol* 73:179, 1992.
21. Rosenberg P, Babick P, Schertzer L, Leung A: The effect of occlusal reduction on pain after endodontic instrumentation, *J Endod* 24:492, 1998.
22. Moos HL, Bramwell JD, Roahen JO: A comparison of pulpectomy alone versus pulpectomy with trephination for the relief of pain, *J Endod* 22:422, 1996.
23. Nist E, Reader A, Beck M: Effect of apical trephination on postoperative pain and swelling in symptomatic necrotic teeth, *J Endod* 27:415, 2001.

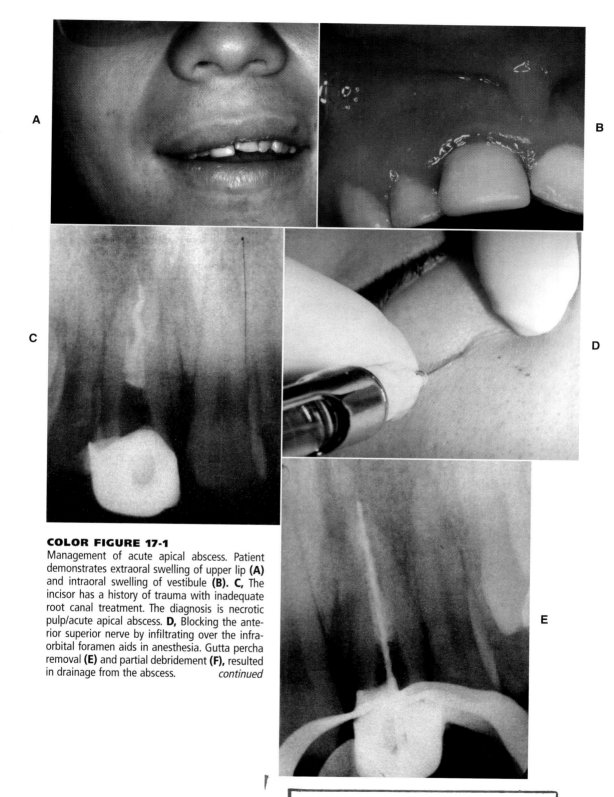

COLOR FIGURE 17-1
Management of acute apical abscess. Patient demonstrates extraoral swelling of upper lip **(A)** and intraoral swelling of vestibule **(B)**. **C,** The incisor has a history of trauma with inadequate root canal treatment. The diagnosis is necrotic pulp/acute apical abscess. **D,** Blocking the anterior superior nerve by infiltrating over the infraorbital foramen aids in anesthesia. Gutta percha removal **(E)** and partial debridement **(F)**, resulted in drainage from the abscess. *continued*

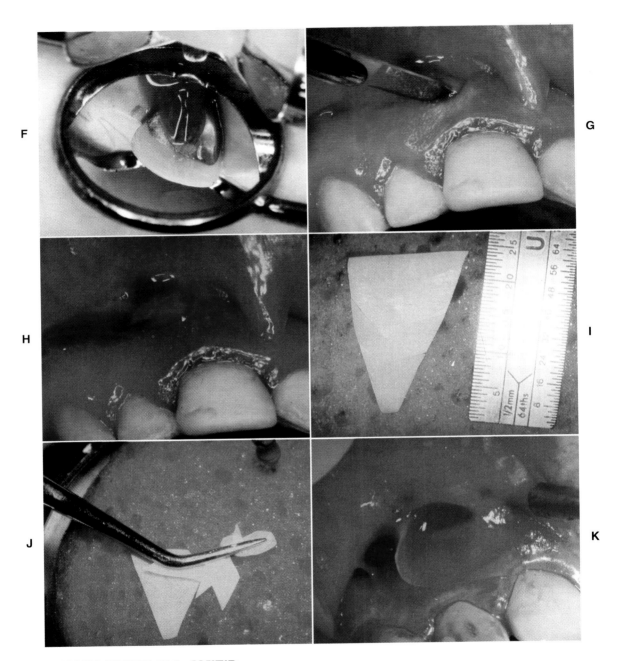

COLOR FIGURE 17-1, CONT'D

Incision of the soft tissue swelling **(G)** released serosanguinous, purulent exudation **(H).** A self-retentive "Christmas Tree" rubber dam drain is cut **(I),** rolled and placed with cotton pliers **(J),** and inserted in the incision **(K).** The drain may be removed in 1 to 2 days by the patient or by the dentist. This removal of necrotic debris and drainage of purulence usually results in rapid resolution.

24. Barnett EM, Jacobsen G, Evans G, et al: Herpes simplex encephalitis in the temporal cortex and limbic system after trigeminal nerve inoculation, *J Infect Dis* 169: 782, 1994.

25. Fouad A, Rivera E, Walton R: Penicillin as a supplement in resolving localized acute apical abscess, *Oral Surg Oral Med Oral Pathol* 81:590, 1996.

26. Henry M, Reader A, Beck M: Effect of penicillin on postoperative endodontic pain and swelling in symptomatic necrotic teeth, *J Endod* 27:117, 2001.

27. Prescription for the future: Responsible use of antibiotics in endodontics, *Am Assoc Endod Newslett,* Spring/Summer, P1, 1999.

28. Pallasch TJ: Antibiotics: myths and reality, *Calif Dent Assoc J* 14:40, 1986.

29. Peterson L: Principles of management and prevention of odontogenic infections. In Peterson L, editor: *Contemporary oral and maxillofacial surgery,* ed 3, St Louis, 1998, Mosby.

30. Touyz LZG, Marchand S: The influence of postoperative telephone calls on pain perception: a study of 118 periodontal surgical procedures, *J Orofac Pain* 12:219, 1998.

31. Morse DR: Infection-related mental and inferior alveolar nerve paresthesia: literature review and presentation of two cases, *J Endod* 23:457, 1997.

32. Barnett F, Tronstad L: The incidence of flare-ups following endodontic treatment, *J Dent Res* 68 (special issue):1253, 1989.

33. Trope M: Flare-up rate of single-visit endodontics, *Int Endod J* 24:24, 1991.

34. Mata E, Koren LZ, Morse DR, Sinai IH: Prophylactic use of penicillin V in teeth with necrotic pulps and asymptomatic periapical radiolucencies, *Oral Surg Oral Med Oral Pathol* 60:201, 1985.

35. Kvist T, Reit C: Postoperative discomfort associated with surgical and nonsurgical endodontic retreatment, *Endod Dent Traumatol* 16:71, 2000.

36. Torabinejad M, Cymberman JJ, Frankson M, et al: The effectiveness of various medications on postoperative pain following complete instrumentation, *J Endod* 20:345, 1994.

37. Walton RE, Chiappenelli J: Prophylactic penicillin: effect on posttreatment symptoms following root canal treatment of asymptomatic periapical pathosis, *J Endod* 19:466, 1993.

38. Pickenpaugh L, Reader A, Beck M, et al: Effect of prophylactic amoxicillin on endodontic flare-up in asymptomatic, necrotic teeth, *J Endod* 27:53, 2001.

39. Calderon A: Prevention of apical periodontal ligament pain: a preliminary report of 100 vital pulp cases, *J Endod* 19:247, 1993.

40. Liesinger A, Marshall JF, Marshall GJ: Effect of variable doses of dexamethasone on postoperative endodontic pain, *J Endod* 19:35, 1993.

41. Nobuhara WK, Carnes DL, Gilles JA: Anti-inflammatory effects of dexamethasone on periapical tissues following endodontic overinstrumentation, *J Endod* 19:501, 1993.

42. Marshall G, Walton RE: The effect of intramuscular injection of steroid on posttreatment endodontic pain, *J Endod* 10:584, 1984.

43. Krasner P, Jackson E: Management of posttreatment endodontic pain with oral dexamethasone: a double-blind study, *Oral Surg Oral Med Oral Pathol* 62:187, 1986.

44. Trope M: Relationship of intracanal medicaments to endodontic flare-ups, *Endod Dent Traumatol* 6:226, 1990.

45. Seltzer S: Pain. In *Endodontology: biologic considerations in endodontic procedures,* ed 2, Philadelphia, 1988, Lea & Febiger.

46. Harrison JW, Baumgartner JC, Svec TA: Incidence of pain associated with clinical factors during and after root canal therapy. Part 2. Postobturation pain, *J Endod* 9:434, 1983.

47. Torabinejad M, Dorn SO, Eleazer PD, et al: The effectiveness of various medications on postoperative pain following root canal obturation, *J Endod* 20:427, 1994.

18

Mahmoud Torabinejad and Ronald R. Lemon

Procedural Accidents

LEARNING OBJECTIVES

After reading this chapter, the student should be able to:

1 / Recognize procedural accidents and describe the cause(s), prevention, and treatment of the following:

a. Pulp chamber perforation

b. Ledging

c. Separated instrument

d. Coronal or radicular perforation

e. Obturation short of prepared working length

f. Obturation materials expressed beyond apex

g. Incomplete obturation

h. Vertical root fracture

i. Post space preparation mishaps

j. Dental materials or dentin shavings obstructing the canal

OUTLINE

Perforations During Access Preparation
Causes
Prevention
Recognition and Treatment
Prognosis

Accidents During Cleaning and Shaping
Ledge Formation
Creating an Artificial Canal
Root Perforations
Separated Instruments
Other Accidents

Accidents During Obturation
Underfilling
Overfilling
Vertical Root Fracture

Accidents During Post Space Preparation
Indicators
Treatment and Prognosis

Like other complex disciplines of dentistry, an operator may encounter unwanted or unforeseen circumstances during root canal therapy that can affect the prognosis. These mishaps are collectively termed *procedural accidents.* However, fear of procedural accident should not deter a practitioner from performing endodontic therapy if proper case selection and competency issues are observed.

Knowledge of the etiologic factors involved in procedural accidents is essential for their prevention. In addition, methods of recognition and treatment as well as the effects of such accidents on prognosis must be learned. Most problems can be avoided by adhering to the basic principles of diagnosis, case selection, treatment planning, access preparation, cleaning and shaping, obturation, and postpreparation.

Examples of procedural accidents include swallowed or aspirated endodontic instruments, crown or root perforation, ledge formation, separated instruments, underfilled or overfilled canals, and vertically fractured roots. A good practitioner uses his or her knowledge, dexterity, intuition, patience, and awareness of his or her own limitations to minimize these accidents. When an accident occurs during root canal treatment, the patient should be informed about (1) the incident, (2) procedures necessary for correction, (3) alternative treatment modalities, and (4) the effect of this accident on prognosis. Proper medical-legal documentation is mandatory. A successful operator learns from past experiences and applies them to future challenges. In addition, the practitioner who knows his or her limitations will recognize potentially difficult cases and will refer the patient to an endodontist. The beneficiary will be the patient, who will receive the best care.

This chapter will discuss the causes, prevention, and treatment of various types of procedural accidents that may occur at different phases of root canal treatment. The effect of these accidents on short-and long-term prognosis will be also described.

Perforations During Access Preparation

The prime objective of an access cavity is to provide an unobstructed or straight-line pathway to the apical foramen. Accidents such as excess removal of tooth structure or perforation may occur during attempts to locate canals. Failure to achieve straight-line access is often the main etiologic factor for other types of intracanal accidents.

CAUSES

Despite anatomic variations in the configuration of various teeth, the pulp chamber, in most cases, is located in the *center* of the anatomic crown. The pulp system is located in the long axis of the tooth. Lack of attention to the degree of axial inclination of a tooth in relation to adjacent teeth and to alveolar bone may result in either gouging or perforation of the crown or the root at various levels (Figure 18-1). *Failure to direct the bur parallel to the long axis of a tooth will cause gouging or perforation* (see Chapter 12). This problem often occurs when the dentist must use the reflected image from an intraoral mirror to make the access preparation. In these situations, the natural tendency is to direct the bur away from the long axis of the root to improve vision through the mirror. Failure to check the orientation of the access opening during preparation may result in a perforation. The dentist should stop periodically to review the bur-tooth relationship. Aids for evaluating progress include transillumination, magnification, and radiographs.

Searching for the pulp chamber or orifices of canals through an underprepared access cavity may also result in accidents (Figure 18-2). Failing to recognize when the bur passes through a small or flattened (disklike) pulp chamber in a multirooted tooth may also result in gouging or perforation of the furcation (Figure 18-3).

A cast crown often is not aligned in the long axis of the tooth; directing the bur along the misaligned casting may result in a coronal or radicular perforation.

PREVENTION
Clinical Examination

Thorough knowledge of tooth morphology, including both surface anatomy and internal anatomy and their relationships, is mandatory to prevent pulp chamber perforations. Next, loca-

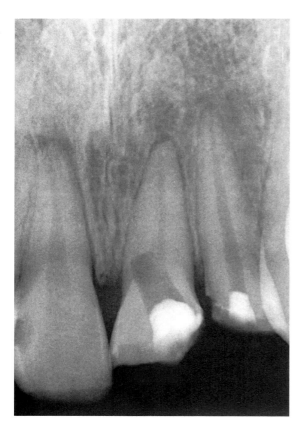

FIGURE 18-1
A misdirected bur created severe gouging and near-perforation during an otherwise routine access cavity preparation.

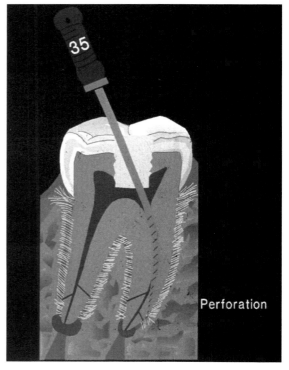

FIGURE 18-2
Inadequate access cavities not only result in compromised preparation and obturation but also may cause procedural accidents such as chamber perforation, canal ledging, and root perforation.

tion and angulation of the tooth must be related to adjacent teeth and alveolar bone to avoid a misaligned access preparation. In addition, radiographs of teeth from different angles provide information about the size and extent of the pulp chamber and the presence of internal changes such as calcification or resorption. *The radiograph is a two-dimensional projection of a three-dimensional object*; varying the horizontal exposure angle will provide at least a distorted view of the third dimension and may be helpful in supplying additional anatomic information.

Operative Procedures

Use of a rubber dam during root canal treatment is usually indicated.[1] However, in situations in which problems are anticipated in locating pulp chambers (e.g., tilted teeth, misoriented castings, or calcified chambers), initiating access without a rubber dam is preferred[2] because it allows better crown-root alignment (see Chapter 12). However, when access is made without rubber dam placement, no intracanal instruments such as files, reamers, or broaches should be used unless they are secured by a piece of floss[2] and a throat pack is placed. Constricted chambers or canals must be sought

patiently, with small amounts of dentin removed at a time.

Another useful method of providing isolation and also visualizing the crown-root alignment is the use of a "split" dam (Figure 18-4). This dam can be applied in the anterior region without a rubber dam clamp (see Chapter 8) or in posterior regions by quadrant isolation if a distal tooth can be clamped. Also, elimination of the metal clamp from the field of operation allows radiographic orientation of coronal access preparation.

To orient the access, a bur may be placed in the preparation hole (secured with cotton pellets) and then radiographed (Figure 18-5). This provides information about depth of access in relation to canal location. Remember, a single canal is located in the center of the root. A direct facial radiograph will show the mesiodistal relationship; a mesial or distal angled film will show the faciolingual location. This procedure is helpful for locating small canals.

Use of a fiberoptic light during access preparation may assist in locating canals. This strong light illuminates the cavity when the beam is directed through the access opening (reflected light) and illuminates the pulp chamber floor (transmitted light). In the latter case, a canal orifice appears as a dark spot. Using magnifying glasses or an operative microscope will also aid in locating a small orifice. Magnification loops (2.5 or greater) are useful especially when combined with transillumination. But the ultimate aid in canal location is the operating microscope. Patients with problems requiring significant magnification for canal location should be referred to an endodontist who has this specialized equipment.

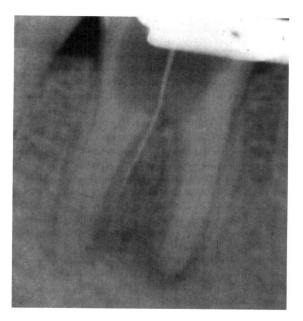

FIGURE 18-3
Failure to recognize when the bur passes through the roof of the pulp chamber if the chamber is calcified may result in gouging or perforation of the furcation. The use of apex locators and angled radiographs is necessary for early perforation detection. Early detection reduces damage and improves repair.

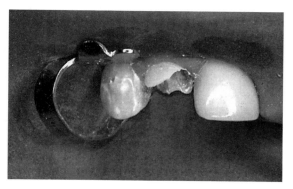

FIGURE 18-4
A rubber dam can be applied in the anterior region without placing the clamp on the tooth that is undergoing root canal therapy or in posterior regions by quadrant isolation if a distal tooth can be clamped.

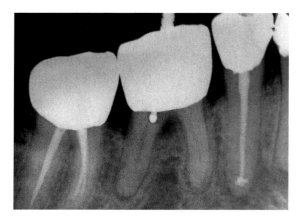

FIGURE 18-5
A small bur is placed during access preparation when orientation is a problem. This provides information about data such as angulation and depth of bur penetration. Continuation of the search without a radiograph to check position would probably have resulted in a perforation into the furcation.

RECOGNITION AND TREATMENT

Perforation into the periodontal ligament or bone usually (but not always) results in immediate and continuous hemorrhage. The canal or chamber is difficult to dry; placement of a paper point or cotton pellet may increase or renew the bleeding. Bone is relatively avascular compared with soft tissue; mechanical perforation may occasionally initially produce only hemorrhage equal to that of pulp tissue.

Perforations must be recognized early to avoid subsequent damage to the periodontal tissues with intracanal instruments and irrigants. Early signs of perforation may include one or more of the following: (1) sudden pain during the working length determination when local anesthesia was adequate during access preparation; (2) sudden appearance of hemorrhage; (3) burning pain or a bad taste during irrigation with sodium hypochlorite; (4) other signs, including a radiographically malpositioned file (see Figure 18-3) or a periodontal ligament reading from an apex locator that is far short of the working length on an initial file entry.

Unusually severe postoperative pain may result from cleaning and shaping procedures performed through an undetected perforation. At a subsequent appointment, the perforation site will be hemorrhagic due to the inflammation of the surrounding tissues. The overall prognosis of the tooth must be evaluated with respect to the strategic value of the tooth, the location and size of the defect, and the potential for repair.

Perforation into the periodontal ligament at any location will have a negative effect on long-term prognosis. The dentist must inform the patient of the questionable prognosis[1] and closely monitor the long-term periodontal response to any treatment. In addition, the patient must know what signs or symptoms indicate failure and, if failure occurs, what the subsequent treatment will be.

Perforations during access cavity preparation present a variety of problems. When a perforation occurs or is strongly suspected, the patient should be considered for referral to an endodontist. In general, a specialist is better equipped to manage these patients. Also, after long-term evaluation, other procedures such as surgery may be necessary if future failure occurs (Figure 18-6).

Lateral Root Perforation

The location and size of the perforation during access are important factors in a lateral perforation. If the defect is located at or above the height of crestal bone, the prognosis for perforation repair is favorable.[3,4] These defects can be easily "exteriorized" and repaired with standard restorative material such as amalgam, glass ionomer, or composite. Periodontal curettage or a flap procedure is occasionally required to place, remove, or smooth excess repair material. In some cases, the best repair is placement of a full crown with the margin extended apically to cover the defect.

Teeth with perforations below the crestal bone in the coronal third of the root generally have the poorest prognosis. Attachment often recedes and a periodontal pocket forms, with attachment loss extending apically to at least the depth of the defect. The treatment goal is to position the apical portion of the defect above crestal bone. Orthodontic root extrusion is generally the procedure of choice for teeth in the aesthetic zone.[5,6] Crown lengthening may be considered when the aesthetic result will not be compromised or when approximal teeth require surgical periodontal therapy. Internal repair of these perforations by mineral trioxide aggregate (MTA) has been shown to provide an excellent seal as compared to other materials.[7]

Furcation Perforation

A perforation of the furcation is generally one of two types: the "direct" or the "stripping" type; each is created and managed differently and the prognoses vary. The *direct perforation* usually occurs during a search for a canal orifice. It is more of a "punched-out" defect into the furcation with

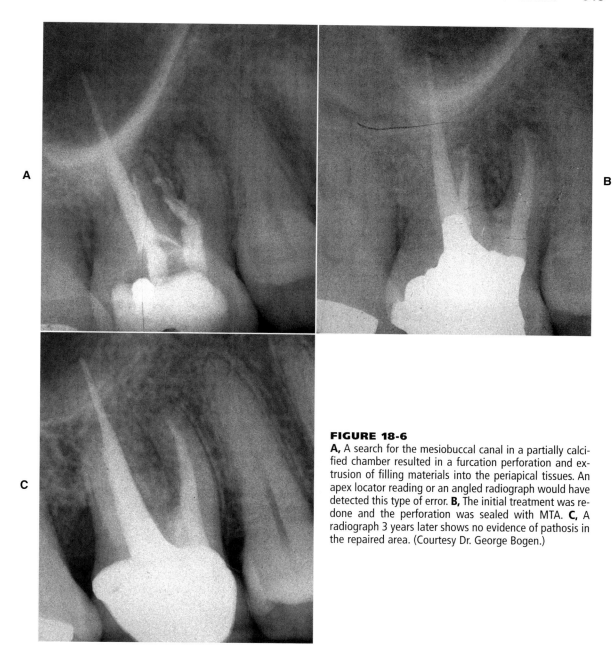

A

B

C

FIGURE 18-6
A, A search for the mesiobuccal canal in a partially calcified chamber resulted in a furcation perforation and extrusion of filling materials into the periapical tissues. An apex locator reading or an angled radiograph would have detected this type of error. **B,** The initial treatment was redone and the perforation was sealed with MTA. **C,** A radiograph 3 years later shows no evidence of pathosis in the repaired area. (Courtesy Dr. George Bogen.)

a bur; therefore, it is usually accessible and may be small and have walls. This type of perforation should be immediately (if possible) repaired with MTA (Figure 18-7), or, if proper conditions exist (dryness), glass ionomer or composite, in an attempt to seal the defect. Prognosis is usually good if the defect is sealed immediately.

A *stripping perforation* involving the furcation side of the coronal root surface results from excessive flaring with files or drills. Whereas direct perforations are usually accessible and therefore can be repaired nonsurgically, stripping perforations are generally inaccessible, requiring more elaborate approaches. The usual sequelae of stripping perforations are inflammation followed by development of a periodontal pocket. Long-term failure results from leakage of the repair material, which produces periodontal breakdown with attachment loss. Skillful use of MTA has significantly improved the prognosis of nonsurgical

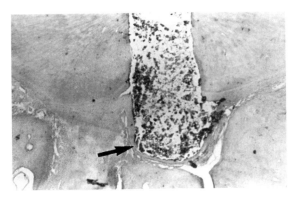

FIGURE 18-7
Immediate repair of perforation in furcation of a dog premolar with MTA results in formation of cementum *(arrow)* adjacent to the material.

repair of stripping perforations compared to other repair materials (Figure 18-8).

Nonsurgical Treatment

If feasible, nonsurgical repair of furcation perforations is preferred to surgical alteration of the tooth[4] (Figure 18-9). Traditionally, materials such as amalgam, gutta-percha, zinc oxide-eugenol, Cavit, calcium hydroxide, freeze-dried bone, and indium foil have been used clinically and experimentally to seal these defects.[8-16] Repair is difficult because of potential problems with visibility, hemorrhage control, and management and sealing ability of the repair materials. In general, perforations occurring during access preparation should be sealed immediately, but the patency of the

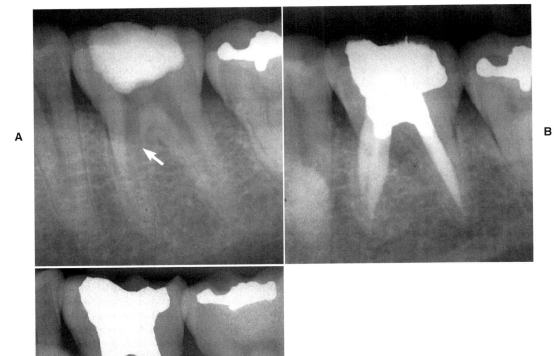

FIGURE 18-8
A, A stripping perforation *(arrow)* is evident in the mesiobuccal root. **B,** The mesial roots were filled with MTA and the distal root with gutta-percha and root canal sealer. **C,** A radiograph made 1 year later shows no periradicular pathosis.

canals must be protected. Immediate repair of the perforations with MTA offers the best results for perforation repair.[16,17]

Surgical Treatment

Surgery requires more complex restorative procedures and more demanding oral hygiene from the patient.[4] Surgical alternatives are hemisection, bicuspidization, root amputation, and intentional replantation. Teeth with divergent roots and bone levels that allow preparation of adequate crown margins are suitable for either hemisection or bicuspidization. Intentional replantation is indicated when the defect is inaccessible or when multiple problems exist, such as a perforation combined with a separated instrument, or when the prognosis with other surgical procedures is poor (Figure 18-10). Dentist and patient must recognize that the prognosis for treatment of surgically altered teeth is guarded because of the increased technical difficulty associated with restorative procedures and demanding oral hygiene requirements. The remaining roots are prone to caries, periodontal disease, and vertical root fracture.

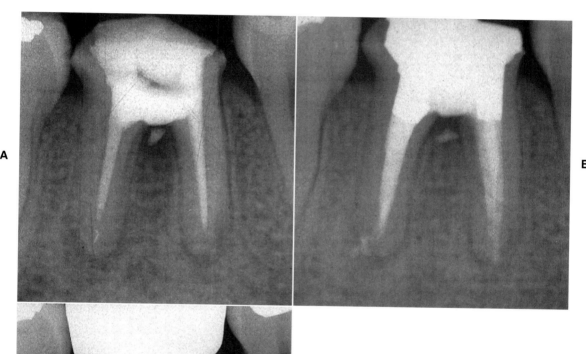

FIGURE 18-9
A, Furcation perforation is evident in the first molar. **B,** The root canal was retreated and the perforation was repaired with MTA. **C,** A radiograph made 26 months later shows no evidence of furcal pathosis.

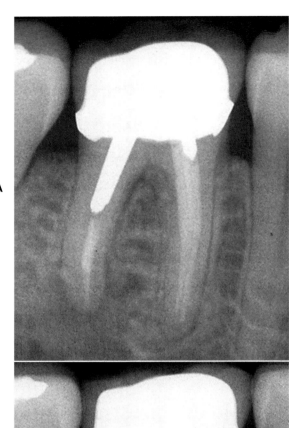

A

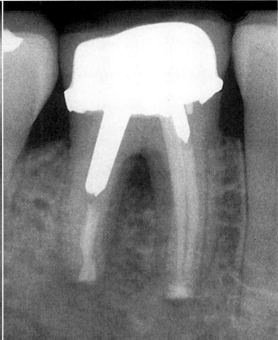

B

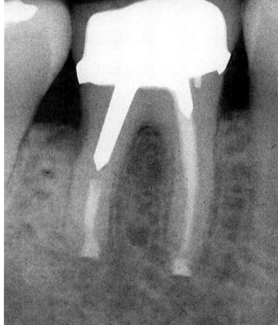

C

FIGURE 18-10
A, A postoperative radiograph 6 years after endodontic treatment. The tooth is percussion sensitive, and periapical lesions are present. A 5-mm probing defect exists on the distolingual root. A fracture is suspected and extract-replant was performed for diagnostic reasons. The tooth was extracted, and no fracture was seen. **B,** The tooth is replanted after a root-end filling with MTA. The cause of failure was probably leakage. **C,** A radiograph 1 year later showed osseous repair. The probing defect healed.

PROGNOSIS

Factors affecting the long-term prognosis of teeth after perforation repair include the location of the defect in relation to crestal bone, the length of the root trunk, the accessibility for repair, the size of the defect, the presence or absence of a periodontal communication to the defect, the time lapse between perforation and repair, the sealing ability of restorative material, and subjective factors such as the technical competence of the dentist and the attitude and oral hygiene of the patient.[4] Early recognition and repair will improve the prognosis by minimizing damage to the periodontal tissues by bacteria, files, and irrigants. Additionally, a small perforation (less than 1 mm) causes less tissue destruction and is more amenable to repair than a larger perforation. Electronic apex locators or angled radiographs with files in place aid in early detection.

An unrecognized or untreated perforation in the furcation usually results in a periodontal defect that communicates through the gingival sulcus within weeks or sometimes days. A preexisting periodontal communication caused by perforation worsens the prognosis; therefore, the time between perforation and repair should be as short as possible.[18,19] Immediate sealing of the defect reduces the incidence of periodontal breakdown. To best determine the long-term prognosis, the dentist must monitor the patient's symptoms, radiographic changes, and, most importantly, periodontal status. Radiographs and periodontal probing during recall examination are the best measures of success or failure of the repair procedure.

Accidents During Cleaning and Shaping

The most common procedural accidents during cleaning and shaping of the root canal system are ledge formation, artificial canal creation, root perforation, instrument separation, and extrusion of irrigating solution periapically. Correction of these accidents is usually difficult and the patient should be referred to an endodontist.

LEDGE FORMATION

By definition, a ledge has been created when the working length can no longer be negotiated and the original patency of the canal is lost. The major causes of ledge formation include (1) inadequate straight-line access into the canal (2) inadequate irrigation and/or lubrication, (3) excessive enlargement of a curved canal with files, and (4) packing debris in the apical portion of the canal.

Prevention of a Ledge

Preoperative Evaluation. Prevention of ledging begins with examination of the preoperative radiograph for curvatures, length, and initial size.

Curvatures. Most important is the coronal third of the root canal. Severe coronal curvature predisposes the apical canal to ledging. Straight-line access to the orifice of the canal can be achieved during access preparation, but accessibility to the apical third of the canal is achieved only with coronal flaring. Severe apical curvatures require a proper sequence of cleaning and shaping procedures to maintain patency (see Chapter 13).

Length. Longer canals are more prone to ledging than shorter canals. Careful attention to maintaining patency is required to prevent ledging.

Initial Size. Canals of smaller diameter are more easily ledged than larger-diameter canals.

In summary, *the canals most prone to ledging are small, curved, and long.* Radiographs are two-dimensional and cannot provide accurate information about the actual shape and curvature of the root canal system. All root canals have some degree of curvature including facial-lingual curves, which may not be apparent on straight facial exposures.

Technical Procedures. Determination of working length in the cleaning and shaping process is a continuation of the access preparation. Optimum straight-line access to the apical third is not achieved until cleaning and shaping have been completed. An accurate working length measurement is a requirement because cleaning and shaping short of the ideal length is a prelude to ledge formation. Frequent recapitulation and irrigation, along with the use of lubricants, are mandatory! Sodium hypochlorite may be used initially for hemorrhage control and removal of debris. However, this agent alone may not be adequate to provide maximum lubrication.

Silicone, glycerine, and wax-based lubricants are commercially available for canal lubrication. Because these materials are viscous, they are carried into the apical regions of the canal with the file. Enhanced lubrication permits easier file insertion, reduces stress to the file, and assists with removal of debris. The lubricant is easily removed with sodium hypochlorite irrigation. Flexible files (nickel-titanium) reduce the chances for ledge formation.

A one-eighth to one-fourth reaming motion with the files should be used in the apical third. A filing motion directed away from the furcation is used to form the funnel shape of the canal and reduce the coronal curvature. Each file must be worked until it is loose before a larger size is used.

Canals with a severe coronal curvature require a passive step-back cleaning and shaping technique (see Chapter 13). A No. 15 file is used at working length. With maximum irrigation or lubrication, the canal is passively and progressively flared in a step-back fashion. The No. 15 file is recapitulated many times to maintain patency. This preflaring technique reduces the coronal curvature and enlarges the canal. Better control of the files is gained for enlarging and cleaning the apical third of the canal as the last step (see "Apical

Clearing" in Chapter 13). Using this technique, the chances of ledge formation are reduced. Rotary files with increased taper will blend and join the shape into a tapering funnel.

Management of a Ledge

Once created, a ledge is difficult to correct. An initial attempt should be made to bypass the ledge with a No. 10 steel file to regain working length. The file tip (2 to 3 mm) is sharply curved and worked in the canal in the direction of the canal curvature. Lubricants are helpful. A "picking" motion is used to attempt to feel the catch of the original canal space, which is slightly short of the apical extent of the ledge. If the original canal is located, the file is then worked with a reaming motion and occasionally an up-and-down movement to maintain the space and remove debris (Figure 18-11), although this may be only partially successful. Once a ledge is created, even if it is initially bypassed, instruments and obturating materials tend to be continually directed into the ledge.

If the original canal cannot be located by this method, then cleaning and shaping of the existing canal space is completed at the new working length. At times, flaring of the canal may allow the ledge to be bypassed by providing improved access to the apical canal. Small, curved files are used in the manner previously described in a final attempt to bypass the ledge. If this is successful, the apical canal space must be sequentially cleaned and flared to an appropriate size. Complete removal or reduction of the ledge facilitates obturation.

Prognosis

Failure of root canal treatment associated with ledging depends on the amount of debris left in the uninstrumented and unfilled portion of the canal. The amount depends on when ledge formation occurred during the cleaning and shaping process. In general, short and cleaned apical ledges have good prognoses. The patient must be informed about the prognosis, the importance of the recall examination, and what signs indicate failure. Future appearance of clinical symptoms or radiographic evidence of failure may require referral for apical surgery or retreatment.

CREATING AN ARTIFICIAL CANAL
Cause and Prevention

Deviation from the original pathway of the root canal system and creation of an artificial canal cause an exaggerated ledge; it is initiated by the factors that cause ledge formation. Therefore, the recommendations for preventing ledge formation should be followed to avoid creating artificial canals. The unfortunate sequence is as follows: A ledge is created and the proper working length is lost. The operator, eager to regain that length, "bores" apically with each file, thus creating an artificial canal. Used persistently, the file eventually perforates the root surface.

Management

Negotiating the original canal that has an exaggerated ledge is normally very difficult. Rarely can the original canal be located, renegotiated, and prepared. To obturate, the dentist should determine whether a perforation exists. Methods include apex locator readings, hemorrhage on paper points while drying, and radiographs with a file in position. If confirmed, the working length is adjusted, an apical stop is created at the adjusted length with larger files, and obturation is begun. If there is no perforation, the canal is obturated with a warm or softened gutta-percha technique in conjunction with a root canal sealer. If there is a perforation, the defect should be repaired internally or surgically (see "Root Perforations" below).

Prognosis

Prognosis depends on the ability of the operator to renegotiate the original canal and the remaining amount of uninstrumented and unfilled portion of the main canal. Unless a perforation exists, teeth in which the original canal can be renegotiated and obturated have a prognosis similar to those without procedure complications. In contrast, when a large portion of the main canal is uninstrumented and unobturated, a poorer prognosis exists, and the tooth must be examined periodically. Failure usually means surgery will be required to resect the uninstrumented and unobturated root canal.

ROOT PERFORATIONS

Roots may be perforated at different levels during cleaning and shaping. Location (apical, middle, or cervical) of the perforation as well as the stage of treatment affects prognosis.[11] The periodontal response to the injury is affected by the level and size of the perforation. Perforation in the early stages of cleaning and shaping affects prognosis significantly.

Apical Perforations

This type of perforation occurs through the apical foramen (overinstrumentation) or through the body of the root (perforated new canal).

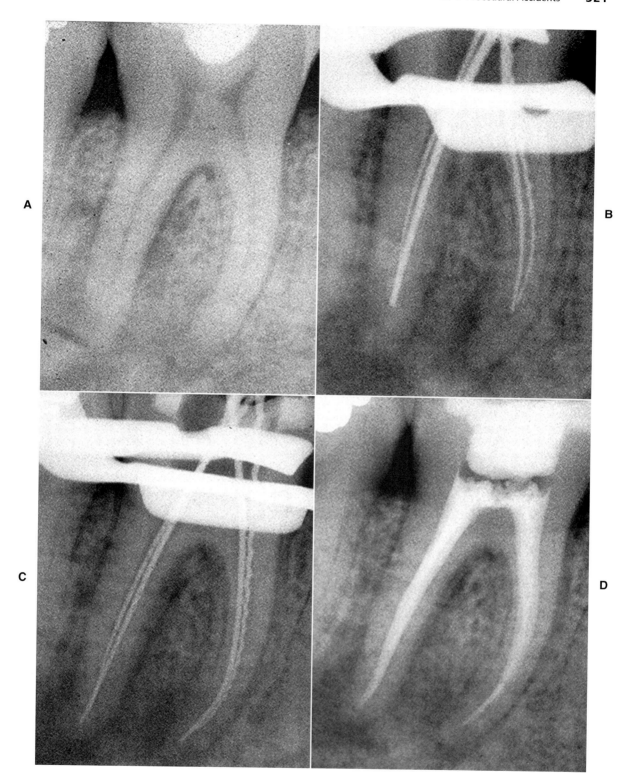

FIGURE 18-11
A, Preoperative radiograph. **B,** Ledges have been formed in the mesial and distal canals with stainless steel files. Ledges can be bypassed only with small, curved stainless steel files. **C,** Ledges are bypassed, and proper length is established. **D,** Final radiograph. Nickel-titanium files can be used only after ledges are removed.

Etiology and Indicators. Instrumentation of the canal beyond the apical constriction results in perforation. Incorrect working length or inability to maintain proper working length causes "zipping"[2] or "blowing out" of the apical foramen. Appearance of fresh hemorrhage in the canal or on instruments, pain during canal preparation in a previously asymptomatic tooth, and sudden loss of the apical stop are indicators of foramen perforation. Extension of the largest (final) file beyond the radiographic apex is also a sign. An electronic apex locator may also confirm this procedural accident.

Prevention. To prevent apical perforation, proper working lengths must be established and maintained throughout the procedure. In curved canals, the flexibility of files with respect to size must be considered. Step-back and flaring procedures straighten the canal somewhat and effectively decrease the working length by as much as 1 to 2 mm, requiring compensation.

Treatment. Treatment includes establishing a new working length, creating an apical seat (taper), and obturating the canal to its new length. Depending on the size and location of the apical foramen, a new working length 1 to 2 mm short of the point of perforation should be established. The canal is then cleaned, shaped, and obturated to the new working length. The master cone must have a positive apical stop at the working length before obturation. Placement of MTA as an apical barrier can prevent extrusion of obturation materials.

Prognosis. Success of treatment depends primarily on the size and shape of the defect. An open apex or reverse funnel is difficult to seal and also allows extrusion of the filling materials. In addition, the feasibility of repairing the perforation surgically may influence the final outcome.

Lateral (Midroot) Perforations

Etiology and Indicators. As discussed earlier, inability to maintain canal curvature is the major cause of ledge formation. Negotiation of ledged canals is not always possible; misdirected pressure and force applied to a file may result in formation of an artificial canal and eventually in an apical or midroot perforation. To avoid these perforations, the same factors mentioned earlier for prevention of ledge formation should be considered: (1) degree of canal curvature and size and (2) inflexibility of the larger files, especially stainless steel files.

Indicators of lateral perforation are similar to those of apical perforation, i.e., fresh hemorrhage in the root canal or sudden pain and deviation of instruments from their original course. Penetration of the instrument out of the root radio-

graphically (or, as indicated by an apex locator) is the ultimate indicator.

Treatment. The optimal goal is to clean, shape, and obturate the entire root canal system of the affected tooth. After the perforation is confirmed, the steps discussed previously for bypassing of ledged canals are followed. If attempts to negotiate the apical portion of the canal are unsuccessful, the operator should concentrate on cleaning, shaping, and obturating the coronal segment of the canal. A new working length confined to the root is established; the canal is then cleaned, shaped, and obturated to the new working length. A low concentration (0.5%) of sodium hypochlorite or saline should be used for irrigation in a perforated canal. Extrusion of concentrated irrigant into the surrounding periodontal tissues would produce severe inflammation.

Prognosis. Success depends partially on the remaining amount of undébrided and unobturated canal. Obturation is difficult because of lack of a stop (matrix); gutta-percha tends to be extruded during condensation. Teeth with perforations close to the apex after complete or partial débridement of the canal have a better prognosis than those with perforations that occur earlier. In addition to the length of uncleaned and unfilled portions of the canal, size and surgical accessibility of perforations are important. In general, small perforations are easier to seal than large ones. Because of surgical accessibility, perforations toward the facial aspect are more easily repaired and therefore these teeth have a better prognosis than those with perforations in other areas.

On recall, both radiographic and periodontal examinations for signs and symptoms are performed; failure generally requires surgery or other approaches. These approaches depend on the severity of perforation, the strategic importance of the tooth, and the location and accessibility of the perforation. Corrective techniques include repair of the perforation site, root resection to the level of the perforation, root amputation, hemisection, replantation, and extraction.

Coronal Root Perforations

Etiology and Indicators. Coronal root perforations occur during access preparation while the operator attempts to locate canal orifices or during flaring procedures with files, Gates-Glidden drills, or Peeso reamers. Perforations during access preparation can be minimized by using the methods described earlier in this chapter. Removal of restorations when possible, use of fiberoptic lights for illumination, magnification, and cautious exploration for calcified canals can prevent most problems during access preparation. Careful flaring (step-back) and conservative use of flaring instruments are required during cleaning and shaping procedures.

Treatment and Prognosis. Repair of a stripping perforation in the coronal third of the root has the poorest long-term prognosis of any type of perforation.[4] The defect is usually inaccessible for adequate repair. An attempt should be made to seal the defect internally, even though the prognosis is guarded. Patency of the canal system must be maintained during the repair process. Referral of the patient to a specialist is recommended.

SEPARATED INSTRUMENTS
Etiology

Limited flexibility and strength of intracanal instruments combined with improper use may result in an intracanal instrument separation. Any instrument may break—steel, nickel-titanium, hand, or rotary. Overuse or excessive force applied to files is the main cause of separation. Manufacturing defects in files are rare.

Recognition

Removal of a shortened file with a blunt tip from a canal and subsequent loss of patency to the original length are the main clues for the presence of a separated instrument. A radiograph is *essential* for confirmation. It is *imperative* that the patient be informed of the accident and its effect on prognosis.[1] As with other procedural accidents, detailed documentation is also necessary for medical-legal considerations.

Prevention

Recognition of the physical properties and stress limitations of files is critical. Continual lubrication with either irrigating solution or lubricants is required. Each instrument is examined before use. If an unwound or twisted file is rotated and viewed, reflections from the chairside light will magnify fluting distortions (Figure 18-12). Small files must be replaced often. To minimize binding, each file size is worked in the canal until it is very loose before the next file size is used.[20] Nickel-titanium files usually do not show visual signs of fatigue similar to the "untwisting" of steel files. Many factors may affect the fatiguing of nickel-titanium files, and they should be discarded before visual signs of untwisting are seen.

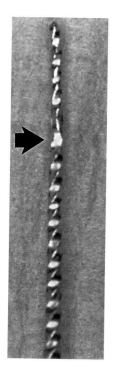

FIGURE 18-12
Each steel file should be inspected for fluting distortion before use in the canal. Only untwisted files will show a shiny spot *(arrow)*. This file must be discarded. Nickel-titanium files usually will not show this distortion and must be discarded after three to six uses.

Treatment

There are basically three approaches: (1) attempt to remove the instrument, (2) attempt to bypass it, and (3) prepare and obturate to the segment. Initial treatment is similar to that discussed earlier for a ledge. Using a small file and following the guidelines described for negotiating a ledge, the operator should attempt to bypass the separated instrument. If this is successful, broaches or Hedström files are used to try to grasp and remove the segment; this usually does not work. Then the canal is cleaned, shaped, and obturated to its new working length (Figure 18-13). If the instrument cannot be bypassed, preparation and obturation should be performed to the coronal level of the fragment.

Prognosis

Prognosis depends on how much undébrided and unobturated canal apical to and including the instrument remains. The prognosis is best when separation of a large instrument occurs in the

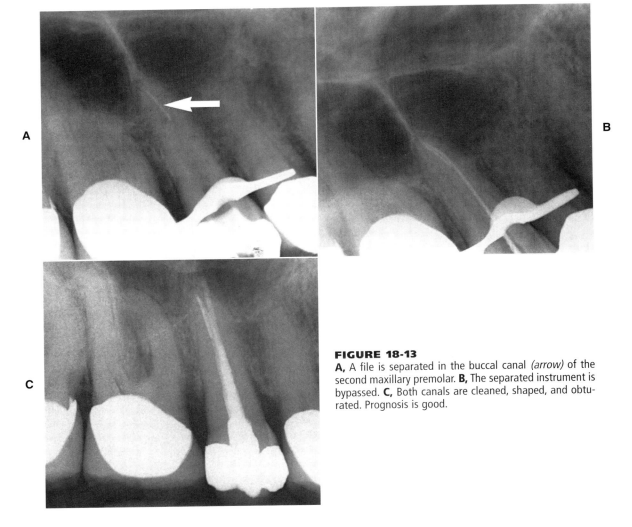

FIGURE 18-13
A, A file is separated in the buccal canal *(arrow)* of the second maxillary premolar. **B,** The separated instrument is bypassed. **C,** Both canals are cleaned, shaped, and obturated. Prognosis is good.

later stages of preparation close to the working length. Prognosis is poorer for teeth with undébrided canals in which a small instrument is separated short of the apex or beyond the apical foramen early in preparation. For medical-legal reasons, the patient must be informed (with documentation in the record) of an instrument separation. Despite the concern of both patient and dentist,[21] clinical studies indicate that the prognosis in most procedures involving broken instruments that are managed properly is favorable.[22]

If the patient remains symptomatic or there is a subsequent failure, the tooth can be treated surgically. Accessible roots are resected with placement of a root-end filling material (Figure 18-14). Accessibility of the root apex for surgical intervention is critical to the final outcome.

OTHER ACCIDENTS
Aspiration or Ingestion

Aspiration or ingestion of instruments is a serious event but is easily avoided with proper precautions. *Use of the rubber dam is the standard of care to prevent such ingestion or aspiration* and subsequent lawsuits.[1]

The disappearance of an instrument that has slipped from the dentist's fingers, followed by violent coughing or gagging by the patient and radiographic confirmation of a file in the alimentary tract or airway, is the chief sign. These patients require immediate referral to a medical service for appropriate diagnosis and treatment. According to a survey by Grossman,[23] 87% of these instruments are swallowed and the rest are aspirated. Surgical removal is required for some

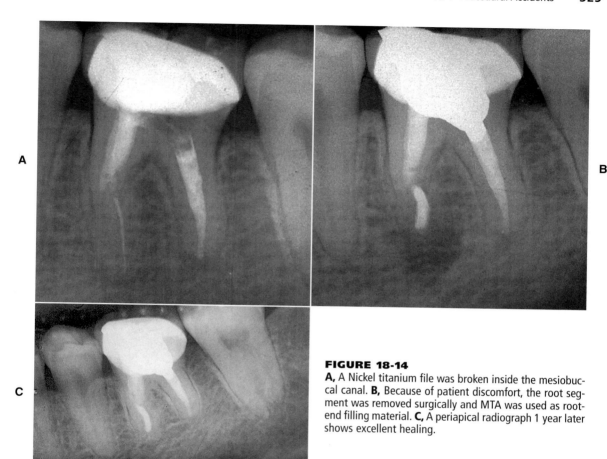

FIGURE 18-14
A, A Nickel titanium file was broken inside the mesiobuccal canal. **B,** Because of patient discomfort, the root segment was removed surgically and MTA was used as root-end filling material. **C,** A periapical radiograph 1 year later shows excellent healing.

swallowed (Figure 18-15) and nearly all aspirated instruments.

Extrusion of Irrigant

Wedging of a needle in the canal (or particularly out of a perforation) with forceful expression of irrigant (usually sodium hypochlorite) causes penetration of irrigants into the periradicular tissues and inflammation and discomfort for patients. Loose placement of irrigation needles and careful irrigation with light pressure or use of a perforated needle[24] precludes forcing of the irrigating solution into the periradicular tissues. Sudden prolonged and sharp pain during irrigation followed by rapid diffuse swelling (the "sodium hypochlorite accident") usually indicates

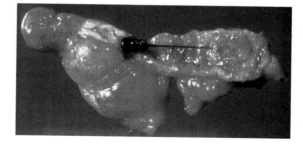

FIGURE 18-15
A swallowed broach lodged in a patent's appendix, resulting in the removal of the appendix and a subsequent lawsuit against a dentist who did not use rubber dam during root canal therapy.

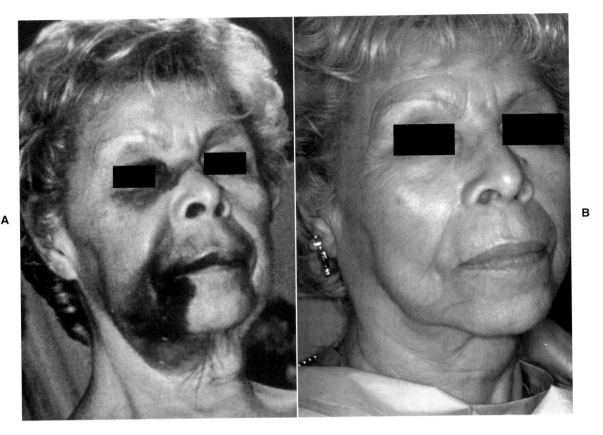

FIGURE 18-16
A, Sodium hypochlorite was inadvertently expressed through an apical perforation in a maxillary canine during irrigation. Hemorrhagic reaction was rapid and diffuse. **B,** No treatment was necessary; the swelling and hematoma disappeared within a few weeks. (Courtesy Dr. James Stick.)

penetration of solution into the periradicular tissues. The acute episode will subside spontaneously with time (Figure 18-16).

Initially there is no reason to prescribe antibiotics or attempt surgical drainage. Treatment is palliative. Analgesics are prescribed, and the patient is reassured. Because the outcome is so dramatic, evaluation is performed frequently to follow progress.

Accidents During Obturation

Appropriate cleaning and shaping are the keys to preventing obturation problems because these accidents usually result from improper canal preparation. In general, adequately prepared canals are obturated without mishap. *The quality of obturation reflects canal preparation.* However, problems do occur.

UNDERFILLING
Etiology

Some causes of underfilling include a natural barrier in the canal, a ledge created during preparation, insufficient flaring, a poorly adapted master cone, and inadequate condensation pressure. Bypassing (if possible) of any natural or artificial barrier to create a smooth funnel is one key to avoiding an underfill. The advent of nickel-titanium rotary files of increased taper has greatly improved the predictability of proper funnel and taper.

Treatment and Prognosis

Removal of underfilled gutta-percha and retreatment is preferred. Forcing gutta-percha apically by increased spreader or plugger pressure can fracture the root. If lateral condensation is the method of obturation, the master cone should be marked to indicate the working length. If dis-

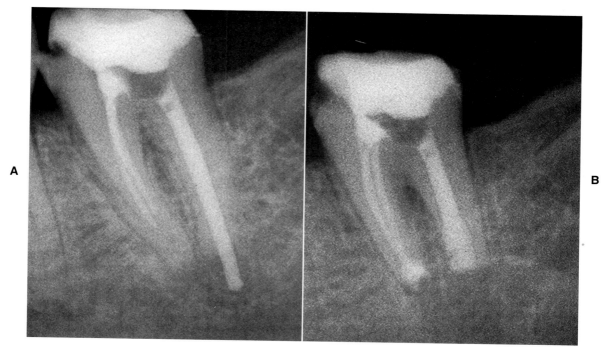

FIGURE 18-17

A, Lack of proper length measurements resulted in overpreparation and then overfill of the distal root and underfill of the mesial root. The tooth remained percussion sensitive. **B,** Surgical curettage, apical root resection, and root-end filling with MTA were necessary to correct the technical deficiencies.

placement of the master cone during condensation is suspected, a radiograph is made *before* excess gutta-percha is removed. Removal can then be accomplished by pulling the cones in the reverse order of placement. Removal of gutta-percha in canals obturated with lateral condensation is easier than removal with other obturation techniques. However, warm gutta-percha techniques allow better obturation of irregularities within the canal.

OVERFILLING

Extruded obturation material causes tissue damage and inflammation. Postoperative discomfort (mastication sensitivity) usually lasts for a few days.

Etiology

Overfilling is usually the sequela of overinstrumentation through the apical constriction or lack of proper taper in prepared canals. When the apex is open naturally or its constriction is removed during cleaning and shaping, there is no matrix against which to condense; uncontrolled

condensation forces extrusion of materials (Figure 18-17). Other causes include inflammatory resorption and incomplete development of the root.

Prevention

To avoid overfilling, guidelines for preventing apical foramen perforation should be followed. Tapered preparation with an apical "matrix" usually prevents overfill. The largest file and master cone at working length should have a positive stop. A customized master cone may be fabricated by briefly applying solvent on the tip. If overfilling is suspected, a radiograph should be made before excess gutta-percha is removed. As with underfilling, the gutta-percha mass may be removed if the sealer has not set.

Treatment and Prognosis

When signs or symptoms of endodontic failure appear, apical surgery may be required to remove the material from apical tissues and place root-end filling material. Long-term prognosis is dictated by the quality of the apical seal, the amount

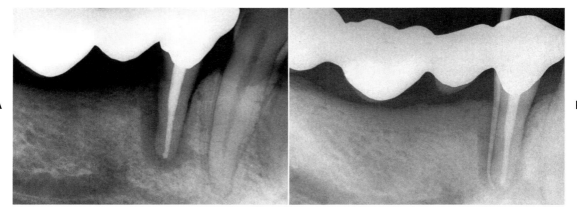

FIGURE 18-18
Indicators of vertical root fracture. **A,** A "tear-drop" lateral radiolucency is noted along the root. **B,** Narrow probing defect extends to the apex.

and biocompatibility of extruded material, host response, and toxicity and sealability of the root-end filling material.

VERTICAL ROOT FRACTURE

Complete vertical root fracture causes untreatable failure. Aspects of vertical root fracture are described in more detail in Chapter 28.

Etiology

Causative factors include root canal treatment procedures and associated factors such as post placement. The main cause of vertical root fracture is post cementation; second in importance is overzealous application of condensation forces to obturate an under- or overprepared canal.[25]

Prevention

As related to root canal treatment procedures, the best means of preventing vertical root fractures are appropriate canal preparation and use of balanced pressure during obturation. A major reason for flaring canals is to provide space for condensation instruments. Finger spreaders produce less stress and distortion of the root than their hand counterparts.[26-28]

Indicators

Long-standing vertical root fractures are often associated with a narrow periodontal pocket or sinus tract stoma as well as with a lateral radiolucency extending to the apical portion of the vertical fracture[29] (Figure 18-18). To confirm the diagnosis, a vertical fracture must be visualized. Exploratory surgery or removal or the restoration is usually necessary to visualize this mishap.

Prognosis and Treatment

Complete vertical root fracture predicts the poorest prognosis of any procedural accident. Treatment is removal of the involved root in multirooted teeth and extraction of single-rooted teeth.

Accidents During Post Space Preparation

To prevent root perforation, gutta-percha may be removed to the desired level with heated pluggers or softened with chloroform and removed by files. This "pilot" post space provides a path of least resistance for sizing drills. When a canal is prepared to receive a post, drills should be used sequentially, starting with a size that fits passively to the desired level. Miscalculation and incorrect preparation may result in perforation at any level. Knowledge of root anatomy is necessary for determining the size and depth of posts.

INDICATORS

The indicators of perforations and vertical root fractures are somewhat similar. Appearance of fresh blood during post space preparation is an indication for the presence of a root perforation. The presence of a sinus tract stoma or probing defects extending to the base of a post is often a sign of root fracture or perforation. Radiographs often show a lateral radiolucency along the root or perforation site.

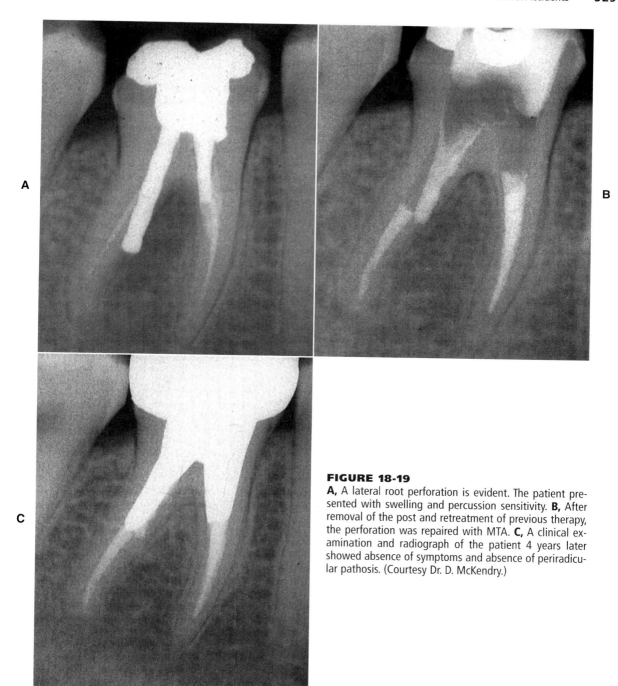

FIGURE 18-19
A, A lateral root perforation is evident. The patient presented with swelling and percussion sensitivity. **B,** After removal of the post and retreatment of previous therapy, the perforation was repaired with MTA. **C,** A clinical examination and radiograph of the patient 4 years later showed absence of symptoms and absence of periradicular pathosis. (Courtesy Dr. D. McKendry.)

TREATMENT AND PROGNOSIS

Prognosis for teeth with vertical root fractures resulting from post space preparation and postinsertion is similar to that for teeth with fractures developing during obturation; the involved root (or tooth) is hopeless and must be removed. As outlined earlier, the prognosis of teeth with root perforation during post space preparation depends on the root size, location relative to epithelial attachment, and accessibility for repair. Management of the post perforation generally is surgical if the post cannot be removed. If the post can be removed, nonsurgical repair is preferred (Figure 18-19). Teeth with small root perforations that are located in the apical region and are accessible for surgical repair have a better prognosis than those with large perforations, close to the gingival sulcus, or inaccessible. Because of the complexity in diagnosis, surgical techniques, and follow-up evaluation, patients with post perforations should be referred to an endodontist.

REFERENCES

1. Cohen S, Schwartz S: Endodontic complications and the law, *J Endod* 13:191, 1987.
2. Weine FS: Access cavity preparation and initiating treatment. In Weine F, editor, *Endodontic therapy,* ed 5, 221, St Louis, 1996, Mosby.
3. Lemon RR: Furcation perforation management: classic and new concepts. In Hardin JF, editor: *Clark's clinical dentistry,* vol 1, Philadelphia, 1990, JB Lippincott.
4. Lemon RR: Nonsurgical repair of perforation defects: internal matrix concept, *Dent Clin North Am* 36:448, 1992.
5. Simon J, Kelly WH, Gordon DG, Ericksen GW: Extrusion of endodontically treated teeth, *J Am Dent Assoc* 97:17, 1978.
6. Lemon RR: Simplified esthetic root extrusion techniques, *Oral Surg Oral Med Oral Pathol* 54:93, 1982.
7. Lee SJ, Monsef M, Torabinejad M: Sealing ability of a mineral trioxide aggregate for repair of lateral root perforation, *J Endod* 19:541, 1993.
8. Nicholls E: Treatment of traumatic perforations of the pulp cavity, *Oral Surg* 15:603, 1962.
9. Stromberg T, Hasselgran G, Bergstedt H: Endodontic treatment of traumatic root perforation in man: a clinical and roentgenological follow up study, *Sven Tandlakidskr* 64:487, 1972.
10. Harris W: A simplified method of treatment for endodontic perforations, *J Endod* 2:126, 1976.
11. Benenati FW, Roane JB, Biggs JT, Simon JH: Recall evaluation of iatrogenic root perforations repaired with amalgam and gutta percha, *J Endod* 12:161, 1986.
12. Sinai J: Endodontic perforations: their prognosis and treatment, *J Am Dent Assoc* 95:90, 1977.
13. Hartwell G, England M: Healing of furcation perforations in primate teeth after repair with decalcified freeze-dried bone: a longitudinal study, *J Endod* 19:357, 1993.
14. Aguirre R, El Deeb ME, El Deeb ME: Evaluation of the repair of mechanical furcation perforations using amalgam, gutta percha, or indium foil, *J Endod* 12:249, 1986.
15. Oswald RJ: Procedural accidents and their repair, *Dent Clin North Am* 23:593, 1979.
16. Pitt Ford TR, Torabinejad M, et al: The sealing ability of a mineral trioxide aggregate for repair of furcal perforations, *Oral Surg* 79:756, 1995.
17. Hong CU, McKendry DJ, Pitt Ford TR, Torabinejad M: Healing of furcal lesions repaired by amalgam or mineral trioxide aggregate, *J Endod* 20:197, 1994.
18. Bhaskar S, Rappaport H: Histologic evaluation of endodontic procedures in dogs, *Oral Surg Oral Med Oral Pathol* 32:26 35, 1971.
19. Selzer S, Sinai I, August D: Periodontal effects of root perforations before and during endodontic procedures, *J Dent Res* 49:332, 1970.
20. Grossman LI: Guidelines for the prevention of fracture of root canal instruments, *Oral Surg Oral Med Oral Pathol* 28:746, 1969.
21. Frank AL: The dilemma of the fractured instrument, *J Endod* 9:515, 1983.
22. Crump MC, Natkin E: Relationship of broken root canal instruments to endodontic case prognosis: a clinical investigation, *J Am Dent Assoc* 80:1341, 1970.
23. Grossman LI: Prevention in endodontic practice, *J Am Dent Assoc* 82:395, 1971.
24. Goldman M, Kronman JH, Goldman LB, et al: New method of irrigation during endodontic treatment, *J Endod* 2:257, 1976.
25. Obermayr G, Walton RE, Leary JM, et al: Vertical root fracture and relative deformation during obturation and post cementation, *J Prosthet Dent* 66:181, 1991.
26. Murgel CA, Walton RE: Vertical root fracture and dentin deformation in curved roots: the influence of spreader design, *Endodont Dent Traumatol* 6:273, 1990.
27. Dang D, Walton R: Vertical root fracture and root distortion: effect of spreader design, *J Endod* 15:294, 1989.
28. Leutchirakarn V, Palamara J, Messer H: Load and strain during lateral condensation and vertical root fracture, *J Endod* 25:99, 1999.
29. Walton RE, Michelich RJ, Smith NG: The histopathogenesis of vertical root fractures, *J Endod* 10:48, 1984.

Evaluation of Success and Failure

LEARNING OBJECTIVES

After reading this chapter, the student should be able to:

1 / Describe a successful root canal treatment.

2 / Describe an unsuccessful root canal treatment.

3 / Describe the most common modalities used to determine success or failure.

4 / State the approximate range of expected outcomes of routine, uncomplicated root canal treatment based on pretreatment conditions.

5 / Describe the factors that influence the outcome of treatment.

6 / Describe how to explain the prognosis to the patient.

7 / Evaluate and estimate prognosis before, during, and after treatment.

8 / Describe the importance of recall appointments.

9 / Recognize signs of unsuccessful root canal treatment.

10 / Identify causes, both endodontic and nonendodontic, that may lead to failure of treatment.

OUTLINE

What Is Success?

Prognosis
  Success Rates
  When to Prognosticate
  How to Prognosticate

Variability of Treatment Results

Factors Influencing Success and Failure

When to Evaluate

Methods of Evaluation
  Clinical Examination
  Radiographic Findings
  Histologic Examination

Causes of Endodontic Failures
  Preoperative Causes
  Operative Causes
  Postoperative Factors

Retreatment of Failures

What is Success?

With a vital pulp, success means that the root canal treatment prevents bacteria from entering the canal system; thereby, the treatment prevents a periradicular lesion from forming. With a necrotic pulp, the treatment is considered successful if it eliminates or significantly reduces bacteria in the root canal system so that an associated periradicular lesion heals.

Unfortunately, not all root canal treatments are successful. Recognition, acceptance, and management of treatments that do not resolve and heal can be difficult and often involve a complex set of factors. Historically the popular belief has been that the success rate for root canal treatment is between 80% and 95%. However general percentages should be taken with caution; rather, *each case should be individually assessed to determine the percentage probability of success.* Several variables affect the outcome of a root canal treatment,[1] many of which will be discussed later in this chapter. Importantly, the clinician should attempt to predict the outcome of each treatment based on the existing situation and current knowledge and then inform the patient about the expected outcome. The status and prediction should be assessed before and immediately after the treatment, and then at reasonable intervals. The importance of communication, both dentist to patient and patient to dentist, is discussed in more detail in Chapter 6.

Prognosis

Prognosis is a key word. This refers to the prediction of whether an endodontic treatment will prevent the development of apical periodontitis or heal it if present. But how are success and failure defined? Interpretation of success varies with the individual practitioner. One dentist's criterion for success may be if the treatment lasts long enough for the patient to pay the bill! And the criterion for failure may be that the patient contacts the dentist complaining of severe symptoms. At the other extreme may be the unreasonably rigorous requirement that no inflammatory cells are present in the periradicular tissues subsequent to treatment. Realistic criteria are somewhere between these two and obviously more toward the latter than the former. It is important to remember that apical periodontitis, which is often a principle indication of a failing endodontic treatment, is frequently asymptomatic; the radiograph is the only way to demonstrate the lesion.[2]

SUCCESS RATES

What is the anticipated outcome of root canal treatment? Studies vary, with reported success rates ranging from a high of 95% to a low of 53%.[1,3,4] There are some known factors that account for at least some of these differences.

Studies on prognosis have analyzed the effects of various factors in relation to success and failure.[5-8] These numerous variables can make interpretation and comparison of prognosis study results difficult. These difficulties include observer bias (with varying criteria for success), bias in interpreting radiographs, varying levels of patient compliance (recall) subjectivity of patient response, host variability in responding to treatment, relative validity and reproducibility of the method of evaluation, degree of control of variables such as sample size, and differences in observation periods. However some of those studies have clearly shown a significant effect of some factors on the ultimate outcome of treatment.

Clearly a very significant factor is the presence of a periradicular lesion associated with the tooth before treatment[5-8] The significance of bacteria in causing and maintaining a periradicular lesion was shown in a classic study by Kakehashi et al.[9] They demonstrated that only root canal systems infected with bacteria would develop periradicular lesions. If there is a periradicular lesion before treatment the prognosis for success is reduced by 10% to 20%.[7,10,11] Elimination or at a least significant reduction in the number of bacteria seems to produce results similar to those expected when noninfected canals are treated.[11,12]

At least two other factors are important in the ultimate outcome of the treatment. Those factors are the technical quality of the root canal filling itself and, more importantly, the effectiveness of the coronal seal.[13] With a poor coronal seal most treatments probably will eventually fail irrespective of the periradicular status of the tooth before treatment or the quality of débridement and obturation.

The advantages of understanding the prognosis for root canal treatment procedures include development of more rational treatment methods, avoidance of factors that result in a higher incidence of failure, and a better understanding of the healing process. To reemphasize and to repeat: generalizations in predicting success and failure are inappropriate when assessing an individual situation; prognosis for each clinical case must be based on the findings and treatment factors relevant to that case.

WHEN TO PROGNOSTICATE

Determining or attempting to predict outcome should be done at three times: *before, during,* and *after* treatment. The prognosis often changes at these intervals, depending on what occurs or what is discovered during or after treatment. Thus, what may have been a favorable prognosis at the beginning may change to a poorer or less favorable prognosis at the conclusion of the procedure.

HOW TO PROGNOSTICATE

Patients must always be informed about the possibility of failure. The outcome prediction (whether made before, during, or after treatment) may be explained in one of two ways. One approach is to generalize about whether the anticipated outcome is favorable, questionable, or unfavorable. A second approach is to make a prediction using percentages; patients usually easily understand this. However, predicting using percentages is somewhat difficult for the dentist, because there are several variables that can affect the ultimate outcome, especially when prognosticating is done before the treatment. By using percentage estimation (particularly if the prognosis is not excellent) patients might have better grasp of the status of their tooth and then participate in the decision about whether to proceed. They need to understand that there is always a possibility of complications during or after treatment. Also, patients can better accept failure if they were informed of that possibility before treatment.

Variability of Treatment Results

Explaining the marked differences in the success rates seen in different prognosis studies is not difficult. There are many variables, alone or in combination, that affect the outcome of treatment; some of these variables are easily identified and others are probably unknown. Thus, no single study has all the answers, and all studies considered as a group are, at best, only overall indicators.[5]

Factors Influencing Success and Failure

An early "classic" comprehensive study performed by Strindberg[5] related treatment outcomes to biologic and therapeutic factors. With time, other variables have been related to success and failure. Few of these variables have been proven to have a clear effect on the final outcome of the root canal treatment. Others are generalities, and their full effects are unknown because of the nature and complexity of the problems. Some of the factors that consistently impact prognosis are (1) apical pathosis, (2) bacterial status of the canal, (3) extent and quality of the obturation, and (4) quality of the coronal restoration.

The presence of bacteria in the canal before obturation predicts a poorer prognosis.[11] In relation to extension of the obturation, healing is less predictable if the filling is too short (more than 2 mm from the radiographic apex) or too long (exiting the apex).[6,14,15] More voids or less density of the obturating materials is also related to lower success rates.[16] And again and importantly, the quality of the coronal restoration is more critically related to the final outcome than the quality of the obturation.[13]

Other variables such as tooth type, age and sex of the patient, technique of obturation, observation period, and type of intracanal medication have been shown to have a slight effect (but usually none) on the results.[17] Medical (health) status or age of the patient has no significant bearing on success or failure.[18] No specific systemic disease or condition has been related to delayed or impaired healing or seems to precipitate failure. Obviously, a patient who is debilitated or whose condition is severely compromised medically may be a poor candidate for root canal treatment.

When to Evaluate

The length of time necessary for adequate postoperative follow-up has been studied. Suggested follow-up periods range from 6 months to 4 years; 6 months is a reasonable interval for a recall evaluation for most patients. However, the important question is, at what point is it unlikely that a treatment outcome will change? In other words, when can it be determined that treatment is successful or has failed and the outcome is unlikely to change so that no further recall is necessary? There is good evidence that a radiographic lesion that is unchanged or has increased in size after 1 year is unlikely to ever resolve; therefore, the treatment is deemed unsuccessful. If at 6 months the lesion is still present but smaller in size, there is an indication that it might heal but additional recall is needed. The larger the periradicular lesion before the root canal treatment, the longer the healing period. Unfortunately, apparent success may revert to failure at a later time (often as a result of coronal leakage), so clinical and radiographic examination of teeth treated with root canals is indicated as a part of routine full-status evaluation of all dental patients.

Methods of Evaluation

The most accurate determinations of healing or nonhealing are based on signs and symptoms and radiographic and histologic examinations. Obviously, at present only clinical findings and radiographic criteria can be readily evaluated by the dentist; current technology precludes histologic examination without surgical intervention.

CLINICAL EXAMINATION

Signs and/or symptoms, *if marked and persistent*, are probably indications of disease and of failure. Importantly, absence of pain or other symptoms does not confirm success. This is because periradicular pathosis without significant symptoms is usually present in teeth before as well as after root canal treatment.[2] There is little correlation between the presence of pathosis and corresponding symptoms; yet when signs and/or symptoms are evident there is a strong likelihood that there is a pathosis.[19]

Persistence of adverse significant signs (e.g., swelling or sinus tract) or symptoms (e.g., spontaneous pain, dull persistent ache, or mastication sensitivity) indicates failure.

RADIOGRAPHIC FINDINGS

According to the findings, the outcome of each treatment could be classified as a success, a failure, or a questionable status. To be able to accurately compare radiographs made at different times, it is important that they are taken in a reproducible fashion and with minimal distortion. The best way to ensure reproducibility is with paralleling radiographic devices (see Chapter 9).

Success is the absence of an apical radiolucent lesion. This means that a resorptive lesion present at the time of treatment has resolved or if there was no lesion present at the time of treatment, none has developed. Thus, success is evident by the elimination or nondevelopment of an area of rarefaction for a minimum of 1 year after treatment (Figure 19-1).

Failure is the persistence or development of radiographically evident pathosis. Specifically, this is a radiolucent lesion that has remained the same, has enlarged, or has developed since treatment (Figure 19-2).

Clinical criteria for success include the following[19]:
1. Absence of pain and swelling.
2. Disappearance of sinus tract.
3. No evidence of soft tissue destruction, including probing defects.

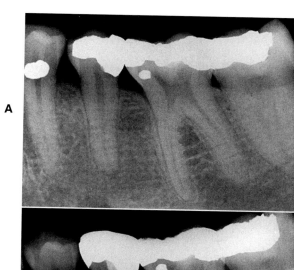
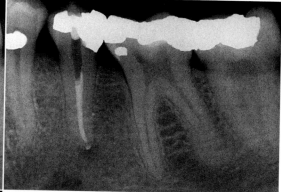
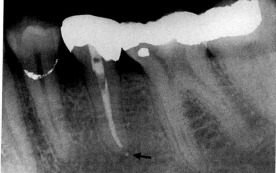

FIGURE 19-1

Success. **A,** Diagnosis of 20: irreversible pulpitis, normal periapex. Pretreatment prognosis: *favorable.* **B,** Obturation 1 month later. As occasionally occurs, periradicular pathosis has developed during the treatment interval, which involved three appointments in the 1-month period. Posttreatment prognosis: *questionable.* **C,** Six-month recall shows resolution and a classification of *success.* Because the periradicular irritation was neither severe nor persistent and because the primary obturating material was contained and condensed within the canal, the slight amount of sealer extruded *(arrow)* neither resorbed nor prevented healing.

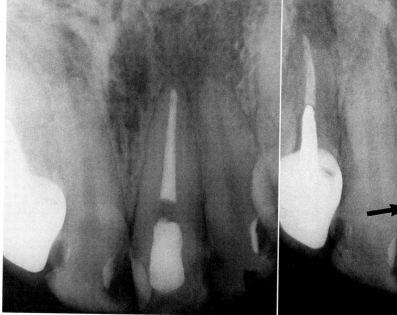
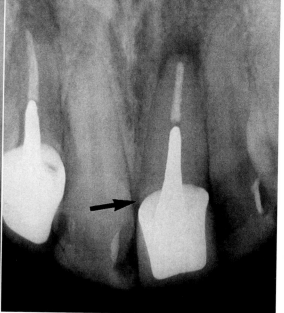

FIGURE 19-2

Failure. **A,** Apparently adequate root canal treatment. Tooth was restored later with a post and core and crown. **B,** Two-year recall. The patient reports persistent discomfort. Periradicular radiolucency indicates *failure,* probably due to coronal leakage at a defective margin *(arrow).* Surgery was required (root end resection and filling) because of restoration.

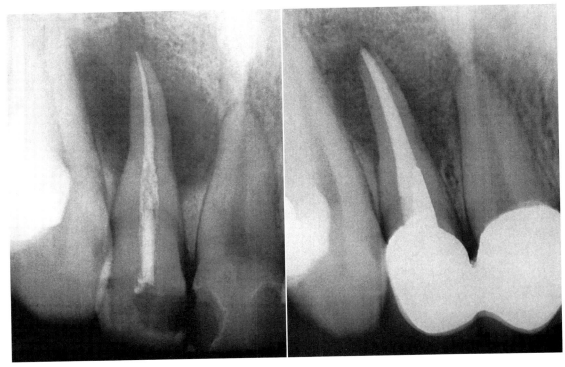

FIGURE 19-3
Questionable. **A,** Inadequate canal preparation, poor obturation, and coronal leakage all contributed to failure. The tooth is suitable for conventional retreatment and restoration. **B,** Twelve-month recall after retreatment. A sinus tract has disappeared, and the patient reports absence of symptoms. The radiolucent lesion is decreasing in size but has not resolved. Because outcome is still *questionable,* additional recall evaluation is necessary.

Questionable status indicates a state of uncertainty. The situation (radiolucent lesion) has neither become larger nor significantly decreased in size. A questionable status is considered to be nonhealing if there is no resolution after more than 1 year (Figure 19-3).

Complete radiographic regeneration of periradicular structures does not always occur. Variations in radiographic appearance that are defined as healed are occasionally seen. Large periradicular lesions present before treatment might not completely regenerate normal bony architecture but rather persist as a slightly larger than normal apical periodontal ligament space. There may also be an unusual trabecular pattern or lack of complete replacement of the cortical plate adjacent to the tooth, giving the appearance of a persistent lesion.

Fallibilities of radiographic interpretation are additional complications. Because radiographs are usually the primary evaluative tools, techniques and interpretation are critical; guidelines must be followed carefully. Consistency in film type, exposure time, cone angulations, film development, and similar radiograph viewing conditions are important. Inconsistency with follow-up radiographs may lead to false assessments of either success or nonhealing. There could be false-positive or false-negative interpretations. For example, an anatomic landmark such as a radiolucent or radiopaque structure may be "pushed" over the apex by a change in cone angulation and may then be misinterpreted as a developing lesion. Also, opacity may obscure a developing lesion. Because of these variations, the validity of evaluating treatment outcome solely with radiographs is unacceptable; other signs and symptoms are considered as well.[20] Periradicular lesions have been "healed" simply by changing radiographic techniques or cone angles. (Figure 19-4).

Personal bias may influence radiographic interpretation.[21,22] Each radiograph must be interpreted objectively and honestly to determine the degree of healing.

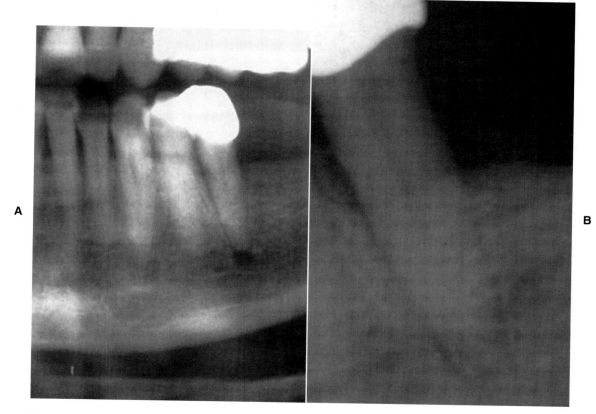

FIGURE 19-4
A, Panoramic radiograph revealed an apical radiolucency on the premolar. **B,** Periradicular film taken 1 week later shows no apparent radiolucency associated with the apex. The tooth responded within normal limits. The likely explanation of the radiolucency on the panoramic film is superimposition of the mental foramen.

HISTOLOGIC EXAMINATION

Routine histologic evaluation of periradicular tissues after root canal treatment is impractical and not possible without surgery.[23] If a treated tooth were to be evaluated histologically, successful treatment would be indicated by reconstitution of periradicular structures and an absence of inflammation.

There is uncertainty about the degree of correlation between histologic findings and radiographic appearance because of the lack of well-controlled, prospective histologic studies. Two histologic investigations of teeth treated with root canals in cadavers reached very different conclusions.[24,25] Brynolf[24] concluded that almost all treated teeth showed some periradicular inflammation despite the appearance of successful treatment on radiographs. In contrast, Green et al.[25] observed that most treated teeth that showed a normal periapex radiographically were indeed free of inflammation histologically. Thus, with cur-rent technology, clinical findings (signs, symptoms, and radiographic evaluation) are the only practical means of assessing degree of healing after root canal treatment.

Causes of Endodontic Failures

Most nonhealing (failures) of root canal treatments is directly or indirectly caused by bacteria somewhere in the root canal system. In general, the most common causes of failure are (1) errors in diagnosis and treatment planning, (2) coronal leakage, (3) lack of knowledge of pulp anatomy, (4) inadequate débridement and/or disinfection of the root canal system, (5) inadequate restorative protection, (6) operative errors, (7) obturation deficiencies or errors, and (8) vertical root fracture.

The various procedures associated with root canal treatment can be divided into three phases: preoperative, operative, and postoperative.

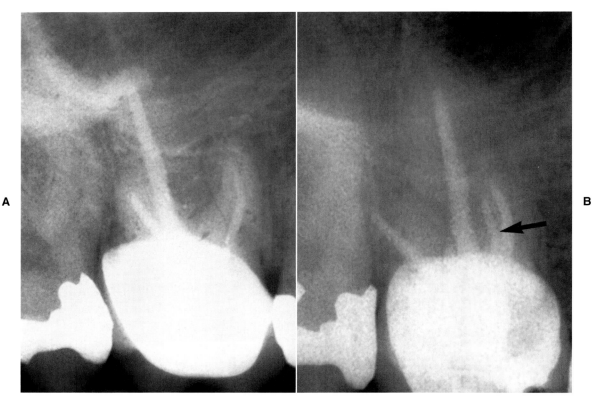

FIGURE 19-5
A, The patient complained of pain in right maxillary teeth when drinking hot liquids. The sensitivity to heat was confirmed to be from tooth 3 by rubber dam isolation and then bathing it with hot water. **B,** The tooth was carefully accessed without anesthesia; vital tissue was located in the mesiolingual canal *(arrow).* The tooth was then anesthetized, and the canal was instrumented and obturated.

PREOPERATIVE CAUSES

Failure of root canal treatment is often traced to misdiagnosis, errors in treatment planning, poor case selection (dentists attempting treatment beyond their skill levels), or treatment of a tooth with a poor prognosis. All of these are preoperative considerations.

Before any invasive dental procedure, including root canal treatment, the dentist should make a "tentative" pulpal and periradicular diagnosis. That diagnosis is based on all available information: history of signs and symptoms, current signs and symptoms, radiographic evaluation, and vitality tests (see Chapter 4). Without evaluating all these factors and forming a diagnosis, there is a risk of inappropriate treatment and/or the wrong tooth being treated. Obviously, the problem would not be resolved.

Not using good radiographic projection, including different mesiodistal angulation to determine various canal system aberrations (extra canals: for example, the mesiolingual canal in maxillary molars and second canals in mandibular incisors), often results in failure, even with correct diagnosis (Figure 19-5).

Coronal or root dentin fractures are also often misdiagnosed or escape early detection. Periodontal defects with associated bone loss often appear after the fracture has been on the crown and root for long enough for the crack to become infected (Figure 19-6).[26-29] However, if there is an isolated, deep probing defect associated with the suspect tooth, vertical root fracture must be considered (Figure 19-7).

OPERATIVE CAUSES

Many failures result from errors in operative procedures. For predictable success, several steps need to be followed. These include chemomechanical cleaning and shaping of the canal space followed by a dense obturation that is confined to the root canal system and then by a quality coronal restoration.

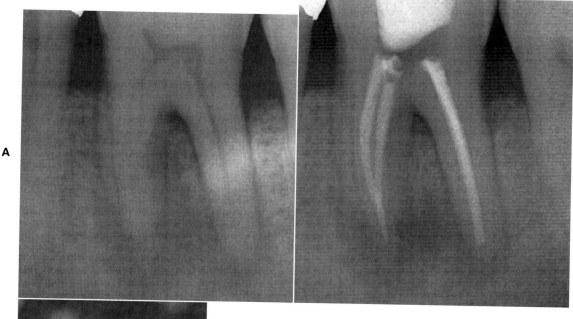

FIGURE 19-6

A, Large periradicular lesion around mesial and distal roots of the first molar. The patient denied any history of symptoms. The tooth was unresponsive to CO_2 snow, but responded normally to percussion and palpation. **B,** Access was attained without anesthesia (test cavity), confirming necrotic pulp. Root canal treatment was performed in two appointments using $Ca(OH)_2$ as an intra-appointment medicament. **C,** After 3 months, severe pain was reported on biting. Extraction revealed a *split tooth* that was probably present before the initial root canal treatment, as there was no restoration or caries, yet the pulp was necrotic.

Mechanical Objectives

An overlooked but important part of successful root canal treatment is a straight-line access preparation that will facilitate débridement and obturation. The access is even more important, with the use of rotary nickel-titanium file systems. If the access is underextended, several mishaps may occur that ultimately will lead to failure. A canal may be missed; the treatment is likely to fail although the located canals were appropriately treated. If the pulp horns are not opened in anterior teeth, debris and sealer may remain in the coronal pulp space. Such remnants often result in discoloration and therefore treatment failure. In addition, with a too small access, instrument maneuverability is limited, resulting in insufficient

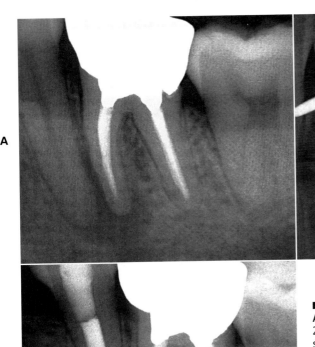

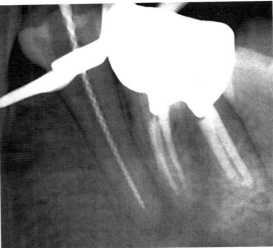

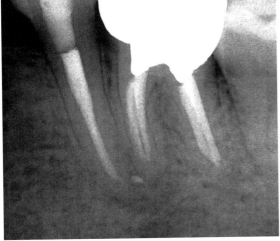

FIGURE 19-7
A, Root canal treatment on the first molar was completed 2 months previously. Discomfort persisted with occasional swelling and drainage into the sulcus in the mesiofacial aspect of the treated tooth. A deep probing defect on the mesiofacial aspect indicated the possibility of a vertical root fracture. However, further testing showed that the second premolar was sensitive to percussion and unresponsive to CO_2 snow and test cavity. **B,** Treatment was initiated on the premolar. **C,** One year after root canal treatment, there is partial periradicular healing around both apexes. Results of periodontal probing were within normal limits. (Courtesy Dr. G. Shuping.)

cleaning and aberrant shaping, or even instrument breakage.

Overextended access cavities, prepared at the expense of dentin, are also a problem. Excessive loss of dentin weakens the tooth, possibly allowing fractures, and increases the risk of perforation.[29,30]

A common error of instrumentation is failure to maintain canal curvature because files cut to the outside of the curve ("transportation" of the canal and/or apex). This alters canal morphology and leaves potentially infected debris in the canal system. Marked deviation or overzealous flaring or over-preparation in the "danger" zone or in the apical $\frac{1}{3}$ may result in perforation (Figure 19-8). These perforations are possible to repair but are difficult to seal nonsurgically.[31] Leakage and/or mechanical irritation may result, and a lesion may develop.[32]

The outcome of a separated instrument (broken endodontic file) in a root canal system depends on the stage of canal preparation and the pretreatment pulp status (vital versus necrotic) (see Figure 19-7).[33,34] The outcome may be unaffected if the instrument can be removed or bypassed.

Confining operative procedures and materials to the canal space enhances repair.[6,35] Overinstrumentation causes some tissue damage, periradicular hemorrhage, and transitory inflammation. Continuous overinstrumentation provokes a persistent inflammatory response capable of resorbing dental and osseous tissues.[36] Overinstrumentation may also transfer microorganisms from the canal into the periapex, possibly compromising the outcome.[37]

Likewise, overextended obturation may lead to treatment failure. In many cases it is probably not the material that causes the periradicular lesion; gutta-percha is relatively inert. Rather, the combination of an inadequate seal probably preceded by

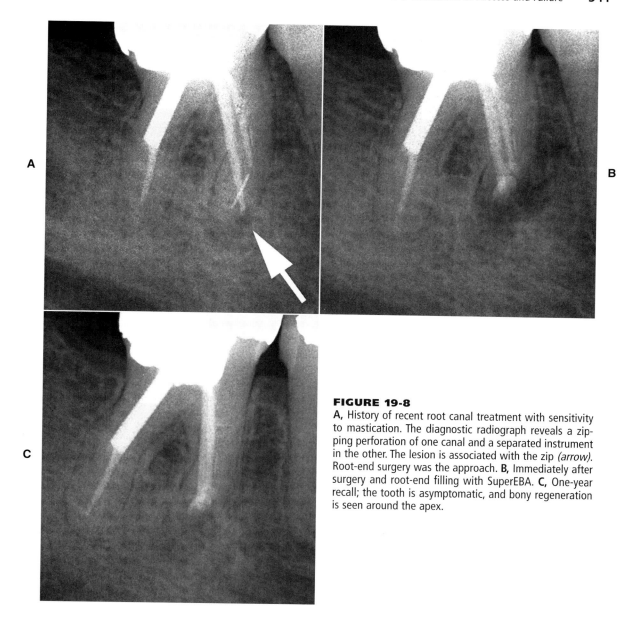

FIGURE 19-8
A, History of recent root canal treatment with sensitivity to mastication. The diagnostic radiograph reveals a zipping perforation of one canal and a separated instrument in the other. The lesion is associated with the zip *(arrow)*. Root-end surgery was the approach. **B,** Immediately after surgery and root-end filling with SuperEBA. **C,** One-year recall; the tooth is asymptomatic, and bony regeneration is seen around the apex.

overinstrumentation causes the failure. The gutta-percha cone slips through the apex because there was inadequate taper or shelf, resulting in inadequate matrix to confine and condense and seal with the gutta-percha. In addition, sealers are irritating or toxic to the periradicular tissue.[23,38,39]

Errors in obturation result from poor canal shaping or selecting an inappropriate obturating technique. A poorly condensed obturation (either underfilled or containing voids) is related to apical and/or coronal percolation.[3,23,40] Either under-obturation or overfilling is likely to result in fail-

ure, particularly in the presence of pulp necrosis and an apical lesion.[41]

Biologic Objectives

Ideally, after preparation the root canal would be free of bacteria.[42] With a vital pulp this means prevention of contamination and with a necrotic pulp, to achieve disinfection. However, as shown experimentally, complete débridement of the canal is virtually impossible.[43,44] Therefore, bacterial counts are minimized by careful instrumentation, with copious NaOCl irrigation.[45] The intracanal medicament, calcium hydroxide, will reduce the number of bacteria,[46] enhance the speed of healing, and reduce inflammation.[47,48] However, there is uncertainty whether use of this medicament ultimately results in a better prognosis.[49]

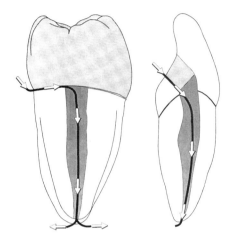

FIGURE 19-9
Coronal leakage. Crown (left) has open margins. Saliva, bacteria, and other irritants have access to canal space. The irritants will percolate through gutta-percha and out of the apex. The same thing may occur with an improperly sealed composite on an anterior tooth (right). (Courtesy Dr. K. Barrieshi.)

POSTOPERATIVE FACTORS

Lack of a coronal seal is probably the most common, but best controllable, problem. Coronal restoration protects and seals the tooth, preventing diffusion of saliva and bacteria apically (Figure 19-9), which results in failed treatment.[13,41-49] There is a definite correlation between poorly restored crowns of endodontically treated teeth and leakage of dye or bacteria or endotoxin through the canals and a poorer prognosis.[13,50-53]

Restoration should occur soon after obturation, using the same disinfection barriers as those used during the root canal treatment, i.e., rubber dam isolation in a saliva-free environment. There should be no space between the coronal filling and the obturation in the cervical area; there is a risk for bacterial contamination through exposed cervical root dentin. Restorative errors also may compromise success. For example, excessive dentin removal for posts weakens the root and increases susceptibility to fracture (Figure 19-10).[29]

Retreatment of Failures

Interestingly, if a failure is retreated by conventional means, the success rate is equivalent to that of initial conventional treatment *if the cause of failure is identified and corrected.*[54] Specific details of retreatment are included in Chapter 20.

A 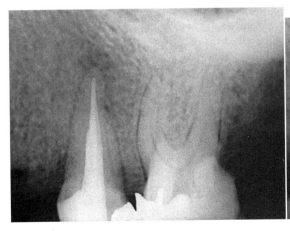 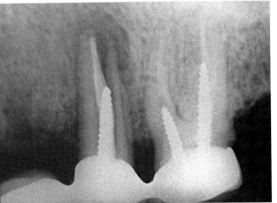 B

FIGURE 19-10
Hopeless prognosis. **A,** Overenlargement has weakened the root. **B,** Then, placement of oversized post combined with earlier condensation forces resulted in a vertical fracture and apical-lateral pathosis. The tooth must be extracted.

REFERENCES

1. Eriksen H: Endodontology epidemiologic considerations, *Endod Dent Traumatol* 7:189, 1991.
2. Lin LM, Pascon EA, Skribner J, et al: Clinical, radiographic, and histologic study of endodontic treatment failures, *Oral Surg Oral Med Oral Pathol* 71:603, 1991.
3. Pekruhn RB: The incidence of failure following single-visit endodontic therapy, *J Endod* 12:68, 1986.
4. Jokinen MA, Kotilainen R, Pockkeus P, et al: Clinical and radiographic study of pulpectomy and root canal therapy, *Scand J Dent Res* 86:366, 1978.
5. Strindberg LZ: The dependence of the results of pulp therapy on certain factors: An analytic study based on radiographic and clinical follow-up examination, *Acta Odontol Scand* 14(Suppl 21):1956.
6. Seltzer S, Bender IB, Turkenkopf S: Factors affecting successful repair after root canal therapy, *J Am Dent Assoc* 67:651 1963.
7. Grahnen J, Hansson L: The prognosis of pulp and root canal therapy, *Odontol Rev* 12:146, 1961.
8. Sjögren U, Hagglund B, Sundqvist G, Wing K: Factors affecting the long term results of endodontic treatment, *J Endod* 16:498, 1990.
9. Kakehashi S, Stanely HR, Fitzgerald RJ: The effects of surgical exposures of dental pulps in germ-free and conventional laboratory rats, *Oral Surg Oral Med Oral Pathol* 20:340, 1965.
10. Mölven O, Halse A: Success rate for gutta-percha and Kloroperka N-Ø root filling made by undergraduate students; radiographic findings after 10-17 years, *Int Endod J* 21:243, 1988.
11. Sjögren U, Figdor D, Persson S, Sundqvist G: Influence of infection at the time of root filling on the outcome of endodontic treatment of teeth with apical periodontitis, *Int Endod J* 30:297, 1997.
12. Sundqvist G, Figdor D, Persson S, Sjögren U: Microbiologic analysis of teeth with failed endodontic treatment and the outcome of conservative retreatment, *Oral Surg Oral Med Oral Pathol* 85:86, 1998.
13. Ray HA, Trope M: Periapical status of endodontically treated teeth in relation to the technical quality of the root filling and the coronal restoration, *Int Endod J* 28:12, 1995.
14. Bergenholtz G, Lekholm U, Milthon R, Engstrom B: Influence of apical overinstrumentation and overfilling on re-treated root canals, *J Endod* 5:310, 1979.
15. Ørstavik D, Hörsted-Bindslev P: A comparsion of endodontic treatment results at two dental schools, *Int Endod J* 26:348, 1993.
16. De Moor RJG, Hommez GMG, De Boever JG, et al: Periapical health related to the quality of root canal treatment in a Belgian population, *Int Endod J* 33:113, 2000.
17. Stabholz A: Success rate in endodontics, *Alpha Omegan* 83:20, 1990.
18. Storms JL: Factors that influence the success of endodontic treatment, *J Can Dent Assoc* 35:83, 1969.
19. Bender IB, Selzer S, Soltanoff W: Endodontic success: a reappraisal of criteria. I and II, *Oral Surg Oral Med Oral Pathol* 22:780, 1966.
20. Swartz DB, Skidmore AE, Griffin JA: Twenty years of endodontic success and failure, *J Endod* 9:198, 1983.
21. Goldman M, Pearson AH, Darzenta N: Endodontic success: who's reading the radiograph? *Oral Surg Oral Med Oral Pathol* 33:432, 1972.
22. Zakariasen KL, Scott DA, Jensen JR: Endodontic recall radiographs: how reliable is our interpretation of endodontic success or failure and what factors affect our reliability? *Oral Surg Oral Med Oral Pathol* 57:343, 1984.
23. Ricucci D, Langeland K: Apical limits of root canal instrumentation and obturation, *Int Endod J* 31:384, 1998.
24. Brynolf I: A histological and roentgenological study of the periapical region of human upper incisors, *Odontol Rev* 18(Suppl 11), 1967.
25. Green TL, Walton RE, Taylor JK, Merrell P: Radiographic and histologic periapical findings of root canal treated teeth in cadavers, *Oral Surg Oral Med Oral Pathol* 83:707, 1997.
26. Ehrmann E, Tyas M: Cracked tooth syndrome: diagnosis, treatment and correlation between symptoms and post-extraction findings, *Aust Dent J* 35:105, 1990.
27. Schweitzer J, Gutmann J, Bliss R: Odontoiatrogenic tooth fracture, *Int Endod J* 22:64, 1989.
28. Yang SF, Rivera EM, Walton RE: Vertical root fracture in nonendodontically treated teeth, *J Endod* 21:337, 1995.
29. Trope M, Maltz DO, Tronstad L: Resistance to fracture of restored endodontically treated teeth, *Endodont Dent Traumatol* 1:108, 1985.
30. Sails S, et al: Patterns of indirect fracture in intact and restored human premolar teeth, *Endodont Dent Traumatol* 3:10, 1987.
31. Hartwell G, England M: Healing of furcation perforations in primate teeth after repair with decalcified freeze-dried bone: a longitudinal study, *J Endod* 19:357, 1993.
32. Seltzer S, Sinai I, August D: Periodontal effects of root perforations prior to and during endodontic procedures, *J Dent Res* 49:332, 1970.
33. Fors UG, Berg JO: Endodontic treatment of root canals obstructed by foreign objects, *Int Endod J* 19:2, 1986.
34. Grossman LI, editor: *Transactions. First International Conference on Endodontics,* Philadelphia, 1953, University of Pennsylvania Press.
35. Wu MK, Wesselink PR, Walton RE: Apical terminus location of root canal treatment procedures, *Oral Surg Oral Med Oral Pathol* 89:99, 2000.
36. Seltzer S, Bender I, Soltanoff I: Biological aspects of endodontics. III. Periapical reactions to root canal instrumentation, *Oral Surg Oral Med Oral Pathol* 26:534, 1968.
37. Seltzer S: *Endodontology,* ed 2, Philadelphia, 1988, Lea & Febiger.
38. Morse DR, Wilcko J, Pullon P, et al: A comparative tissue toxicity evaluation of the liquid components of gutta-percha root canal sealers, *J Endod* 7:545, 1981.
39. Seltzer S: Long-term radiographic and histological observation of endodontically treated teeth, *J Endod* 25:12, 1999.
40. Wu M, DeGee A, Wesselink P, Moorer W: Fluid transport and bacterial penetration along root canal fillings, *Int Endod J* 26:1, 1993.
41. Smith C, Setchell D, Harty F: Factors influencing success of conventional root canal therapy: a five-year retrospective study, *Int Endod J* 26:321, 1993.
42. Grossman LI: Endodontic failures, *Dent Clin North Am* 16:59, 1972.

43. Mandel E, Machtou P, Friedman S: Scanning electron microscope observation of canal cleanliness, *J Endod* 16:279, 1990.

44. Dalton BC, Ørstavik D, Phillips C, et al: Bacterial reduction with nickel-titanium rotary instrumentation, *J Endod* 24:763, 1998.

45. Byström A, Sundqvist G: Bacteriologic evaluation of the effect of 0.5 percent sodium hypochlorite in endodontic therapy, *Oral Surg Oral Med Oral Pathol* 55:35, 1983.

46. Sjögren U, Figdor D, Spangberg L, Sundqvist G: The antimicrobial effect of calcium hydroxide as a short-term intracanal dressing, *Int Endod J* 24:119, 1991.

47. Katebzadeh N, Sigurdsson A, Trope M: Radiographic evaluation of periapical healing after obturation of infected root canals: an in vivo study, *Int Endod J* 33:60, 2000.

48. Katebzadeh N, Hupp J, Trope M: Histological periapical repair after obturation of infected root canals in dogs, *J Endod* 25:364, 1999.

49. Weiger R, Rosendahl R, Löst C: Influence of calcium hydroxide intracanal dressings on the prognosis of teeth with endodontically induced periapical lesions, *Int Endod J* 33:219, 2000.

50. Swanson K, Madison S: An evaluation of coronal microleakage in endodontically treated teeth. Time periods, *J Endod* 13:56, 1987.

51. Magura ME, Kafrawy A, Brown C, Newton C: Human saliva coronal microleakage in obturated root canals. An in vitro study, *J Endod* 17:324, 1991.

52. Khayat A, Lee S-J, Torabinejad M: Human saliva penetration of coronally unsealed obturated root canals, *J Endod* 19:458, 1993.

53. Alves J, Walton R, Drake D: Coronal leakage: endotoxin penetration from mixed bacterial communities through obturated post-prepared root canals, *J Endod* 24:587, 1998.

54. Bergenholtz G, Lekholm U, et al: Retreatment of endodontic fillings, *Scand J Dent Res* 87:217, 1979.

Orthograde Retreatment

LEARNING OBJECTIVES

After reading this chapter, the student should be able to:

1 / Describe differences from initial treatment.

2 / State rationale and indications.

3 / Discuss considerations for case selection.

4 / Identify restrictive clinical conditions.

5 / Identify patients with difficult problems who should be referred.

6 / Describe a basic armamentarium and techniques.

7 / Communicate benefits and risks, alternative treatments, and reasons for referral.

OUTLINE

Unique Considerations

Case Selection
Diagnosis
Selection of Treatment
Treatment of Existing Disease
Prevention of Disease

Retreatment Techniques
Access—Crowns
Access—Post and Core
Canal Obstructions
Completion of Retreatment
Degree of Difficulty

Short-Term and Long-Term Treatment Outcome

Communication and Referral

C ross-sectional studies of populations in various countries, including the United States, indicate that, overall, *treatment failure,* characterized by endodontic disease (apical periodontitis), is seen in more than 30% of root canal treated teeth.[1] Most patients can relate to the concept of disease-treatment-healing, whereas failure, apart from being a negative and relative term, does not imply the necessity to pursue treatment. Therefore, use of the term "disease" will minimize ambiguity and facilitate communication between the clinician and the patient. In this chapter, *post-treatment disease* is used rather than *treatment failure,* although the latter term appears in this textbook's other chapters.

Post-treatment disease (apical periodontitis associated with root canal-treated teeth) is primarily caused by infection of the root canal system.[2,3] Microorganisms may either have survived the previous treatment or invaded the filled canal space after treatment, mainly because of coronal leakage.[4,5] Less often, specific microorganisms (*Actinomyces* species in particular) may have become established in the periradicular tissue.[6]

The affected teeth can be treated either by retreatment (orthograde) or by apical surgery (retrograde). These two approaches differ significantly in rationale—retreatment is an attempt to *eliminate* root canal microorganisms, whereas surgery is an attempt to *confine* the microorganisms within the canal. The main benefit of retreatment, therefore, is better curtailment of the root canal infection. Being limited in this regard, surgery is a compromise unless microorganisms are assumed to be harbored periapically, retreatment is unfeasible or restricted, or a retreatment attempt has failed.[7]

Retreatment is distinguished from initial root canal treatment by unique considerations and techniques.[8] Because of the complexity, retreatment is often performed by the endodontist. However, the general dentist must understand retreatment in order to support diagnosis, case selection, and treatment or referral as appropriate and to communicate with the patient and endodontist. The objective of this chapter is to provide an understanding of retreatment.

Unique Considerations

Retreatment and initial root canal treatment share similar biologic principles and objectives. However, the following are unique to retreatment:[8]

1. An extensive restoration may have to be sacrificed and remade.
2. Retreatment may be performed to prevent potential disease.[7-9]

3. Morphologic alterations resulting from the previous treatment may present unusual technical and therapeutic challenges.[10]
4. Root filling and possibly restorative materials must be removed from the canals.
5. The healing rate is generally slower than that after initial treatment, because of greater difficulty in eliminating the infection.[1]
6. Patients may be more apprehensive than with the "routine" initial treatment; effective communication is required.

These considerations distinguish retreatment from initial root canal treatment and make patient selection complicated.[8] As a result, clinicians faced with post-treatment disease frequently hesitate to intervene despite the presence of pathosis.[11-14]

To foster confidence and appropriate management, definitive criteria are required to select cases for tooth extraction, retreatment, and apical surgery.

Case Selection

Retreatment is usually performed to treat existing disease, presenting with definitive signs and symptoms. However, even in the absence of disease, retreatment may be indicated to prevent future emergence of disease.[7,8]

DIAGNOSIS

The presence or absence of periradicular disease is determined according to clinical and radiographic findings, as discussed in Chapter 19. Differential diagnosis of nonendodontic disease is also considered.[15] In this regard, the *case history* is reviewed by examining previous radiographs when available and by noting past symptoms, time elapsed since previous treatment (to avoid premature diagnosis of post-treatment disease), and previous attempts to retreat or to perform apical surgery (may suggest vertical fracture).

SELECTION OF TREATMENT

After diagnosis, the most appropriate treatment modality is selected based on the criteria outlined below. In the past, the clinician selected and then performed the treatment. Currently, however, *the patient ultimately selects the treatment*, based on information communicated by the clinician. The following section is consistent with this concept.

TREATMENT OF EXISTING DISEASE

Post-treatment disease definitely requires intervention, even when symptoms are absent.[8] When treatment is preferred over extraction, both retreatment and apical surgery should be considered. Comparing the two modalities, retreatment offers a greater benefit—a better ability to eliminate the disease's etiology (root canal infection) with minimal invasion—and a smaller risk—significantly less postoperative discomfort and a lesser chance of injuring nerves, sinuses, or other structures.[16] Therefore, retreatment is generally considered the treatment of choice; however, it is not always feasible.

At times, retreatment can be more time consuming and costly than surgery, particularly when an extensive restoration must be replaced. Also, the ability to attain the goals of retreatment may be restricted.[8] Furthermore, clinicians' capabilities to perform retreatment and surgery may vary considerably. *In summary,* retreatment is generally selected because of its greater benefit and smaller risk compared with apical surgery. Therefore, case selection is based on considerations that either preclude retreatment or restrict its feasibility in a way that decreases the potential benefits and increases the potential risks; the modified benefit-risk balance may not outweigh that of apical surgery.

Patient Considerations

Patients' (and clinicians') attitudes toward dental disease and the necessity to treat it differ significantly.[17] Moreover, the motivation to retain every tooth and pursue the best long-term treatment outcome may vary, as do the motivation and ability to allocate time and finances. Because these general attitudes influence the patient's preferences of treatment, they are primary considerations in the process of case selection (Box 20-1).

Motivation to retain the tooth. The considerable effort associated with both retreatment and surgery is justifiable by the potential to retain the tooth. For the unmotivated patient, extraction is selected.

Motivation to pursue the best long-term outcome. For the patient who is receptive to a compromised long-term outcome, apical surgery is selected when retreatment is expected to be very involved.

Time. For the time-restricted patient who is receptive to a compromise to minimize time commitment, the quicker apical surgery procedure is selected. However, the associated postoperative discomfort and recovery can cause loss of work time and income.[16]

Finances. For the financially restricted patient who is willing to compromise in order to minimize cost, apical surgery is selected when the combined cost of retreatment and restoration is

---

BOX 20-1

Patient Considerations Governing Case Selection in the Management of Existing Disease After Root Canal Treatment

	No	Consideration	Yes	
Extraction	←	Motivation to retain tooth	→	Retreatment or surgery
Surgery	←	Motivation to pursue best long-term outcome	→	Retreatment
Retreatment	←	Time concerns	→	Surgery
Retreatment	←	Financial concerns	→	Surgery

---

higher. Again, the potential loss of income associated with postoperative recovery is considered.[16]

Tooth Considerations

When the patient indicates a preference for retreatment, the tooth and surrounding tissues are scrutinized to identify clinical conditions that might adversely affect the prognosis, either by decreasing the benefits or by increasing the risks of retreatment. In selected situations, the modified benefit-risk balance no longer justifies the preference of retreatment over surgery.

Site of infection. Root canal infection is best eliminated by retreatment.[1] Periapical (extraradicular) infection independent of the root canal flora is best eliminated by apical surgery.[18] In contrast, when a vertical root fracture is present, infection cannot be eliminated with either procedure.[19] Therefore, differential diagnosis is required to establish the likely site of infection. This difficult task is facilitated by recognizing the typical manifestation of extraradicular infection (one or more sinus tracts), and that of vertical crack/fracture (isolated, narrow defect along the root), and by comparing older and recent radiographs (see Chapter 28).[6,19]

Root canal obstacles. For retreatment to eliminate canal infection, the canal must be renegotiated throughout. Therefore, obstacles to total renegotiation reduce the potential benefit of retreatment, while attempts to overcome the obstacles increase the risk of procedural complications. The principal obstacles are (Figure 20-1): *calcification, complex morphology* of the root canal system, *suspected ledge*, and *separated instrument.* The feasibility of overcoming these obstacles must be assessed; again, the benefit-risk balance may change in favor of surgery.

A post may obstruct the canal. Because posts can usually be removed (see discussion later in this chapter), they do not influence the benefit-risk balance as described above.

Perforation. Perforation of the pulp chamber or root can be a pathway of infection to worsen the prognosis.[1] Therefore, retreatment in conjunction with internal repair of the perforation is usually warranted (Figure 20-2). Nevertheless, when healing is not expected or does not occur, surgery may be required. The surgical procedure includes external repair of the perforation (see Chapter 18).

Restorative, periodontal, and esthetic factors. Teeth considered to have a hopeless prognosis for either restoration or periodontal healing should be extracted. With compromised periodontal support, surgery may result in an unfavorable crown-root ratio; therefore, retreatment is selected. With an extraoral sinus tract, surgery may be an adjunct to retreatment to minimize scarring associated with the healing of the sinus.

Clinician Considerations

Clinicians vary in capability as well as availability of armamentarium and time that can be spent on involved treatment of one tooth; their confidence levels regarding specific treatment procedures vary accordingly. When the patient's treatment preference conflicts with that of the clinician, the patient should be referred to another dentist who can perform the preferred procedure. When referral is unfeasible, however, it is appropriate to select the treatment with which the clinician is most confident.

Capability. Capability is a combination of training, skill, and experience. Endodontists usually are more capable of treating post-treatment disease than general dentists. Occasionally, however, an endodontist may not be equally adept at both retreatment and apical surgery. When referral is not an option, the procedure is selected that can be performed best by the endodontist.[8]

Armamentarium. Use of special instruments can optimize the benefit-risk balance of both retreatment and apical surgery. Without the option of referral, if the instruments required to perform

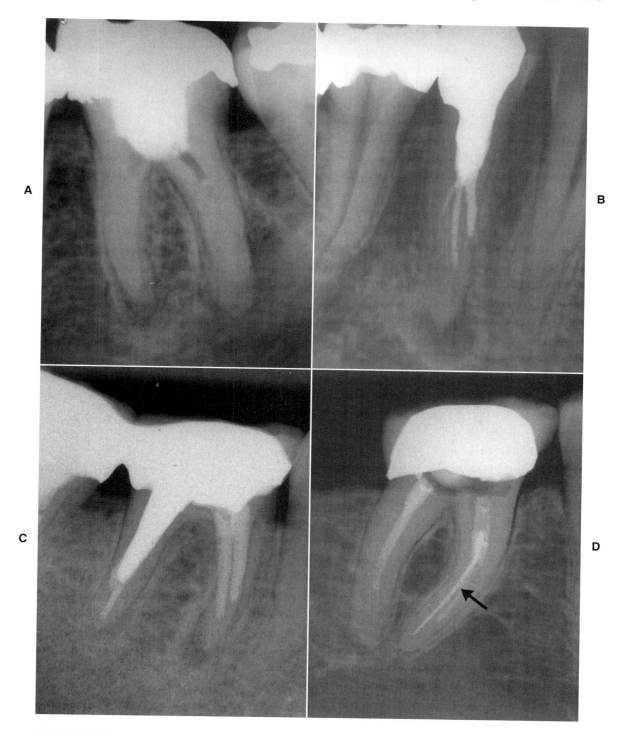

FIGURE 20-1

Root canal obstacles that may compromise retreatment. **A,** Calcific metamorphosis. **B,** Complex morphology. **C,** Suspected ledges. **D,** Separated instrument *(arrow)*. These obstacles restrict renegotiation of the canal and increase the risk of perforation.

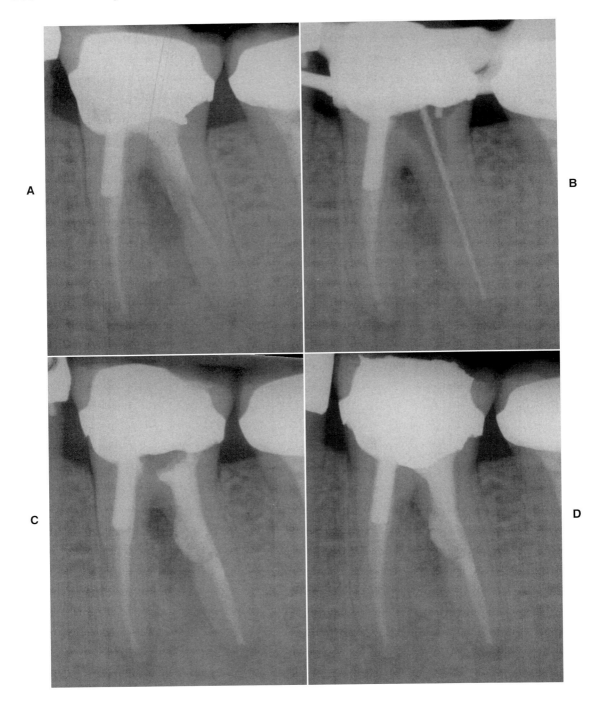

FIGURE 20-2

Retreatment in conjunction with an internal perforation repair. **A,** Distal root perforation into the furcation; there is post-treatment disease. **B,** Distal access through the crown without disturbing the mesial root. **C,** Completed retreatment and perforation seal with mineral trioxide aggregate (MTA). **D,** Progressive healing at 4 months.

only one procedure are available to the attending endodontist, that procedure is usually selected.[8]

Time availability. In specific circumstances (geographically remote areas, community clinics), an excessive practice load may prevent the clinician from undertaking an elaborate retreatment of one tooth with a complex problem. In these circumstances only and without an option for referral, surgery is selected.[8]

Previous Treatment Attempts

If a previous retreatment or apical surgery procedure did not result in healing, the quality of that procedure should be evaluated. If the initial case selection was appropriate and the quality can be significantly improved, the same procedure is repeated. Otherwise, the alternative is selected, which may better address the site of the infection (Figure 20-3).

PREVENTION OF DISEASE

Root canal–treated teeth may appear to be disease-free, yet harbor microorganisms in the canal.[3] The apparent absence of disease suggests a balance between the intracanal microorganisms, their environment, and the host; a change in this balance can result in infection and disease. Another possibility is coronal leakage. The microorganisms invade the filled canal and cause infection within weeks or months, even if the root canal is well filled.[5]

The factors that may affect emergence of post-treatment disease are the following:

1. *Coronal restoration:* If the endodontic system (pulp chamber, canals) has been exposed to coronal leakage or secondary caries, replacing the restoration may modify the canal environment. This modification may result in availability of oxygen and substrate to favor pathogenic microbial strains, which may then establish infection (Figure 20-4).
2. *Post restoration:* There is a risk of canal contamination during post space preparation or post cementation.
3. *Compromised host resistance:* Theoretically, weakened host resistance can modify the balance and prompt infection. This factor, however, has not been thoroughly investigated and its incidence is unknown.

Considerations controlling prevention of post-treatment disease include the following: (1) adequacy of the root filling; (2) adequacy of the coronal seal; and (3) need for a new restoration (post and crown/bridge restorations represent a particular concern, because they will restrict the option of retreatment should disease emerge). The likelihood of emergence of post-treatment disease appears to be highest when both the root filling and the coronal seal are suspect and a new restoration is needed. In these cases retreatment is indicated, because it offers the benefit of preventing post-treatment disease. However, when a new restoration is not needed and only the root filling is suspect, emergence of post-treatment disease is less likely, and the benefit of retreatment is smaller. For these patients only follow-up is indicated; retreatment (and possible complications) can be avoided.[7,8]

Retreatment Techniques

To perform retreatment, obstructions must be overcome to fully renegotiate the canal. These include the coronal restoration, post and core, and root filling materials. Other occasional obstructions, such as separated instruments, may also have to be dealt with.

ACCESS—CROWNS

Many retreatments require removal of a crown. On the other hand, a crown may be retained if satisfactory.[20] In these cases, retreatment can be performed through the crown; rubber dam isolation and temporization are facilitated, function and esthetics are maintained, and additional cost of replacement is avoided. However, visibility may be obscured of key factors such as perforations, coronal extension of silver points, small canal orifices, and vertical cracks. Also, with the crown in place, the risk of irreparable errors during access is increased.[21] If crown margins are poorly adapted, leakage and microbial contamination may occur during retreatment and between appointments (Figure 20-5).

To avoid complications, *crowns are removed for retreatment* when marginal leakage or a cracked tooth is suspected or when future remake of the crown is planned. However, to facilitate function, esthetics, and isolation in selected teeth, the crown may be retained temporarily with appropriate steps to prevent complications.

Satisfactory crowns should be retained. Usually, a wider-than-usual access is prepared through the crown and repaired later (see Figure 20-2). For selected teeth, the crown may be removed intact

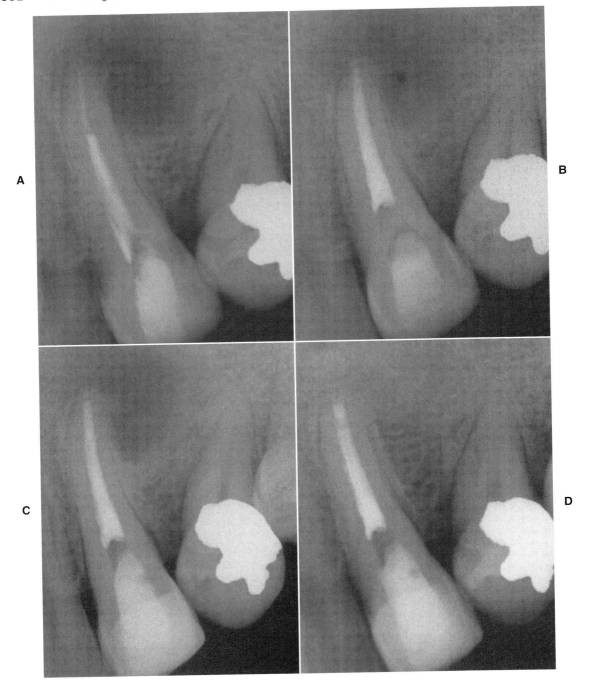

FIGURE 20-3
Persistent disease after retreatment. **A,** Post-treatment disease in lateral incisor. **B,** Completed retreatment. **C,** Disease persists at 1 year; because healing is unlikely after another retreatment, root-end surgery is indicated. **D,** Complete healing at 6 months after surgery.

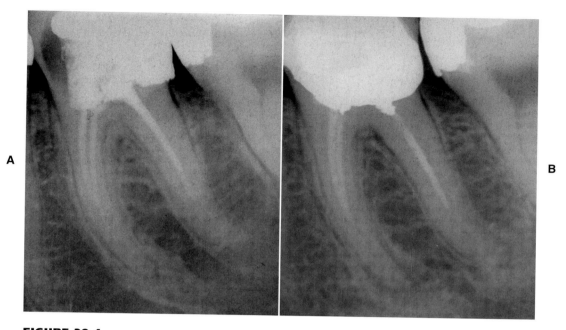

FIGURE 20-4
Delayed emergence of post-treatment disease. **A,** Absence of disease 10 years after inadequate initial treatment in mandibular first molar. Restoration is required. **B,** Post-treatment disease at 6 months after restoration was performed. Retreatment was not performed and is now indicated, necessitating access through new crown.

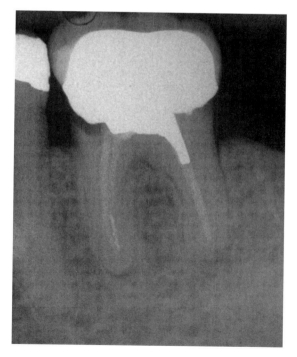

FIGURE 20-5
Recurrent caries at the margins of the existing crown will allow leakage and microbial contamination during retreatment and between appointments. The crown must be removed before retreatment.

and reused later (Figure 20-6). Removal of permanently cemented crowns may cause fracture of tooth structure; special devices must be used cautiously during this procedure. Crown removal is avoided when the type of cement and amount of supporting tooth structure are unknown.

ACCESS—POST AND CORE

Many retreatments require removal of a post and core. Long and large posts are often strongly retained; attempts to remove them must preclude risks of root fracture or post breakage.[22] A technique for post removal with minimal risk is outlined below.

Retention

Post retention must first be weakened (Figure 20-7, *A* and *B*).[20] The core is drilled away (cast core is reduced), leaving just the post extending from the canal. The cement is then broken up with piezoelectric ultrasonic vibration on the post for 10 to 20 minutes.[23] Pointed tips are used to ultrasonically trough around the post.[24]

Extraction of Post

If the post has not been loosened and removed by vibration, it must be extracted with special

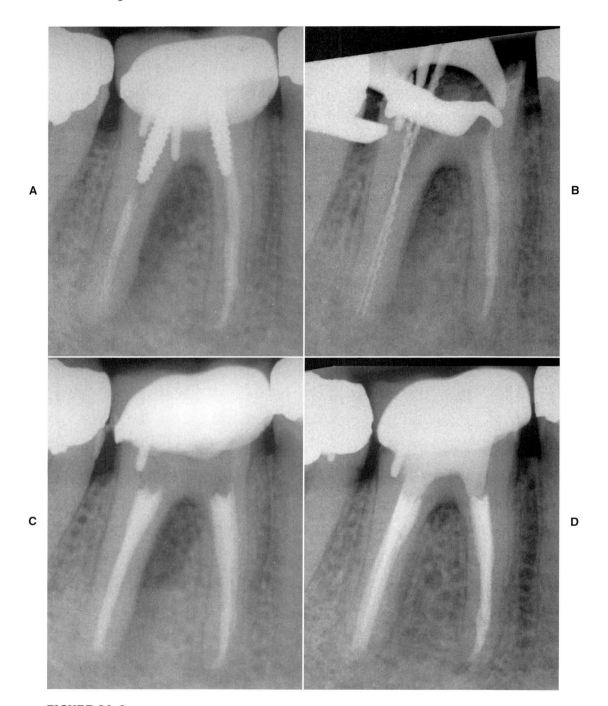

FIGURE 20-6
Crown removed before retreatment and then reused after retreatment. **A,** Crown removal is required to examine the possibility of vertical root fracture or pin perforation with post-treatment disease. **B,** Crown was removed with no fracture or perforation. Note the previously untreated distal canal. **C,** Original crown is recemented after retreatment. **D,** Complete healing at 1 year. A defect is now visible at the distal crown margin; the crown should be replaced.

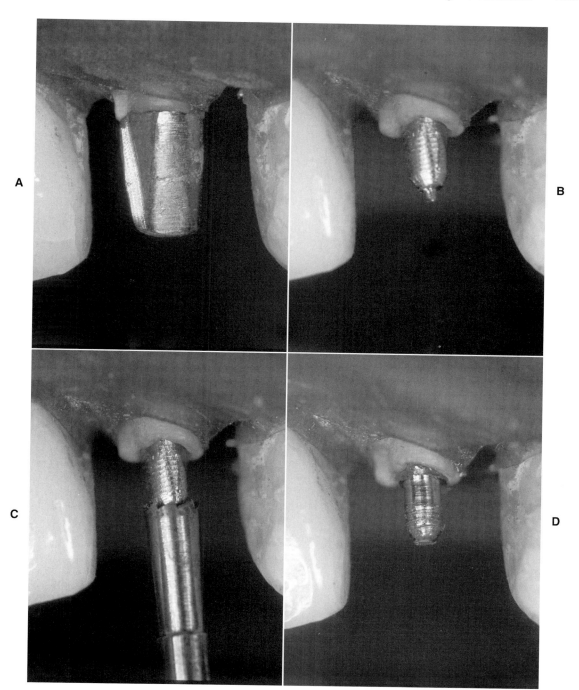

FIGURE 20-7

Extraction of a cast post and core. **A,** Rubber dam is applied. **B,** To weaken retention, core diameter is reduced to estimated post size, followed by ultrasonic vibration. **C,** Post diameter is standardized with a trepan bur (shown), then tapped with the extractor. **D,** Tapped post ready for extraction.

Continued

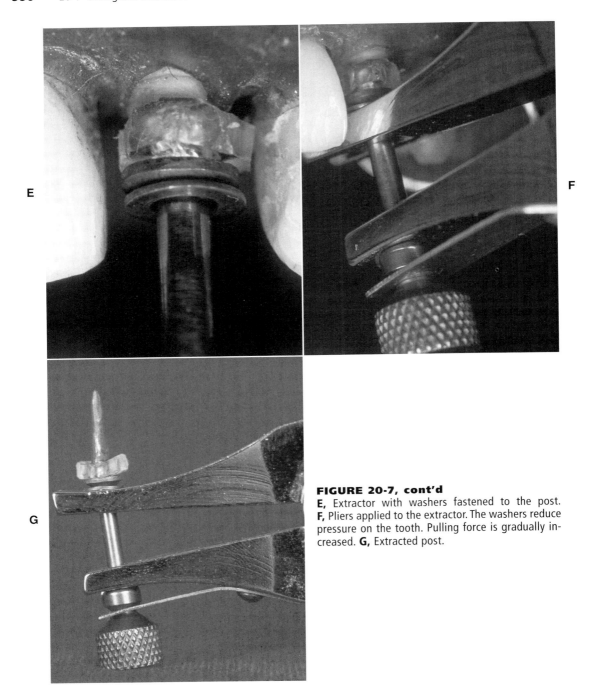

FIGURE 20-7, cont'd
E, Extractor with washers fastened to the post.
F, Pliers applied to the extractor. The washers reduce pressure on the tooth. Pulling force is gradually increased. **G,** Extracted post.

instruments (Figure 20-7, C through G).[22,24,25] The post is bored with a trepan and then tapped and firmly engaged with the matching size extractor. Special pliers are applied to the extractor. The tooth is used as the fulcrum, while rubber (and possibly steel) washers are placed as a cushion to reduce pressure. This technique is effective and relatively safe (Figure 20-8).[26] In se-lected situations, posts can be removed through an in-crown access (Figure 20-9).

Avoiding Post Removal

In a multirooted tooth, retreatment may be indicated specifically in canal(s) other than the one retaining the post. If post removal is considered risky, access can be established through the core only to the retreated canal(s), without disturbing the post (Figures 20-10 and 20-2).[20]

CANAL OBSTRUCTIONS

Canal patency is regained by eliminating the root filling and occasionally separated instruments. To be successful, this procedure requires a nonrestrictive straight-line access.[27] Previous access is evaluated; often it must be extended before elimination of canal obstructions is attempted.

The basic techniques for removing most obstructions are outlined in the following sections for general understanding; further details are available in reference articles.

Gutta-Percha

Gutta-percha is eliminated with rotary instruments and hand files. Solvent is used selectively. A "crown-down" sequence (progressing from larger to smaller instruments, coronal to apical) is preferable.[28]

Rotary instruments. A variety of instruments can effectively remove gutta-percha, when rotated at 350 to 1000 rpm (exceeds the safety limits of nickel titanium).[29,30] In the coronal portion of the canal, wide-taper rotary instruments such as Gates-Glidden burs are used with minimal apical pressure. This expedites the procedure, forms a receptacle for solvent, and improves access (Figure 20-11).[24,28,29] Use of heated instruments creates only a limited space without improving access.[24]

Further apically, nickel titanium rotary files can be used.[24,29,30] Caution is required to avoid separation; pressure is very light, and drilling must cease when gutta-percha debris stops surfacing.

Solvent. Solvent softens gutta-percha and helps prevent canal transportation. Therefore, it is used specifically for dense root fillings and curved canals.[27] However, because of toxicity, solvent must not be extruded periapically.[31]

Gutta-percha and sealers are soluble to a varying degree in chloroform, carbon disulfide, benzene, xylene, essential oils, methyl chloroform, halothane, and white rectified turpentine.[32-34] Being highly volatile, chloroform is the most effective.[33] It is safe for use in dentistry; however, in high concentrations its vapor is potentially hazardous.[35-37] Therefore, chloroform is dripped directly into the canal orifice, avoiding excessive flooding of the chamber. The operating team wears protective masks, and the patient's nose is covered with the rubber dam.

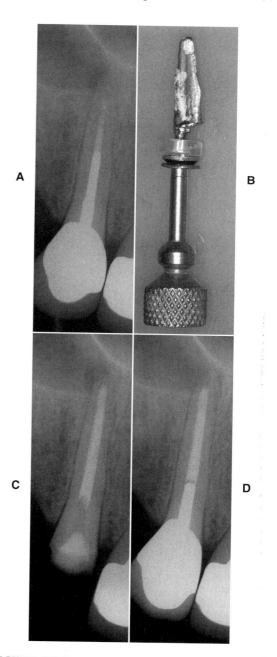

FIGURE 20-8
Retreatment in tooth with a well-retained post. **A,** Long cast post and crown in maxillary canine with post-treatment disease. **B,** Proximal view of the post and extractor. Note the parallel design of this strongly retained post. **C,** Completed retreatment. **D,** Complete healing at 6 months.

Hand files. These are used mainly in the apical portion of the canal.[20,28] When gutta-percha cones are poorly condensed or overextended, solvent is avoided. A reamer or file is used first to negotiate a pathway along the root filling. A larger file is

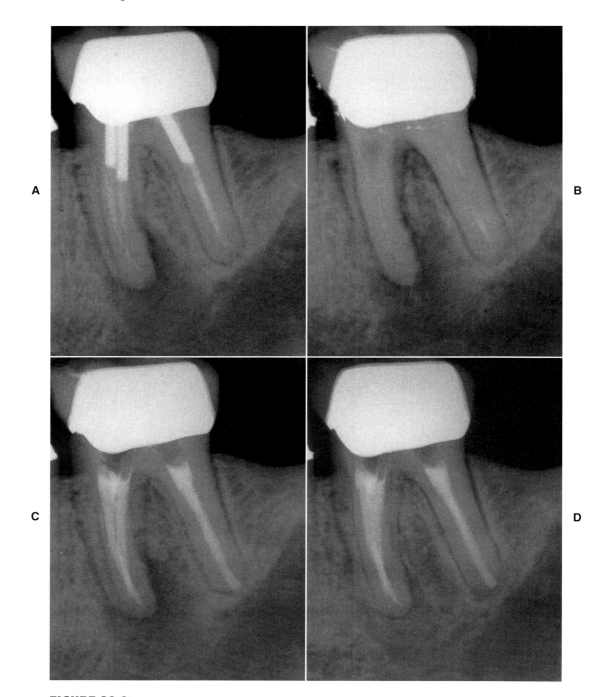

FIGURE 20-9
Retreatment and post removal through crown. **A,** Three prefabricated posts in molar with post-treatment disease. **B,** Access for retreatment of mesial canals is through the crown and core. **C,** Completed retreatment. **D,** Progressive healing at 6 months.

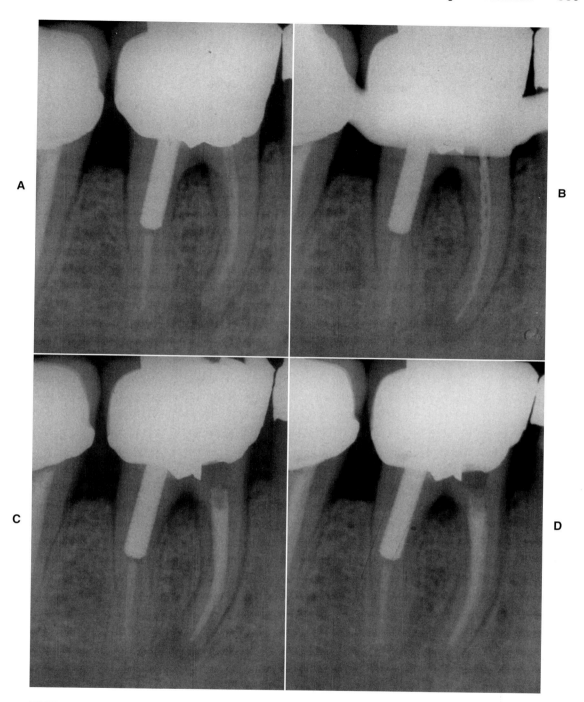

FIGURE 20-10
Retreatment avoiding post removal in a multirooted tooth. **A,** Post-treatment disease associated with the mesial root of the mandibular first molar. Removal of oversized post from the distal root is risky, with minimal benefit from retreatment of the distal canal. **B,** Access is through the crown and core with retreatment of mesial canals. **C,** Completed retreatment. **D,** Complete healing at 6 months.

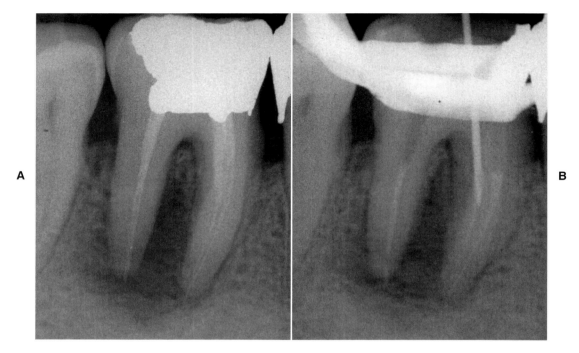

FIGURE 20-11
Initial removal of gutta-percha. **A,** Poorly condensed root fillings. **B,** Coronal portion of gutta-percha is removed with a Gates-Glidden bur. Access is improved, and a receptacle for solvent is formed.

then carefully "screwed" into the filling mass and pulled back, often retrieving all the gutta-percha cones.[27] With overextended cones, the file may have to be extended periapically to avoid separation of the cone at the apical foramen (Figure 20-12).[27] Overextended cones may separate at the apex and cannot be retrieved.

Pastes and Cements

Pastes and cements of varying hardness are used as the principal root filling materials in certain regions of the world. To assess its hardness, the material must be evaluated clinically.[20] Some filling pastes are very hard and insoluble.

Soft-setting pastes. Canals filled with soft-setting pastes may be penetrated with files.[27] A "crown-down" sequence is used to gradually eliminate the paste from the entire canal.[28]

Hard-setting cements. Resin-type cements should be exposed to solvents such as tetrachlorethylene, xylene, eucalyptol, or eugenol.[24] If softened, the cement is managed like soft-setting pastes.[20] If not, the cement is broken down with moderate ultrasonic vibration, using special pointed tips (Figure 20-13) under light apical pressure.[24,27] To prevent perforation, the procedure is frequently

monitored with radiographs or an operating microscope.[24] This procedure is time consuming.[38]

As a last resort, the cement is drilled out with long-shank, small round burs (Mueller burs are useful).[27] This is a very exacting procedure; frequent radiographic or microscopic control is imperative to prevent perforation.[27] The cement is intermittently probed with a sharp endodontic explorer to identify spaces that would permit renegotiating the canal with instruments.[27]

Metallic Objects—Silver Points and Separated Instruments

Metallic objects may often be retrieved or bypassed.[27] These procedures depend on accessibility and canal anatomy.[20] Accessibility is gradually more restricted from the orifice level apically, particularly in curved canals.[39] Bypass is most feasible in oval canals.[39]

Retrieval from the chamber. Extension of the silver point into the chamber is key to retrieval.[27] Ultrasonic vibration is carefully applied to reduce retention and free the point from the surrounding core cement.[24] After being loosened, the point is grasped and retrieved with small pliers or special extractors.[27]

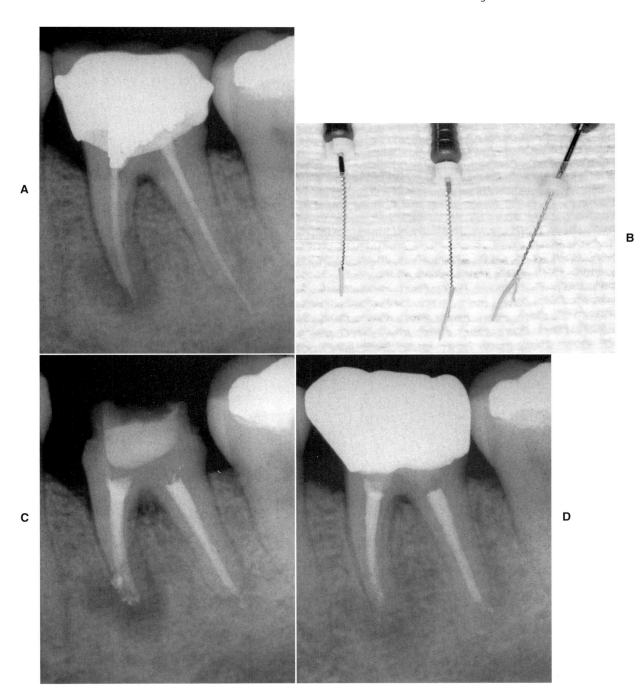

FIGURE 20-12
Removal of overextended gutta-percha. **A,** Root filling extends beyond the apices; there is post-treatment disease. **B,** After initial use of burs (see Figure 20-11), the gutta-percha cones were engaged with files and retrieved. Solvent was avoided. **C,** Completed retreatment. **D,** Progressive healing at 6 months.

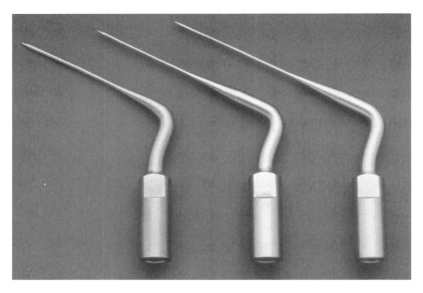

FIGURE 20-13
Ultrasonic tips for breaking up hard-setting cements and loosening separated instruments under the operating microscope.

An amalgam core is separated from the surrounding dentin with ultrasonic tips or burs and dislodged as a whole.[20] If the silver points are embedded in the core, they may be retrieved (Figure 20-14).

Bypass. The canal is first flared with Gates-Glidden burs. Hand files are then used with solvent to prepare a pathway around the metallic object and possibly retrieve it.[20,24] Ultrasonic files or pointed tips (see Figure 20-13) can be used to vibrate the object, which may dislodge (Figure 20-15) or shatter.[24,39] If the object is bypassed but not retrieved, it will be enclosed in the root filling.[39] This procedure can be very time consuming and possibly complicated by additional file separation, perforation, or apical displacement of the object.[39] Visualization is optimized with the operating microscope.[24]

Extraction from the canal. As a last resort, objects can be extracted with special devices.[20] Most available devices include end-cutting trepans and extracting tubes, with or without a locking mechanism (Figure 20-16).[22,24,27] A trough is cut around the object with ultrasonic tips or the trepans. A matching extracting tube is applied, locked, ultrasonically vibrated, and withdrawn. This is an exacting procedure; frequent radiographic or microscopic control is imperative to prevent perforation (Figure 20-17).

Because the extraction procedure requires considerable sacrifice of root dentin, it is safe only in large, straight roots.[27] It is also time consuming,

particularly in posterior teeth.[27,39] For these reasons, extraction is not the first choice for retrieval of metallic objects.[39]

If the object is not bypassed or retrieved, by necessity, only the accessible canal portion is retreated. Prognosis is better when there is no root canal infection and periradicular disease.[1]

COMPLETION OF RETREATMENT

After renegotiating the canal, treatment is completed using routine procedures. However, elimination of root canal infection in retreatment is more challenging than in initial treatment, primarily because there may be therapy-resistant microorganisms, such as *Enterococcus faecalis*.[1-3] Also, microorganisms may persist under residual root filling "patches," which usually remain during retreatment.[30,40,41] Finally, canal wall surfaces may remain untouched during retreatment.[40]

The following are important for management of post-treatment disease:

1. A wide, direct access is needed for better instrumentation.
2. The canal is enlarged somewhat beyond its previous size (see examples in figures) to reduce residue of root filling materials.
3. Calcium hydroxide is used for canal disinfection; therefore, two or more visits are required.

When retreatment is performed to prevent post-treatment disease, the canal enlargement is

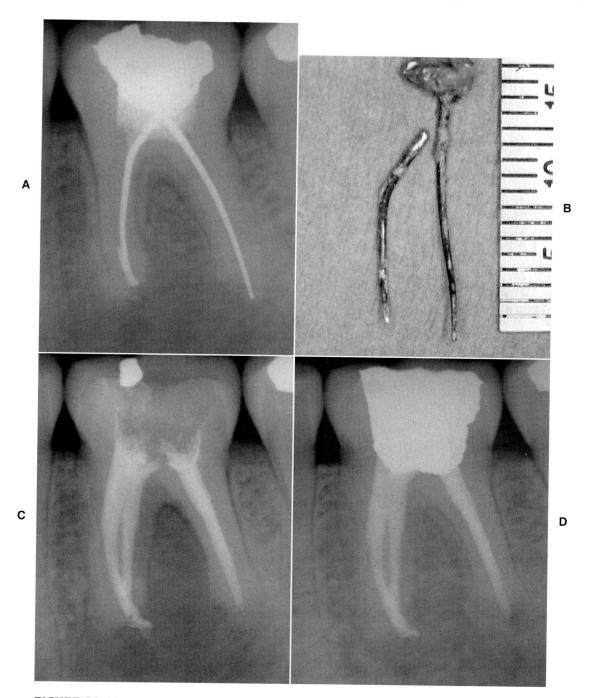

FIGURE 20-14
Retrieval of silver points extending into the pulp chamber. **A,** Silver points in molar with post-treatment disease. The points may be embedded in the amalgam partial core. **B,** The amalgam core was dislodged with one point embedded. The underlying cement was dispersed ultrasonically, and the second point was retrieved with small pliers. **C,** Completed retreatment, with sealer extruded. **D,** Complete healing at 6 months.

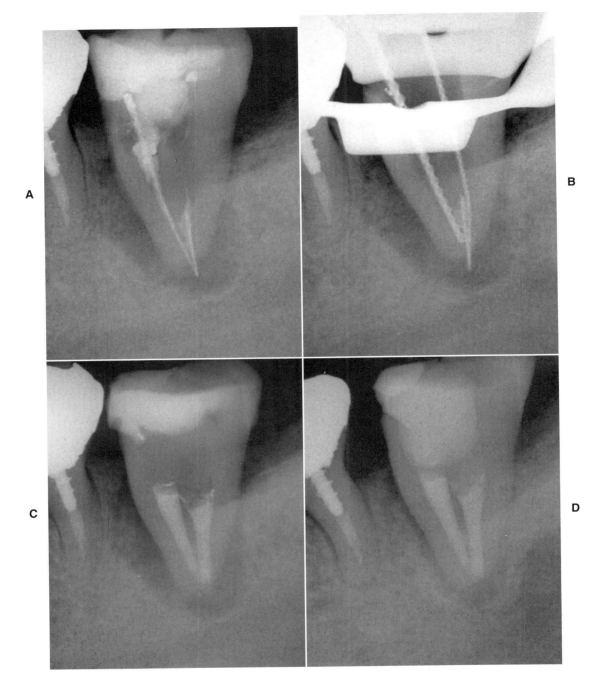

FIGURE 20-15
Retrieval of Thermafil carriers. **A,** Poorly adapted Thermafil root fillings; there is extensive post-treatment disease. **B,** Mesial carrier is removed with ultrasonic vibration. Distal carrier is bypassed. **C,** Completed retreatment after the distal carrier was retrieved. **D,** Incomplete healing at 1 year.

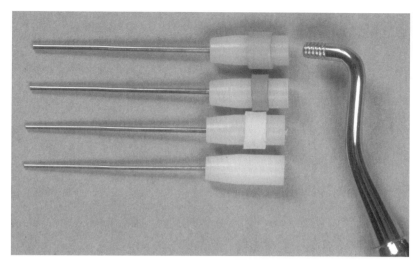

FIGURE 20-16
Hollow tubes to extract separated silver points and instruments from root canals. Cyanoacrylate glue is used in lieu of a locking mechanism.

moderate and use of intracanal medication is less critical. Therefore, retreatment can be completed in one visit, when feasible.

As a final step, the canal is obturated and the tooth is restored. Outcome assessment is similar to that for initial root canal treatment, as outlined in Chapter 19.

DEGREE OF DIFFICULTY

Clinical conditions that require particular expertise are listed below, with indication of the degree of difficulty (*e* = extreme; *m* = moderate). To avoid complications, these conditions should be managed by endodontists.

Crown: Removal of the crown intact (*e*); retreatment through an in-crown access (*m*).
Post: Cast post (*e*); oversized prefabricated post (*e*); retreatment avoiding post removal (*e*); regular-sized prefabricated post (*m*).
Root filling: Overextended gutta-percha (*e*); well-compacted gutta-percha (*m*); gutta-percha in a curved or ledged canal (*m*); hard-setting cement (*e*); silver point with coronal extension (*m*); silver point with restricted accessibility (*e*); separated instrument (*e*).

Short-Term and Long-Term Treatment Outcome

In the short term, retreatment with existent post-treatment disease may be associated with postoperative discomfort, including pain and swelling.[16] This is an additional reason why retreatment for existent disease should not be completed in one visit.[42]

The long-term outcome of retreatment depends largely on regaining canal patency. The healing rate after retreatment for existent disease is 74%, which is lower than after initial treatment.[1,2] The probability of healing is higher when factors facilitating infection (untreated or poorly treated canal) are identified and can be addressed satisfactorily during retreatment.[9] The healing rate after retreatment for prevention of disease is higher, comparable to initial treatment.[1]

Communication and Referral

Retreatment is more frequently associated with procedural complications than is initial treatment.[43] Effective communication requires that the patient be informed of potential problems *before retreatment is initiated* to avoid frustration, discontent, and possible litigation. This communication includes explanation of the benefits, risks, potential restrictive factors as well as the short- and long-term outcome. Both retreatment and subsequent restorative procedures are then authorized by the patient.[43]

Even when the patient is referred to the endodontist, explanation by the generalist is still essential; it allows the patient to consider the option of referral and consultation with the

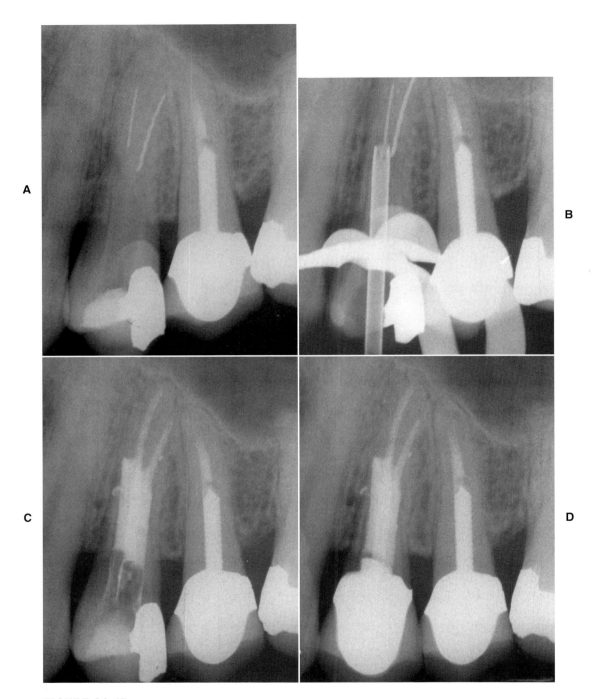

FIGURE 20-17

Extraction of separated files. **A,** Both canals are blocked by separated files. **B,** Trepan bur is used to cut a trough around each separated file. The trepan bur must remain centered to avoid perforation. **C,** Completed retreatment after both files were extracted. Note the sacrifice of root dentin. **D,** Complete healing at 1 year.

endodontist. Furthermore, the patient will have realistic expectations.

The referral should be in writing and include all pertinent information: case history, previous radiographs, and an outline of the restorative/prosthetic treatment plan, particularly for the tooth to be retreated. Emergency procedures performed by the referring dentist are also mentioned. Midtreatment referrals (aborted retreatment attempt by the generalist), frequently associated with complications, are to be avoided.[43]

REFERENCES

1. Friedman S: Treatment outcome and prognosis of endodontic therapy. In Ørstavik D, Pitt Ford TR, editors, *Essential endodontology: prevention and treatment of apical periodontitis,* Oxford, 1998, Blackwell Science.
2. Sundqvist G, Figdor D, Persson S, Sjögren U: Microbiologic analysis of teeth with failed endodontic treatment and the outcome of conservative retreatment, *Oral Surg Oral Med Oral Pathol* 85:86, 1998.
3. Molander A, Reit C, Dahlén G, Kvist T: Microbiological status of root filled teeth with apical periodontitis, *Int Endod J* 31:1, 1998.
4. Sjögren U, Figdor D, Persson S, Sundqvist G: Influence of infection at the time of root filling on the outcome of endodontic treatment of teeth with apical periodontitis, *Int Endod J* 30:297, 1997.
5. Friedman S, Komorowski R, Maillet W, et al: Resistance of coronally induced bacterial ingress by an experimental glass ionomer cement root canal sealer *in vivo, J Endod* 26:1, 2000.
6. Sakellariou PL: Periapical actinomycosis: report of a case and review of the literature, *Endod Dent Traumatol* 12:151, 1996.
7. Taintor JF, Ingle JI, Fahid A: Retreatment versus further treatment, *Clin Prev Dent* 5:8, 1983.
8. Friedman S, Stabholz A: Endodontic retreatment: case selection and technique. Part 1: Criteria for case selection, *J Endod* 12:28, 1986.
9. Bergenholtz G, Lekholm U, Milthon R, et al: Retreatment of endodontic fillings, *Scand J Dent Res* 87:217, 1979.
10. Lewis RD, Block RM: Management of endodontic failures, *Oral Surg Oral Med Oral Pathol* 66:711, 1988.
11. Reit C, Grondahl H-G: Endodontic retreatment decision making among a group of general practitioners, *Scand J Dent Res* 96:112, 1988.
12. Hülsmann M: Retreatment decision-making by a group of general dental practitioners in Germany, *Int Endod J* 27:125, 1994.
13. Petersson K, et al: Follow-up study of endodontic status in an adult Swedish population, *Endod Dent Traumatol* 7:221, 1991.
14. Friedman S, Lustmann J, Shaharabany V: Treatment results of apical surgery in premolar and molar teeth, *J Endod* 17:30, 1991.
15. Crump M: Differential diagnosis in endodontic failure, *Dent Clin North Am* 23:617, 1979.
16. Kvist T, Reit C: Postoperative discomfort associated with surgical and nonsurgical endodontic retreatment, *Endod Dent Traumatol* 16:71, 2000.
17. Reit C, Kvist T: Endodontic retreatment behavior: the influence of disease concepts and personal values, *Int Endod J* 31:358, 1998.
18. Tronstad L, Kreshtool D, Barnett F: Microbiological monitoring and results of treatment of extraradicular endodontic infection, *Endod Dent Traumatol* 6:129, 1990.
19. Pitts DL, Natkin E: Diagnosis and treatment of vertical root fracture, *J Endod* 9:338, 1983.
20. Stabholz A, Friedman S: Endodontic retreatment: case selection and technique. Part 2: treatment planning for retreatment, *J Endod* 14:607, 1988.
21. Metzger Z, Shperling I: Iatrogenic perforation of the roots of restoration-covered teeth, *J Endod* 7:232, 1981.
22. Goon WWY: Managing the obstructed root canal space: rationale and techniques, *Calif Dent Assoc J* 19:51, 1991.
23. Johnson WT, Leary JM, Boyer DB: Effect of ultrasonic vibration on post removal in extracted human premolar teeth, *J Endod* 22:487, 1996.
24. Machtou P, Friedman S: Advances in endodontic retreatment, *Alpha Omegan* 90:47, 1997.
25. Machtou P, Sarfati P, Cohen AG: Post removal prior to retreatment, *J Endod* 15:552, 1989.
26. Altshul JH, Marshall G, Morgan LA, Baumgartner JC: Comparison of dentinal crack incidence and of post removal time resulting from post removal by ultrasonic or mechanical force, *J Endod* 23:683, 1997.
27. Friedman S, Stabholz A, Tamse A: Endodontic retreatment: case selection and technique. Part 3: retreatment techniques, *J Endod* 16:543, 1990.
28. Mandel E, Friedman S: Endodontic retreatment: a rational approach to root canal reinstrumentation, *J Endod* 18:565, 1992.
29. Hülsmann M, Stotz S: Efficacy, cleaning ability and safety of different devices for gutta-percha removal in root canal retreatment, *Int Endod J* 30:227, 1997.
30. Sae-Lim V, Rajamanickam I, Lim BK, Lee HL: Effectiveness of ProFile .04 taper rotary instruments in endodontic retreatment, *J Endod* 26:100, 2000.
31. Barbosa SV, Burkard DH, Spangberg LW: Cytotoxic effects of gutta-percha solvents, *J Endod* 20:6, 1994.
32. Wennberg A, Ørstavik D: Evaluation of alternatives to chloroform in endodontic practice, *Endod Dent Traumatol* 5:234, 1989.
33. Wourms DJ, Campbell AD, Hicks ML, Pelleu GB: Alternative solvents to chloroform for gutta-percha removal, *J Endod* 16:539, 1990.
34. Whitworth JM, Boursin EM: Dissolution of root canal sealer cements in volatile solvents, *Int Endod J* 33:19, 2000.
35. McDonald MN, Vire DE: Chloroform in the endodontic operatory, *J Endod* 18:301, 1992.
36. Margelos J, Verdelis K, Eliades G: Chloroform uptake by gutta-percha and assessment of its concentration in air during the chloroform-dip technique, *J Endod* 22:547, 1996.
37. Chutich MJ, Kaminski EJ, Miller DA, Lautenschlager EP: Risk assessment of the toxicity of solvents of gutta-

percha used in endodontic retreatment, *J Endod* 24:213, 1998.

38. Jeng HW, ElDeeb ME: Removal of the hard paste fillings from the root canal by ultrasonic instrumentation, *J Endod* 13:295, 1987.

39. Nagai O, Yani N, Kayaba Y, et al: Ultrasonic removal of broken instruments in root canals, *Int Endod J* 19:298, 1986.

40. Wilcox LR, Swift ML: Endodontic retreatment in small and large curved canals, *J Endod* 17:313, 1991.

41. Baldassari-Cruz LA, Wilcox LR. Effectiveness of gutta-percha removal with and without the microscope, *J Endod* 25:627, 1999.

42. Trope M: Flare-up rate of single-visit endodontics, *Int Endod J* 24:24, 1991.

43. Selbst AG: Understanding informed consent and its relationship to the incidence of adverse treatment events in conventional endodontic therapy, *J Endod* 16:387, 1990.

Preventive Endodontics: Protecting the Pulp

LEARNING OBJECTIVES

After reading this chapter, the student should be able to:

1 / Describe anatomic and functional relationships between dentin and pulp.

2 / Understand unique physiologic and structural characteristics of the pulp and how these affect pulp response to injury.

3 / Discuss the effects of vasoconstrictor-containing local anesthetics on pulpal hemodynamics.

4 / Discuss the formation and role of tertiary dentin in pulp protection.

5 / Comprehend the sensory function of the pulp.

6 / Recognize reparative potential of the pulp.

7 / Describe permeability of dentin and under what conditions permeability can be modified.

8 / Identify and determine etiologic factors responsible for pulp pathosis.

9 / Recognize effects of chemical components of various restorative materials on the pulp.

10 / Appreciate the significance of microleakage and the smear layer on pulp responses.

11 / Discuss how bacterial growth beneath restorations can affect the pulp.

12 / Provide a rationale for cavity varnishes, liners, bases, and hybridization of dentin.

13 / Understand "thermal shock" and its significance.

14 / Be aware of potentially injurious effects of polishing of restorations, removal of metallic restorations, and placement of pins.

15 / Understand the relationship between postrestorative pain and injury to the pulp.

16 / Discuss the possible effects of orthodontic tooth movement on the pulp.

17 / Discuss the management of deep carious lesions without pulp exposure.

18 / Discuss management of carious as well as accidental pulp exposure.

19 / Discuss the potential for periapical repair after treatment of deep carious lesions.

20 / Summarize preventive measures that should be observed during dental restorative procedures.

OUTLINE

Pulp-Dentin Complex

Unique Characteristics of the Pulp

Reduced Blood Flow Associated with Local Anesthetics

Tertiary (Reparative) Dentin

Sensory Function of the Pulp

Repair Potential of the Pulp

Dentin Permeability

Pulp Pathosis

Effects of Restorative Procedures
  Cavity and Crown Preparation Factors

Effects of Restorative Materials
  Role of Bacteria
  Microleakage
  Exothermic Materials
  Hygroscopic Materials
  Toxicity of Materials
  Biologic Properties of Specific Materials
  Protectants
  Additional Factors
  Postrestorative Hypersensitivity
  Summary of Protective Measures

Orthodontic Procedures

Management of the Vital Pulp
  Effect of Natural Causes of Pathoses

Maintenance of a Vital Pulp
  Indirect Pulp Capping
  Direct Pulp Capping
  Pulpotomy
  Periapical Repair after Treatment of Deep
    Carious Lesions

The goal of this chapter is to consider preventive measures to protect the dentin and pulp from injury. Why should the dentist be concerned about pulpal protection? What is so important about this minuscule tissue?

In addition to its primary responsibility for dentin formation, the pulp serves as a sensory organ. Certain stimuli cause sensory receptors in the pulp to trigger protective reflexes (such as jaw opening) that serve to protect the tooth from fracture. If it becomes necessary to remove the pulp, the impact of endodontic treatment on tooth strength should be considered. To perform pulpectomy, the access cavity that must be prepared results in the removal of mineralized tooth structure. If removal is excessive, the cusps are weakened and prone to fracture. Root canal treatment may also compromise an existing restoration, thus necessitating its replacement. Involved then are both the cost of root canal treatment and the potential discomfort and inconvenience to the patient. Maintaining the pulp and dentin intact (and healthy) is obviously a desirable objective. Vital pulp therapy as an alternative to pulpectomy deserves serious consideration.

Pulp-Dentin Complex

The dental pulp is an ectomesenchymal-differentiated tissue that produces the dentin component of mammalian teeth. The term *dentin-pulp complex* emphasizes the intimate anatomic and physiologic relationships between dentin and pulp. The odontoblast processes and nerves that reside within the dentinal tubules make dentin a living tissue. Consequently, when performing clinical procedures, the clinician *must* view vital dentin the same as other living tissues.

Unique Characteristics of the Pulp

The pulp is a loose, fibrous connective tissue resembling other connective tissues. However, the pulp is unique in that it lacks a collateral circulation because its blood supply is limited to the few arterioles entering the apical foramen. In addition, the pulp is rigidly encased in hard tissue, thus placing it in a low compliance environment similar to brain, bone marrow, and nail beds. These tissues respond somewhat differently to noxious stimuli than do other tissues such as skin. In most tissues the cardinal signs of inflammation include redness, heat, swelling, pain, and loss of function.

Swelling results from reactive hyperemia and increased vascular permeability; these vascular reactions lead to the accumulation of edema fluid within the tissue. As tissue pressure increases, the tissue swells, which tends to ease the tissue pressure. Being encased in dentin, the pulp is unable to swell. Elevated tissue pressure is a major factor in pain associated with acute inflammatory reactions. For this reason, pain is generally more severe in tissues in a low-compliance (unyielding) environment. Thus, pulpal edema or abscess formation is more likely to be painful than comparable lesions in a more compliant tissue, such as gingiva and oral mucosa.

When the pulp is subjected to injury, a significant increase in intrapulpal pressure occurs.[1] Blood pressure is greatest in arterial vessels and progressively falls in magnitude in arterioles, capillaries, postcapillary venules, and venules, in that order. Because of the rigidity of dentin, the pulp does not expand; a sharp rise in intrapulpal pressure could result in compression of venules, thus increasing vascular hindrance (resistance to blood flow). This "strangulation" hypothesis holds that space for additional blood and tissue fluid is provided by compression of venules, since pressure in the venules is lower than in the arterioles and capillaries. According to this hypothesis, compression of venules would produce increased vascular resistance and passive congestion, which in turn would result in hypoxia; pulp tissue would eventually become necrotic because of a lack of oxygen.

Marked compression of venules is unlikely, since the pulp is rich in proteoglycans. These molecules have the ability to bind water, thus making the pulp a resilient tissue. Consequently, pulpal venules are in a relatively compliant environment, which should protect them from abrupt pressure changes. It has been demonstrated that pressure changes in one part of the pulp do not necessarily produce pressure changes in other parts.[2]

By applying Starling's Law, when interstitial tissue pressure exceeds intravascular pressure, fluid is forced back into the venules. Additionally, lymphatics are capable of removing excess fluid. This removal of fluid seems to be efficient, because increased tissue pressure in the pulp may actually begin to decrease while blood flow is still increasing. These phenomena have been elucidated by Heyeraas and Kvinnsland,[3] a "must-read" publication.

If the strangulation hypothesis were valid, inflamed pulps would undergo infarction. An infarct is an area of ischemic necrosis produced by either occlusion of the arterial supply or its venous drainage. *Pulpal infarcts are uncommon and*

are usually due to trauma to the vessels entering the pulp rather than to intrapulpal inflammation.

How then do pulps die? Much depends on the cause of the injury, the most common being bacterial infection. Often infection involves the presence of pyogenic bacteria, in which case pulpal death is associated with suppuration (liquefactive necrosis). Bacteria that do not evoke suppurative inflammation can damage tissues in other ways. For example, endotoxin, even in low concentrations, adversely affects the function and metabolic processes of cells.[4] The cell types particularly influenced by endotoxin are fibroblasts, phagocytes, platelets, and B-lymphocytes. In high concentration, endotoxin will kill cells.

Activation of the immune system by antigenic bacterial products usually has deleterious effects on cells. For example, macrophages that are activated by the immune system are important in mediation of tissue destruction by secreting a wide variety of biologically active products, including toxic oxygen metabolites, nitric oxide, and proteases. The immune system can also stimulate fibroblasts, macrophages, and synovial cells to secrete metalloproteinases, which can act on a variety of extracellular components, including proteoglycans, laminin, fibronectin, and amorphous collagens. Activation of the immune system can also trigger the proliferation of fibroblasts and production of collagen fibers. Ultimately, this results in pulpal fibrosis with the replacement of normal constituents of the pulp and diffuse calcification.

Reduced Blood Flow Associated with Local Anesthetics

Vasoconstrictors added to local anesthetics may have a profound effect on pulpal blood flow, depending upon where the solution is injected. A periodontal ligament (PDL) injection of an anesthetic such as 2% lidocaine with epinephrine 1:100,000 significantly reduces pulpal blood flow (Figure 21-1).[5,6] Fortunately, the rate of oxygen consumption in the pulp is relatively low; if necessary, pulp cells can anaerobically produce energy through the pentose phosphate pathway of carbohydrate metabolism.[7] Therefore, a healthy pulp may survive episodes of ischemia lasting for 1 hour or more. An ischemic pulp subjected to severe injury may hemorrhage when subjected to trauma, such as that associated with full crown preparation without the use of an adequate coolant. However, under experimental conditions, deep cavity preparation after PDL injection with 2% lidocaine and epinephrine failed to evoke pulpal hemorrhage or other evidence of damage.[8]

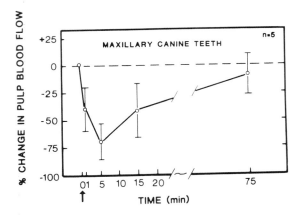

FIGURE 21-1
Effects of infiltration anesthesia (2% lidocaine with 1:100,000 epinephrine) on pulpal blood flow in the maxillary canine teeth of dogs. The *arrow* indicates the time of injection. The bar depicts SD. (From Kim S, Edwall L, Trowbridge H, Chien S: *J Dent Res* 63:650, 1984.)

Tertiary (Reparative) Dentin

Tertiary dentin formation is a fundamental defense mechanism. This is nature's way to seal off cut or diseased dentinal tubules at the pulp surface, thereby diminishing the effects of attrition, dental caries, and other forms of trauma (Figure 21-2). Primary (developmental) dentin is formed during tooth development whereas physiologic (regular) secondary dentin is deposited circumpulpally throughout the life of a vital tooth, thus causing the pulp chamber to become progressively smaller with age. Tertiary (reparative) dentin forms at the pulpal end of those tubules that are in communication with irritants such as attrition of tooth structure and dental caries.

Does tertiary dentin protect the pulp? Yes, in most cases. There is usually no continuity between the tubules in primary dentin and those in tertiary dentin.[9] Furthermore, the walls of the tubules along the junction between primary and tertiary dentin are thickened and often occluded.[10] Consequently, this junctional zone limits the diffusion of irritants into the pulp. Poor-quality tertiary dentin does not afford this protection. When the pulp becomes inflamed as a result of irritation, the tertiary dentin that is formed often contains voids where soft tissue has been entrapped, thus giving the dentin the appearance of Swiss cheese (Figure 21-3). High-speed cutting techniques using water-spray as a coolant decrease tertiary formation by minimizing trauma to the pulp.[11]

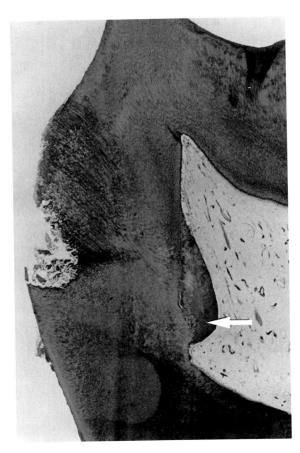

FIGURE 21-2
Tertiary dentin *(arrow)* deposited beneath caries. (From Trowbridge HO: *J Endod* 7:52, 1981.)

There is a misconception that calcium hydroxide stimulates tertiary formation when applied as a cavity liner or base. However, evidence would suggest that this notion has no validity.[12] There is no significant difference in the amount or thickness of tertiary dentin under silicate, amalgam, calcium hydroxide, zinc oxide-eugenol (ZnOE), or composites when placed in cavities of comparable depth.[13] Tertiary dentin probably forms in response to the trauma inflicted by cavity preparation rather than to the restorative material. As an agent used to cap mechanical exposures, calcium hydroxide does provide a consistent, yet transient antimicrobial environment for dentin "bridge" formation. However, the long-term sealing efficacy of calcium hydroxide is very poor; continual microleakage results in recurrent caries, bacterial penetration through the "bridge," pulp infection, and eventual necrosis.[14,15]

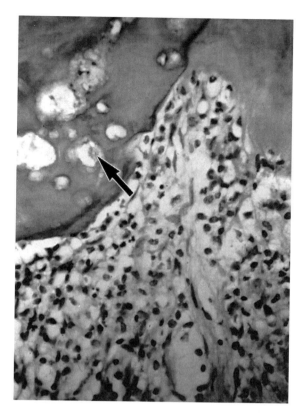

FIGURE 21-3
Poor quality tertiary dentin containing voids *(arrow)*. This form of dentin is often referred to as "Swiss cheese" dentin. Note the presence of inflammatory cells in the pulp.

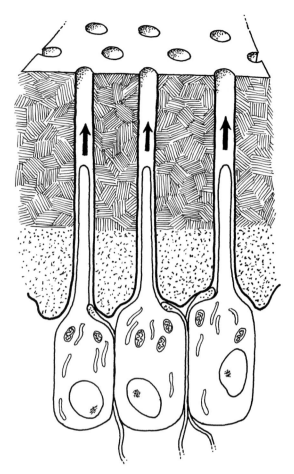

FIGURE 21-4
Hydrodynamics. Fluid movement *(arrows)* in dentinal tubules resulting from drying of exposed dentin. The movement of fluid may stimulate the receptors at the base of the tubules, causing pain.

Sensory Function of the Pulp

Beyond 150 μm into the dentin from the pulp the vital tubule complex is essentially devoid of nerve fibers, yet the dentinoenamel junction (DEJ) is a sensitive area. Dentinal tubules contain odontoblast processes and fluid derived from pulpal blood vessels. Stimuli are conducted from the outer surface of the tooth to nerve fibers in the underlying pulp via the fluid within the dentinal tubules. According to the hydrodynamic theory of dentin sensitivity, exposure of the tooth surface to cold or heat causes contraction or expansion of fluid in the tubules, thus creating hydraulic forces.[16] Application of a hypertonic solution, air blasts, or a probe to freshly exposed dentin causes a rapid outward flow of fluid in the dentinal tubules (Figure 21-4). This rapid fluid movement serves as a transducer mechanism by deforming mechanoreceptive sensory nerve endings located in the tubules and underlying pulp, thus eliciting pain signals.

Repair Potential of the Pulp

Theoretically, the pulp is as well equipped to cope with injury as any other organ of the body. It is well vascularized and has an ample supply of connective tissue cells capable of initiating repair. In addition, the pulp may produce tertiary dentin and thus withdraw from irritation. However, teeth are subjected to various forms of trauma, which may limit the pulp's ability to respond to injury. In periodontally involved teeth, for example, the pulp may have fewer fibroblasts, blood vessels, more collagen fibers, and dystrophic calcifications than normal pulp (Figure 21-5). Connective tissue repair may be compromised in a pulp thus affected. However, whether these pulps are less resistant to injury has yet to be determined.

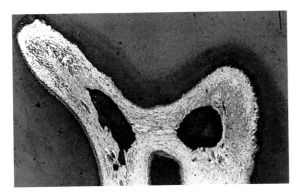

FIGURE 21-5
Pulp of periodontally involved tooth. Note fewer than normal cells and blood vessels and the presence of collagen fibers and dystrophic calcifications.

Dentin Permeability

Dentin is permeable because of the dentinal tubules. Solutes can move through dentin in either direction, that is, toward the pulp or toward the oral cavity. When bacteria invade tooth structure as a result of caries or restorative procedures, substances they release diffuse through the tubules toward the pulp along a concentration gradient; when these bacterial products reach the pulp, they evoke inflammation. Potentially irritating substances of bacterial origin include enzymes, byproducts of cell respiration, proteases, endotoxin, fragments of cell walls, and ammonia. Most of these substances are also antigens and elicit an immunologic response. Thus, the permeability of dentin influences the degree to which the pulp is subjected to inflammatory and immunologic stimuli.

With caries, dentinal tubules beneath the carious lesion will often become partially occluded by mineral deposits, a condition known as dentinal sclerosis. Other causes of dentinal sclerosis include attrition, erosion, and fracture of tooth structure. This sclerosis reduces the permeability of dentin.

Dentin permeability is of particular interest when the effects of restorative procedures on the pulp are considered. Restorations that do not provide an impervious seal permit leakage to occur between the restoration and tooth structure, thus allowing bacteria to colonize the cavity. Without adequate precautions, toxic bacterial products may diffuse from cavity to pulp and evoke inflammation. For this reason, cavity varnishes and liners were developed to attempt to block the openings of the dentinal tubules and prevent the ingress of irritating substances.

Other factors may also limit permeability. For example, hours after cavity preparation, the permeability of dentin may decrease considerably.[17] This dramatic reduction appears to result from accumulation of plasma proteins in the tubules.[18] The precise mechanism responsible for the ingress of proteins into the tubules is unknown. Apparently, trauma associated with cavity preparation results in inflammation and an increase in vascular permeability. This allows plasma proteins to pass out of small blood vessels and diffuse into the dentinal tubules. The clinical significance of this interesting phenomenon requires further research.

Pulp Pathosis

Specific causes of pulp disease include bacterial infection and injury resulting from impact trauma, dentin fracture, attrition, abrasion, erosion, and dental treatment. Bacterial infection most commonly results from caries, but pulps may also become infected as a result of tooth fracture, restorative procedures, and very severe periodontal disease (Figure 21-6). Diagnosis and treatment of periodontal disease are important if the pulp is to be maintained in a healthy condition.

In this chapter attention is focused on dental treatment procedures as a cause of pulp disease and how pulpal injury can be minimized or prevented.

Effects of Restorative Procedures

Among the various forms of dental treatment, restorative procedures are the greatest cause of pulpal injury. Trauma to the pulp cannot always be avoided, particularly with excavation of a deep carious lesion or preparation of teeth for full crowns. However, the astute clinician, by being aware of the dangers involved in each step of the restorative process, can minimize or avoid injury, as outlined in the following discussion.

CAVITY AND CROWN PREPARATION FACTORS
Depth of Cavity

Dentin permeability increases exponentially with increasing cavity depth, as both diameter and density of dentinal tubules increase as the cavity deepens (Figure 21-7). Thus, the deeper the cavity, the greater the tubular surface area into which potentially toxic substances can penetrate and diffuse to the pulp. The length of the dentinal

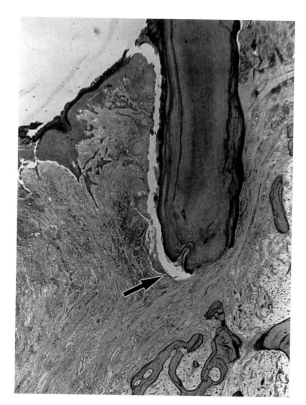

FIGURE 21-6
Severe periodontal disease. Apical migration of pocket epithelium *(arrow)* has resulted in exposure of the apical foramen of this tooth; this will often result in severe damage to the pulp. The space between the tooth and pocket epithelium is a fixation artifact.

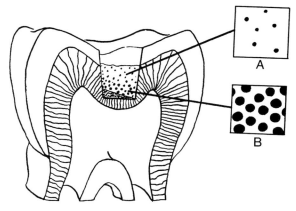

FIGURE 21-7
Difference in size and number of tubules in the dentinal floor of a shallow *(A)* and a deep *(B)* cavity preparation. (From Trowbridge HO: *Dentistry* 82:22, 1982.)

tubules beneath the cavity is also of importance. The farther substances have to diffuse, the more they will be diluted and buffered by the dentinal fluid. A remaining dentin thickness of 2 mm is usually sufficient to shield the pulp from most forms of irritation. However, there is always the threat of microleakage; it is wise to seal vital dentin regardless of the thickness of remaining dentin.

As stated earlier, cavity depth determines the extent to which amputation of odontoblast processes results in injury to the cell body. If processes are severed close to the odontoblast cell body, the cell is likely to suffer irreversible injury. In general, the deeper the cavity preparation, the more damage and death of ontoblasts.[12,19]

Frictional Heat

Frictional heat is produced whenever a revolving bur or stone is brought into contact with tooth structure. Until the 1950s the method of enamel and dentin preparation involved heavy torque, low rotational speeds, and steel burs that were not cooled with water. Consequently, vital dentin was often scorched, and pulps were injured as a result of noxious heat.

Dentin is an effective insulator; for this reason judicious cutting is not likely to damage the pulp unless the thickness of dentin between preparation and pulp is less than 1.0 mm. Even then, the response should be mild. Perhaps the greatest amount of frictional heat is generated with a large diamond stone when teeth are prepared for a full crown. The heat generated may also have a desiccating effect by "boiling" away dentinal tubule fluid at the dentin surface.

"Blushing" of dentin during cavity or crown preparation is thought to be due to frictional heat resulting in vascular injury (hemorrhage) in the pulp. The dentin takes on an underlying pinkish hue soon after the operative procedure. Crown preparation performed without the use of a coolant leads to a marked reduction in pulpal blood flow, presumably because of vascular stasis and thrombosis.[20]

In the absence of infection or other complicating factors, damaged pulps usually undergo repair.[21] However, a pulp that has already been compromised by caries or is ischemic after a PDL injection of a vasoconstrictor-containing local anesthetic may be more vulnerable to thermal injury than an otherwise healthy pulp.

The amount of heat produced during cutting is determined by sharpness of the bur, the amount of pressure exerted on the bur or stone, and the length of time the cutting instrument contacts tooth structure. The safest way to prepare tooth structure is to use ultra-high speeds of rotation (100,000 to 250,000 rpm), an efficient water cooling system, light pressure, and intermittent cutting. During cutting at high speeds, the revolving bur creates an area of turbulence that tends to deflect a stream of water. Therefore, an air-water spray with sufficient volume and pressure must be used if the coolant is to overcome the rotary turbulence. The bur-dentin interface should be constantly wet.

Cavity preparation with a low-speed handpiece, sharp bur, and light, intermittent pressure is only slightly more injurious than cutting at high speeds. Hand instruments and low-speed cutting are relatively safe ways to finish a cavity preparation, rather than using a high-speed handpiece with the water coolant shut off.

Injury to Odontoblasts

Odontoblasts are vulnerable and, unfortunately, may be subjected to many insults. In addition to desiccation, heat, and vibration, they may be exposed to bacterial toxins, acids, caustic sterilizing agents, and other chemical irritants. Even in carefully prepared cavities, intracellular changes within odontoblasts located beneath the cavity may occur, including disruption of mitochondria and rough endoplasmic reticulum.[22] When cellular injury is reversible, the organelles return to normal within a few days.

Drying of Dentin

A prolonged blast of compressed air to freshly exposed vital dentin will cause a rapid outward movement of fluid in patent dentinal tubules. Tubule diameter is extraordinarily small; midway between the pulp and the DEJ the mean diameter of the tubules is only 1.5 mm.[23] The smaller the bore of a capillary tube, the greater the capillary pressure. Therefore, removal of fluid from the tubules by a blast of air activates strong capillary forces. These in turn lead to a rapid outward flow of dentinal fluid. Fluid removed from the tubules at the dentin surface is replaced by fluid from the pulp.

As discussed above, rapid outward flow of fluid in the dentinal tubules stimulates mechanoreceptors in the subjacent pulp, thus producing pain. Rapid outward fluid movement may also result in *odontoblast displacement*; odontoblasts are dislodged from the odontoblast layer and pulled outward into the tubules (Figure 21-8). Within a short time the displaced cells undergo autolysis and disappear. Providing the pulp has not been

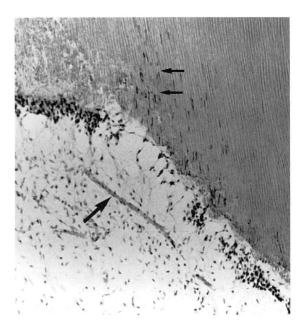

FIGURE 21-8
Nuclei of odontoblasts *(small arrows)* that have been displaced into dentinal tubules. Note intact capillary *(large arrow)*. Had desiccation produced trauma to the subodontoblast zone, the capillary would have been disrupted.

severely injured, either by caries or other factors, displaced odontoblasts are replaced by new cells that are derived from odontoprogenitor cells in the underlying cell-rich zone of the pulp.[24] In this way the odontoblast layer is reconstituted by "replacement" odontoblasts capable of producing tertiary dentin (Figure 21-9). However, vigorous drying of dentin alone does not result in severe injury to the underlying pulp.[25] Loss of odontoblasts is often followed by the formation of tertiary dentin (Figure 21-10).

Recently, drying agents containing lipid solvents such as acetone and ether have appeared on the market. Because of their rapid rate of evaporation, application of such substances (including alcohol) to exposed dentin produces strong hydrodynamic forces in the tubules, often causing odontoblast displacement.[26] Therefore, cavities should be dried with cotton pellets and short blasts of air rather than harsh chemicals. Prolonged air-drying should be avoided.

Cavity Cleansing

The traditional method of cleansing cavity walls of saliva and cutting debris is to flush the cavity with a stream of water. However, flushing with water is ineffective in removing the *smear layer*,

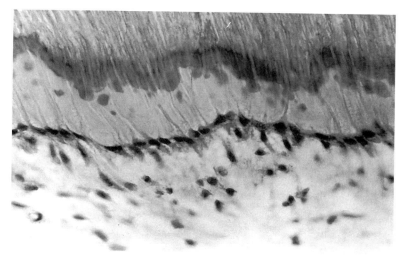

FIGURE 21-9
Layer of replacement odontoblasts. (From Trowbridge HO: *J Endod* 7:52, 1981.)

which consists of fragments of microscopic mineral crystals and organic matrix produced when tooth structure is cut with a bur or chisels. This layer may interfere with the adherence of adhesive restorative materials such as dentin bonding agents, although some newer bonding agents reportedly bond to the smear layer. Acidic cavity cleansing products and chelating agents have been used to remove the smear layer.

Complete dissolution of the smear layer opens the dentinal tubules, significantly increasing the permeability of dentin. If the dentin is left unsealed, diffusion of irritants to the pulp may intensify and prolong the severity of pulp reactions.[27,28] However, the smear layer does have some desirable properties. By blocking the orifices of dentinal tubules, the smear plugs greatly decrease the permeability of dentin, thus limiting the diffusion of substances to the pulp.[26] While the smear layer is impervious to bacteria, thus preventing microorganisms from gaining access to the dentinal tubules, it is not a barrier to bacterial products, the primary cause of pulpal irritation.[29]

Acid Etching

Organic and inorganic acids are often used to etch the enamel and dentin to enhance the retention of adhesive resin systems. Even with the development of acidic gels for enamel etching, acid may flow onto dentin. Acid etching of dentin *greatly* increases dentin permeability. Thus, if microleakage develops in a cavity in which the walls have been acid etched and poorly sealed, irritants

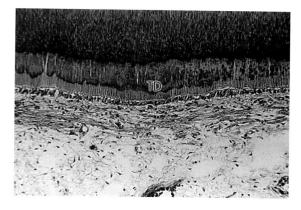

FIGURE 21-10
Formation of tertiary dentin *(TD)* resulting from loss of primary odontoblasts during a restorative procedure. The tertiary dentin is being formed by replacement odontoblasts.

are likely to reach the pulp. However, in the absence of microleakage, acid etching of dentin in itself does not appear to produce injury to the pulp.[30,31] The reason is that when dentin is demineralized by acid, calcium and phosphate ions are released, thus producing a buffering action. Data show that even when placed in deep cavities, acid etchants produce only a small increase in hydrogen ion concentration in the pulp.[32]

Cavity Disinfection

Until the 1950s, potent antimicrobial agents such as phenol, thymol, beechwood creosote, and silver nitrate were routinely used for cavity disinfection. These caustic substances are not recommended; agents that destroy bacteria also injure the pulp. Although milder germicides such as benzalkonium chloride and 9-aminoacridine are probably well tolerated by the pulp, their clinical effectiveness is untested.[33,34]

Making of Impressions

Rubber base and hydrocolloid materials do not injure the pulp when they are used for impressions of cavity and crown preparations. However, heated modeling compound may be damaging; the combination of heat and pressure can be deleterious.[35] Devastating temperatures of up to 52°C have been recorded in the pulp during impressions with modeling compound in copper bands.[36]

Fabrication of Provisional Resinous Crowns

Heat generated during the exothermic polymerization of autopolymerizing resinous materials may injure the pulp.[37] The use of cooling procedures is strongly recommended when provisional crowns are directly fabricated. Before cementing provisional crowns, the crown preparation should be carefully lined with temporary cement to minimize microleakage. It is important to have the cement in place for a short period of time; temporary cements are not stable and will eventually wash out.

Cementation of Castings

During cementation of crowns, inlays, and bridges, strong hydraulic forces may be exerted on the pulp as cement compresses the fluid in the dentinal tubules. In deep preparations this can result in a separation of the odontoblast layer from the predentin, which is a mild injury. To reduce this pressure, vents in the casting will allow cement to escape. This also facilitates seating of the casting and relieves pressure on the pulp.

Occasionally pain occurs during or after cementation of castings. Pain may occur when either zinc phosphate or glass ionomer cements are used, but generally the discomfort does not last very long.[38]

Effects of Restorative Materials

With regard to the biologic impact of restorative materials on the pulp, the physical properties are considerably more important than the chemical

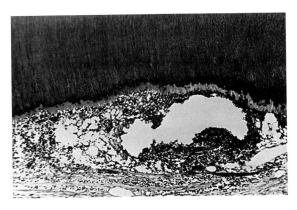

FIGURE 21-11
Pulpal abscess that has developed as a result of severe microleakage around a restoration.

components. For many years it was thought that certain restorative materials were more irritating than others. However, the cause of irritation remained speculative. Presumably, restorative materials contain toxic chemicals that leach from the restoration and diffuse through the dentinal tubules to injure the pulp. Until recently this explanation was universally accepted, but more sophisticated investigative techniques and better interpretation of research results have provided new insights into the cause of pulpal injury.

ROLE OF BACTERIA

There is strong evidence that microleakage resulting in bacterial colonization of cavity walls is the major cause of pulpal injury. Histobacterial stains have been used to relate the response of pulps to restorative materials. A high correlation was found between the presence of bacteria beneath restorations and inflammation in the underlying pulp.[21,39] Development of an abscess is not uncommon when microleakage is severe (Figure 21-11).

Germ-free animal studies also implicated bacteria as a factor in pulpal injury resulting from restorative procedures. When acidic cements were applied to exposed pulps in molars of germ-free and conventional rats, there was no pulpal inflammation in the germ-free group.[40] In the pulps of conventional animals, bacteria were observed in association with inflammation and necrosis.

Another means of studying the role of bacteria is "surface-sealing" of restorations. Surface sealing involves the removal of the outer part of a restoration and replacement with ZnOE. This material prevents bacteria from penetrating the gap between the restoration and the walls of the cavity. Such surface-sealing experiments have

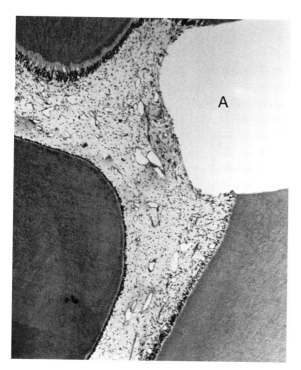

FIGURE 21-12
Specimen from a surface-sealing experiment showing pulp 7 days after placement of amalgam *(A)* against exposed pulp tissue. Note absence of pulpal inflammation. (From Cox CF, Keall CL, Keall HJ, Ostro E: *J Prosthet Dent* 57:1, 1987.)

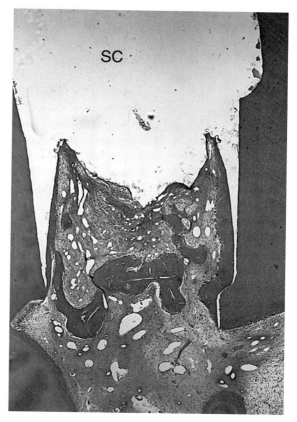

FIGURE 21-13
Surface-sealing experiment demonstrating 14-day response of the pulp to silicate cement *(SC)*, which was occupying the space. In the absence of bacterial leakage new dentin matrix has been deposited adjacent to remaining dentin walls as well as to the silicate interface. (From Cox CF, Keall CL, Keall HJ, Ostro E: *J Prosthet Dent* 57:1, 1987.)

shown that potentially irritating restorative materials such as amalgam, composite resins, silicate cement, and zinc phosphate cement produce only a thin zone of contact necrosis with no significant inflammation when placed on exposed human and primate pulps (Figures 21-12 and 21-13).[41] Cox et al.[31] usually observed dentin bridge formation when composite resins, silicate cement, and zinc phosphate cement were placed in contact with the pulp.

Some bacteria may remain in the smear layer after the tooth has been restored.[42] However, microorganisms require nutrients to maintain their viability; if denied substrate they eventually die.[43] Evidence suggests that bacteria will grow beneath a restoration *only* in the presence of microleakage.[44]

MICROLEAKAGE

Microleakage is a major problem in restorative dentistry. Until the advent of more advanced dentin bonding adhesive systems, most materials did not adapt to tooth structure well enough to provide a leak-proof marginal seal. Or, if there was good adaptation at the time of insertion, shrinkage resulting from physical or chemical changes within the material commonly caused gaps to open, resulting in microleakage.[27] This is exemplified by shrinkage of certain acrylic resins during polymerization. If a restorative material has a higher coefficient of thermal expansion than tooth structure, a decrease in temperature will cause contraction gaps to develop.

Another cause of microleakage is elastic deformation of tooth structure produced by masticatory forces.[45] In other words, the enamel and dentin surrounding the rigid restoration flex and move, resulting in gaps (an "unzipping" from occlusal to cervical). This is particularly apt to increase leakage in deep MOD restorations.[46] Masticatory forces may have a marked effect on leakage in class V cavities restored with composite. In one primate study, leakage was greater in teeth in functional occlusion than in adjacent teeth without antagonists.[47]

Skill of the operator also influences microleakage. The quality of the preparation and the way the material is inserted can greatly influence adaptation. In the case of amalgam alloy, the method of insertion and plasticity of the mix are the most important factors in determining the extent of microleakage.[48] In this respect, computer-driven amalgamators provide better amalgam trituration than the older mechanical units.

Moisture control is also important because certain restorative materials may develop marginal leakage if they are contaminated with saliva, blood, or water during placement.

None of the older permanent resin-based, esthetic restorative materials mentioned previously consistently provided a long-term marginal seal. Recently developed dentin bonding and adhesive agents have been shown to couple (hybridize*) within vital dentin.[49] These new materials show promise in preventing microleakage. Without a long-term seal of the remaining dentin or dentin bridges, microleakage will occur, leading to bacterial colonization and eventual pulpal inflammation (Figure 21-14). It is for this reason that adhesive systems such as 4-meta are recommended.

EXOTHERMIC MATERIALS

Some luting cements generate heat during setting; it has been suggested that this might cause pulpal injury. The most exothermic luting material is zinc phosphate (ZnOP) cement.[50] However, during setting an intrapulpal temperature increase of only 2°C was recorded. Heat of this magnitude is not sufficient to injure the pulp.

HYGROSCOPIC MATERIALS

Some hygroscopic materials may potentially cause injury by withdrawing fluid from dentin. However, little relationship exists between the hydrophilic properties of materials and their effect on the pulp.[50] Moisture absorbed by materials is probably

---

*Hybridization is the mechanical penetration of adhesive polymers with both collagen and carbonate dentin substrate. Specifically, the polymers infiltrate the intertubular, peritubular, and dentinal tubule complex to provide a seal against microleakage. In addition, the hybrid layer provides a bonding substrate in preparation for placement of the definitive restoration.

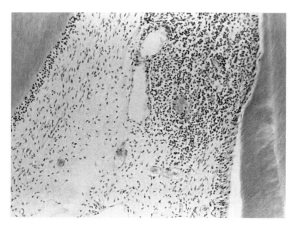

FIGURE 21-14
Eight-week response after restoring with a composite resin. Inflammatory reaction adjacent to tertiary dentin indicating continued irritation. (From Heys RJ, Heys DR, Fitzgerald M: *Int Endod J* 18:260, 1985.)

much less than that removed from dentin during cavity drying, a procedure that produces an insignificant amount of pulpal inflammation.[25]

TOXICITY OF MATERIALS

Certain restorative materials are composed of chemicals that have the potential to irritate the pulp. However, when placed in a cavity, the intervening dentin usually neutralizes or prevents leachable ingredients from reaching the pulp in a high enough concentration to cause injury. For example, eugenol in ZnOE is potentially irritating, but very little can diffuse to the pulp.[51] Phosphoric acid is a component of silicate and zinc phosphate cements. For decades it was thought that injury was due to the high concentration of hydrogen ions reaching the pulp. However, the buffering capacity of dentin greatly limits the ability of hydrogen ions to reach the pulp.[52]

BIOLOGIC PROPERTIES OF SPECIFIC MATERIALS
Zinc Oxide–Eugenol

Zinc oxide–eugenol (ZnOE) has many uses in dentistry, having had a long history as a temporary filling material, cavity liner, cement base, and luting agent for provisional cementation of castings. Before the introduction of calcium hydroxide, ZnOE was the material of choice for direct pulp capping.

Eugenol, biologically the most active ingredient in ZnOE, is a phenol derivative and is toxic

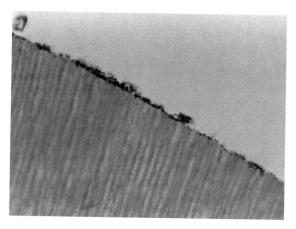

FIGURE 21-15
Positive bacterial staining reaction showing bacteria on cavity wall beneath composite resin restoration. These bacteria produce by-products that may diffuse through tubules to cause pulpal inflammation. (From Heys RJ, Heys DR, Fitzgerald M: *Int Endod J* 18:260, 1985.)

when placed in direct contact with tissue. It also possesses antibacterial properties. Eugenol's usefulness in pain control is attributed to its ability to block the transmission of nerve impulses.[53] Researchers have found that a thin mix of ZnOE significantly reduces intradental nerve activity when placed in a deep cavity preparation in cats' teeth; however, a dry mix of ZnOE has no effect.[54]

It is the physical and chemical properties of ZnOE that are beneficial in preventing pulpal injury and in reducing postoperative tooth sensitivity. Importantly, it provides a good biologic seal; also its antimicrobial properties enable it to suppress bacterial growth, thus reducing formation of toxic metabolites that might result in pulpal inflammation. Of the restorative materials tested, only ZnOE consistently inhibited bacterial growth beneath restorations.[44]

Zinc Phosphate Cement

Zinc phosphate is a popular luting and basing agent. It has a high modulus of elasticity and therefore is commonly used as a base beneath amalgam restorations. The phosphoric acid liquid phase was formerly thought to injure the pulp. However, recent studies have shown that this is not the case.[31] Cementation of castings with ZnOP is well tolerated by the pulp.[55] Researchers reported that ZnOP is more likely to produce pulpal sensitivity at the time of cementation and 2 weeks after cementation than glass ionomer.[38] However, 3 months after cementation there was no difference in sensitivity.

Polycarboxylate Cement

When placed in cavities or used as a luting cement, zinc polycarboxylate does not irritate the pulp.[56] In cementing well-fitting crowns and inlays, neither polycarboxylate nor ZnOP cements contract enough to permit the ingress of bacteria. Consequently, it is unnecessary to apply a varnish or liner to cavity walls; doing so only reduces cement adhesion.

Restorative Resins

Early adhesive bonding and resin composite systems contracted during polymerization, resulting in gross microleakage and bacterial contamination of the cavity. Bacteria on cavity walls and within axial dentin are associated with moderate pulpal inflammation (Figure 21-15).[57] Over a period of time, some composites absorb water and expand; this tends to compensate for initial contraction. To limit microleakage and improve retention, the enamel margins are beveled and acid etched to facilitate mechanical bonding. When compared with unfilled resins, the newer resin composites present a coefficient of thermal expansion similar to that of tooth structure. With recently developed hydrophilic adhesive bonding composite systems, the problem of marginal leakage appears to have been diminished.[58]

Glass Ionomer Cements

Glass ionomer cement originally was used as an esthetic restorative material. Biocompatibility studies[59,60] show that these cements generally have no effect on the pulp. However, when used as a bulk filling material, glass ionomer leaks; a cavity liner is strongly suggested with this type of cement.[61]

Through the use of finely ground powders and light-curing technology, glass ionomer luting cements have evolved to rival the use of other luting agents. The results of a microleakage study showed that glass ionomer cements provide a good marginal seal when used to cement castings in vitro.[62] Although many reports of pulpal sensitivity have been associated with the use of glass ionomer cements, there appear to be no sensitivity differences between glass ionomer and ZnOP cements. Endodontic problems are infrequent.[38]

Amalgam

Amalgam alloy is the most widely used dental material for restoring posterior teeth. A problem with older, lathe-cut amalgams was shrinkage during setting, which resulted in microleakage.

Over time, this initial microleakage decreases as corrosion products accumulate between restoration and cavity walls.[63] Newer high-copper spherical amalgam alloys show slight to moderate pulpal inflammation that diminishes with time, also probably because of progressive corrosion (which is slower than lathe-cut amalgams) and reduction in microleakage.[64]

PROTECTANTS
Cavity Varnishes, Liners, and Bases

An attempt has been made to minimize the effects of microleakage through the use of cavity varnishes and liners. Varnishes are solutions of organic solvent and resin. Liners are a suspension of materials such as calcium hydroxide, polystyrene, and ZnOE in a volatile organic liquid or aqueous solution. When the solvent evaporates, a thin film of residue forms a coating on the dentin to hopefully seal tubule openings. Thicker cements (bases) may also be used to line the cavity; in shallow cavities thick bases take up too much space, interfere with retention, weaken the restoration, and provide no protection.[65]

Varnishes provide a partial short-term barrier to irritants that might injure the pulp.[66,67] When applied to dentin, they neither bond nor form an impervious coating. Application of two or three coats is necessary to minimize the voids. Although the varnish layers eventually disintegrate, they compensate for the initial contraction of amalgam and thus reduce microleakage until corrosion products fill the contraction gaps. Pashley et al.[68] determined that varnishes, liners, and bases all reduced dentin permeability—varnishes the least and bases the most.

"Insulating" Effect of Bases

A common misconception is the necessity of placing an insulator beneath metallic restorations to protect the pulp from thermal shock (hypersensitivity). Dentin is an excellent insulator; additional thermal insulation is rarely if ever needed. In fact, thick cement bases are no more effective than just a thin layer of varnish in preventing thermal sensitivity, indicating that postrestorative sensitivity is at least partly due to microleakage.[69]

According to the hydrodynamic theory of dentin sensitivity, rapid heating or cooling of the tooth causes fluid in the dentinal tubules to expand or contract, resulting in rapid movement of fluid in the dentinal tubules.[16,70] Presumably this fluid movement produces pressure changes that activate mechanosensitive nerve endings located in the underlying pulp, thus producing pain.

When a tooth is restored with amalgam, gaps open around the restoration as the material sets, and fluid accumulates in these gaps. Unless dentin is sealed, fluid in the contraction gaps communicates directly with fluid in the underlying tubules. When the restoration is subjected to ice-cold foods or liquids, fluid in the contraction gaps and dentinal tubules contracts, resulting in hydrodynamic activation of sensory nerve fibers and sharp pain. Newer adhesive dentin bonding systems minimize microleakage; therefore, fluid in the marginal gap is separated from the fluid in the dentinal tubules, thus reducing the volume of fluid affected by temperature change.[58]

Inflammation may also relate to postoperative hypersensitivity. Traumatic cavity preparation often produces an acute inflammatory reaction in the pulp. This results in an elevation in intrapulpal pressure and activation of inflammatory mediators such as bradykinin and prostaglandin E_2, which may produce a state of hyperalgesia. Until the inflammation resolves, the pulp may respond to stimuli that would not normally evoke pain signals.[71] Hyperalgesia is more profound in low-compliance tissues such as the pulp and nail bed.

ADDITIONAL FACTORS
Heat of Polishing

Enough frictional heat may be generated during polishing of a restoration to seriously injure the pulp. Continuous polishing of amalgam restorations with rubber cups at high speeds causes a damaging temperature increase of up to 20°C in the pulp; heat of this magnitude may produce tissue necrosis. For safety, polishing with rubber wheels or rubber cups should be at low speeds using intermittent pressure and a coolant.[72,73]

Removal of Metallic Restorations

The use of burs to remove metallic restorations may also produce very high levels of frictional heat, exposing the pulp to injury. A coolant such as water spray or a combination of water and air avoids a burn lesion in the pulp. It is also advisable to use intermittent grinding using light pressure.

Pins

Pins to retain amalgam or other material require caution; pulp damage may result from pinhole preparation or pin placement. Coolants do not reach the depth of the pin preparation. During pinhole preparation there is always the risk of pulp exposure. Furthermore, friction-locked pins often produce microfractures that may extend through dentin to the pulp, subjecting it to irritation and the effects of microleakage.[74]

POSTRESTORATIVE HYPERSENSITIVITY

Many patients complain of hypersensitivity after a restorative procedure.[75] Pain may be a warning signal that the pulp has been injured. Often (but not always) a relationship exists between tooth sensitivity and pulpal inflammation.[66] Discomfort is usually of short duration; if pain is persistent or spontaneous, the injury probably resulted in irreversible pulpitis. Many patients receiving restorative treatment experience some degree of postoperative discomfort. Hypersensitivity to cold is common; sensitivity to heat is less so.

Pain evoked by biting pressure indicates injury to the periodontal ligament resulting from hyperocclusion. Hyperocclusion is not injurious to the pulp but may cause a transient hypersensitivity, which usually resolves with occlusal adjustment.

SUMMARY OF PROTECTIVE MEASURES

Most injuries to the pulp from restorative procedures are avoided with certain precautions.

Heat produced during cavity preparation is minimized using light, intermittent cutting, an efficient water-cooling system, and a handpiece with high speeds rather than high torque. Preparations should be finished using hand instruments or with low speed and sharp burs.

Desiccation of dentin is avoided by drying the preparation with cotton pellets and short air blasts from an air syringe; prolonged air blasts are damaging. Newer hydrophilic primers bond and hybridize vital dentin while some surface moisture is still present.

Chemicals on freshly exposed dentin may diffuse to the pulp and produce injury. Therefore, caustic drying, cleansing, and sterilizing agents such as alcohol, acetone, phenol, and silver nitrate should be avoided and are ineffective anyway.

Physical as well as chemical properties should be considered when a restorative material is selected. These include aspects such as coefficient of thermal expansion, modulus of elasticity, contraction during polymerization, and adaptation to tooth structure.

Unstable, soluble liners and bases (most contain calcium hydroxide) should not be used on the floor of a deep cavity. Within a few years recurrent caries may develop beneath such liners and bases.

Microleakage must be minimized; it is a much greater threat than the toxic ingredients of materials per se. Because gaps form around restorations, a bonded hybridized adhesive, varnish, or liner should be used in conjunction with most restorative materials to prevent microleakage.[76]

Polishing of metallic restorations is a potential source of noxious heat. Intermittent polishing with an adequate air-water coolant will reduce the risk of pulpal injury.

Long-term assessment is critical whenever there is doubt as to the pulp response to previous pathosis or to the restorative procedure.

Orthodontic Procedures

Fortunately, tooth movement is not a common cause of pulp pathosis, although pulp necrosis is an occasional complication.[77] Forces involved in tooth movement may produce changes in pulpal blood flow.[78] Also, oxygen utilization by pulp cells is depressed after application of orthodontic forces.[79] Subsequent to arch wire activation, teeth often are hypersensitive to cold for a few days, suggesting that sensory structures are transiently affected.[80] At times, orthodontically treated teeth with vital pulps do not respond to the electric pulp test.[81] This condition may result from altered blood flow or injury to the sensory nerve fibers entering the apex.

Management of the Vital Pulp

EFFECT OF NATURAL CAUSES OF PATHOSES

Caries

Caries is a localized, progressive destruction of tooth structure and the most common cause of pulp disease. It is now generally accepted that for caries to develop, specific bacteria must become established on the tooth surface. Products of bacterial metabolism, notably organic acids and proteolytic enzymes, cause the destruction of enamel and dentin. Bacterial metabolites diffusing from the lesion to the pulp are capable of eliciting an immune response and inflammatory reaction. Eventually, extensive dentin involvement results in bacterial infection of the pulp, particularly after carious exposure.

Removal of gross caries and preparation for restoration are generally accomplished with rotary instruments. Hand instruments are avoided near the pulpal wall to prevent accidental mechanical pulp exposure. Final removal of carious dentin is generally accomplished with a large, sharp round bur at slow speed to remove the last layer of softened and discolored dentin.

Erosion, Abrasion, and Attrition

With increasing frequency, our senior citizens are retaining their natural teeth. Consequently, dentists are dealing with an increasing incidence of age-related dental problems. In addition to root caries, older teeth exhibit the typical signs of wear and tear. *Erosion* results from the effects of oral or gastric acids on enamel and dentin from the constant "sipping" of acidic drinks. *Abrasion* lesions generally occur from improper oral habits such as the use of toothpicks, pins, or other hard objects or from overaggressive tooth brushing with abrasive toothpastes, often in an attempt to whiten the teeth. The result of this is the creation of facial cervical defects. *Attrition* lesions appear in those teeth with malocclusions or with certain oral habits of individuals, resulting in the grinding away of enamel and vital dentin. Previously, these lesions were restored with unsightly materials such as gold foil, amalgam, silicate, or resin composite systems. However, with recent improvements in composite systems, permanent restorations that are functionally and aesthetically acceptable are now available.

Maintenance of a Vital Pulp

Maintaining an intact healthy pulp is preferable to root canal treatment or other endodontic procedures that are complex, expensive, and time consuming. When dealing with a deep carious lesion, some authors advocate indirect pulp capping, a procedure that avoids pulp exposure during the removal of carious dentin. Another approach is to remove all carious dentin, even if it means producing a carious exposure and then covering the exposed pulp tissue with a biocompatible liner (direct pulp capping). Others advocate a procedure involving surgical removal of inflamed pulp tissue (pulpotomy); the remaining tissue is then covered with dressing that hopefully allows healing. The success rate of these procedures is variable and depends upon proper diagnosis and clinical judgment, but primarily on the status of the pulp before the procedure.

INDIRECT PULP CAPPING

This procedure is used in the management of deep carious lesions where removal of all carious dentin would probably result in pulp exposure. Proponents believe that accidental mechanical exposure is to be avoided so the pulp is not subjected to additional injury. Indirect pulp capping is considered only if there is no history of pulpalgia or signs of irreversible pulpitis. After all of the

softened, mushy dentin is removed, either ZnOE or calcium hydroxide is placed on the remaining carious dentin to suppress bacteria.[82,83] It is felt that indirect pulp capping causes less damage than exposure and allows pulpal inflammation to undergo resolution. After several weeks, the temporary filling and ZnOE or calcium hydroxide liner may be removed and replaced with a definitive restoration.

Indirect pulp capping remains a matter of considerable controversy. Some dentists feel that this form of treatment is not warranted under any circumstances, arguing that it is not possible to perform a diagnosis of the pulp unless all carious dentin is removed. If caries has exposed pulp, allowing a large number of bacteria to invade, irreversible pulpitis has already developed. Others reason that the biologic principles of restorative dentistry dictate that all carious dentin must be removed, even if it means exposing the pulp. Still others believe that if irreversible pulpitis has not already developed, indirect pulp capping is likely to be successful.[82] Evidence supports the latter view.

DIRECT PULP CAPPING

There are two considerations for direct pulp capping: accidental mechanical pulp exposure and exposure caused by caries. Accidental exposure may be caused by injudicious cavity or crown preparation, placement of pins or retention points. These two types of exposure differ in that the condition of the pulp is normal in the case of accidental mechanical exposure whereas it is likely to be inflamed beneath a deep carious lesion.

The long-term success rate of direct pulp capping is approximately 80%.[84,85] The degree of bleeding indicates the prognosis.[86] The application of 10% sodium hypochlorite for "chemical surgery" of the exposed pulp tissue has been advocated.[87] Control of bleeding is a must! Once bleeding has stopped, a pulp-capping agent can be applied to the exposure site, followed by placement of a permanent restoration. With the advent of adhesive systems, investigators have found that, under experimental conditions, mechanically exposed pulps can be successfully capped with adhesive resins.[88] Long-term success of capping of carious exposures is lower. Failure tends to increase with longer observation periods.[89]

Until recently, calcium hydroxide has remained the standard for treatment of mechanical exposures. This material was thought to stimulate differentiation of new odontoblast-like cells, which would then form tertiary dentin. However, studies have shown that neither the calcium ion nor the hydroxyl ion is necessary for "dentin bridge" formation.[12] However, calcium hydroxide is an effective material when placed in direct contact with vital pulp tissue. It provides a short-term antimicrobial effect, and certain commercial calcium hydroxide liners provide a hard-set interface upon which fibroblasts are able to proliferate and differentiate into cells capable of elaborating dentin matrix.

PULPOTOMY

Pulpotomy is an alternative to direct pulp capping or root canal treatment when carious pulp exposures occur in young permanent incisors. Pulpotomy involves the removal of all carious dentin and then ablation of pulp tissue to the level of the radicular pulp.[90,91] The vital pulp stump is capped with a calcium hydroxide liner and the tooth is temporarily restored with intermediate restorative material (IRM). Several months later the liner and IRM are replaced by a hybridized adhesive seal bonded into the remaining enamel and dentin and the cavity is filled with a permanent restorative material. This procedure has been shown to be successful providing there is no bacterial microleakage.[92,93]

Partial pulpotomy has been used to successfully treat cariously exposed pulps in permanent molars.[91,94] This procedure involves the removal of coronal pulp tissue to the level of healthy tissue, which may at times be difficult to determine. Bleeding should be within normal limits and easily controlled.

There are two potential problems with pulpotomy as a permanent endodontic treatment. It is not possible to determine whether all diseased tissue has been removed, as inflammation or necrosis may extend into one or more of the root canals and cause the pulpotomy to fail. However, the apparent clinical success of total and partial pulpotomy makes them a viable alternative to pulpectomy.

PERIAPICAL REPAIR AFTER TREATMENT OF DEEP CARIOUS LESIONS

Endodontic treatment is usually indicated where deep carious lesions have resulted in periapical bone resorption. It is likely that these small apical radiolucencies represent bone resorption in response to chemical mediators diffusing from an inflamed coronal pulp. There have been reports of resolution of periapical pathosis and preservation of pulp vitality after pulpotomy or direct or indirect pulp capping.[95,96] Careful case selection is critical to success. Jordan and Suzuki[82] found that only young patients benefited from this procedure. There are no reports of success in patients

older than age 24. The tooth to be treated must be vital on pulp testing and lack a history of spontaneous pain. Presumably the pulps of young teeth are better able to respond favorably to pulp capping procedures because of a richer blood supply and greater degree of cellularity.

REFERENCES

1. Van Hassel HJ: Physiology of the human dental pulp, *Oral Surg Oral Med Oral Pathol* 32:126, 1971.
2. Narhi M: Activation of dental pulp nerves of the cat and the dog with hydrostatic pressure, *Proc Finn Dent Soc* 74(suppl 5):1, 1978.
3. Heyeraas KJ, Kvinnsland I: Tissue pressure and blood flow in pulpal inflammation, *Proc Finn Dent Soc* 88(suppl 1):393, 1992.
4. Taussig MJ: *Processes in pathology and microbiology*, ed 2, Oxford, 1984, Blackwell Scientific.
5. Kim S, Edwall L, Trowbridge H, Chien S: Effects of local anesthetics on pulpal blood flow in dogs, *J Dent Res* 63:650, 1984.
6. Ahn J, Pogrel MA: The effects of 2% lidocaine with 1:100,000 epinephrine on pulpal and gingival blood flow, *Oral Surg Oral Med Oral Pathol* 85:197, 1998.
7. Fisher AK, Walters VE: Anaerobic glycolysis in bovine dental pulp, *J Dent Res* 47:717, 1968.
8. Plamondon T, Walton R, Graham G, et al: Pulp response to the combined effect of cavity preparation and PDL injection, *Oper Dent* 15:86, 1990.
9. Wang YN, Ashrafi SH, Weber DF: Scanning electron microscope observations of casts of human dentinal tubules along the interface between primary and secondary dentin, *Anat Rec* 211:149, 1985.
10. Scott JN, Weber DF: Microscopy of the junctional region between human coronal primary and secondary dentin, *J Morphol* 154:133, 1977.
11. Stanley HR, Swerdlow H: Accelerated handpiece speeds. The potential abuse of high speed techniques, *Dent Clin North Am* 4:621, 1960.
12. Lee S, Walton R, Osborne J: Pulp response to bases and cavity depths, *Am J Dent* 5:63, 1992.
13. Cox CF, White KC, Ramus DL: Reparative dentin; factors affecting its deposition, *Quintessence Int* 23:257, 1992.
14. Cox CF, Bergenholtz G, Heys DR: Pulp capping of dental pulp mechanically exposed to the oral microflora: a 1-2 year observation of wound healing in the monkey, *J Oral Pathol* 14:156, 1985.
15. Cox CF, Sübay RK, Ostro E, et al: Tunnel defects in dentin bridges: their formation following direct pulp capping, *Oper Dent* 21:4, 1996.
16. Trowbridge HO, Franks M, Korostoff E, Emling R: Sensory response to thermal stimulation in human teeth, *J Endod* 6:405, 1980.
17. Pashley DH, Kepler EE, Williams EC, Okabe A: Progressive decrease in dentine permeability following cavity preparation, *Arch Oral Biol* 28:853, 1983.
18. Pashley DH, Galloway SE, Stewart FP: Effects of fibrinogen in vivo on dentine permeability in the dog, *Arch Oral Biol* 29:725, 1984.

19. About I, Murray P, Franquin J-C, et al: Effect of cavity restoration variables on odontoblast cell numbers and dentinal repair, *J Dent* 29:109, 2001.

20. Kim S: Dynamic changes in the pulpal circulation in response to dental procedures and materials: macro-circulation and microcirculation studies. In Rowe NH, editor: *Dental pulp: reactions to restorative materials in the presence or absence of infection*, Ann Arbor, Mich, 1982, University of Michigan.

21. Brännström M: *Dentin and pulp in restorative dentistry*, p. 67, London, 1982, Wolf Medical Publications.

22. Chiego DJ, Sheets JA, Edwards CA, Avery JK: Ultrastructural changes in odontoblastic organelles after cavity preparations. (abstract) *J Dent Res* 66(special issue):287, 1987.

23. Garberoglio R, Brännström M: Scanning electron microscopic investigation of human dentinal tubules, *Arch Oral Biol* 21:355, 1976.

24. Fitzgerald M, Chiego DJ Jr, Heys DR: Autoradiographic analysis of odontoblast replacement following pulp exposure in primate teeth, *Arch Oral Biol* 35:707, 1990.

25. Brännström M: The effect of dentin desiccation and aspirated odontoblasts on the pulp, *J Prosthet Dent* 20:165, 1968.

26. Pashley DH: Smear layer: physiological considerations, *Oper Dent* 9(suppl 3):13, 1984.

27. Stanley HR, Going RE, Chauncey HH: Human pulp response to acid pretreatment of dentin and to composite restoration, *J Am Dent Assoc* 91:817, 1975.

28. Cox CF: Microleakage related to restorative procedures, *Proc Finn Dent Soc* 88:83, 1992.

29. Michelich VJ, Schuster GS, Pashley DH: Bacterial penetration of human dentin in vivo, *J Dent Res* 59:1398, 1980.

30. Snuggs HM, Cox CF, Powell CS, White KC: Pulp healing and dentinal bridge formation in an acidic environment, *Quintessence Int* 24:501, 1993.

31. Cox CF, Keall CL, Keall HJ, Ostro E: Biocompatibility of various surface-sealed dental materials against exposed pulps, *J Prosthet Dent* 57:1, 1987.

32. Wang J-D, Hume WR: Diffusion of hydrogen ion and hydroxyl ion from various sources through dentine, *Int Endod J* 21:17, 1988.

33. Brännström M: Communication between the oral cavity and the dental pulp associated with restorative treatment, *Oper Dent* 9:57, 1984.

34. Stark MM, Nicholson RJ, Soelberg KB: Direct and indirect pulp capping, *Dent Clin North Am* 20:341, 1976.

35. Seltzer S, Bender IB: *The dental pulp*, ed 3, Philadelphia, 1984, JB Lippincott.

36. Grajower R, Kaufman E, Stern N: Temperature of the pulp chamber during impression taking of full crown preparations with modelling compound, *J Dent Res* 54:212, 1975.

37. Castelnuovo J, Tjan AH: Temperature rise in pulpal chamber during fabrication of provisional resinous crowns, *J Prosthet Dent* 78:441, 1997.

38. Johnson GH, Powell LV, Derouen TA: Evaluation and control of post-cementation sensitivity: zinc phosphate and glass ionomer luting cements, *J Am Dent Assoc* 124:39, 1993.

39. Volinovic O, Nyborg H, Brännström M: Acid treatment of cavities under resin fillings: bacterial growth in dentinal tubules and pulpal reactions, *J Dent Res* 52:1189, 1973.

40. Watts A: Bacterial contamination and the toxicity of silicate and zinc phosphate cements, *Br Dent J* 146:7, 1979.

41. Cox CF, Sübay RK, Suzuki S, et al: Biocompatibility of various dental materials: pulp healing with a surface seal, *Int J Periodontics Restorative Dent* 16:241, 1996.

42. Brännström M: Smear layer: pathological and treatment considerations, *Oper Dent* (suppl) 3:35, 1984.

43. King JB, Crawford JJ, Lindahl RL: Indirect pulp capping: a bacteriologic study of deep carious dentine in human teeth, *Oral Surg Oral Med Oral Pathol* 20:663, 1965.

44. Bergenholtz G, Cox CF, Loesche WJ, Syed SA: Bacterial leakage around dental restorations: its effect on the pulp, *J Oral Pathol* 11:439, 1982.

45. Hood JAA: Biomechanics of the intact, prepared and restored tooth: some clinical implications, *Int Dent J* 41:25, 1991.

46. Granath L-E, Möller B: Leakage around restorations, principles of testing and biologic implications. In Van Amerongen AJ, Dippel HW, Spanauf AJ, Vrijhoef MMA, editors: *Proceedings of the International Symposium on Amalgam and Tooth-Colored Restorative Materials*, Nijmegen, The Netherlands, 1975, University of Nijmegen.

47. Qvist V: The effect of mastication on marginal adaptation of composite restorations in vivo, *J Dent Res* 62:904, 1983.

48. Mahler DB, Nelson LW: Factors affecting the marginal leakage of amalgam, *J Am Dent Assoc* 108:51, 1984.

49. Nakabayashi N, Ashizawa M, Nakamura M: Identification of a resin-dentin hybrid layer in vital human dentin created in vivo: durable bonding to vital dentin, *Quintessence Int* 23:135, 1992.

50. Plant CG, Jones DW: The damaging effects of restorative materials. Part 1. Physical and chemical properties, *Br Dent J* 140:373, 1976.

51. Hume WR: An analysis of the release and the diffusion through dentin of eugenol from zinc oxide-eugenol mixtures, *J Dent Res* 63:881, 1984.

52. Silver D, Trowbridge H, Greco M, Yankell S: In vitro assessment of permeability of dentin to acid, *J Dent Res* 67(special issue):276, 1988.

53. Kozam G: The effect of eugenol on nerve transmission, *Oral Surg Oral Med Oral Pathol* 44:799, 1977.

54. Trowbridge H, Edwall L, Panopoulos P: Effect of zinc oxide-eugenol and calcium hydroxide on intradental nerve activity, *J Endod* 8:403, 1982.

55. Brännström M, Nyborg H: Pulpal reaction to polycarboxylate and zinc phosphate cements used with inlays in deep cavity preparations, *J Am Dent Assoc* 94:308, 1977.

56. Jendresen M, Trowbridge H: Biologic and physical properties of a zinc polycarboxylate cement, *J Prosthet Dent* 28:264, 1972.

57. Heys RJ, Heys DR, Fitzgerald M: Histological evaluation of microfilled and conventional composite resins on monkey dental pulps, *Int Endod J* 18:260, 1985.

58. Kitasako Y, Najajima M, Pereira PNR, et al: Monkey pulpal response and microtensile bond strength beneath a one-application resin bonding system in vivo, *J Dent* 28:193, 2000.

59. Nordenvall K-J, Brännström M, Torstensson B: Pulp reactions and microorganisms under ASPA and concise composite restorations, *J Dent Child* 46:449, 1979.

60. Kawahara H, Imanishi Y, Oshima H: Biological evaluation on glass ionomer cement, *J Dent Res* 58:1080, 1979.

61. Alperstein KS, Graver HT, Herold RCB: Marginal leakage of glass-ionomer cement restorations, *J Prosthet Dent* 50:803, 1983.

62. Graver HT, Alperstein K, Trowbridge H: Microleakage of castings cemented with glass ionomer cements, *Oper Dent* 15:2, 1990.

63. Phillips RW, Gilmore HW, Swartz ML, Schenker SI: Adaptation of restorations in vivo as assessed by Ca^{45}, *J Am Dent Assoc* 62:9, 1961.

64. Heys DR, Cox CF, Heys RJ, et al: Histopathologic and bacterial evaluation of conventional and new copper amalgams, *J Oral Pathol* 8:65, 1979.

65. Cox CF, Suzuki S: Re-evaluation of pulp protection: calcium hydroxide liners vs. cohesive hybridization, *J Am Dent Assoc* 125:823, 1994.

66. Edwards DJ: The response of the human dental pulp to the use of a cavity varnish beneath amalgam fillings, *Br Dent J* 145:39, 1978.

67. Yates JL, Murray GA, Hembree JH: Cavity varnishes applied over insulating bases: effect on microleakage, *Oper Dent* 5:43, 1980.

68. Pashley DH, O'Meara JA, Williams EC, Kepler EE: Dentin permeability: effects of cavity varnishes and bases, *J Prosthet Dent* 53:511, 1985.

69. Piperno S, Barouch E, Hirsch SM, Kaim JM: Thermal discomfort of teeth related to presence or absence of cement bases under amalgam restorations, *Oper Dent* 7:92, 1982.

70. Trowbridge HO: Intradental sensory units: physiological and clinical aspects, *J Endod* 11:489, 1985.

71. Johnson RH, Dachi SF, Haley, JV: Pulpal hyperemia—a correlation of clinical and histologic data from 706 teeth, *J Am Dent Assoc* 81:108, 1970.

72. Grajower R, Kaufman E, Rajstein J: Temperature in the pulp chamber during polishing of amalgam restorations, *J Dent Res* 53:1189, 1974.

73. Hatton J, Holtzmann D, Ferrillo P, et al: Effect of handpiece pressure and speed on intrapulpal temperature rise, *Am J Dent* 7:108, 1994.

74. Felton DA, Webb EL, Kanoy BE, Cox CF: Pulpal response to threaded pin and retentive slot techniques: a pilot investigation, *J Prosthet Dent* 66:597, 1991.

75. Silvestri AR Jr, Cohen SN, Wetz JH: Character and frequency of discomfort immediately following restorative procedures, *J Am Dent Assoc* 95:85, 1977.

76. Sübay R, Cox C, Kaya H, et al: Human pulp reactions to dentine bonded amalgam restorations: a histologic study, *J Dent* 28:327, 2000.

77. Popp TW, Artun J, Linge L: Pulpal response to orthodontic tooth movement in adolescents: a radiographic study, *Am J Orthod Dentofacial Orthop* 101:228, 1992.

78. Brodin P, Linge L, Aars H: Instant assessment of pulpal blood flow after orthodontic force application, *J Orofac Orthop* 57:306, 1996.

79. Hamersky P, Weimar A, Taintor J: The effect of orthodontic force application on the pulpal tissue respiration rate in the human premolar, *Am J Orthod* 77:368, 1980.

80. Sailus J, Trowbridge H, Greco M, Emling R: Sensitivity of teeth subjected to orthodontic forces (abstract 556), *J Dent Res* 66(special issue):556, 1987.

81. Hall CJ, Freer TJ: The effects of orthodontic force application on pulp test responses, *Aust Dent J* 43:359, 1998.

82. Jordan RE, Suzuki M: Conservative treatment of deep carious lesions, *J Can Dent Assoc* 37:337, 1971.

83. Leung RL, Loesche WJ, Charbeneau GT: Effect of Dycal on bacteria in deep carious lesions, *J Am Dent Assoc* 100:193, 1980.

84. Horsted P, Sondergaard B, Thylstrup A, et al: A retrospective study of pulp capping with calcium hydroxide compounds, *Endod Dent Traumatol* 1:29, 1985.

85. Fuks AB, Bielak S, Chosak A: Clinical and radiologic assessments of direct pulp capping and pulpotomy in young permanent teeth, *Pediatr Dent* 24:244, 1982.

86. Matsuo T, Nakanishi T, Shimizu H, Ebisu S: A clinical study of direct pulp capping applied to carious-exposed pulps, *J Endod* 22:551, 1996.

87. Tsuneda Y, Hayakawa T, Yamamoto H, et al: A histopathological study of direct pulp capping with adhesive resins, *Oper Dent* 20:223, 1995.

88. Walton RE: Pulp capping with adhesive resins, *J Esthet Dent* 10:272, 1998.

89. Barthel C, Rosenkranz B, Leuenberg A, Roulet J-F: Pulp capping of carious exposures: treatment outcome after 5 and 10 years. A retrospective study, *J Endod* 26:525, 2000.

90. Cvek M, Granath LE, Cleaton-Jones P, Austin J: Hard tissue barrier formation in pulpotomized monkey teeth capped with cyanoacrylate or calcium hydroxide for 10 and 60 minutes, *J Dent Res* 66:1166, 1987.

91. Mejare I, Cvek M: Partial pulpotomy in young permanent teeth with deep carious lesions, *Endod Dent Traumatol* 9:238, 1993.

92. Fuks AB, Gavra S, Chosack A: Long-term followup of traumatized incisors treated by partial pulpotomy, *Pediatr Dent* 15:334, 1993.

93. Sübay KR, Suzuki S, Suzuki S, et al: Human pulp response after partial pulpotomy with two calcium hydroxide products, *Oral Surg Oral Med Oral Pathol* 3:330, 1995.

94. Nosrat IV, Nosrat CA: Reparative hard tissue formation following calcium hydroxide application after partial pulpotomy in cariously exposed pulps of permanent teeth, *Int Endod J* 31:221, 1998.

95. Jordan RE, Suzuki M, Skinner DH: Indirect pulp-capping of carious teeth with periapical lesions, *J Am Dent Assoc* 97:37, 1978.

96. Caliskan MK: Pulpotomy of carious vital teeth with periapical involvement, *Int Endod J* 28:172, 1995.

Thomas R. Pitt Ford and Shahrokh Shabahang

Management of Incompletely Formed Roots

LEARNING OBJECTIVES

After reading this chapter, the student should be able to:

1 / Describe and differentiate between the open and closed apices.

2 / Discuss methods of diagnosis and selection of appropriate treatment.

3 / Identify situations in which a tooth with an open apex requires vital pulp therapy or root-end closure and root canal therapy.

4 / Explain why nonsurgical root canal treatment and periapical surgery are technically difficult and inappropriate in a tooth with an open apex.

5 / Describe the prognosis for vital pulp therapy and root-end closure.

6 / Describe how to perform vital pulp therapy by pulpotomy.

7 / Describe how to perform root-end closure.

8 / Recognize the success or failure of treatment of an open apex.

9 / Select appropriate treatment when failure has occurred.

10 / Recognize when a patient should be considered for referral.

OUTLINE

Definition of Terms
    Open Apex
    Vital Pulp Therapy
    Root-End Closure
Diagnosis and Treatment Planning
    Subjective Examination
    Objective Examination
    Treatment Planning
    Case Selection and Referrals
Indications and Contraindications
    Vital Pulp Therapy
    Root-End Closure
Treatment Techniques
    Vital Pulp Therapy
    Root-End Closure
    Coronal Restoration
    Root-End Closure with MTA
Follow-Up
    Successful Treatment
    Failed Treatment

A n immature tooth that develops pulpal disease presents special problems. When the apex is not closed but is wide open, routine root canal treatment procedures cannot be performed and results are unpredictable. This chapter discusses the endodontic management of teeth with open apices and with pulp and/or periradicular pathoses. The diagnosis and treatment planning, case selection, techniques of management, and outcomes of treatment are also discussed. Included are those situations and reasons why patients needing open apex treatment should be considered for referral.

Definition of Terms

OPEN APEX

An open apex is found in the developing roots of immature teeth and, in the absence of pulp or periradicular disease, is normal. Apical closure occurs approximately 3 years after eruption. However, when the pulp undergoes necrosis before root growth is complete, dentin formation ceases, and root growth is arrested. Therefore, the canal and the apex remain wide (Figures 22-1 and 22-2); the root may also be shorter. An open apex may develop also as a result of extensive resorption of a mature apex after orthodontic treatment, or from periradicular inflammation (Figure 22-3), or as part of healing after trauma. The normal mature permanent tooth often has an apical constriction of the canal approximately 0.5 to 1.0 mm from the anatomic apex.[1] An immature root has an apical opening that is comparatively very large. The walls of the canal in an immature root with an open apex are thinner than those of a mature root. They may diverge (see Figure 22-1), be parallel (see Figure 22-2), or converge slightly, depending on the stage of root formation.

VITAL PULP THERAPY

Vital pulp therapy, previously called *apexogenesis,* is defined as treatment of a vital pulp in an immature tooth to permit continued dentin formation and apical closure. The current, more general terminology refers to maintenance of pulp vitality to allow continued development of the entire root and not just the apex. The objective is to maintain the vitality of the radicular pulp.

A vital pulp of an immature tooth may present with a small coronal exposure after trauma; normal formation of root dentin will continue by means of a shallow pulpotomy. Most immature teeth with crown fractures and exposed pulps

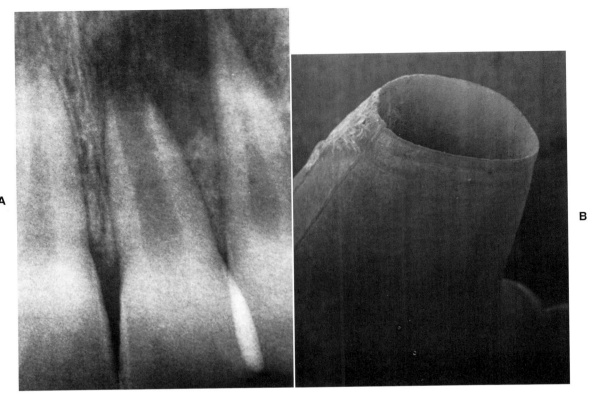

FIGURE 22-1
A, Incisor (history of luxation injury) with an open apex (divergent walls), necrotic pulp, and apical pathosis. Root-end closure is indicated. **B,** Apical region of an immature central incisor extracted from a 7-year-old. Besides being wide open, the apical dentin walls are egg-shell thin. These teeth are difficult to treat; long-term prognosis would be questionable. (Courtesy Dr. L. Baldassari-Cruz.)

have vital pulps in which inflammation is limited to the pulp surface.[2] Treatment that allows the root to continue developing may also be indicated in immature teeth with a small carious pulpal exposure; success is dependent on the extent of pulpal damage and on the restorability of the tooth. A large carious or traumatic exposure may require a pulpotomy at the level of the cervical constriction to retain radicular pulp viability.

ROOT-END CLOSURE

Root-end closure, previously referred to as apexification, is defined as the process of creating an environment within the root canal and periapical tissues after pulp death that allows a calcified barrier to form across the open apex. This barrier has been characterized as dentin, cementum, bone, and osteodentin (Figure 22-4). The usual result is blunting of the end of the root and very little, if any, increase in root length.

Creation of the proper environment for formation of the calcified barrier involves cleaning and removal of debris and bacteria, as well as the placement of a material to induce apical closure. Different materials have been used successfully to induce root-end closure. Most favored has been a paste of calcium hydroxide and water. The addition of other medicaments to calcium hydroxide has been suggested, but with no beneficial effect on root-end closure.[3] Calcium hydroxide has been used as a temporary obturating material; it is bactericidal with an alkaline pH that may be responsible for stimulating apical calcification.[4] Complete débridement to remove bacteria and necrotic tissue from the root canal system is an essential factor responsible for apical closure.[5] Recently, placement of an apical plug of mineral trioxide aggregate (MTA) has been shown to be more effective and convenient than the use of calcium hydroxide.[6]

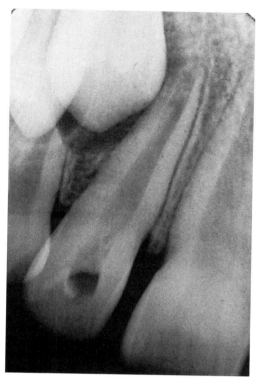

FIGURE 22-2
Incisor with a necrotic pulp, but with substantial dentin formation and an open apex (parallel walls). An access opening has been made into the pulp chamber. Root-end closure is indicated. Long-term prognosis is good.

Diagnosis and Treatment Planning

The essentials of diagnosis and treatment planning are reviewed here; details of diagnosis and treatment planning are discussed in Chapter 4. Before treatment of an incompletely formed root is started, tests are essential. A common cause of pulp damage is trauma, but damage may also result from caries, mechanical exposure, or a developmental anomaly (e.g., dens invaginatus). Depending on the diagnosis and findings, vital pulp therapy, root-end closure and obturation, nonsurgical root canal treatment, or possibly periapical surgery may be appropriate.

SUBJECTIVE EXAMINATION
History

There is often a history (usually much earlier) of a traumatic injury (blow) that may or may not in-

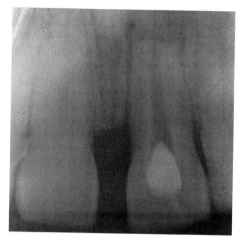

FIGURE 22-3
Resorbed apex (now open) caused by periapical inflammation resulting from pulpal necrosis.

volve a crown fracture. If fractured, the tooth may have been restored with composite resin retained by etched enamel; however, the tooth may since have become discolored or may show symptoms indicating pulp necrosis.

Symptoms

The symptoms most helpful in diagnosis relate primarily to duration of pain. Duration may vary, but if pain is spontaneous or persists after stimulus in a tooth with a vital pulp, irreversible pulpitis is likely. Of course, both irreversible pulpitis and necrosis are often asymptomatic. If the pain has a throbbing character and the tooth is tender to touch, either apical periodontitis or a symptomatic abscess with a necrotic pulp is likely. Confirmation of these findings by performing objective tests is necessary.

OBJECTIVE EXAMINATION
Visual Examination

Both hard and soft tissues are examined. If pain is due to irreversible pulpitis, there should be an etiologic factor to explain it, such as a deep restoration, history of trauma, tooth fracture, or caries. The crown may be discolored. Apical redness, tenderness, or swelling may indicate the presence of a symptomatic periradicular abscess, whereas a sinus tract indicates an asymptomatic periradicular abscess (suppurative apical periodontitis).

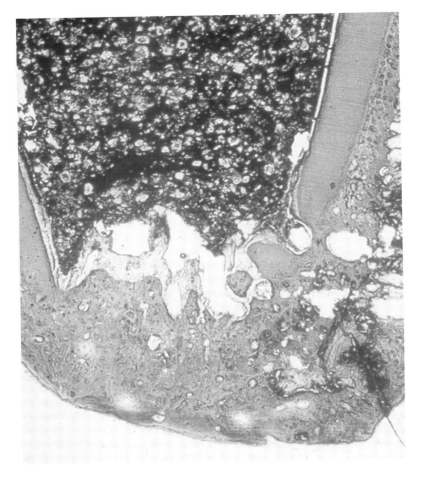

FIGURE 22-4
Histology of apical barrier after root-end closure of an open-apex tooth treated with MTA. Osteodentin deposition is shown as an irregular cellular calcified tissue unlike dentin or bone. Note the numerous spaces (sponge-like) that contain tissue remnants.

Percussion

Pain on pressure is diagnostic only when a significant painful response is elicited from the affected tooth. Digital pressure is preferred; tapping with a mirror handle to elicit pain is unreliable and unpleasant for the patient.

Thermal Testing

Thermal testing is widely used with open apices but may be complicated by a lack of neural development or by an exaggerated response caused by apprehension in a young patient. No response to repeated thermal testing, as compared to a positive response in the contralateral control tooth, may indicate the presence of a necrotic pulp; this can be confirmed by other tests. A problem (with an open or closed apex) after a luxation injury is that nerves may be damaged while the blood supply remains intact, and, therefore, the pulp is healthy but unresponsive.

Electric Pulp Testing

Electric pulp testing is unreliable in traumatized young teeth with wide open apices because of the injury and because sensory nerves may not yet have developed fully. Results must therefore be interpreted with caution; lack of response does not necessarily indicate pulpal necrosis. The presence of a response may also be inaccurate because the child may overreact or be unreliable.

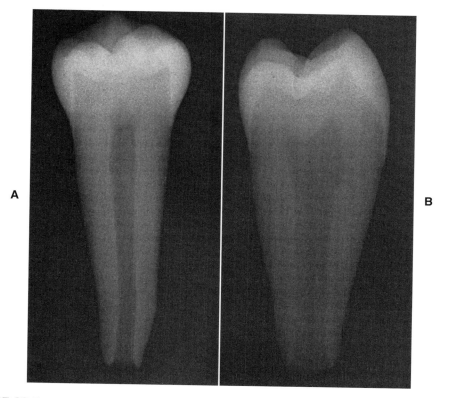

FIGURE 22-5
A, The apex appears to be near parallel as seen from the facial aspect. **B,** From the proximal aspect, the apical walls diverge.

Radiographic Findings

It is normal for a radiolucent area with a corticated margin to surround the developing open apex of an immature tooth with a healthy pulp. It is sometimes difficult to differentiate this from the pathologic radiolucency (usually there is not a corticated bony margin) resulting from a necrotic pulp. Comparison with the periapex of the contralateral tooth is helpful, especially in conjunction with the results of other diagnostic tests. When a sinus tract is present, a radiograph with a gutta-percha point in the tract may indicate the source.

A radiograph provides only a two-dimensional image and does not reveal the third dimension, which is important in teeth with an open apex. Only the mesiodistal aspect is seen in a routine radiograph. Although the apical opening appears almost closed, it is more open when seen from the proximal aspect (Figure 22-5). Thus, conventional radiographs may result in selection of inappropriate routine root canal treatment when vital pulp therapy or root-end closure is indicated instead.

If there is doubt about the apical anatomy, an angled radiograph is helpful (see Chapter 9).

TREATMENT PLANNING

Pulpal status and degree of root development are the major factors in treatment planning (Figure 22-6). If the pulpal diagnosis is reversible pulpitis, the treatment of choice is vital pulp therapy, regardless of the degree of root development. Depending on the extent of pulpal damage, pulp capping or shallow or conventional pulpotomy may be indicated.

If the diagnosis is irreversible pulpitis or pulp necrosis, the amount of root development will determine the proper treatment. If the apex is closed, root canal therapy can be performed. However, in a tooth with incomplete root development, root-end closure must be performed before the obturation. A number of other factors must also be considered. The patient may become impatient or disinterested, especially when many visits are required. The risk of root fracture is high

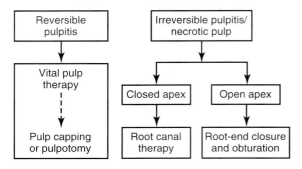

FIGURE 22-6
Case selection decision tree.

in immature teeth, especially in thin-walled roots; other treatment options require consideration.[7] Alternative treatments include (1) apical plug, (2) root canal treatment, (3) periapical surgery, and (4) extraction.

Vital Pulp Therapy

A patient with a tooth suitable for vital pulp therapy after trauma should be seen immediately or preferably not more than a few days later, although teeth with long exposure times have been successfully treated.[2] As with any traumatic injury, a thorough general, facial, and oral examination should be carried out; these aspects are discussed in detail in Chapter 25. Normally, the crown fracture involves the pulp, which is vital and can be seen directly. Radiographs do not usually show apical pathosis.

Another possible indication for vital pulp therapy is a tooth with an open apex that has a carious exposure.

Root-End Closure

The patient may or may not be having pain and may have suffered previous trauma. The pulp is necrotic, usually accompanied by periradicular inflammation.

Apical Plug

The advantage of placing an apical plug is elimination of repeated placement of calcium hydroxide. It is often difficult to recall some of these patients because of relocation. It would be advantageous to be able to complete the treatment in two appointments so that the risk of contamination caused by loss of the temporary seal would be reduced and the outcome would be more predictable.[6,8]

Root Canal Treatment

The presence of an open apex is a major problem in routine root canal treatment. Obtaining a well-condensed obturation to the desired level is very difficult. The likely result is extrusion of excess material periapically as well as large voids within the material.

Surgery

Surgical intervention is possible but is best avoided in children. If surgery is necessary, it should be performed by an endodontist. The procedure is complicated by the short root and thin fragile walls at the root end, which compromise the strength of the tooth. If surgery is indicated, MTA is the preferred root-end filling material.[9] Root-end resection should be minimized or avoided because it reduces the length of an already short root.

Extraction

If the tooth has a very poor prognosis, extraction must be considered, together with the orthodontic implications. The space may be allowed to close or may be maintained with a prosthesis; a multidisciplinary assessment is required. A removable provisional partial denture is often the immediate replacement. For the longer term, an adhesive or conventional bridge or an implant is a possibility. *Remember* that adjacent teeth will also require assessment as suitable abutments because they may also have suffered from trauma.

CASE SELECTION AND REFERRALS

The need to refer patients requiring vital pulp therapy is not great. Generally, after traumatic exposure, treatment (shallow pulpotomy) is straightforward and predictable. In contrast, general dentists should be selective about treating teeth needing root-end closure; treatment is time consuming and unpredictable. There may be complications such as displacement (leakage) of the temporary restoration or root fracture. In addition, the average practitioner has limited experience with such situations. When treatment is technically difficult, such as in patients with very immature or badly fractured teeth that cannot be properly isolated, the dentist should consider referral.

Expense is another factor; the patient (or parent) must be aware that these procedures require much more time and more appointments than conventional root canal treatment. The specialist who has more experience can manage these problems more efficiently.

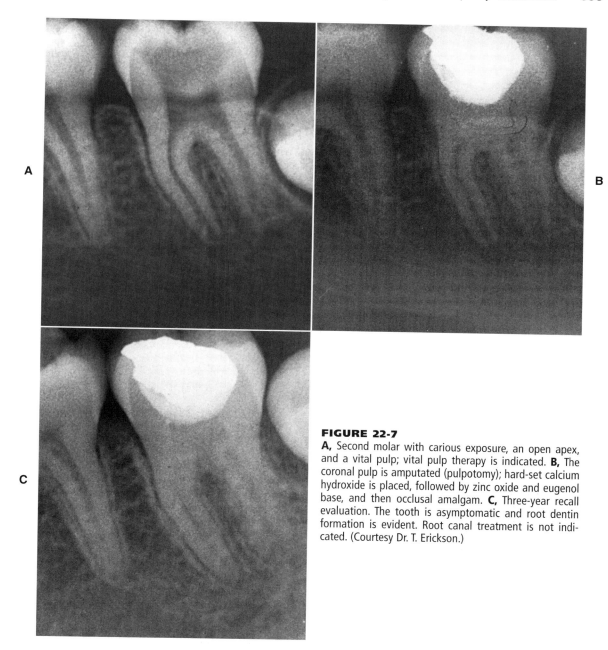

FIGURE 22-7
A, Second molar with carious exposure, an open apex, and a vital pulp; vital pulp therapy is indicated. **B,** The coronal pulp is amputated (pulpotomy); hard-set calcium hydroxide is placed, followed by zinc oxide and eugenol base, and then occlusal amalgam. **C,** Three-year recall evaluation. The tooth is asymptomatic and root dentin formation is evident. Root canal treatment is not indicated. (Courtesy Dr. T. Erickson.)

Indications and Contraindications

VITAL PULP THERAPY
Indications

Vital pulp therapy (Figure 22-7) is indicated for an immature tooth with incomplete root formation and with damage to the coronal pulp but whose radicular pulp is presumed to be healthy. The crown must be fairly intact and restorable.

Contraindications

Contradictions include the following:
1. Avulsed and replanted or severely luxated tooth
2. Severe crown-root fracture that requires intraradicular retention for restoration
3. Tooth with an unfavorable horizontal root fracture (i.e., close to the gingival margin)
4. Carious tooth that is unrestorable
5. Necrotic pulp

Prognosis

The prognosis is good when pulp capping or shallow pulpotomy (Cvek technique[2]) is done correctly after a traumatic exposure. A completely formed root is then produced that can support an appropriate restoration. Subsequent root canal treatment is unlikely to be necessary. Conventional pulpotomy is slightly less successful, particularly in anterior teeth because of tissue damage when the coronal pulp is severed.

Complications

Complications should be few. Microbial contamination through a leaking or lost temporary or permanent restoration may cause pulpal necrosis and periradicular pathosis. If this occurs before complete root development, root-end closure would be necessary; if contamination occurs after root formation, root canal treatment is required.

ROOT-END CLOSURE
Indications

Root-end closure is required for a restorable immature tooth with pulp necrosis.

Contraindications

Contraindications include the following:
1. All vertical and most horizontal root fractures
2. Replacement resorption (ankylosis)
3. Very short roots
4. Marginal periodontal breakdown
5. Vital pulps

Prognosis

Generally, root-end closure procedures have a good success rate.[10-12] However, very immature teeth (thin dentin walls) are at high risk for root fracture either during or after treatment; the incidence of fracture depends on the stage of root development. Also, barrier formation occurs more rapidly when the apical opening is less wide.[12]

Treatment Techniques
VITAL PULP THERAPY

Either pulp capping, shallow pulpotomy, or conventional pulpotomy (Figure 22-8) is indicated for crown fracture of an anterior tooth involving exposure of the pulp and an open apex.[13] Conventional pulpotomy is difficult to perform in an immature incisor, which has a large pulp in the cer-

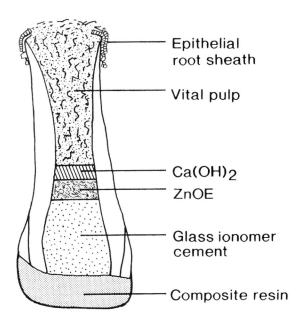

FIGURE 22-8
Conventional pulpotomy. Pulp is amputated at the cervical level and covered with calcium hydroxide and then a sealing layer of fortified zinc oxide-eugenol (ZnOE) cement and glass ionomer cement. The incisal is restored with composite resin.

vical region. Pulp capping or shallow or conventional pulpotomy is suitable in posterior teeth.

Techniques

Pulp capping. After anesthesia is obtained and a rubber dam is applied, the exposed pulp is rinsed with 2.5% sodium hypochlorite (NaOCl). Heavy bleeding from the exposure site can be controlled with a cotton pellet moistened with NaOCl. MTA powder is mixed with sterile water and placed in the access cavity with a large plastic amalgam carrier and then patted against the exposures site(s) with a moist cotton pellet. A moist cotton pellet is placed on the MTA, and then a temporary filling is placed. In compliant patients, the cavity is filled with MTA, and then a wet piece of gauze is placed between the treated and opposing teeth for 3 to 4 hours. Because MTA cannot be used as a permanent filling material, the coronal 3 to 4 mm of MTA is removed after setting and the cavity is restored permanently.[8] Pulp status is evaluated clinically and radiographically every 3 to 6 months.

Shallow pulpotomy. Shallow pulpotomy was developed in Scandinavia.[2,14] In crown-fractured teeth, the pulp is vital and often inflamed on the exposed surface; the pulp may become hyperplastic with time. Because the inflammation is superficial (2 to 3 mm deep), only the inflamed tissue is removed, leaving a small wound surface. The procedure is outlined in Chapter 25.

There is a high success rate when the technique is carefully performed and the essential overlying seal is produced and maintained.[2] This is a permanent procedure; normally, root canal treatment is not required subsequently. The technique has also been used for managing carious exposures; however, success depends on careful case selection and treatment.[15] In the pulp capping or shallow pulpotomy technique, MTA has been recommended instead of calcium hydroxide.[8,16]

Pulpotomy with calcium hydroxide. The technique (see Figure 22-8) involves the following steps:

1. After local anesthesia, rubber dam isolation, and surface disinfection, a conventional access cavity is made with a high-speed bur using copious water spray coolant. Water spray and gradual reduction minimize embedding of dentinal debris in the pulp.[5]
2. Strands of pulp and debris are removed coronal to the amputation site. Amputation of the coronal pulp at the cervical level is performed with a sharp spoon excavator or a large sterile round metal or diamond bur. Creation of a clean wound without damaging the underlying pulp is difficult with an excavator. Low-speed burs may cause contusion and tearing of the remaining pulp, leading to calcific metamorphosis.
3. Bleeding of the cut pulp stump is controlled with local anesthetic, sodium hypochlorite, or saline on a cotton pellet applied with gentle pressure. Caustic chemicals or medicaments should not be used so that the health of the radicular pulp is maintained.
4. Calcium hydroxide powder is mixed with sterile water, saline, or anesthetic solution to a thick consistency. The paste is carefully placed on the pulp stump surface 1 to 2 mm thick.[16]
5. A layer of zinc oxide–eugenol cement must be placed over the calcium hydroxide for two reasons: first, to protect against leakage of bacteria from saliva around the final restoration, and second, to provide a rigid base against which a final restoration can be placed.
6. A permanent well-sealing restoration is essential. Temporary restorations invariably deteriorate and leak over a period of time, resulting in bacterial contamination and subsequent pulp necrosis. Acid-etched composite resin is recommended for anterior teeth and amalgam for posterior teeth. The composite resin should be placed below the cement-enamel junction to reduce the incidence of subsequent tooth fracture.[17]

Pulp capping or pulpotomy with mineral trioxide aggregate. The technique involves the following steps:

1. After local anesthesia and rubber dam isolation is obtained, access to the pulp chamber is made, and depending on the extent of pulpal damage, pulp capping or pulpotomy is performed. Control of bleeding is obtained as described for pulpotomy with calcium hydroxide.
2. The MTA is prepared immediately before use by mixing the powder with sterile water or saline at a ratio of 3:1 on a glass or paper slab. The mixture is placed on the exposed pulp or pulp stump surface and patted with a moist cotton pellet. The amount of moisture in the MTA can be manipulated by adding more water or absorbing excess moisture with a small dry piece of gauze.[8]
3. Because MTA sets in the presence of moisture over a 3-hour period, a wet cotton pellet is placed over the material and the rest of the cavity is filled with temporary filling material. Alternatively the entire cavity can be filled with MTA and protected by a wet piece of gauze for 3 to 4 hours.[8]
4. The coronal 3 to 4 mm of MTA is removed, and a final restoration is placed 1 week later.[8]

Recall Schedule

The patient is usually scheduled for recall appointments at 3- to 6-month intervals to monitor pulp vitality and apical growth. The total follow-up time varies, depending on the initial degree of root maturation. If the root were in a very early stage of development, root formation could take 2 to 3 years. Recall appointments should then be done for at least 4 years.

Absence of symptoms does not indicate absence of disease. Monitoring of signs and symptoms, periodic pulp testing, and radiographs are required to determine pulp and periapical status. One advantage of pulp capping or shallow pulpotomy over conventional pulpotomy is of the ability to test the pulp.

Possible Outcomes

The ideal result is continued apical growth of the root with a normal or nearly normal apex (Figure 22-9). Treatment failure is cessation of growth and apical disease, requiring root-end closure or root canal treatment.

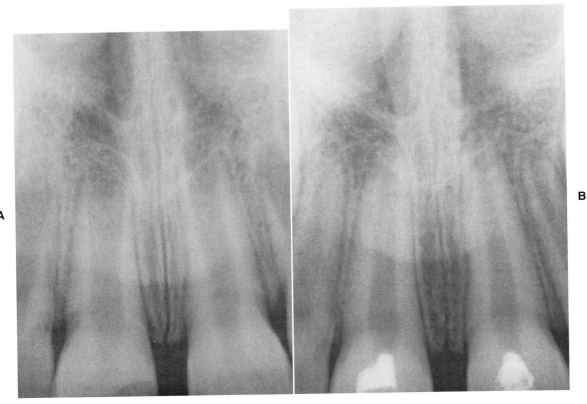

FIGURE 22-9
Preoperative (**A**) and postoperative (**B**) radiographs demonstrate continued root development after pulpotomy procedures on both incisors. If these are restored with good sealing restorations, the pulps should remain healthy; root canal treatment would be unnecessary.

Pulp capping or shallow pulpotomy. After root formation, vital tissue may be maintained for long periods of time, usually indefinitely. Histologic examination of pulps of some crown-fractured teeth after pulp capping or shallow pulpotomy has usually shown normal tissue.[18] The tissue response to MTA has been excellent (Figure 22-10).[16] Histologic evidence does not support the use of routine pulp extirpation and root filling after apical closure. Cvek[2] reported a very high clinical success rate.

Conventional pulpotomy. Conventional pulpotomy can also be permanent treatment. However, after conventional pulpotomy, the success rate is lower and calcific metamorphosis is a common occurrence.[19] When there is evidence of this type of calcification, a case has been made for root canal treatment, although this is probably unwarranted; calcific metamorphosis is not pathosis. One problem with calcific metamorphosis is that if the pulp becomes necrotic and root canal treatment is necessary, canals may not be negotiable, and surgery may be necessary.

Treatment of Failures

After pulpotomy, teeth must be evaluated periodically with subjective and objective tests and radiographs. If failure occurs after root formation is complete, conventional root canal treatment is indicated. If failure (pulp necrosis) occurs before apical closure, root-end closure is required.

ROOT-END CLOSURE

This is the induction of a calcified barrier (or the creation of an artificial barrier) across an open apex.[20-22] The factors most critical to success are thorough débridement of the pulp space and a complete coronal seal. The material placed in the canal to allow barrier formation is less important than has been believed historically, although calcium hydroxide has been commonly used in the mistaken belief that it stimulates hard tissue formation. Calcium hydroxide does provide a suitable medium, however, to permit apical closure.

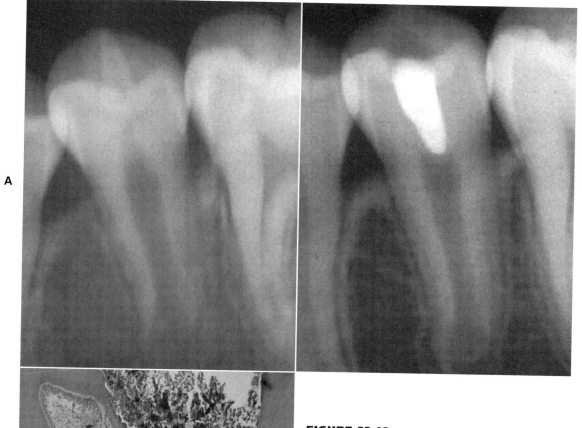

FIGURE 22-10
A, Premolar with dens evaginatis resulting in pulp exposure. **B,** One-year postoperative radiograph after pulpotomy with MTA demonstrating evidence of a dentin barrier. **C,** Histologic section of the MTA-pulp interface. A continuous layer of hard tissue bridge is interposed between the MTA and underlying healthy pulp.

Technique

The technique of creating this environment is divided into three general phases: access, instrumentation, and placement of calcium hydroxide or MTA. The steps for root-end closure with calcium hydroxide are the following:

1. After isolation, a large access is made to allow removal of all necrotic tissue.
2. Necrotic pulp or a large part of it (unless liquefied) is removed by inserting, rotating, and withdrawing a large barbed broach or a large Hedström file.
3. Working length is determined slightly short of the radiographic apex.

4. Instrumentation is performed with a gentle circumferential filing motion, beginning with a relatively large file and progressing up through the file sizes. The use of Hedström files is not advocated because their sharp flutes may perforate the thin fragile walls of dentin. The aim is to maximize cleansing, aided by copious irrigation with sodium hypochlorite and to minimize dentin removal. Instrumentation beyond the apex is avoided because of damage to the tissue that will ultimately form the barrier.
5. Large sterile paper points or cotton rolled on a broach are used to dry the canal.

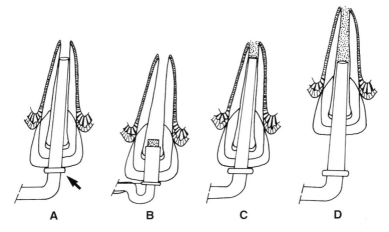

FIGURE 22-11
Placement of calcium hydroxide in the canal with amalgam carrier and pluggers. **A,** The plugger is prefitted 2 to 3 mm short of the apex, and the depth is marked with a rubber stop *(arrow).* **B,** A 3- to 4-mm section of a calcium hydroxide pellet is placed with an amalgam carrier. **C,** The material is pushed apically with the plugger and verified radiographically. **D,** Successive increments are placed and condensed. (Modified from Webber R: *Dent Clin North Am* 28:688, 1984.)

6. Calcium hydroxide powder with barium sulfate added for radiopacity (9:1 ratio) is mixed with saline (or local anesthetic or glycerine) to form a stiff paste. This or a manufactured paste of calcium hydroxide is introduced with either an amalgam carrier or the manufacturer's syringe in the canal at the working length (Figure 22-11). An alternative material, particularly in larger canals, is dry powder; pellets of packed powder are made by packing calcium hydroxide into an amalgam carrier.[23] Displacing too much material periapically should be avoided. Subsequent increments should fill the canal without voids.

7. A radiograph verifies that the canal space is filled (Figure 22-12). If voids exist, calcium hydroxide is recondensed before temporization. Although extrusion of calcium hydroxide apically should be minimized, there are no apparent long-term adverse effects.

Coronal Seal

An effective temporary seal between visits is critical.[5] Fortified zinc oxide-eugenol cement (IRM) is preferred. In selected instances it may be covered by composite resin to restore the missing tooth structure.

Recall Schedule

The patient is recalled in 4 to 6 weeks. Inflamed periapical tissue fluids may have dissolved the cal-

cium hydroxide; if so, the material will not appear dense radiographically. In such cases the tooth is reopened, the calcium hydroxide is washed out and repacked, and a temporary filling is placed. If at recall, the calcium hydroxide appears dense and there are no clinical signs or symptoms of disease, it need not be replaced. Recall is then scheduled for 3 and 6 months; the calcium hydroxide is changed only if radiographic density significantly decreases.

If healing (bony resolution) has progressed well after 1 year, the calcium hydroxide is removed. A hard tissue barrier is often not visible radiographically but is detected tactically.[10] The hard tissue barrier is probed with a medium-sized file or observed by an operating microscope. If a small file does not pass through an opening, sufficient closure has occurred, permitting successful obturation. If the apex is still open, the canal is irrigated thoroughly, the calcium hydroxide replaced, and the patient recalled in 3 months.

Obturation

The canal is cleaned and irrigated copiously and then dried. A modified lateral condensation technique is often necessary. When the canal is large, even large standardized gutta-percha cones will not fit snugly. A large cone of gutta-percha is warmed and softened slightly over a flame or in hot water, introduced into the canal, and adapted to the shape of the apical canal and barrier.[24] Then accessory points are laterally con-

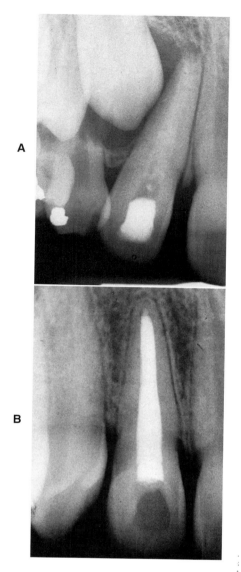

A

B

FIGURE 22-12
Root-end closure. **A,** Calcium hydroxide adequately fills the canal space. A zinc oxide–eugenol cement temporary filling seals the access. **B,** Incisor after 12 months and successful root-end closure. Apical barrier formation is complete, allowing dense, laterally condensed gutta-percha obturation.

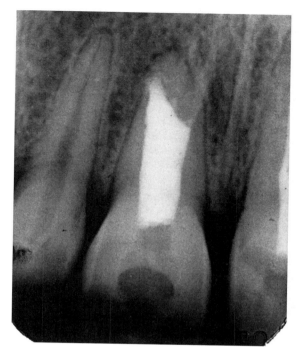

FIGURE 22-13
Unusual root-end closure. A barrier has formed, leaving a wide, divergent canal space. Obturation was accomplished with thermoplasticized gutta-percha. Access was restored with glass ionomer.

ered by an appropriate system (Figure 22-13). After obturation recall appointments should be scheduled annually up to 4 years.

CORONAL RESTORATION

After obturation, the pulp chamber should be partially filled with composite resin to strengthen the tooth and reduce the risk of fracture.[17]

ROOT-END CLOSURE WITH MTA[25]

The steps for root-end closure with MTA are the following:

1. After local anesthesia is obtained and a rubber dam is applied, a large access is made to allow débridement of the canal(s) with intracanal instruments and sodium hypochlorite.
2. Calcium hydroxide paste is placed in the canal for a period of 1 week to disinfect the root canal system.
3. After the calcium hydroxide is rinsed from the canal at the subsequent appointment, a mixture of MTA powder with sterile water is carried into the canal with an amalgam carrier. The mix is condensed to

densed using an appropriate sealer. A warmed spreader may improve condensation.

A master cone may be customized by warming several cones and rolling and fusing them between two glass slabs.[3] Then they are introduced and condensed into the canal as just described. Another method of softening gutta-percha is to dip the master gutta-percha cone briefly in chloroform or other suitable solvent. Alternatively, the canal may be filled with warm gutta-percha deliv-

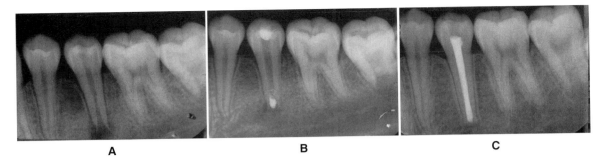

FIGURE 22-14
Root-end closure with MTA. **A,** Preoperative radiograph demonstrating a radiolucent periradicular lesion. **B,** Interoperative placement of an apical plug of MTA. **C,** Radiograph 6 months after obturation demonstrates healing.

the apical extent using pluggers or paper points to create a 3- to 4-mm apical plug (see Figure 22-13).[8]

4. The MTA placement is radiographically examined. If ideal extension is not accomplished, the MTA is rinsed out with sterile water and the procedure is repeated.[8]

5. To ensure proper setting of MTA, a moist cotton pellet is placed in the canal over the material and the tooth is temporized.[8]

6. The remainder of the canal is obturated with gutta-percha and sealer or bonded composite resin and the final restoration is placed in the access cavity (Figure 22-14).[8]

Follow-up

SUCCESSFUL TREATMENT
Vital Pulp Therapy

Successfully treated teeth (Figure 22-15) have the following characteristics:
1. Presence of a vital pulp
2. Absence of signs or symptoms of pulp or periapical disease: no pain, swelling, sinus tract, radiolucency, or deep probing defects
3. Continued growth of the root and canal narrowing, indicating dentin formation
4. A bridge of calcification (may not be visible radiographically) beneath the filling material

Root-End Closure

Successfully treated teeth are characterized by the following:
1. Absence of signs or symptoms of periradicular pathosis
2. Presence of a calcific barrier across the apex as demonstrated by radiographs or, more often, by careful tactile probing with a file typically with a short and blunt root

Root-End Closure with MTA

Successfully treated teeth (see Figure 22-14) are characterized by the following:
1. Absence of signs or symptoms of periradicular pathosis
2. Presence of a calcific barrier across the root apex as demonstrated by radiographs

FAILED TREATMENT
During Treatment

Vital pulp therapy for continued root development and root-end closure usually fails because of one common cause: bacterial contamination. This is manifested by the absence of apical closure. Generally, the source of bacteria is loss of the coronal seal or inadequate débridement (with root-end closure). One or more of the following are also present:
1. Symptoms (pain, tenderness to pressure)
2. Signs (sinus tract, swelling, probing defects, periapical radiolucency)
3. No evidence of root-end closure either radiographically or by tactile examination or resorption of a previously formed apical barrier[26]
4. Continual loss of calcium hydroxide from the canal space, indicating persistent periradicular inflammation
5. Down-growth of granulomatous tissue into the canal, manifested by bleeding when files are placed short of the apex

After Treatment

After apparently successful treatment, all patients should be recalled at 12-month intervals for 4 years for clinical and radiographic evaluation. Conventional pulpotomy may show short-term clinical success but long-term failure. Failure usually results from bacterial contamination through microleakage around the restoration

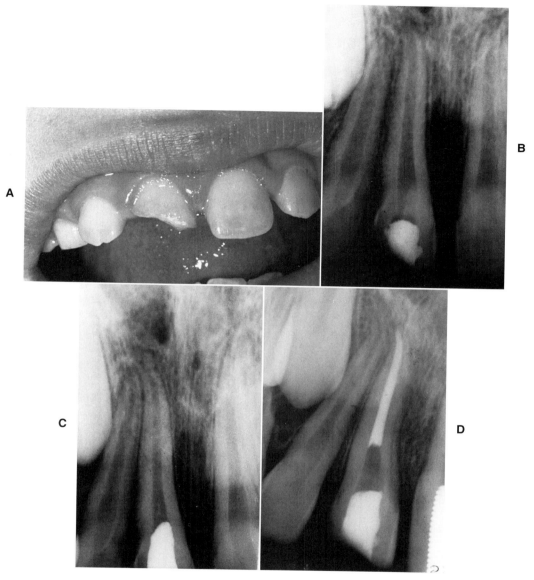

FIGURE 22-15
Vital pulp therapy. **A,** Trauma resulted in fracture and large pulp exposure. Pulp is vital. **B,** Conventional pulpotomy was performed. **C,** Apical development 11 months later. **D,** Irreversible pulpitis subsequently developed, requiring root canal treatment. (Courtesy Dr. G. Parsons.)

and through the porous bridge at the pulpotomy site. This is likely if the zinc oxide-eugenol base did not seal and cover the calcium hydroxide.

Some root-end closures that were initially successful may eventually fail, even though a calcified barrier was present across the apex and a proper root canal filling was placed. Infected necrotic material trapped in the barrier may contribute to these failures, particularly if treatment was not performed under strict aseptic conditions. A further reason for failure is an undetected vertical or horizontal root fracture.[10]

REFERENCES

1. Kuttler Y: A precision and biologic root canal filling technique, *J Am Dent Assoc* 56:38, 1958.
2. Cvek M: A clinical report on partial pulpotomy and capping with calcium hydroxide in permanent incisors with complicated crown fracture, *J Endod* 4:232, 1978.

3. Gutmann JL, Heaton JF: Management of the open (immature) apex. 2. Non-vital teeth, *Int Endod J* 14:173, 1981.
4. Binnie WH, Mitchell DF: Induced calcification in the subdermal tissues of the rat, *J Dent Res* 52:1087, 1973.
5. Torneck C, Smith JS, Grindall P: Biologic effects of endodontic procedures on developing incisor teeth. II. Effect of pulp injury and oral contamination, *Oral Surg Oral Med Oral Pathol* 35:378, 1973.
6. Shabahang S, Torabinejad M, Boyne P, et al: A comparative study of root-end induction using osteogenic protein-1, calcium hydroxide, and mineral trioxide aggregate in dogs, *J Endod* 25:1, 1999.
7. Morse DR, O'Larnic J, Yesilsoy C: Apexification: review of the literature, *Quintessence Int* 21:589, 1990.
8. Torabinejad M, Chivian N: Clinical applications of mineral trioxide aggregate, *J Endod* 25:197, 1999.
9. Torabinejad M, Pitt Ford T, McKendry D, et al: Histologic assessment of mineral trioxide aggregate as a root-end filling in monkeys, *J Endod* 23:225, 1997.
10. Cvek M: Prognosis of luxated non-vital maxillary incisors treated with calcium hydroxide and filled with gutta-percha. A retrospective clinical study, *Endod Dent Traumatol* 8:45, 1992.
11. Kleier D, Barr E: A study of endodontically apexified teeth, *Endod Dent Traumatol* 7:112, 1991.
12. Finucane D, Kinirons M: Non-vital immature permanent incisor factors that may influence treatment outcome, *Endod Dent Traumatol* 15:273, 1999.
13. Gutmann JL, Heaton JF: Management of the open (immature) apex. 1. Vital teeth, *Int Endod J* 14:166, 1981.
14. Granath L, Hagman G: Experimental pulpotomy in human bicuspids with reference to cutting technique, *Acta Odontol Scand* 29:155, 1971.
15. Mejare I, Cvek M: Partial pulpotomy in young permanent teeth with deep carious lesions, *Endod Dent Traumatol* 9:238, 1993.
16. Pitt Ford TR, Torabinejad M, Abedi HR, et al: Using mineral trioxide aggregate as a pulp-capping material, *J Am Dent Assoc* 127:1491, 1996.
17. Katebzadeh N, Dalton BC, Trope M: Strengthening immature teeth during and after apexification, *J Endod* 24:256, 1998.
18. Cvek M, Lundberg M: Histological appearance of pulps after exposure by a crown fracture, partial pulpotomy, and clinical diagnosis of healing, *J Endod* 9:8, 1983.
19. Hallett GEM, Porteous JR: Fractured incisors treated by vital pulpotomy, *Br Dent J* 115:279, 1963.
20. Cvek M: Treatment of non-vital permanent incisors with calcium hydroxide. I. Follow-up of periapical repair and apical closure of immature roots, *Odontol Rev* 23:27, 1972.
21. Frank AL: Therapy for the divergent pulpless tooth by continued apical formation, *J Am Dent Assoc* 72:87, 1966.
22. Heithersay GS: Stimulation of root formation in incompletely developed pulpless teeth, *Oral Surg Oral Med Oral Pathol* 29:620, 1970.
23. Krell KV, Madison S: The use of the Messing gun in placing calcium hydroxide powder, *J Endod* 11:233, 1985.
24. Cvek M: Endodontic management of traumatized teeth. In Andreasen JO, Andreasen FM, editors, *Textbook and color atlas of traumatic injuries to the teeth*, ed 3, p 517, Copenhagen, 1993, Munksgaard.
25. Shabahang S, Torabinejad M: Treatment of teeth with open apices using mineral trioxide aggregate, *Pract Periodontics Aesthet Dent* 12:315, 2000.
26. Capurro M, Zmener O: Delayed apical healing after apexification treatment of non-vital immature tooth: a case report, *Endod Dent Traumatol* 15:244, 1999.

Bleaching Discolored Teeth: Internal and External

LEARNING OBJECTIVES

After reading this chapter, the student should be able to:

1 / Identify the cause and nature of tooth discoloration.

2 / Describe means of preventing coronal discolorations.

3 / Differentiate between dentin and enamel discolorations.

4 / Evaluate the prognosis of bleaching treatments.

5 / Select the appropriate bleaching agent and technique according to the cause of the discoloration.

6 / Describe, step by step, the internal "walking bleach" technique.

7 / Describe briefly an external bleaching technique for intrinsic developmental discolorations (for example, tetracycline).

8 / Describe, step-by-step, an external bleaching technique for extrinsic developmental discolorations (for example, fluorosis).

9 / Describe briefly a mouthguard vital bleaching technique.

10 / Recognize the potential adverse effects of bleaching and discuss means of prevention.

OUTLINE

Causes of Discoloration
    "Natural" or Acquired Discolorations
    Iatrogenic or Inflicted Discolorations

Endodontically Related Discolorations
    Obturating Materials
    Remnants of Pulpal Tissue
    Intracanal Medicaments
    Coronal Restorations

Bleaching Materials
    Hydrogen Peroxide
    Sodium Perborate
    Carbamide Peroxide
    Other Oxidizing Agents

Internal (Nonvital) Bleaching Techniques
    Thermocatalytic Technique
    Walking Bleach
    Final Restoration
    When to Bleach

Complications and Safety
    External Resorption
    Coronal Fracture
    Chemical Burns

External (Vital) Bleaching Techniques
    Intrinsic Discolorations
    Extrinsic Discolorations

Mouthguard Bleaching
    Bleaching Technique
    Alternative Techniques
    Prognosis
    Safety

Laser Bleaching

When and What to Refer

D iscoloration of anterior teeth is a cosmetic problem that is often significant enough to induce patients to seek corrective measures. Although restorative methods such as crowns and veneers are available, discoloration can often be corrected totally or partially by bleaching. Bleaching procedures are more conservative than restorative methods, relatively simple to perform, and less expensive. Procedures may be internal (within the pulp chamber) or external (on the enamel surface) and involve various approaches (see Color Figures 23-1 to 23-3 after page 436).

To better understand bleaching techniques, it is important to know the causes of discoloration, location of the discoloring agent, and the treatment modalities available.[1] Also important is the ability to predict the outcome of treatment; that is, how successfully can various discolorations be treated and how long will the esthetic result last. In other words, before attempting to correct discoloration, a diagnosis must be made (determine the cause and location of the discoloration), treatment planning must be done (internal and/or external bleaching and technique), and a prognosis arrived at (anticipated short-term and long-term success). Patients must be informed of these factors before undergoing the procedure; they should not anticipate esthetic results that may not occur. Any discoloration treatment must be tempered by the explanation that substantial improvement may or may not occur. However, internal bleaching is worth a try; with proper and careful technique, no irreversible damage to the crown or root occurs.

This chapter reviews discoloration and its correction. Discussed are the causes and management of discoloration as related to (1) location of discoloration, (2) approach used for correction, and (3) anticipated short-term and long-term success of bleaching. Specially discussed are the following aspects of discoloration and bleaching procedures:

1. Causes and location of discoloration.
2. Commonly used bleaching agents.
3. Internal bleaching techniques (usually in conjunction with or after root canal treatment).
4. External bleaching techniques (usually in teeth with a vital pulp).
5. Predictability and permanence of each procedure.
6. Possible complications and safety of the various procedures.

Causes of Discoloration

Discolorations occur during or after enamel and dentin formation. Some discolorations appear after tooth eruption, and others are the result of dental procedures. The first group, natural (acquired) discolorations, may be on the surface or incorporated into tooth structure. Sometimes they result from flaws in enamel or a traumatic injury. The second group, iatrogenic (inflicted) discolorations, which result from dental procedures, are usually incorporated into tooth structure and are preventable.

"NATURAL" OR ACQUIRED DISCOLORATIONS
Pulp Necrosis

Bacterial, mechanical, or chemical irritation of the pulp may result in necrosis. Tissue disintegration byproducts are then released; these colored compounds may permeate tubules to stain surrounding dentin. The degree of discoloration is directly related to how long the pulp has been necrotic. The longer the discoloration compounds are present in the pulp chamber, the greater the discoloration. This type of discoloration can be bleached internally, usually with both short-term and long-term success.

Intrapulpal Hemorrhage

Generally, intrapulpal hemorrhage is associated with an impact injury to a tooth, which results in disrupted coronal blood vessels, hemorrhage and lysis of erythrocytes. It has been theorized that blood disintegration products, presumably as iron sulfides, permeate tubules to stain surrounding dentin. Discoloration tends to increase with time.

If the pulp becomes necrotic, the discoloration usually remains. If the pulp survives, the discoloration may resolve, and the tooth reverts to its original shade. Sometimes, mainly in young individuals, the tooth remains discolored even if the pulp responds to vitality tests.

Internal bleaching of discoloration after intrapulpal hemorrhage is usually successful both short and long term.[2,3]

Calcific Metamorphosis

Calcific metamorphosis is extensive formation of tertiary (irregular secondary) dentin in the pulp chamber or on canal walls. This phenomenon usually follows an impact injury that did not result in pulp necrosis. There is temporary disruption of blood supply with partial destruction of odontoblasts. These are usually replaced by cells that rapidly form irregular dentin on the walls of the pulp space. As a result, the crowns of these teeth gradually decrease in translucency and may acquire a yellowish or yellow-brown discoloration (Figure 23-1). The pulp usually remains vital and does not require root canal treatment.[4]

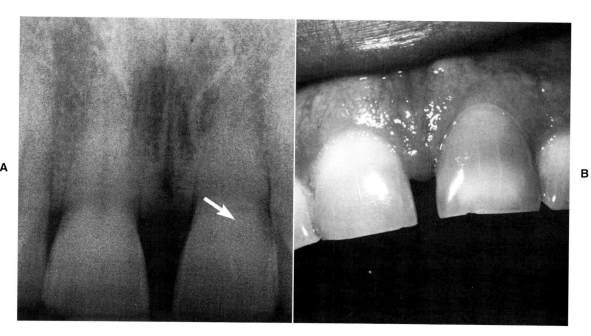

FIGURE 23-1
Calcific metamorphosis. Impact trauma resulted in reversible pulp damage with (**A**) extensive tertiary dentin formation *(arrow)* and (**B**) lost translucency and darkening of the crown. These teeth present difficulties with root canal treatment and internal bleaching.

If the patient desires color correction, external bleaching should be attempted first. If this is unsuccessful, root canal treatment is performed (sometimes with difficulty), and internal bleaching is done. This may be carried out whether the pulp is vital or necrotic. Such teeth are bleached with fair esthetic prognosis.

Age

In older patients, color changes in the crown occur physiologically as a result of extensive dentin apposition as well as thinning of and optical changes in enamel. Food and beverages also have a cumulative discoloring effect because of the inevitable cracking and other changes on the enamel surface and in the underlying dentin. In addition, previously applied restorations that degrade over time cause further discoloration. There is an increasing demand for bleaching among these older patients.

Developmental Defects

Discolorations may result from developmental defects or from substances incorporated into enamel or dentin during tooth formation.

Endemic fluorosis. Ingestion of excessive amounts of fluoride during tooth formation produces defects in mineralized structures, particularly enamel matrix, with resultant hypoplasia. The severity and degree of subsequent staining generally depend on the degree of hypoplasia, which depends in turn on the amount of fluoride ingested during odontogenesis.[5] The teeth are not discolored on eruption but may appear chalky. Their surface, however, is porous, and gradually absorbs stains from chemicals in the oral cavity.

Because the discoloration is in the porous enamel, such teeth are bleached (or corrected) externally. Success depends mainly on the degree and duration of the discoloration. Some regression and reoccurrence of discoloration tend to occur but can be corrected with future rebleaching.

Systemic drugs. Administration or ingestion of certain drugs or chemicals (many of which have not been identified) during tooth formation may cause discoloration, which is occasionally severe.

The most common as well as the most dramatic discoloration of this type occurs after tetracycline ingestion, usually in children. Discoloration is usually bilateral, affecting multiple teeth in both arches. It may range from yellow through brownish to dark gray, depending on the amount, frequency, and type of tetracycline and the patient's age (stage of development) during administration. Tetracycline discoloration has been classified into three groups according to

severity.[6] First-degree discoloration is light yellow, light brown, or light gray and occurs uniformly throughout the crown without banding. Second-degree discoloration is more intense and is also without banding. Third-degree discoloration is very intense and the clinical crown exhibits horizontal color banding. This type of discoloration usually predominates in the cervical region.

Tetracycline binds to calcium, which then is incorporated into the hydroxyapatite crystal in both enamel and dentin. Most of the tetracycline is found in dentin. Chronic sun exposure of teeth with the incorporated drug may cause formation of a reddish-purple tetracycline oxidation byproduct, resulting in further discoloration of permanent teeth.

A phenomenon of adult-onset tetracycline discoloration is also reported.[7] This type of discoloration occurs occasionally in mature teeth in patients receiving long-term tetracycline therapy, usually given for control of cystic acne. The discoloration is gradual and generally is not severe.

Two approaches have been used for bleaching tetracycline discoloration. The first, which involves bleaching the external enamel surface, is of limited usefulness and is generally unsuccessful in the long term.[8] The second, root canal treatment followed by internal bleaching, is a more predictable procedure and has proved successful, in both the short and long term.[9,10] These techniques are discussed in more detail later in this chapter.

Defects in tooth formation. Defects in tooth formation are confined to the enamel and are either hypocalcific or hypoplastic. Enamel hypocalcification is common, appearing as a distinct brownish or whitish area, often on the facial aspect of a crown. The enamel is well formed and intact on the surface and feels hard to the explorer. Both the whitish and the brownish spots are amenable to bleaching with the pumice and acid technique (described later in this chapter) with good results.

Enamel hypoplasia differs from hypocalcification in that the enamel in the former is defective and porous. This condition may be hereditary (amelogenesis imperfecta) or may result from environmental factors. In the hereditary type, both deciduous and permanent dentitions are involved. Defects caused by environmental factors may involve only one or several teeth. Presumably during tooth formation the matrix is altered and does not totally or properly mineralize. The porous enamel readily acquires stains from the oral cavity. Depending on the severity and extent of hypoplasia and the nature of the stain, these teeth may be bleached (or corrected by the acid-pumice method) from the enamel surface with some degree of success.[11] The bleaching effect may not be permanent, and stains may recur with time. These stains may, however, be recorrected. As stated earlier, it is most important to inform the patient of the likely reoccurrence of discoloration of these teeth.

Blood dyscrasias and other factors. Various systemic conditions may cause massive lysis of erythrocytes. If this occurs in the pulp at an early age, blood disintegration products are incorporated into and discolor the forming dentin. An example of this phenomenon is the severe discoloration of primary teeth that usually follows erythroblastosis fetalis. This disease in the fetus or newborn results from Rh incompatibility factors, which lead to massive systemic lysis of erythrocytes. Large amounts of hemosiderin pigment then stain the forming dentin of the primary teeth. This type of lysis is now uncommon because of new preventive measures. This discoloration is not correctable by bleaching.

High fever during tooth formation may result in linear defined hypoplasia. This condition, known as chronologic hypoplasia, is a temporary disruption in enamel formation that results in a banding-type of surface defect that acquires stain. Porphyria, a metabolic disease, may cause deciduous and permanent teeth to show a red or brownish discoloration. Thalassemia and sickle cell anemia may cause intrinsic blue, brown, or green discolorations. Amelogenesis imperfecta may result in yellow or brown discolorations. Dentinogenesis imperfecta can cause brownish violet, yellowish, or gray discoloration. These conditions are also not amenable to bleaching and should be corrected restoratively.

Other staining factors related to systemic conditions or ingested drugs are rare and may not be identifiable.

IATROGENIC OR INFLICTED DISCOLORATIONS

Discolorations caused by various chemicals and materials used in dentistry are usually avoidable. Many of these stains are very difficult to correct by bleaching.

Endodontically Related Discolorations

OBTURATING MATERIALS

Obturating materials are the most common and severe cause of single tooth discoloration. Incomplete removal of materials from the pulp chamber upon completion of treatment often results in dark discoloration. Such discoloration can be prevented by removing all obturation materials to a level just cervical to the gingival margin. Primary offenders are sealer remnants, whether of the zinc oxide-eugenol type or plastics.[12] The prognosis of bleaching in such cases depends on the constituents of the sealer. Sealers with metallic components often do not bleach well, and any bleaching effect tends to regress with time.

REMNANTS OF PULPAL TISSUE

Pulp fragments remaining in the crown, usually in pulp horns, may cause gradual discoloration. Pulp horns must be "opened up" and exposed during access to ensure removal of pulpal remnants and to prevent retention of sealer at a later stage. Internal bleaching in such cases is usually successful.

INTRACANAL MEDICAMENTS

Most medicaments, but not all, have the potential to cause internal discoloration of the dentin.[13] Phenolic or iodoform-based intracanal medications, sealed in the root canal space, are in direct contact with dentin, sometimes for long periods, allowing for their penetration and oxidization. These compounds have a tendency to discolor the dentin gradually. Fortunately, most discolorations are not marked and they are readily and permanently corrected by bleaching. Iodoform-induced discolorations tend to be more severe.

CORONAL RESTORATIONS

Restorations are generally of two types, metallic or composite. The reasons for discoloration (and therefore, the appropriate correction) are quite different.

Metallic Restorations

Amalgam is the worst offender because its dark-colored elements may turn dentin dark gray. If used to restore a lingual access preparation, amalgam often discolors the crown. Such discolorations are difficult to bleach and tend to reoccur with time. However, bleaching them is worth a try.

Discoloration from inappropriately placed metal pins and prefabricated posts in anterior teeth may sometimes occur. This is due to metal that can be seen through the composite or tooth structure. Occasionally, discoloration from amalgam is also caused by visibility of the restoration through translucent tooth structure. In such cases, replacement of old metallic restorations with an esthetically pleasing composite will suffice.

Composite Restorations

Microleakage of composites causes discoloration. Open margins may permit chemicals to penetrate between the restoration and tooth structure to stain the underlying dentin. In addition, composites may become discolored with time and alter the shade of the crown. These conditions can sometimes be corrected by replacing the old composite with a new well-sealed esthetic restoration. In many cases, internal bleaching is carried out first with good results.

Bleaching Materials

Bleaching chemicals may act as either oxidizing or reducing agents. Most bleaching agents are oxidizers and many preparations are available. Commonly used agents are solutions of hydrogen peroxide of different strengths, sodium perborate, and carbamide peroxide. Sodium perborate and carbamide peroxide are chemicals compounds that are gradually degraded to release low levels of hydrogen peroxide. Hydrogen peroxide and carbamide peroxide are mainly indicated for external bleaching, whereas sodium perborate is mostly used for internal bleaching. All have proved effective.

HYDROGEN PEROXIDE

Hydrogen peroxide is a powerful oxidizer that is available in various strengths, but 30% to 35% stabilized solutions (Superoxol, Perhydrol) are the most common. These high-concentration solutions must be handled with care because they are unstable, lose oxygen quickly, and may explode unless they are refrigerated and kept in a dark container.[14] Also, these are caustic chemicals and will burn tissue on contact.

SODIUM PERBORATE

This agent is available in powder form or in various commercial proprietary combinations. When fresh, it contains about 95% perborate, corresponding to 9.9% available oxygen. Sodium perborate is stable when dry, but in the presence of acid, warm air, or water it decomposes to form sodium metaborate, hydrogen peroxide, and nascent oxygen.[15] Various types of sodium perborate preparations are available: monohydrate, trihydrate, and tetrahydrate. They differ in

oxygen content, which determines their bleaching efficacy.[16] Commonly used sodium perborate preparations are alkaline, and their pH depends on the amount of hydrogen peroxide released and the residual sodium metaborate.[17]

Sodium perborate is more easily controlled and safer than concentrated hydrogen peroxide solutions. Therefore, it should be the material of choice for internal bleaching.

CARBAMIDE PEROXIDE

Carbamide peroxide, also known as urea hydrogen peroxide, is available in concentrations varying between 3% and 15%. Popular commercial preparations contain about 10% carbamide peroxide and have an average pH of 5 to 6.5. They usually also include glycerin or propylene glycol, sodium stannate, phosphoric or citric acid, and flavor. In some preparations Carbopol, a water soluble resin, is added to prolong the release of active peroxide and to improve shelf life. Ten percent carbamide peroxide breaks down into urea, ammonia, carbon dioxide, and approximately 3.5% hydrogen peroxide.

Carbamide peroxide systems are for external bleaching and have been associated with varying degrees (usually slight) of damage to teeth and surrounding mucosa.[18,19] They may adversely affect the bond strength of composite resins and their marginal seal.[18,20,21] Therefore, these materials must be used with caution and usually under strict supervision of the dentist.

OTHER OXIDIZING AGENTS

In the past, a preparation of sodium peroxyborate monohydrate (Amosan R), which releases more oxygen than does sodium perborate, was recommended for internal bleaching.[22] Today, its clinical use is less common.

Sodium hypochlorite is a common root canal irrigant that is available commercially as a 3% to 5.25% household bleach. Although used as a household bleaching agent, it does not release enough oxidizer to be effective and is not recommended for routine bleaching.

Other nonperoxide bleaching agents were also suggested for clinical use; however, these have been no more effective than traditional agents.[23,24]

Internal (Nonvital) Bleaching Techniques

The methods most commonly used to bleach teeth in conjunction with root canal treatment are the *thermocatalytic* technique and the so-called *walking bleach* technique.[15,22] These techniques are somewhat different, but both produce similar results.[2,3] The walking bleach technique is preferred because it requires the least chair time and is more comfortable and safer for the patient. The walking bleach technique is described in detail later in this chapter. Whatever technique is used, the active ingredient is the oxidizer, which is available in different chemical forms. The least potent form is preferred.

Indications for internal bleaching technique are (1) discolorations of pulp chamber origin, (2) dentin discolorations, and (3) discolorations that are not amenable to external bleaching. Contraindications are (1) superficial enamel discolorations, (2) defective enamel formation, (3) severe dentin loss, (4) presence of caries, and (5) discolored composites.

THERMOCATALYTIC TECHNIQUE

The thermocatalytic technique involves placing the oxidizing agent in the pulp chamber and then applying heat. Heat may be supplied by heat lamps, flamed instruments, or electrical heating devices, which are manufactured specifically to bleach teeth.

Potential damage from the thermocatalytic approach includes the possibility of external cervical root resorption because of irritation to cementum and periodontal ligament, possibly from the oxidizing agent in combination with heat.[25,26] Therefore, the application of heat during bleaching should be limited. The thermocatalytic technique has not proved more effective than other methods and is not recommended for routine internal bleaching.

A thermocatalytic variation is ultraviolet photooxidation. Ultraviolet light is applied to the labial surface. A 30% to 35% hydrogen peroxide solution is placed in the chamber on a cotton pellet, followed by a 2-minute exposure to ultraviolet light. Supposedly, this causes the release of oxygen similar to that seen in other thermocatalytic bleaching techniques.[27,28]

There has been little clinical experience in the use of ultraviolet photo-oxidation. Probably, it is no more effective than the walking bleach technique and requires more chair time.

WALKING BLEACH

The walking bleach technique should be used in all situations requiring internal bleaching. Not only is it as effective as the techniques previously described, but it also is the safest and requires the least chair time (Box 23-1).[29-32]

It is commonly believed that "overbleaching" is desirable because of future reoccurrence of discoloration. However, bleaching a tooth to a lighter shade than its neighbors should be performed with caution; the overbleached tooth may not discolor again.[33] A tooth that is too light may be as unesthetic as one too dark.

Repeat treatments are similar. If early bleaching does not provide satisfactory results, the following additional procedures may be attempted. (1) A thin layer of stained facial dentin is removed with a small round bur (see step 7). (2) The walking bleach paste is strengthened by mixing the sodium perborate with increasing concentrations of hydrogen peroxide (3% to 30%) instead of water. The more potent oxidizer may enhance the bleaching effect, but with the possibility of subsequent root resorption.[25,26]

Recently, 10% carbamide peroxide was suggested for internal bleaching.[34] This agent, however, is probably not superior to sodium perborate.

Although usually the final results are excellent, occasionally only partial lightening is achieved. Surprisingly, the patient often is very pleased and satisfied with a modest improvement and does not expect perfection.[35] Therefore, internal bleaching is worth the attempt.

FINAL RESTORATION

The pulp chamber and access cavity are restored at the final visit (Figure 23-2, *E*). Although it has been proposed that substances (such as acrylic monomer or silicones) be placed in the chamber to fill the dentinal tubules, this is beneficial. Furthermore, these substances may themselves lead to discoloration with time. However, it is important to restore the chamber carefully and to seal the lingual access to augment the new shade and prevent leakage. The ideal method for filling the chamber after tooth bleaching has not been determined. However, by no means should the chamber be filled totally with composite, because this causes a loss of translucency and an actual darkening of the tooth.[36]

It is easy and effective to fill the chamber with a light-colored gutta-percha temporary stopping, glass ionomer, or a light shade of zinc phosphate cement and then to restore the lingual access with a light-cured acid-etched composite (Figure 23-2, *E*).[37] An adequate depth of composite should be ensured to seal the cavity and provide some incisal support. Light curing from the labial, rather than the lingual, surface is recommended, because this results in shrinkage of the composite resin toward the axial walls, reducing

---

BOX 23-1

Walking Bleach Technique

The steps involved in walking bleach are the following (Figure 23-2):

1. As stated earlier, the patient is familiarized with the probable causes of staining, the procedure to be followed, the expected outcome, and the possibility of future reoccurrence of discoloration (regression). To avoid disappointment or misunderstanding, effective communication before, during, and after treatment is absolutely necessary.

2. Radiographs are made to assess the status of the periapical tissues and the quality of root canal treatment. Treatment failure or questionable obturation requires retreatment before bleaching.

3. The quality and shade of any restoration present are assessed; if defective, the restoration is replaced. Often, tooth discoloration results from leaking or discolored restorations. Also, the patient is informed that the bleaching procedure may temporarily (or permanently) affect the color of the restoration, requiring its replacement.

4. Tooth color is evaluated with a shade guide, and clinical photographs are taken at the beginning of and throughout the procedure. These provide a point of reference for future comparison by both dentist and patient.

5. The tooth is isolated with a rubber dam. Interproximal wedges may also be used for better isolation. If Superoxol is used, protective cream (such as petroleum jelly, Orabase, or cocoa butter) must be applied to the gingival tissues before dam placement. This protection is not required with sodium perborate use.

6. The restorative material is removed from the access cavity (Figure 23-2, *B*). Refinement of access and removal of all old obturating materials from the pulp chamber comprise the most important stage in the bleaching process. There must be a check that pulp horns or other "hidden" areas are opened.

   A chamber totally filled with composite presents a major problem. First, this material is resistant to cutting with burs. Second, its shade is often indistinct from that of dentin. However, all composite must be removed to allow the bleaching agent to contact and penetrate the dentin. Care must be taken during removal to avoid inadvertent cutting of sound dentin. The operating microscope or magnifying loupes are beneficial.

7. (Optional) This step may be necessary if the discoloration seems to be of metallic origin or if on the second or third appointment bleaching alone does not seem to be sufficient. A thin layer of stained dentin is carefully removed toward the facial aspect of the chamber with a round bur in a slow-speed handpiece (Figure 23-2, *B*). This will remove much of the discoloration (which is concentrated in the pulpal surface area). It may also open the dentinal tubules for better penetration by the bleaching agents.

8. All materials should be removed to a level just below the gingival margin. Appropriate solvents (such as orange solvent, chloroform, or xylol on a cotton pellet) are used to dissolve remnants of the common sealers.

9. If Superoxol is used, a sufficient layer of protective cement barrier (such as polycarboxylate, zinc phosphate, glass ionomer, intermediate restorative material (IRM), or Cavit at least 2 mm thick) is applied on the obturating material. This is essential to minimize leakage of bleaching agents.[29] The barrier should protect the dentin tubules and conform to the external epithelial attachment.[30] It should not extend incisal to the gingival margin (Figure 23-2, *C*).

   Acid etching of dentin internally with phosphoric (or other) acid to remove the smear layer and open the tubules is not effective.[31] The use of any caustic chemical in the chamber is unwarranted because periodontal ligament irritation or external root resorption may result. The same reservation applies to solvents such as ether or acetone before application of the bleaching agent. The application of concentrated hydrogen peroxide with heat (thermocatalytic) has been suggested as the next step. As mentioned earlier, this is questionable from a safety standpoint.

10. The walking bleach paste is prepared by mixing sodium perborate and an inert liquid such as water, saline, or anesthetic solution to a consistency of wet sand (approximately 2 g/ml). Although sodium perborate mixed with 30% hydrogen peroxide will bleach faster, in most cases the long-term results are similar to those of sodium perborate mixed with water, and therefore the former mixture should not be used routinely.[2,3,15,32] Another advantage of sodium perborate and inert liquid is that the protective cement barrier and gingival protection are unnecessary. With a plastic instrument, the chamber is packed with the paste. Excess liquid is removed by tamping with a cotton pellet. This also compresses and pushes the paste into the recesses (Figure 23-2, *C*).

11. Excess oxidizing paste is removed from undercuts in the pulp horns and gingival area with an explorer. A cotton pellet is not used but a thick mix of Cavit or zinc oxide-eugenol (preferably IRM) is applied directly against the paste and into the undercuts. The temporary filling is packed carefully to a thickness of at least 3 mm to ensure a good seal (Figure 23-2, *D*).

12. The rubber dam is removed. The patient is informed that the bleaching agent works slowly and that significant lightening may not be evident for 2 or more weeks. It is common to see no change initially, but dramatic results occur in successive days or weeks or after a future reapplication.

13. The patient is scheduled to return approximately 2 to 6 weeks later, and the procedure is repeated. If at any future appointment (third or fourth), progressive lightening is not evident, further walking bleach treatments with a sodium perborate and water solution may not prove beneficial.[32]

the rate of microleakage.[38] Proper restoration is essential for long-term successful bleaching results. Coronal microleakage of lingual access restorations is a problem[39]; a leaky restoration may lead to reoccurrence of discoloration.

Residual peroxides of bleaching agents, mainly hydrogen peroxide and carbamide peroxide, may affect the bonding strength of composites to the tooth.[21,40] Therefore, it is not recommended that the tooth be restored with composite immediately

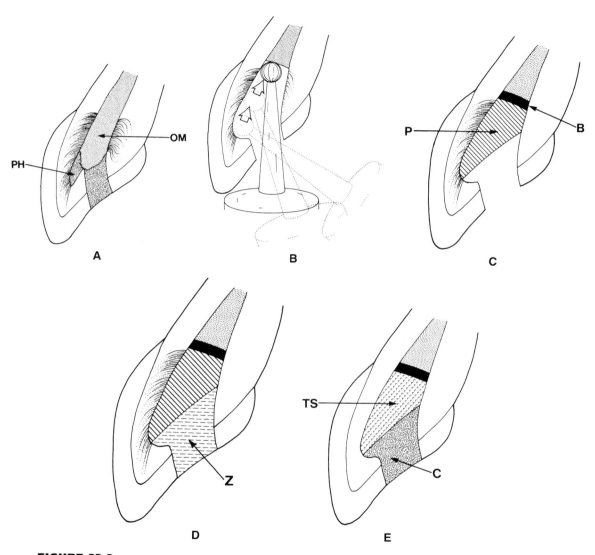

FIGURE 23-2

Walking bleach. **A,** Internal staining of dentin caused by remnants of obturating materials *(OM)* in the chamber, as well as by materials and tissue debris in pulp horns *(PH)*. **B,** Coronal restoration is removed completely, access preparation is improved, and gutta-percha is removed to just below the cervical margin. Next, the pulp horns are cleaned with a round bur (shaving a thin layer of dentin from the facial wall is optional and may be attempted at later appointments if discoloration persists). **C,** A protective cement base *(B)* is placed over the gutta-percha, not extending above the cervical margin. After removal of sealer remnants and materials from the chamber with solvents, a paste *(P)* composed of sodium perborate and water (mixed to the consistency of wet sand) is placed. The incisal area is undercut to retain the temporary restoration. **D,** A thick mix of zinc oxide–eugenol type temporary filling *(Z)* seals access. **E,** At a subsequent appointment, when the desired shade has been reached, a permanent restoration is placed. A suggested method is to fill the chamber with white temporary stopping *(TS)* or with light polycarboxylate or zinc phosphate base. Acid-etched composite *(C)* restores lingual access and extends into the pulp horns for retention and to support of the incisal. (From Walton RE: Bleaching procedures for teeth with vital and nonvital pulps. In Levine N, editor: *Current treatment in dental practice*, Philadelphia, 1986, WB Saunders.)

after bleaching but only after an interval of a few days. The use of catalase has also been proposed for fast elimination of residual peroxides from the access cavity[41]; this merits further investigation.

Another suggestion is that packing calcium hydroxide paste in the chamber for a few weeks before the final restoration is placed would reverse the acidity caused by bleaching agents and prevent resorption. This procedure is ineffective and unnecessary.[17,26]

WHEN TO BLEACH

Internal bleaching may be performed at various intervals after root canal treatment (Figures 23-3 and 23-4). The appearance of the discolored tooth may be improved soon after treatment. However, the walking bleach technique may be initiated at the same appointment as the endodontic obturation. In fact, this may motivate the patient to accept bleaching because the appearance of the discolored tooth may be improved soon after treatment. Bleaching may also be attempted successfully many years after discoloration has occurred (Figures 23-5 and 23-6). Such teeth show no markedly greater tendency toward reoccurrence of discoloration than teeth stained for shorter periods.[33] However, it is probable that a shorter discoloration period tends to improve the chances for successful bleaching as well as to reduce the likelihood of reoccurrence of discoloration.[42]

Other factors that may influence long-term success have also been evaluated clinically. The patient's age and the rate of discoloration have no major effect on the long-term stability of bleaching.[33]

Complications and Safety

Patient safety is always the major concern in any procedure. Some possible adverse effects produced by chemicals and bleaching procedures are listed in the following section.

EXTERNAL RESORPTION

Clinical reports[43-45] and histologic studies[25,26] have shown that internal bleaching may induce external root resorption. The oxidizing agent, particularly 30% hydrogen peroxide, may be the culprit. However, the exact mechanism by which periodontium or cementum is damaged has not been elucidated. Presumably, the irritating chemical diffuses through the dentinal tubules[46] and reaches the periodontium through defects in the cementoenamel junction.[47] Chemicals combined with heat are likely to cause necrosis of the cementum, inflammation of the periodontal ligament, and root resorption.[25,26] The process is liable to be enhanced in the presence of bacteria.[48] Previous traumatic injury and young age may also act as predisposing factors.[43]

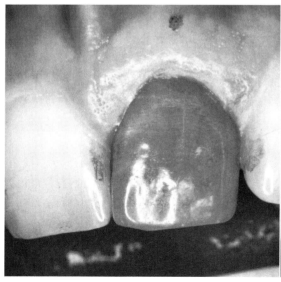 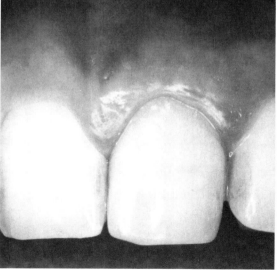

FIGURE 23-3
A, Discoloration as a result of a traumatic injury followed by pulp necrosis. **B,** After root canal treatment, a paste of sodium perborate and water to a consistency of wet sand was sealed in the chamber. After 21 days of "walking bleach" the tooth regained its original shade. (Courtesy Dr. A. Claisse.)

Therefore, injurious chemicals and procedures should be avoided if they are not essential for bleaching. Also, below the cervical margin, oxidizing agents should not be exposed to more of the pulp space and dentin than is absolutely necessary to obtain a satisfactory clinical result.

CORONAL FRACTURE

Increased brittleness of the coronal tooth structure, particularly when heat is applied, is also thought to result from bleaching. This may be due to desiccation of the dentin and enamel. Clinical experience suggests that bleached teeth are no more susceptible to fracture, although this has not been proven conclusively.

CHEMICAL BURNS

As mentioned earlier, sodium perborate is safe, but 30% hydrogen peroxide is caustic and will cause chemical burns and sloughing of gingiva. When this strong chemical is used, the soft tissues should be coated with an isolating cream. Animal studies suggest that catalase applied to oral tissues before hydrogen peroxide treatment fully prevents the associated tissue damage.[49]

External (Vital) Bleaching Techniques

Results of the so-called vital bleaching technique (application of oxidizer to the enamel surface of a tooth with vital pulp) are much less predictable.

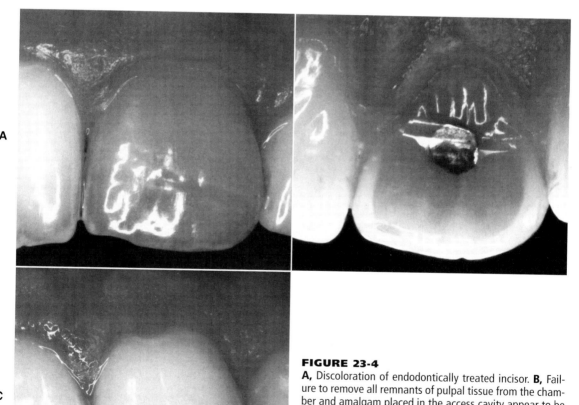

A

B

C

FIGURE 23-4
A, Discoloration of endodontically treated incisor. **B,** Failure to remove all remnants of pulpal tissue from the chamber and amalgam placed in the access cavity appear to be the causes of discoloration. **C,** Removal of amalgam, intracoronal bleaching, and placement of a new composite restored esthetics. (Courtesy Dr. A. Claisse.)

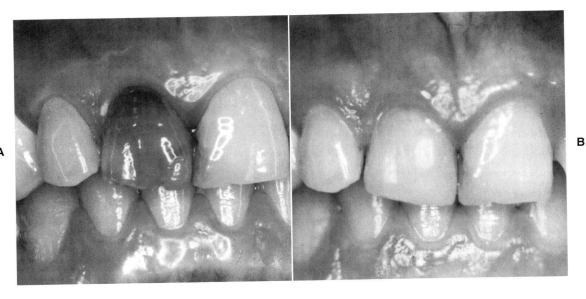

FIGURE 23-5
A, Discoloration as a result of trauma and subsequent treatment. The patient was involved in an accident caus-ing coronal fracture. Root canal treatment was done, but gutta-percha and sealer were not completely removed from the chamber. An additional discoloration factor was the defective leaking restoration. **B,** Two appointments of "walking bleach" and placement of a new well-sealed composite restored esthetics. (Courtesy Dr. M. Israel.)

More variables are present with this technique than with internal bleaching. When discolora-tions are in dentin, bleaching agents placed on rel-atively impermeable enamel have less chance of reaching the stain. If discoloration is on the enamel surface or the enamel is defective and porous, a better result is expected.

Many techniques have been advocated for external bleaching of vital teeth. Some condi-tions and types of discoloration are potentially treatable by this method; others are not. Criti-cal factors are the location and nature of the discoloration.

Indications for these bleaching methods usually are (1) light enamel discolorations, (2) endemic fluorosis discolorations, and (3) age-related dis-colorations. Contraindications are (1) severe dark discolorations, (2) severe enamel loss, (3) close proximity of pulp horns, (4) presence of caries, (5) hypersensitive teeth, and (6) poor coronal restorations.

INTRINSIC DISCOLORATIONS

Intrinsic discolorations are those incorporated into tooth structure during tooth formation.[50] Significantly, most of these discolorations are in dentin and are relatively difficult to treat ex-ternally.[51] A good example is staining due to tetracycline, which is incorporated into the min-eral structure of the developing tooth. The in-corporated tetracycline imparts its color to the dentin.

Tetracycline

Both external and internal bleaching techniques have been advocated as means of improving the appearance of tetracycline discolored teeth. As noted earlier, the internal technique is more effec-tive.[10,11,51,52] However, the best resolution for tetra-cycline discolorations is prevention.

External bleaching. Techniques advocated for applying oxidizing agents to enamel surface are largely based on case reports. Long-term follow-up studies in humans are limited and partial suc-cess has been seen only for light-yellow stained teeth in young patients. The more prevalent darker discolorations have generally shown little response to surface bleaching, although at its in-troduction the vital bleaching technique gener-ated considerable optimism.

Animal studies of tetracycline-stained teeth demonstrated that success is minimal.[9,51] External bleaching was done after dogs were given large doses of discoloring tetracycline. Although a sig-nificantly lighter shade of the enamel surface could be obtained, the original dark color soon reappeared.[51] Techniques used in these studies were similar to those proposed for humans.

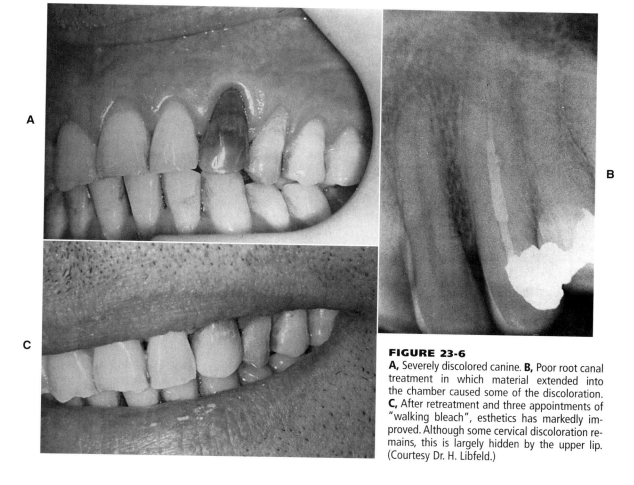

FIGURE 23-6
A, Severely discolored canine. **B,** Poor root canal treatment in which material extended into the chamber caused some of the discoloration. **C,** After retreatment and three appointments of "walking bleach", esthetics has markedly improved. Although some cervical discoloration remains, this is largely hidden by the upper lip. (Courtesy Dr. H. Libfeld.)

Technique. Basically the technique involves application of 30% hydrogen peroxide to the enamel surface combined with the application of heat (+125° F) (commercial instruments are available). Supposedly, higher temperature (+142° F) and repeated applications as well as numerous treatments are beneficial.[53] Photobleaching dentin by shortwave ultraviolet light has also been suggested.[28]

Results obtained over time must be evaluated with clinical photographs. Regression to the original shade confirms that bleaching has been ineffective and that repetition of the procedure is not indicated. As stated earlier, success is more common with yellowish or cream discoloration but not gray discoloration.

Safety. The benefits of these bleaching techniques are questionable, and the effect of the bleaching solution or heat on the underlying pulp is a matter of concern. Various studies have shown that bleaching agents may penetrate the pulp chamber through enamel and dentin and alter the activity of certain pulpal enzymes.[54,55] Although long-term irreversible effects on the pulp were usually not demonstrated, the procedure must be approached with caution.[56,57]

Internal bleaching. Internal bleaching of tetracycline-stained teeth has been shown clinically[10,58,59] and experimentally[52] to lighten severe discolorations. Effects persist for long periods, perhaps indefinitely.

The technique involves root canal treatment followed by an internal walking bleach technique, as outlined earlier in this chapter (Figure 23-7). If the procedure is explained to patients, they may accept this approach with gratifying results.

Other Intrinsic Discolorations

Other drugs or ingested chemicals are incorporated into teeth that are forming and cause discoloration; there are no reports of attempts to bleach these teeth. Presumably attempts to lighten teeth with dentinal discolorations by the

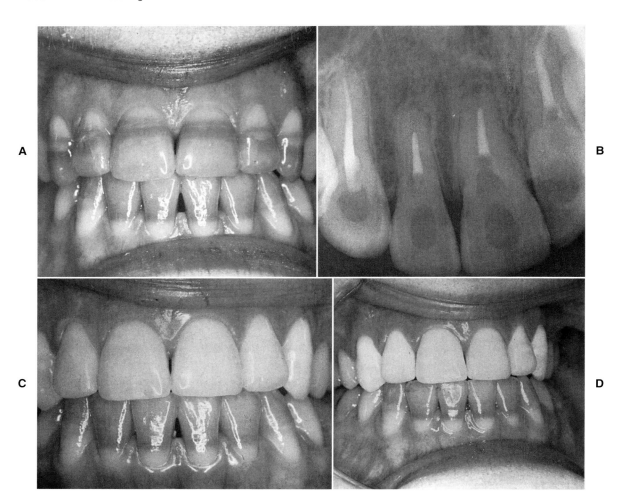

FIGURE 23-7
A, Characteristic grayish discoloration and banding of tetracycline discolorations. Cervical regions on maxillary and mandibular teeth show no discoloration; tetracycline was not administered during those periods of tooth development. **B,** Root canal treatments have been completed on the maxillary anterior teeth, with subsequent "walking bleach" procedures. **C,** After the necessary number of bleaching appointments, the teeth are restored permanently. Note the marked contrast with the mandibular incisors, which remain untreated. **D,** A 4-year follow-up shows no regression and no recurrence of discoloration. (Courtesy Dr. H. Wayne Mohorn.)

external application of bleaching agents would be only marginally effective.

EXTRINSIC DISCOLORATIONS

These discolorations are more superficial and are obviously more amenable to external bleaching. The success of bleaching, however, depends more on the depth of the stain in the enamel rather than on the color of the stain itself.

Superficial Defects

Although a number of conditions may result in hypoplasia of enamel accompanied by porosity, the most common and often the most disfiguring is endemic fluorosis. This hypoplastic defect may result in various degrees and colors of superficial stains.

Mechanism of discoloration. Ingestion of high levels of fluoride during tooth formation disrupts the ameloblasts and leads to hypoplasia of the forming enamel.[60] After tooth eruption, the porous enamel is gradually discolored. The discoloration may vary from chalky white through light yellow and brown to almost black, depending on the degree of fluorosis (enamel porosity) and the type of chemical stain.

The appearance of all such discolorations may be improved with bleaching or other measures, some dramatically. Although a variety of tech-

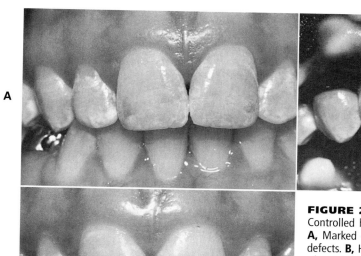

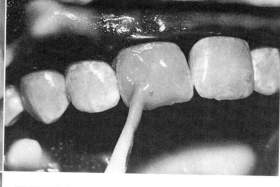

FIGURE 23-8
Controlled hydrochloric acid–pumice abrasion technique. **A,** Marked discoloration results from surface hypoplastic defects. **B,** Hydrochloric acid 18% is mixed with fine flour of pumice to form a thick paste, which is applied to the surface with a crushed orangewood stick. The paste is worked into the enamel with a swirling motion for 5 seconds; this is followed by a water rinse. Paste is reapplied as necessary. Finally, acid is neutralized with sodium bicarbonate. **C,** The desired improvement was obtained in a single appointment. There was no regression. (Courtesy Dr. S. Goepferd.)

niques involving different chemicals and procedures have been suggested, probably the most effective is the "controlled hydrochloric acid-pumice abrasion" technique.[11] This is not a true bleaching (oxidizing) technique but decalcification and removal of a thin layer of stained enamel. This technique has been modified somewhat since its development in the mid 1980s.[11,61]

Acid-pumice technique. The procedure is as follows (Figure 23- 8):
1. The teeth to be treated are photographed to serve as a permanent record and as a basis for future comparison.
2. The gingiva is protected, and the teeth are carefully isolated with an inverted rubber dam and ligatures. The rubber dam is extended over the patient's nostrils.
3. Exposed areas of the patient's face and eyes are covered with a suitable drape or towel for added safety from acid spatter.
4. A 36% hydrochloric acid solution is mixed with an equal volume of distilled water to make an 18% hydrochloric acid solution. A substantial amount of fine flour of pumice is added to form a thick paste. In another dappen dish, sodium bicarbonate and water are mixed to a thick paste, which will be used later for acid neutralization. Ready-made commercial products are also available.

5. The hydrochloric acid and pumice paste is applied to the enamel surface with a piece of wooden tongue blade or crushed orangewood stick. Exerting firm pressure, the paste is worked into the enamel surface with a swirling motion for 5 seconds. The enamel surface is then rinsed for 10 seconds with water.
6. The paste is reapplied until the desired color is achieved.
7. The surface is neutralized with sodium bicarbonate and water. The rubber dam is removed, and the teeth are pumiced with a fine prophylactic paste to smooth the abraded surface. Usually the desired shade is obtained in a single appointment. If not, the stains may be too deep and not amenable to lightening.

Alternative techniques. Another traditional approach, the McInnes technique,[62] is essentially similar to the previous one but uses a solution composed of five parts of 30% hydrogen peroxide, five parts of 36% hydrochloric acid, and one part of diethyl ether. The solution is applied directly to the stained areas for 1 to 2 minutes with cotton applicators. While the surface is wet, a fine cuttle disc is run over the stained surfaces for 15 seconds. This process is repeated several times.

Additional appointments may be necessary to bleach the tooth to the desired shade. The number of appointments increases with the severity of the stain.

Comparison of techniques. The acid-pumice method does not actually bleach the stain as in the McInnes technique, which uses hydrogen peroxide. The acid-pumice technique is probably the most effective and requires the least amount of chair time.

Prognosis. The acid-pumice abrasion technique is relatively permanent if initial lightening is achieved. Many patients have been followed for long periods of time with no reoccurrence of discoloration.[11]

Safety. There are two areas in which safety is a concern: the effects on enamel (excessive decalcification) and chemical burns of soft tissue.

With care and judicious application of acid in either of the hydrochloric acid techniques, an insignificant amount of enamel is removed. Chemical burns of the gingiva by either concentrated acid or hydrogen peroxide may be easily prevented by coating the gingiva with isolating materials, inverting the rubber dam, and ligating the teeth. There are minimal to no pulpal effects, at least with the McInnes technique.[63] Other studies using radioactive labels demonstrated an absence of penetration of such agents into the pulp chamber as well as a decrease in enamel permeability.[64]

Mouthguard Bleaching

This technique is generally used for mild discolorations. It has been basically advocated as a home bleaching technique, and there are wide variations in materials, bleaching agents, and frequency and duration of treatment.[65] Numerous products are available for both home and in-office use. Most are composed of either 1.5% to 10% hydrogen peroxide or 10% to 15% carbamide peroxide, which degrades slowly to release hydrogen peroxide. Higher concentrations of the active ingredient are also available and may reach up to 50%, levels that are very toxic and contraindicated. The carbamide peroxide products are more commonly used, although carbamide peroxide (20%) and hydrogen peroxide (7.5%) have been shown to be equally effective and safe.[66]

BLEACHING TECHNIQUE

Owing to a lack of consensus about treatment techniques, step-by-step instructions shown in Box 23-2 should be used only as a general guideline.

ALTERNATIVE TECHNIQUES

A modification of technique has been suggested in which the discolored tooth is first treated

---

BOX 23-2

Bleaching Procedure

1. The patient is familiarized with the probable causes of discoloration, the procedure to be followed, and the expected outcome.
2. Prophylaxis is performed, and the color of the teeth is assessed with a shade guide. Photographs are taken at the beginning of and throughout the procedure.
3. An alginate impression is made of the arch to be treated. The guard is outlined in the cast model. It should completely cover the teeth in the arch; second molars do not need to be covered unless required for retention. Two layers of die relief are placed on the buccal aspects of the cast teeth to form a small reservoir for the bleaching agent. A vacuum-formed soft plastic matrix approximately 2 mm thick is fabricated and trimmed with crown and bridge scissors to 1 mm past the gingival margins; this is then adjusted with an acrylic trimming bur.
4. The mouthguard is inserted to ensure proper fit. The guard is removed and the bleaching agent applied in the space of each tooth to be bleached. The mouthguard is then reinserted over the teeth, and excess bleaching agent is removed.

5. The patient is familiarized with the use of the bleaching agent and with the method of wearing the guard. The procedure is usually performed for 3 to 4 hours a day, and the bleaching agent is replenished every 30 to 60 minutes. Some practitioners recommend wearing the guard during sleep for better long-term esthetic results; this is of little benefit because the oxidizer is exhausted fairly rapidly.
6. The patient is informed about possible thermal sensitivity and minor irritation of soft tissues; use of the guard is discontinued if it is uncomfortable.
7. Treatment continues for 4 to 24 weeks. The patient is recalled every 2 weeks to monitor lightening or complications. Evidence of tissue irritation, oral lesions, enamel etching, and leaky restorations is sought. If complications occur, treatment is stopped and the patient is reevaluated for the feasibility of its continuation at a later date. Note that incisal edges often bleach more than the remainder of the crown.

by enamel microabrasion (acid-pumice) and later by home bleaching (carbamide peroxide mouth-guard system).[66] This method enhances the esthetic results of the enamel microabrasion technique.

PROGNOSIS

Long-term esthetic results of mouthguard bleaching are still unknown although short-term effectiveness is very good.[67,68] Reoccurrence of discoloration occurs no more often than with the other techniques.

SAFETY

The techniques, if well controlled, are relatively safe and have little effect on sound enamel.[69] Adverse effects such as unpleasant taste, burning sensation in the oral tissues, and tooth sensitivity may be associated with these products. Effects are usually temporary and disappear within several days. However, accidental ingestion of large amounts of bleaching gel is of concern. Animal studies have indicated that ingestion of large amounts of bleaching gel is toxic and may cause irritation to the gastric and respiratory mucosa.[70] Bleaching gels containing carbopol, which retards the rate of oxygen release from peroxide, are usually more toxic.

Mouthguard bleaching is contraindicated in patients with hypersensitive teeth, bruxism, or allergic reactions to any of the bleaching product components. Gingival irritation is apparently minor.[71] Although peroxide may penetrate the pulp in teeth with esthetic restorations, the amount and effect are probably insignificant.[55]

Some studies suggest that certain damage to composite resins may occur.[18,20,21] Therefore, patients must be informed that old composites may require replacement after bleaching. It was also reported that bleaching agents enhance the liberation of mercury from amalgam restorations, thus possibly increasing exposure of patients to toxic byproducts.[72-74] Although bleaching gels are mainly applied to anterior teeth, excessive gel may inadvertently make contact with amalgam restorations placed in premolar and molar teeth. Coverage of amalgam restorations with a protective layer (such as Copalite) before gel application may be beneficial.[75]

To date, few conclusive experimental or clinical studies on the safety of prolonged use of these bleaching agents are available. Therefore, caution should be exercised in prescribing and applying them. Of major concern are the products marketed directly to the public (over the counter), often without professional control. The use of these materials should be discouraged.

Laser Bleaching

This relatively new technique uses laser energy for bleaching vital teeth.[76,77] The bleaching effect is achieved by a laser-induced chemical oxidation process, which rapidly breaks down the hydrogen peroxide to oxygen and water. Two types of lasers are usually used: the argon laser, which emits visible blue light at a wavelength of 480 nm; and the CO_2 laser, which emits invisible infrared light at a wavelength of 10,600 nm. The argon laser is absorbed by dark colors and therefore can easily remove yellow-brown discolorations. The CO_2 laser, which has no affinity to colors, emits heat and thus enhances the bleaching effect initiated by the argon laser. These lasers are designed to work in conjunction with patented commercial catalysts that are applied on the external surfaces of the discolored teeth. The combination of catalyst and peroxide is potentially damaging; exposed soft tissues, eyes, and clothing must be carefully protected.

Combined use of argon and CO_2 lasers can effectively reduce intrinsic stains in dentin. The argon laser can remove stain molecules without overheating the pulp but becomes less effective as the tooth whitens. The CO_2 laser interacts directly with the catalyst-peroxide combination and removes the stain regardless of tooth color.

Some laser bleaching techniques involve hydrogen peroxide formulations at high concentrations (up to 50%). Although such techniques lightened teeth faster, severe postoperative tooth sensitivity was a common complication. Also, 50% hydrogen peroxide is a caustic chemical.

Laser bleaching is a relatively new technique. Sufficient controlled long-term studies of safety and efficacy are currently lacking.

When and What to Refer

Most bleaching procedures can be performed by general dentists, particularly if the cause of the discoloration is diagnosed. If the general practitioner cannot make this identification, referral to a specialist should be considered.

The practitioner may also wish to refer patients whose tooth discoloration does not respond to conventional methods of bleaching, either external or internal. Unidentified factors may be preventing the bleaching chemicals from effectively reaching the stain. The specialist may be able to identify and correct these factors.

REFERENCES

1. Walton R: Bleaching procedures for teeth with vital and nonvital pulps. In Levine N, editor: *Current treatment in dental practice,* Philadelphia, 1986, WB Saunders.

2. Rotstein I, Zalkind M, Mor C, et al: In vitro efficacy of sodium perborate preparations used for intracoronal bleaching of discolored non-vital teeth, *Endod Dent Traumatol* 7:177, 1991.

3. Rotstein I, Mor C, Friedman S: Prognosis of intracoronal bleaching with sodium perborate preparations in vitro: 1 year study, *J Endod* 19:10, 1993.

4. Jacobsen I, Kerkes K: Long-term prognosis of traumatized permanent anterior teeth showing calcifying processes in the pulp cavity, *Scand J Dent Res* 85:588, 1977.

5. Driscoll W, Herschel S, Meyers R, et al: Prevalence of dental caries and dental fluorosis in areas with optimal and above-optimal water fluoride concentrations, *J Am Dent Assoc* 107:42, 1983.

6. Jordan R, Boskman L: Conservative vital bleaching treatment of discolored dentition, *Compend Contin Educ Dent* 5:803, 1984.

7. Chiappinelli J, Walton R: Tooth discoloration resulting from long-term tetracycline therapy: a case report, *Quintessence Int* 23:539, 1992.

8. Corcoran J, Zillich R: Bleaching of vital tetracycline stained teeth, *J Mich Dent Assoc* 56:340, 1974.

9. Walton R, O'Dell N, Lake F: Internal bleaching of tetracycline stained teeth in dogs, *J Endod* 9:10, 1983.

10. Abou-Rass M: Long-term prognosis of intentional endodontics and internal bleaching of tetracycline-stained teeth, *Compend Contin Educ Dent* 19:1034, 1998.

11. Croll T: Enamel microabrasion: observations after 10 years, *J Am Dent Assoc* 128:45S, 1997.

12. Van der Burgt T, Plasschaert A: Bleaching of tooth discoloration caused by endodontic sealers, *J Endod* 12:231, 1986.

13. Kim S, Abbott P, McGinley P: Effects of Ledermix paste on discoloration of mature teeth, *Int Endod J* 33:227, 2000.

14. Hardman P, Moor D, Petteway G: Stability of hydrogen peroxide as a bleaching agent, *Gen Dent* 33:121, 1985.

15. Spasser H: A simple bleaching technique using sodium perborate, *NY State Dent J* 27:332, 1961.

16. Weiger R, Kuhn A, and Löst C: In vitro comparison of various types of sodium perborate used for intracoronal bleaching, *J Endod* 20:338, 1994.

17. Rotstein I, Friedman S: pH variation among materials used for intracoronal bleaching, *J Endod* 17:376, 1991.

18. Swift E, Perdigao J: Effects of bleaching on teeth and restorations, *Compend Contin Educ Dent* 19:815, 1998.

19. Li Y: Tooth bleaching using peroxide-containing agents: current status of safety issues, *Compend Contin Educ Dent* 19:783, 1998.

20. Crim GA: Post-operative bleaching: effect on microleakage, *Am J Dent* 5:109, 1992.

21. Titley K, Torneck C, Ruse N: The effect of carbamide-peroxide gel on the shear bond strength of a microfil resin to bovine enamel, *J Dent Res* 71:20, 1992.

22. Nutting E, Poe G: Chemical bleaching of discolored endodontically treated teeth, *Dent Clin North Am* 15:655, 1970.

23. Marin P, Heithersay G, Bridges T: A quantitative comparison of traditional and non-peroxide bleaching agents, *Endod Dent Traumatol* 14:64, 1998.

24. Kaneko J, Inoue S, Kawakami S, Sano H: Bleaching effect of sodium percarbonate on discolored teeth in vitro, *J Endod* 26:25, 2000.

25. Madison S, Walton R: Cervical root resorption following bleaching of endodontically treated teeth, *J Endod* 16:570, 1990.

26. Rotstein I, Friedman S, Mor C, et al: Histological characterization of bleaching-induced external root resorption in dogs, *J Endod* 17:436, 1991.

27. Howell R: Bleaching discolored root-filled teeth, *Br Dent J* 148:159, 1980.

28. Lin L, Pitts D, Burgess L: An investigation into the feasibility of photobleaching tetracycline-stained teeth, *J Endod* 14:293, 1988.

29. Rotstein I, Zyskind D, Lewinstein I, Bamberger N: Effect of different protective base materials on hydrogen peroxide leakage during intracoronal bleaching in vitro, *J Endod* 18:114, 1992.

30. Steiner D, West J: A method to determine the location and shape of an intracoronal bleach barrier, *J Endod* 20:304, 1994.

31. Casey L, Schindler W, Murata S, Burgess J: The use of dentinal etching with endodontic bleaching procedures, *J Endod* 15:535, 1989.

32. Holmstrup G, Palm A, Lambjerg-Hansen H: Bleaching of discoloured root-filled teeth, *Endod Dent Traumatol* 4:197, 1988.

33. Howell R: The prognosis of bleached root-filled teeth, *Int Endod J* 14:22, 1981.

34. Vachon C, Vanek P, Friedman S: Internal bleaching with 10% carbamide peroxide in vitro, *Pract Periodontics Aesthet Dent* 10:1145, 1998.

35. Glockner K, Hulla H, Eberleseder K, Stadtler P: Five-year follow-up of internal bleaching, *Braz Dent J* 10:105, 1999.

36. Freccia W, Peters D, Lorton L: An evaluation of various permanent restorative materials' effect on the shade of bleached teeth, *J Endod* 8:265, 1982.

37. Rivera E, Vargas M, Ricks-Williamson L: Considerations for the aesthetic restoration of endodontically treated anterior teeth following intracoronal bleaching, *Pract Periodontics Aesthet Dent* 9:117, 1997.

38. Lemon R: Bleaching and restoring endodontically treated teeth, *Curr Opin Dent* 1:754, 1991.

39. Wilcox L, Diaz-Arnold A: Coronal microleakage of permanent lingual access restorations in endodontically treated anterior teeth, *J Endod* 15:584, 1989.

40. Titley K, Torneck C, Ruse N, Krmec D: Adhesion of a resin composite to bleached and unbleached human enamel, *J Endod* 19:112, 1993.

41. Rotstein I: Role of catalase in the elimination of residual hydrogen peroxide following tooth bleaching, *J Endod* 19:567, 1993.

42. Brown G: Factors influencing successful bleaching of the discolored root-filled tooth, *Oral Surg Oral Med Oral Pathol* 20:238, 1965.

43. Harrington G, Natkin E: External resorption associated with bleaching of pulpless teeth, *J Endod* 5:344, 1979.
44. Friedman S, Rotstein I, Libfeld H, et al: Incidence of external root resorption and esthetic results in 58 bleached pulpless teeth, *Endod Dent Traumatol* 4:23, 1988.
45. Heithersay GS, Dahlstrom SW, Marin PD: Incidence of invasive cervical resorption in bleached root-filled teeth, *Aust Dent J* 39:82, 1994.
46. Rotstein I, Torek Y, Misgav R: Effect of cementum defects on radicular penetration of 30% H_2O_2 during intracoronal bleaching, *J Endod* 17:230, 1991.
47. Newvald L, Consolaro A: Cementoenamel junction: microscopic analysis and external cervical resorption, *J Endod* 26:503, 2000.
48. Heling I, Parson A, Rotstein I: Effect of bleaching agents on dentin permeability to *Streptococcus faecalis*, *J Endod* 21:540, 1995.
49. Rotstein I, Wesselink PR, Bab I: Catalase protection against hydrogen peroxide-induced injury in rat oral mucosa, *Oral Surg Oral Med Oral Pathol* 75:744, 1993.
50. Skinner H, Nalbandian J: Tetracyclines and mineralized tissues: review and perspectives, *Yale J Biol Med* 48:377, 1975.
51. Walton R, O'Dell N, Myers D, et al: External bleaching of tetracycline stained teeth in dogs, *J Endod* 8:536, 1982.
52. Lake F, O'Dell N, Walton R: The effect of internal bleaching on tetracycline in dentin, *J Endod* 11:415, 1985.
53. Seale N, Thrash W: Systematic assessment of color removal following vital bleaching of intrinsically stained teeth, *J Dent Res* 64:457, 1985.
54. Cooper J, Bokmeyer T, Bowles W: Penetration of the pulp chamber by carbamide peroxide bleaching agents, *J Endod* 18:315, 1992.
55. Gokay O, Yilmaz F, Akin S, et al: Penetration of the pulp chamber by bleaching agents in teeth restored with various restorative materials, *J Endod* 26:92, 2000.
56. Cohen S: Human pulpal response to bleaching procedures on vital teeth, *J Endod* 5:134, 1979.
57. Robertson W, Melfi R: Pulpal response to vital bleaching procedures, *J Endod* 6:645, 1980.
58. Anitua E, Zabalegui B, Gil J, et al: Internal bleaching of severe tetracycline discolorations: four-year clinical evaluation, *Quintessence Int* 21:783, 1990.
59. Aldecoa E, Mayordomo F: Modified internal bleaching of severe tetracycline discoloration: A 6-year clinical evaluation, *Quintessence Int* 23:83, 1992.
60. Walton R, Eisenmann D: Ultrastructural examination of dentine formation following multiple fluoride injections, *Arch Oral Biol* 20:485, 1975.
61. DeAbranjo F, Zia V, Dutra C: Enamel color change by microabrasion and resin-based composite, *Am J Dent* 13:6, 2000.
62. McInnes JW: Removing brown stain from teeth, *Ariz Dent J* 12:13, 1966.
63. Baumgartner JC, Reid DE, Pickett AB: Human pulpal reaction to the modified McInnes bleaching technique, *J Endod* 9:12, 1983.
64. Griffen R, Grower M, Ayer W: Effects of solutions used to treat dental fluorosis on permeability of teeth, *J Endod* 3:139, 1977.
65. Haywood V, Heymann H: Nightguard vital bleaching, *Quintessence Int* 20:173, 1989.
66. Reinhardt J, Eivins S, Swift E, Denehy G: A clinical study of nightguard vital bleaching, *Quintessence Int* 24:379, 1993.
67. Mokhlis G, Mateo B, Cochren M, Eckert G: A clinical evaluation of carbamide peroxide and hydrogen peroxide whitening agents during daytime use, *J Am Dent Assoc* 131:1269, 2000.
68. Blankenau R, Goldstein R, Haywood V: The current status of vital tooth whitening techniques, *Compend Contin Educ Dent* 20:781, 1999.
69. Potocnik I, Kosec L, Gaspersic D: Effect of 10% carbamide peroxide bleaching gel on enamel microhardness, microstructure, and mineral content, *J Endod* 26:203, 2000.
70. Redmond A, Cherry D, Bowers D Jr: Acute illness and recovery in adult female rats following ingestion of a tooth whitener containing 6% hydrogen peroxide, *Am J Dent* 10:268, 1997.
71. Schultz J, Morrissette D, Gasior E, et al: Clinical changes in the gingiva as a result of at home bleaching, *Compend Contin Educ Dent* 14:1362, 1993.
72. Hummert T, Osborne J, Norling B, Cardenas H: Mercury in solution following exposure of various amalgams to carbamide peroxide, *Am J Dent* 6:305, 1993.
73. Rotstein I, Mor C, Arwaz J: Changes in surface levels of mercury, silver, tin and copper of dental amalgam treated with carbamide peroxide and hydrogen peroxide, *Oral Surg Oral Med Oral Pathol* 83:506, 1997.
74. Rotstein I, Dogan H, Avron Y, et al: Mercury release from dental amalgam following treatment with 10% carbamide peroxide in vitro, *Oral Surg Oral Med Oral Pathol* 89:216, 2000.
75. Rotstein I, Dogan H, Avron Y, et al: Protective effect of Copalite surface coating on mercury release from dental amalgam following treatment with carbamide peroxide, *Endod Dent Traumatol* 16:107, 2000.
76. Garber D: Dentist-monitored bleaching: a discussion of combination and laser bleaching, *J Am Dent Assoc* 128(suppl.):26S, 1997.
77. Reyto R: Laser tooth whitening, *Dent Clin North Am* 42:755, 1998.

24

Neville J. McDonald and Mahmoud Torabinejad

Endodontic Surgery

LEARNING OBJECTIVES

After reading this chapter, the student should be able to:

1 / Discuss the role of endodontic surgery as compared with nonsurgical root canal therapy.

2 / Recognize situations in which surgery is not the treatment of choice.

3 / Define the terms *incision for drainage, apical curettage, root-end resection, root-end preparation and filling, root amputation, hemisection,* and *bicuspidization.*

4 / Discuss the indications for each procedure listed in Objective 3.

5 / Discuss the prognosis for each procedure listed in Objective 3.

6 / Recognize the medical or dental situations in which endodontic surgery is contraindicated or, if performed, has a questionable outcome.

7 / State the principles of flap design.

8 / Diagram the various flap designs and describe the indications, advantages, and disadvantages of each.

9 / Describe, in brief, the step-by-step procedures involved in periradicular surgery, including those for incision and reflection, access to the apex, apical curettage, root-end resection, root-end preparation and filling, flap replacement, and suturing.

10 / List the more commonly used root-end filling materials.

11 / Review the basic principles of suturing.

12 / Describe general patterns of soft and hard tissue healing.

13 / Write out postsurgical instructions to be given to the patient concerning bleeding, pain, swelling, diet, and suture removal.

14 / List and describe conditions that indicate referral to a specialist for evaluation and/or treatment.

OUTLINE

Incision for Drainage
 Indications
 Contraindications
 Procedure

Periradicular Surgery
 Indications
 Contraindications
 Sequence of Procedures

Healing
 Soft Tissue
 Hard Tissue

Corrective Surgery
 Indications
 Techniques

Root Amputation, Hemisection, and Bicuspidization
 Definitions
 Indications and Contraindications
 Techniques
 Prognosis

Conditions That Indicate Referral

Nonsurgical root canal therapy is a highly successful procedure if the diagnosis is correct and technical aspects are carefully performed.[1,2] There is a common belief that if root canal therapy fails, surgery is indicated for correction. This is not necessarily true; most failures are best corrected by retreatment. Studies have shown that more than two thirds of retreatments after original root canal therapy are successful.[3,4] However, in some situations surgery is necessary to retain a tooth that would otherwise be extracted.[5]

This chapter describes both the indications and the procedures used for endodontic surgery. Experienced clinicians and specialists should perform most of these procedures. However, general practitioners should be skilled in diagnosis and treatment planning and should be able to recognize what procedures are appropriate in different situations. In other words, clinicians must be aware of what procedures are available, in order to present these procedures to patients as treatment options. Included in this chapter are descriptions of incision for drainage, periradicular surgery, corrective surgery, root amputation, hemisection, and bicuspidization.

Incision for Drainage

Incision for drainage releases purulent and or hemorrhagic exudate from a soft tissue swelling. The objectives are to evacuate exudate and purulence, which are potent and toxic irritants. Removal speeds healing and reduces discomfort resulting from the irritants and from the buildup of pressure. Performance of most intraoral incisions is generally within the ability of general practitioners.

INDICATIONS

The best treatment for swelling originating from an acute apical abscess of pulpal origin is to establish drainage through the offending tooth (see Color Figure 24-1, *A*, following page 436). Often, adequate drainage cannot be accomplished through the tooth itself; the second choice is to obtain soft tissue drainage. Occasionally drainage is performed through the soft tissue even if it has also been obtained through the tooth. The reason is that there may be two (or more) separate, noncommunicating abscesses—one at the apex and another in a submucosal location or in an anatomic space. So, if necessary and feasible, such supplemental drainage is indicated.

Drainage through the soft tissue is accomplished most effectively when the swelling is fluctuant. A fluctuant swelling is a fluid-containing mass in which a wavelike sensation or motion is felt as pressure is applied (see Color Figure 24-1, *B*). The feeling is similar to that experienced when pushing on a water balloon or a small plastic packet of catsup. Incising a fluctuant swelling releases purulence immediately and provides rapid relief. If the swelling is nonfluctuant or indurated (firm), the outcome is somewhat less predictable and often results in drainage of only blood and serous fluids. Although the results may not be as dramatic or complete as those achieved by incising a fluctuant swelling, incising a nonfluctuant swelling releases pressure and facilitates healing by reducing irritants and increasing circulation in the area.

CONTRAINDICATIONS

There are relatively few contraindications to the use of incisions. Diffuse swellings are not usually incised. Patients with prolonged bleeding or clotting times must be treated cautiously, and hematologic screening is often indicated. An abscess in an anatomic space may require more involved treatment; the patient should be referred to an oral and maxillofacial surgeon for an extraoral or aggressive intraoral incision.

PROCEDURE
Anesthesia

Profound anesthesia is difficult to achieve in the presence of inflammation, swelling, and exudate because of hyperalgesia. Direct subperiosteal infiltration not only is ineffective but also may be quite painful. Standard infiltration may not be totally effective either. Therefore, regional block anesthesia techniques are preferred. Mandibular blocks for posterior areas, bilateral mental blocks for the anterior mandible, posterior superior alveolar blocks for the posterior maxilla, and infraorbital blocks for the premaxilla are preferred choices. These may be supplemented by regional infiltration.

If regional block anesthesia is not sufficient, one of the following methods may be used. The first technique is infiltration starting peripheral to the swelling. The solution is injected *slowly* with limited pressure and depth; this is followed by additional injections in previously anesthetized tissue, moving progressively closer to the center of the swelling. This procedure results in improved anesthesia without extreme discomfort.

A second technique is the use of topical ethyl chloride.[6] A stream of this agent is directed onto the swelling from a distance, permitting the liquid to volatilize on the tissue surface. Within seconds, the tissue at the site of volatilization turns white.

The incision is quickly accomplished with continued ethyl chloride spray. This topical anesthesia is a supplement to block anesthesia when a quick incision is required. If none of these procedures work, the incision for drainage may be done with intravenous sedation.

Incision

After anesthesia, the incision is made horizontally or vertically with a No. 11, 12, or 15 blade. Vertical incisions are parallel with the major blood vessels and nerves and leave very little scarring. The incision should be made firmly through periosteum to bone. If the swelling is fluctuant, pus usually flows immediately, followed by blood. Occasionally, there is only a serosanguineous exudate, which is acceptable. If the swelling is nonfluctuant, the predominant flow is hemorrhagic.

Drainage

After the initial incision, a small closed hemostat may be placed in the incision and then opened to enlarge the draining tract.[7] This procedure is indicated with more extensive swellings; the initial incision and subsequent enlargement usually provide the needed drainage. If a drain is necessary because of limited initial drainage, a self-retentive I-shaped or "Christmas tree" drain cut from a rubber dam or a piece of iodoform gauze is placed (suturing is optional) in the incision (see Color Figure 24-1, *C*). The drain should be removed after 2 to 3 days; if it is not sutured, the patient may remove the drain at home.

Periradicular Surgery

This surgery is commonly performed to remove a portion of the root with undébrided canal space or to retroseal the canal when a complete seal cannot be obtained with an orthograde (through the crown) approach. Occasionally, periradicular curettage without root resection is needed.

INDICATIONS

The main indications for periradicular surgery (PS) are (1) nonsurgical root canal therapy is unfeasible, (2) retreatment of failed root canal therapy is impossible or would not produce a better result, or (3) biopsy is indicated.

In the following situations, periapical surgery may be necessary:
- Anatomic problems
- Procedural accidents requiring surgery

- Irretrievable materials in the root canal
- Persistent symptoms
- Horizontal apical fracture
- Biopsy

Anatomic Problems

A non-negotiable canal, blockage, or severe root curvature may prevent adequate cleaning and shaping or obturation. Nonsurgical root canal therapy or retreatment (if possible) before surgery improves the surgical success rate.[8,9] However, if neither is feasible, removal of the uninstrumented and unfilled portion of the root or apical surgery may be necessary (Figure 24-1). Anatomic perforation of the root apex through the bone (fenestration), although uncommon, may necessitate apical surgery after root canal treatment. Occasionally, even after an apparently adequate obturation, inflammation and discomfort continue if the root apex protrudes outside the bony cortical plate. This condition is corrected by beveling the root apex and placing it within the bone.

Occasionally, adequate root canal therapy is compromised by extensive apical root resorption. It may then be necessary to expose the root, then remove and repair the resorbed area.

Procedural Accidents

Separated instruments, ledging, perforations, and gross overfills may cause failure of root canal treatment which will require surgical intervention. Slight to moderate overfilling is not in itself an indication for surgery; if symptoms persist or develop or if nonhealing is shown radiographically, surgery is usually necessary.

Irretrievable Materials in the Root Canal

Retreatment is recommended for treatment failures when retreatment is possible. However, irretrievable posts or dowels or root filling materials such as silver cones, amalgam, or nonabsorbable pastes often prevent retreatment, or their removal would result in further damage to the root structure. The best alternative is a surgical approach, including placement of a root-end filling material (Figure 24-2).

Persistent Symptoms

Most symptoms disappear after complete cleaning and obturation of root canals. However, if symptoms persist after meticulous performance of these procedures endodontic surgery should be considered to identify the cause(s) for the persistence of the symptoms. The main cause for persistent pain is the presence of inflammation because of the inability of the operator to completely clean the root canal(s). Exploratory surgery may identify undetected vertical root fractures, additional apical and lateral foramina (possible missed canals), perforations,

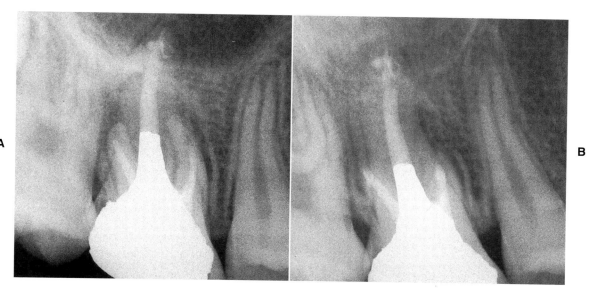

FIGURE 24-1
A, A non-negotiable ledge in present in the mesiobuccal root of the first maxillary molar. **B,** Periradicular surgery (root-end resection and filling) corrected this accident and deficiencies in the distobuccal root.

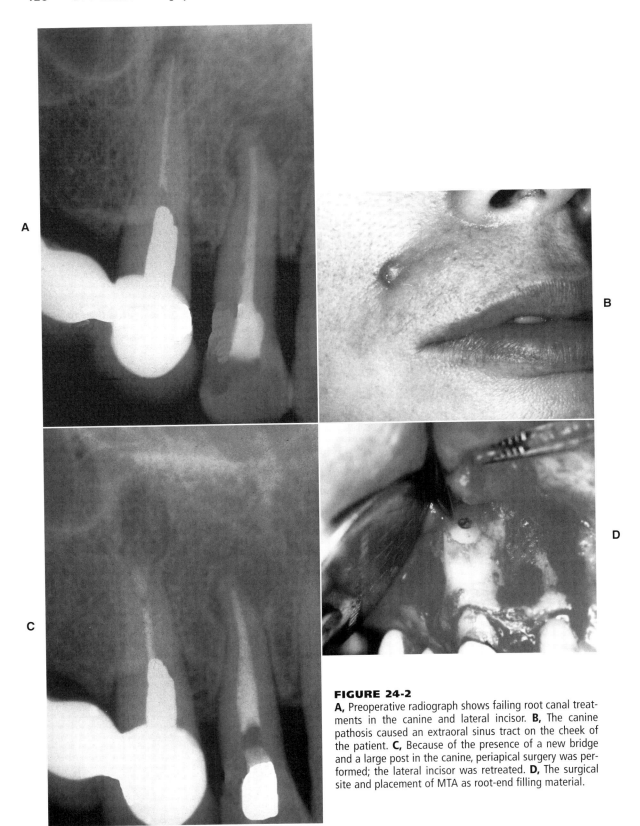

FIGURE 24-2
A, Preoperative radiograph shows failing root canal treatments in the canine and lateral incisor. **B,** The canine pathosis caused an extraoral sinus tract on the cheek of the patient. **C,** Because of the presence of a new bridge and a large post in the canine, periapical surgery was performed; the lateral incisor was retreated. **D,** The surgical site and placement of MTA as root-end filling material.

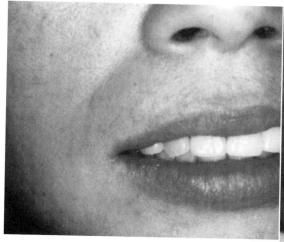

E

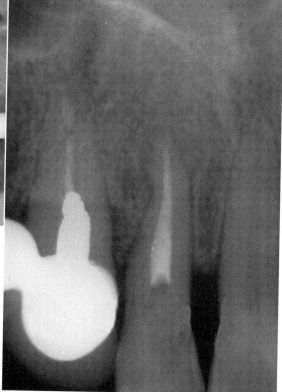

F

FIGURE 24-2, cont'd
E, The sinus tract disappeared 6 weeks after the surgery.
F, A 5-year recall shows complete resolution of the lesion
in the canine. (Courtesy Dr. C. Hong.)

apical ramifications, overfills, or other causes of failure. Once the cause has been determined a proper treatment plan can be initiated. Surgery should be performed only after causes that are correctable without surgery are ruled out. Examples of such causes are missed canals, cracked teeth, occlusal trauma, referred pain (from another tooth), or inadequate débridement or obturation.

Horizontal Apical Fracture

Although most traumatic horizontal apical fractures usually heal without intervention, occasionally the apical canal becomes necrotic and cannot be treated. In these cases, the apical segment of the root must be removed.

Biopsy

Although most pathoses are of pulpal origin, nonpulpal lesions do exist (see Chapter 3). Findings include the presence of a vital pulp in a tooth with a radicular radiolucency (Figure 24-3), undefined periapical lesions in teeth with vital pulps in patients with a history of previous ma-

lignancy, lip paresthesia, or anesthesia. These conditions are indications for biopsy.

CONTRAINDICATIONS

Contraindications are relatively few. There are four major categories[7]: (1) anatomic factors, (2) medical or systemic complications, (3) indiscriminate use of surgery, and (4) unidentified cause of treatment failure.

Anatomic Factors

Inaccessibility of the surgical site owing to tooth location, spaces such as maxillary sinus or nasal fossa, unusual bony configuration, or proximity of neurovascular bundles may be a contraindication or at least require caution or special approaches. For example, a thick external oblique ridge associated with a mandibular molar or apices contiguous with the mandibular canal may compromise surgical access. These factors are also related to operator skill. Other situations that may contraindicate periradicular surgery or modify the approaches used include very short root length (precluding root-end resection),

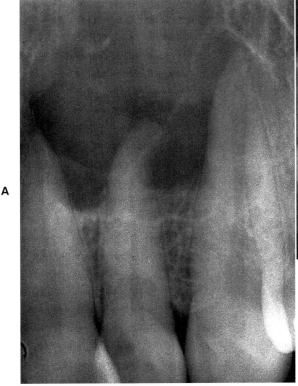

A

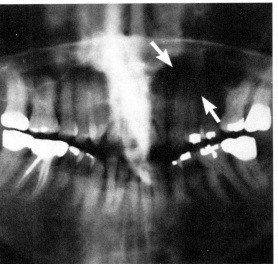

B

FIGURE 24-3
A, Presence of vital pulps in the left anterior teeth and a multilocular large radiolucency indicated the probability of a lesion of a nonpulpal origin. **B,** A panoramic radiograph shows the extent of this lesion *(arrows).* A biopsy revealed the presence of a keratocyst.

severe periodontal disease (hopeless prognosis, even with surgery), or unrestorable teeth.

Medical or Systemic Complications

Serious systemic health problems or extreme apprehension makes the patient a poor candidate for surgery. Surgery may also be contraindicated in patients with blood disorders, terminal disease, uncontrolled diabetes, or severe heart disease, or for those who are immunocompromised.

Indiscriminate Use of Surgery

As previously stated, surgery is not indicated when a nonsurgical approach would probably result in successful treatment. The practice of managing all accessible periapical pathoses or large periradicular lesions surgically is unethical and not rational. In these situations, root canal treatment resolves the problem without subjecting the patient to additional trauma.

Unidentified Cause of Treatment Failure

Importantly, surgery to correct a treatment failure for which the cause cannot be identified is unlikely to be successful.

SEQUENCE OF PROCEDURES

The typical sequence of procedures used in periradicular surgery (with modifications according to the situation) is the following:

1. Flap design
2. Incision and reflection
3. Apical access
4. Periradicular curettage
5. Root-end resection
6. Root-end cavity preparation
7. Root-end filling
8. Flap replacement and suturing
9. Postoperative care and instructions
10. Suture removal and evaluation

Flap Design

The first stage requires exposure of the surgical site by incising and reflecting the overlying soft tissues of gingiva, mucosa, and periosteum. A properly designed and carefully reflected flap gives good surgical access and results in improved healing. The following are general guidelines and principles[10,11]:

1. Adequate blood supply to the reflected tissue is maintained with a wide flap base.
2. Incisions over bony defects or over the periradicular lesion should be avoided; these

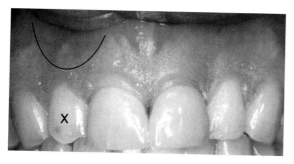

FIGURE 24-4
A submarginal curved (semilunar) flap is shown in the attached gingiva to perform periapical surgery on the right lateral incisor *(X)*. This design has deficiencies and usually is not indicated.

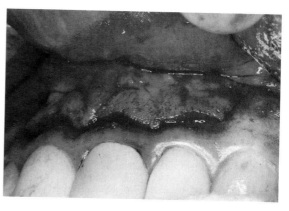

FIGURE 24-5
A scalloped submarginal horizontal incision (Ochsenbein-Luebke) is made in the attached gingiva with two accompanying vertical incisions to perform surgery on the right central incisor.

might cause postsurgical soft tissue fenestrations or nonunion of the incision.

3. The flap should be designed for maximum access by avoiding limited tissue reflection. The actual bone resorption is larger than the size observed radiographically.

4. Acute angles in the flap are avoided. Sharp corners are difficult to reposition and suture and may become ischemic and slough, resulting in delayed healing and possibly scar formation.

5. Incisions and reflections include periosteum as part of the flap. Any remaining pieces or tags of cellular nonreflected periosteum will hemorrhage, compromising visibility.

6. The interdental papilla must not be split (incised through). The interdental papilla should be either fully included or excluded from the flap; dividing may result in sloughing of the tissue.

7. Vertical incisions must be extended to allow the retractor to rest on bone and not crush portions of the flap.

8. A minimal flap, which should include at least one tooth on either side of the intended tooth, should be used.

Although there are numerous flap designs, two meet most periradicular surgery needs: the submarginal (curved, triangular, and rectangular) and the full mucoperiosteal (triangular and rectangular) flaps.

Submarginal curved flap. Also known as the semilunar flap, this flap is a slightly curved, half-moon-shaped, horizontal incision made in oral mucosa, or in the attached gingiva with the convexity nearest the free gingival margin (Figure 24-4). It is simple and easily reflected and provides access to the apex without impinging on the tissue surrounding the crowns. Its disadvantages include restricted access with limited visibility, tearing of the

incision corners when attempting to improve access by stretching the tissue, and leaving the incision directly over the lesion if the surgical defect is larger than anticipated. The incision often heals with scarring.[5,12] The submarginal curved flap is limited by the presence of the frenum, muscle attachments, or canine and other bony eminences. Because of its many problems, this design is generally not indicated.

Submarginal triangular and rectangular flaps. The triangular or rectangular flaps are known as modified submarginal curved flaps. A scalloped horizontal incision (Ochsenbein-Luebke) is made in the attached gingiva with one or two accompanying vertical incisions (Figure 24-5). This flap is used most successfully in maxillary anterior teeth with crowns. Prerequisites are at least 4.0 mm of attached gingiva and good periodontal health.

This flap design provides better access and visibility compared with the submarginal curved flap and less risk of incising tissue over a bony defect and no recession of marginal gingiva postsurgically. Disadvantages are possible scarring and hemorrhaging from the cut margins to the surgical site.[13] It also provides less visibility than the full mucoperiosteal flap.

Full mucoperiosteal flap. The full mucoperiosteal (sulcular) flap consists of an incision at the gingival crest with full elevation of the interdental papillae, free gingival margin, attached gingiva, and alveolar mucosa. It may have either a single (triangular) or double (rectangular) vertical releasing incision (Figure 24-6 and Color Figure 24-1, *D*). It allows maximal access and visibility, precludes incising over a bony defect, and has fewer tendencies for hemor-

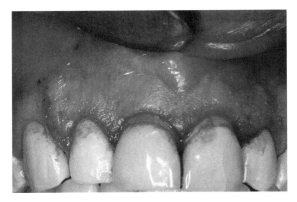

FIGURE 24-6
A triangular full mucoperiosteal (sulcular) flap with one vertical incision is made to access the right central incisor.

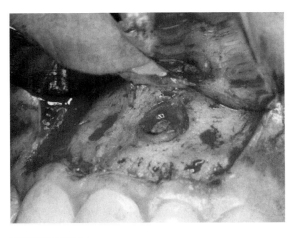

FIGURE 24-7
The flap is reflected with a periosteal elevator and held with a retractor to allow visibility and access to the surgical site. The retractor must be placed on sound bone.

rhage. This design permits periodontal curettage, root planing, and bony reshaping and heals with minimal scar formation. Its disadvantages include the difficulty of replacement, suturing, and making alterations (height and shape) to the free gingival margin, as well as possible gingival recession postsurgically and exposing the crown margins.[12,14]

Incision and Reflection

A firm incision is made with a No. 15 or another suitable blade. To prevent tearing during reflection, the incision must be made through periosteum to bone. The tissue is reflected with a sharp periosteal elevator beginning in the vertical incision and then raising the horizontal component. Because periosteum is reflected as part of the flap, the elevator must firmly contact bone as the tissue is peeled back, using firm controlled force. The tissue is reflected to a level that will provide adequate access and visibility of the surgical site while allowing a retractor to be placed on sound bone (Figure 24-7).

Access to Apex

In many cases because of the presence of a lesion, bone has been resorbed, and either a soft tissue lesion is visible, or firm probing with an explorer will locate the apical lesion. If the opening is small, the bone can be removed by a sharp round bur until the apex is visible. If there is limited bone destruction, after placement of a radiopaque object near the apex a radiograph should be taken to locate the apex. Removal of bone with a bur is performed in the presence of copious sterile saline irrigation.[10,11,15]

Periradicular Curettage

Removal of pathologic soft tissue surrounding the apex is necessary because it does the following:
1. Provides access and visibility of the apex
2. Removes inflamed tissue
3. Provides a biopsy specimen for histologic examination
4. Reduces hemorrhage

The tissue should be carefully peeled out, ideally in one piece, with a suitably sized sharp curette (see Color Figure 24-1, *E*). This process should leave a clean bony cavity. When the lesion is very large, portions of tissue can be left without compromising the blood supply to an adjacent tooth. This should not affect periradicular healing.

Root-End Resection

Root-end resection involves beveling of the apical portion of the root. This step is often an integral part of periradicular surgery and serves the following two purposes:
1. It removes the untreated apical portion of the root and enables the operator to determine the cause of failure.
2. It provides a flat surface to prepare a root end cavity and pack it with a root-end filling material.

Apical sectioning is done with a tapered fissure bur in a high-speed handpiece and copious sterile saline irrigation (Figure 24-8). The bevel should be made at approximately 45 degrees in a facial-lingual direction, with the least amount of bevel to give maximum visibility to the root apex.[10,11] In

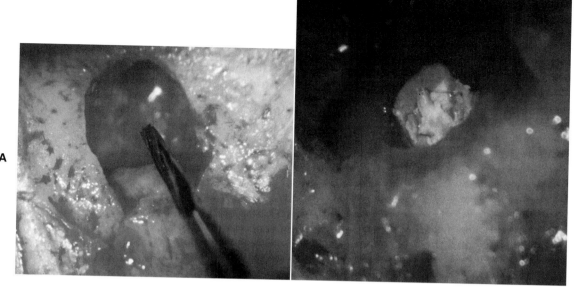

FIGURE 24-8
Root-end resection (apicoectomy). **A,** A fissure bur is used to remove the apical portion of the root. **B,** The entire resected portion should be visible.

general, the amount of root removed depends on the reason for performing the root-end resection. However, resection must be sufficient to do the following:

1. Provide access to the palatal-lingual root surface
2. Place the canal in the center of the sectioned root
3. Expose additional canals or fractures

Root-End Cavity Preparation and Filling

Root-end cavity preparation and filling are indicated when the apical seal appears to be inadequate. A class I type preparation is made with ultrasonic tips to a minimum depth of 3 mm into the canal[10,11,13,16,17] (Figure 24-9). More complicated apical root anatomy may require other types of preparation.[10] The ultrasonic instrument offers advantages of control and ease of use and permits less apical root beveling and uniform depth of preparation.[16,17] In addition, the ultrasonic tips follow the direction of the canals and clean the canal surfaces better than burs.[18]

A *root-end filling material* is then inserted into the prepared cavity (Figure 24-10). These materials should have the following characteristics

1. Well sealing
2. Well tolerated by the periradicular tissue
3. Nonresorbable
4. Easily inserted

5. Unaffected by moisture
6. Radiographic visibility
7. Ability to allow regeneration of periradicular tissues

Many materials have been used as root-end filling materials.[19-24] Amalgam, SuperEBA, IRM, mineral trioxide aggregate (MTA) and ProRoot MTA, are acceptable and the most commonly used materials.

Flap Replacement and Suturing

After a root-end filling material is placed and a radiograph is made, the flap should be placed into its original position and held it in place for 5 minutes using moderate digital pressure with moistened gauze. This allows expression of hemorrhage from under the flap, initial adaptation, and easier suturing and produces less postoperative swelling and bleeding.

Suturing is commonly done with silk, although other materials are acceptable.[25,26] There are many suturing techniques, including interrupted, continuous mattress, and sling sutures.[11] Interrupted sutures are commonly used (Figure 24-11, *A*). In these, the needle passes first through reflected and then through attached tissue. The sutures are tied with a simple surgeon's knot. The knot should not be placed over the incision line because it collects debris and bacteria, which will promote inflammation and

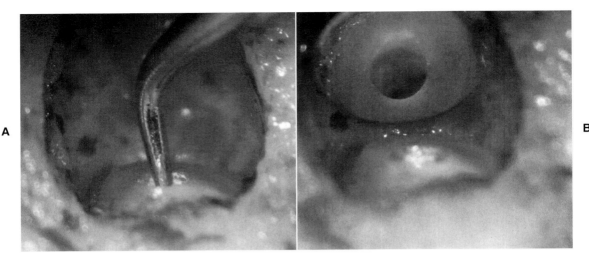

FIGURE 24-9
Root-end cavity preparation. An ultrasonic unit using specialized tips (**A**) is used to create a class I preparation in the apical portion of the root canal (**B**). (Courtesy Dr. R. Rubinstein.)

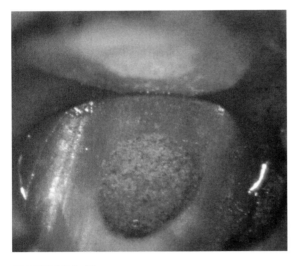

FIGURE 24-10
Root-end filling placement. MTA (3 mm) is placed in the root-end cavity preparation to provide a fluid-tight apical seal. (Courtesy Dr. R. Rubinstein.)

infection. The sutures are usually removed 3 to 7 days after surgery (Figure 24-11, *B*); shorter times are preferred.

Postoperative Care and Instructions

Both oral and written postoperative instructions should be given to the patient. Instructions should be written in simple, straightforward language. They should minimize patient anxiety aris-

ing from normal postoperative sequelae by describing how to promote healing and comfort.

The following instructions are for patients. The items in parentheses identified as "Note" are intended for the practitioner, not the patient.

1. Some swelling and discoloration are common. Use an ice pack with moderate pressure on the outside of your face (20 minutes on, 5 minutes off) until you go to bed tonight. (Note: Ice and pressure [primarily] decrease bleeding and swelling and provide an analgesic effect.)

2. Some oozing of blood is normal. If bleeding increases, place a moistened gauze pad or facial tissues over the area and apply finger pressure for 15 minutes. If bleeding continues, call our office.

3. Do not lift up your lip or cheek to look at the area. The stitches are tied and you may tear them out.

4. Starting tomorrow, dissolve 1 teaspoon of salt in a glass of warm water and *gently* rinse your mouth three or four times daily. Rising with a mouthwash can promote healing. Careful brushing is important, but vigorous brushing may damage the area. Tonight you should brush and floss all areas except the surgery site. Tomorrow night *carefully* brush the surgery site.

5. Eat a diet of soft food and chew on the opposite side of your mouth. Drink lots of fluids and eat foods such as cottage cheese and yogurt, eggs, and ice cream. (Note: Proper diet and fluid intake are essential

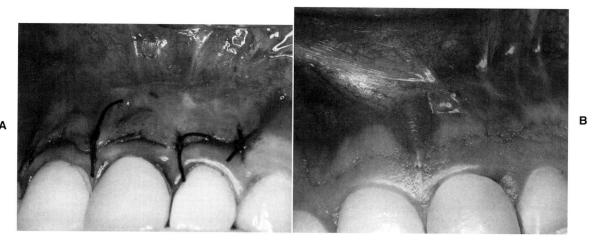

FIGURE 24-11
A, Interrupted sutures are commonly used to hold the soft tissue flap in its original location. **B,** Sutures are removed 3 to 7 days after surgery.

after surgery. Patients often lose their appetite after the procedure, so they need to be encouraged to drink fluids and to eat.)

6. Some discomfort is normal. If pain medication was prescribed, follow the instructions. If no medication was prescribed, take your preferred nonprescription pain remedy if needed. If this is not sufficient, call our office. (Note: Surprisingly, pain is usually minimal after endodontic surgery, and strong analgesics are not required.)

7. Do not smoke for the first 3 days after the procedure. (Note: Smoking has been shown to adversely affect healing; this is an opportunity to counsel a patient to quit permanently.)

8. If you experience excessive swelling or pain or if you have a fever, call our office immediately. (Note: Excessive swelling, pain, or fever may indicate the presence of an infection [very rare] that requires antibiotic or other therapy. The patient must be evaluated.)

9. Keep your appointment to have the stitches removed. (Note: Sutures are removed 3 to 7 days after surgery.)

10. Call our office if you have any concerns or questions.

Suture Removal and Evaluation

Sutures are carefully removed by cutting with small scissors. The sutures are removed only if the flap margins are in contact and are adhering to the underlying tissues. Usually, anesthesia is unnecessary for this procedure.

Healing

Surgery involves the manipulation of soft and hard tissues. Handling of both soft tissues (periosteum, gingiva, periodontal ligament, and alveolar mucosa) and hard tissues (dentin, cementum, and bone) is accomplished by incision, dissection, and excision.

SOFT TISSUE

Healing involves clotting, inflammation, epithelialization, connective tissue healing, and maturation and remodeling of both connective tissue and bone.[27] Clotting and inflammation consist of both chemical and cellular phases. The clotting mechanism is important because it is based on the conversion of fibrinogen to fibrin; under pressure, the clot should be a thin layer. Failure of a clot to form results in leakage of blood into the wound site. The inflammatory components of healing are a complex network of both extrinsic and intrinsic elements.[27]

Initial epithelial healing consists of the formation of the epithelial barrier, made up of layers of epithelial cells that depend on the underlying connective tissue for nutrients. This epithelial layer migrates along the fibrin surface until it makes contact with epithelial cells from the opposite border of the wound, forming an epithelial bridge.

The connective tissue component comes from fibroblasts, which are differentiated from ecto-mesenchymal cells and are attracted to the wound site by cellular and humoral mediators. Adjacent blood vessels provide nutrients for the fibroblasts and their precursors, which elaborate collagen, initially type III, followed by type I. Macrophages are an important part of these processes. As healing matures, there is a decrease in the amount of inflammation and numbers of fibroblasts, accompanied by deaggregation and reaggregation of collagen with formation of collagen fibers into a more organized pattern.[27-30]

HARD TISSUE

As with soft tissue, the hard tissue response is based on the fibroblast, which results in synthesis of ground substance, cementum, and bone matrix formation.[31] New cementum deposition from cementoblasts begins about 12 days after surgery; eventually a thin layer of cementum may cover resected dentin and even certain root end filling materials (see Color Figure 24-1, *F*). The exposed dentin acts as an inductive force with new cementum forming from the periphery to the center.

Osseous healing begins by the proliferation of endosteal cells into the coagulum of the wound site. At 12 to 14 days, woven trabeculae and osteocytes appear, leading to early maturation of the collagen matrix at about 30 days. This process occurs from inside to outside, ending in the formation of mature lamellar bone,[32-35] which is visible radiographically (Figure 24-12).

Corrective Surgery

These procedures are especially designed to correct pathologic or iatrogenic entities (procedure errors) that have damaged the root and are not correctable via the pulp space (internally).

INDICATIONS
Procedural Errors

Correction of root perforations often presents a more difficult challenge than procedures that merely involve periradicular surgery. Typically these accidents occur during access, canal preparation, or restorative procedures (usually post placement). They require restorative as well as endodontic management (Figure 24-13). See Chapter 18 for more detail. The location of the perforation is often the factor that determines the

success of treatment. If the defect is on the proximal root surfaces in close proximity to adjacent teeth, repair is a problem; access to the site is difficult without damaging adjacent teeth. This is particularly true of the lingual surface of mandibular teeth. However, defects on the facial surface are easier to treat.

Resorptive Perforations

Resorptive root perforations typically occur as sequela to trauma or internal bleaching procedures. The defects may be localized to the root surface or communicate with the canal.

TECHNIQUES

Repair of these defects poses unique problems. Often a defect on the root surface wraps onto the palatal or lingual surface, compromising access and hemostasis. Repair can be accomplished with various materials. If the field can be kept dry, glass ionomer, dentin-bonding agent with composite resin, or MTA (white ProRoot MTA) can be used. Esthetically pleasing materials are preferred for facial repairs because dark materials such as amalgam or gray ProRoot MTA may stain the teeth. If a post perforates the root, it must be shortened so that it is well within the root structure. Then the defect is repaired with ProRoot MTA.

Repairs in the cervical portion of the root are often difficult to manage and maintain because communication with the gingival sulcus leads to periodontal breakdown. This often means that periodontal treatment (such as crown lengthening), orthodontic extrusion, or a combination thereof is necessary in conjunction with the repair.

Root Amputation, Hemisection, and Bicuspidization

The three categories described previously, incision for drainage, periradicular surgery and corrective surgery, involve cutting bone, soft tissue, and root. This last category involves resecting the root(s) and/or crown.[36]

DEFINITIONS

Root amputation is the removal of one or more roots of a multirooted tooth. The involved root(s) is (are) separated at the junction of and into the crown (Figure 24-14). In general, this procedure is

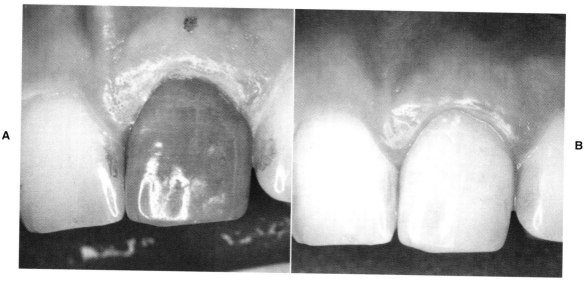

COLOR FIGURE 23-1
Internal bleaching. **A,** Pulp necrosis resulting from a traumatic injury caused severe dentin discoloration. **B,** After internal bleaching with a "walking bleach" paste the tooth regained its original shade. (Refer to Figure 23-3.)

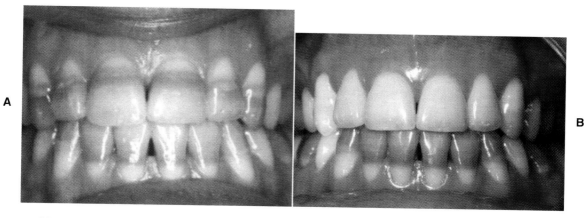

COLOR FIGURE 23-2
Internal bleaching. **A,** Tetracycline discoloration caused a marked esthetic problem. **B,** Root canal treatment followed by "walking bleach" results in a permanent, pleasing shade change. (Refer to Figure 23-7, *A* and *C*.)

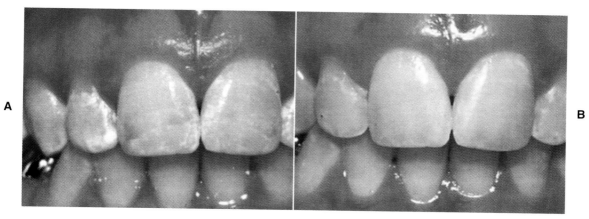

COLOR FIGURE 23-3
External bleaching. **A,** Enamel hypoplasia resulted in surface stains. **B,** An acid-pumice burnishing of the enamel surface removes much of the discoloration (Refer to Figure 23-8, *A* and *C*.)

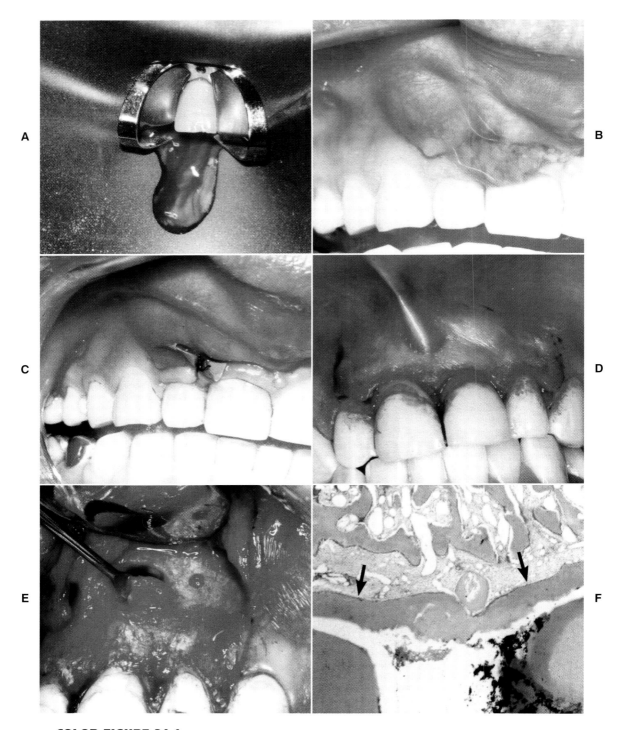

COLOR FIGURE 24-1

A, Establishment of drainage through an offending tooth. **B,** A fluctuant swelling is the result of an abscess from the lateral incisor. **C,** An incision for drainage is made horizontally into the swelling. A rubber drain is sutured in place to prevent closure of the incision. **D,** A rectangular flap with a sulcular and two vertical incisions is created to perform periapical surgery on the left central incisor. **E,** Apical curettage. Removal of diseased tissue at the apex enhances visualization of the apex and surrounding bone. This tissue may be submitted for histologic evaluation. **F,** Complete periapical healing and formation of cellular cementum *(arrows)* adjacent to mineral trioxide aggregate when it is used as a root-end filling material in monkeys.

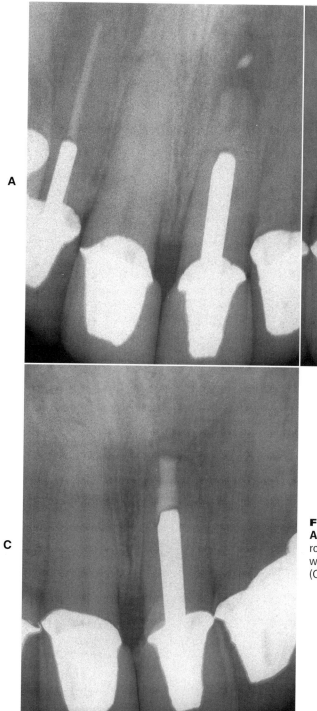

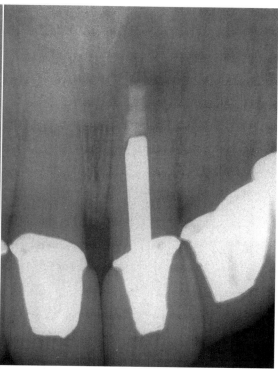

FIGURE 24-12
A, Failed root canal treatment requiring surgery. **B,** The root end is resected, and a cavity is prepared and is filled with MTA. **C,** One-year recall shows complete healing. (Courtesy Dr. R. Rubinstein.)

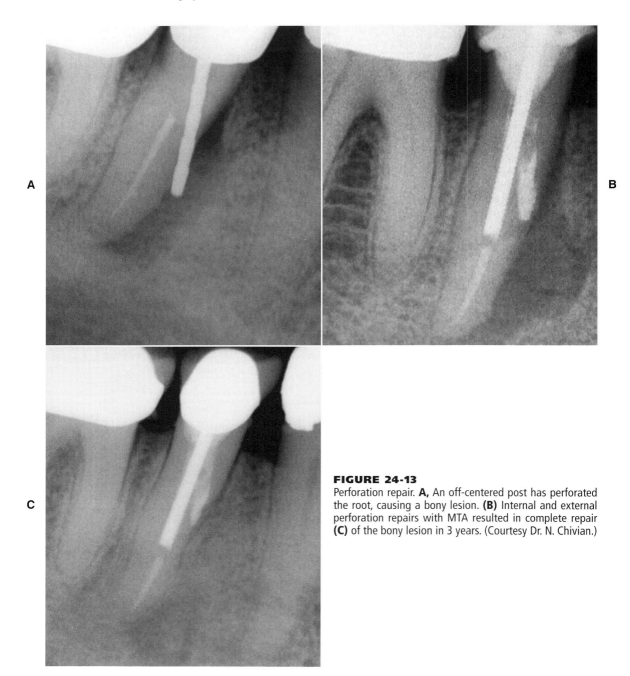

FIGURE 24-13
Perforation repair. **A,** An off-centered post has perforated the root, causing a bony lesion. **(B)** Internal and external perforation repairs with MTA resulted in complete repair **(C)** of the bony lesion in 3 years. (Courtesy Dr. N. Chivian.)

performed in maxillary molars, but it can be performed in mandibular molars.

Hemisection is the surgical division of a multirooted tooth. In mandibular molars the tooth is divided buccolingually through the bifurcation (Figure 24-15). In maxillary molars the cut is made mesiodistally, also through the furcation. The defective or periodontally involved root and its coronal crown are then removed.[37]

Bicuspidization is a surgical division (as in hemisection, usually a mandibular molar), but the crown and root of both halves are retained. If severe bone loss or destruction of tooth structure is confined primarily to the furcation area, hemisection and furcal curettage may allow retention of both halves (Figure 24-16). Each half may be restored to approximate a bicuspid, hence the term *bicuspidization*.

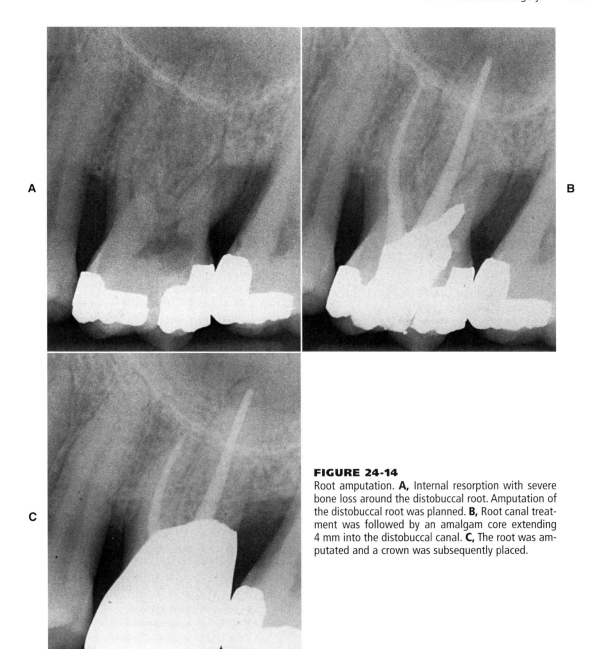

FIGURE 24-14
Root amputation. **A,** Internal resorption with severe bone loss around the distobuccal root. Amputation of the distobuccal root was planned. **B,** Root canal treatment was followed by an amalgam core extending 4 mm into the distobuccal canal. **C,** The root was amputated and a crown was subsequently placed.

INDICATIONS AND CONTRAINDICATIONS
Indications for Root Amputation or Hemisection

Indications include the following:
- The presence of severe bone loss in a non-surgical treatable periodontally involved root or furcation

- Roots that are untreatable because of broken instruments, perforations, caries, resorption, vertical fractures, or calcified canals
- Strategically important root(s) and accompanying crown

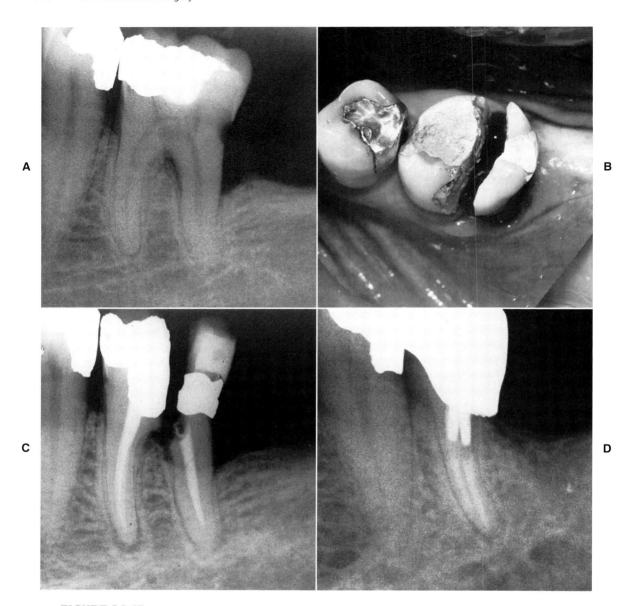

FIGURE 24-15
Hemisection. **A,** Furcation caries and bone loss have compromised the distal root. **B,** After root canal treatment, the crown was divided through the furcation (**C**). **D,** Twenty-month recall, after posts and core and a crown were placed. The extraction socket has healed and the tooth is stable.

Contraindications for Root Amputation or Hemisection

Contraindications include the following:
- Insufficient bony support for the remaining root(s)
- Root fusion or proximity such that root separation is not possible
- Strong abutment teeth available (the involved tooth should be extracted and a prosthesis fabricated)
- Inability to complete root canal treatment on the remaining root(s)

Indications for Bicuspidization

Indications include the following:
- Furcation perforation
- Furcation pathosis from periodontal disease
- Buccolingual cervical caries or fracture into furcation

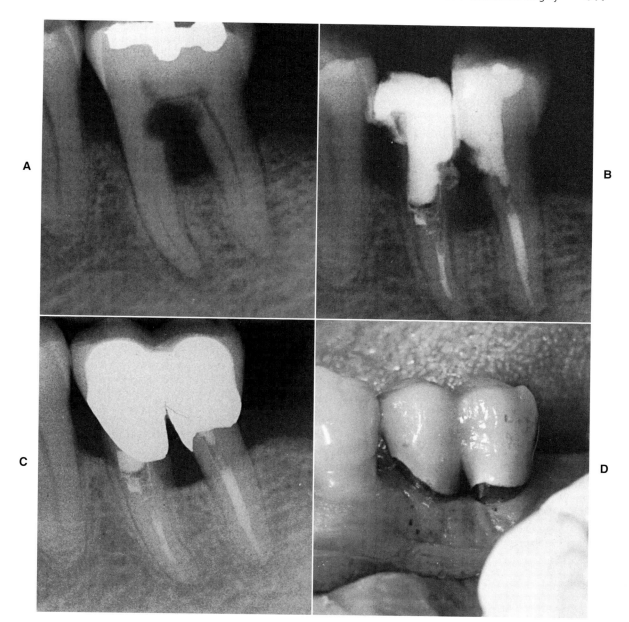

FIGURE 24-16
Bicuspidization. **A,** Caries in the furcation and furcal bone loss are evident, but there is adequate support for both roots. **B,** Root canal treatment and bur separation through furcation and crown. **C,** Restoration with a porcelain fused to metal crown splinting the two roots. **D,** Good home care and a good gingival response at 30-month re-call with no probing defects. Note that the furcation is open to facilitate special oral hygiene procedures. (Courtesy of Dr. R. Walton.)

Contraindications for Bicuspidization

Contraindications include the following:

- Deep furcation (thick floor of pulp chamber)
- Unrestorable half
- Periodontal disease (each half must be periodontally sound)

- Inability to complete root canal treatment on either half
- Root fusion
- Severe periodontal disease

TECHNIQUES

Root amputation is performed by making an angled cut from the furcation to the proximal aspect to separate the root from the crown. The crown remains intact, and the root is removed. Therefore, the crown is cantilevered over the extracted root segment and remains in contact with the approximating tooth. A second approach is to use an angled vertical cut in which the crown above the root to be amputated is recontoured, decreasing the occlusal forces and making the procedure easier. As the crown is shaped, the bur is gradually angled into the root, resulting in good anatomic contour.

Hemisection involves making a vertical cut through the crown into the furcation. This results in complete separation of the hemisected section (crown and root) from the tooth segment that is retained. The defective half of the tooth is extracted.

Bicuspidization is performed after a vertical cut is made through the crown into the furcation with a fissure bur. This procedure results in complete separation of the roots and creation of two separate crowns. After healing of tissues the teeth can be restored to form two separate premolars.

(These techniques may or may not require flap reflection. Often, if the root is periodontally involved, it is removed without a flap. If bony recontouring is indicated, a flap is necessary before root resection is carried out. A sulcular flap design is often possible without a vertical releasing incision. However, when in doubt, a flap should be raised; doing so will always help.)

PROGNOSIS

Each case is unique and has a different prognosis according to the situation. Varying results have been reported for root removal.[38] Success is defined by tooth retention with absence of pathosis. Success depends on the following factors:

- Case selection
- Cutting and preparing the tooth without creating additional damage
- Restoration
- Good oral hygiene
- Development of caries (most common cause of failure)
- Root fractures
- Excessive occlusal forces
- Poor restorative procedures
- Untreatable endodontic problems
- Periodontal disease (second most common cause of failure)

The major factor affecting success is the patient's oral hygiene, even if these procedures are performed correctly, and the tooth is restored properly. The patient must be willing and able to perform extra procedures to prevent plaque accumulation, particularly in the area adjacent to what was once the furcation. Failure to do so could possibly result in untreatable caries or periodontal disease. The dentist must work carefully with the patient to render this area plaque-free. A procedure that appears to be a success at 5 years may fail later. Thus the judgment of success or failure should be guarded and should extend over many years.

Conditions That Indicate Referral

Although the procedures described in this chapter may appear straightforward, endodontic surgery requires advanced training, experience, and considerable surgical skill. There is concern about standard of care and litigation. This, coupled with the availability of experienced specialists, means that general dentists must carefully examine their own expertise and accurately assess the difficulty of the situation before they attempt a surgical procedure. These procedures are often the last hope for retaining the tooth and require the highest level of skill and expertise and use of optical aids, special instruments and materials to enhance success. Lack of training may result not only in the loss of the tooth but also in damage to adjacent structures, paresthesia from nerve injury, sinus perforations, soft tissue fenestrations, and postoperative complications such as hemorrhage and infection.

In many situations, access to the surgical site is limited and potentially hazardous. Long-standing large lesions may impinge on adjacent structures, requiring special techniques for resolution (Figure 24-17). The neurovascular bundle near the apexes of mandibular molars, premolars, and maxillary palatal roots predisposes the patient to postsurgical paresthesia or excessive hemorrhage. The treatment of endodontic problems in these areas requires careful preoperative assessment and considerable surgical skill. The presence of thick cortical bone and bony eminences throughout the mandible and in the palate, frenum, and muscle attachments, fenestrations of the cortical bone, and the various sinus cavities all require considerable surgical skill and experience in gaining access to most teeth.

Most important is the need for appropriate diagnosis, treatment planning, case assess-

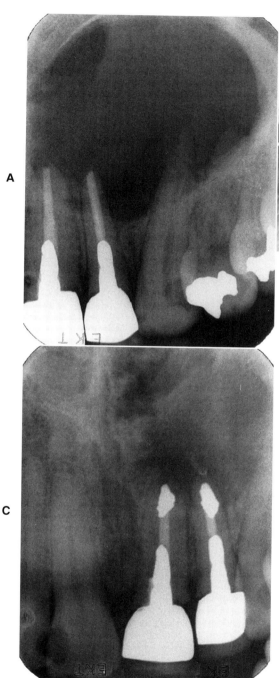

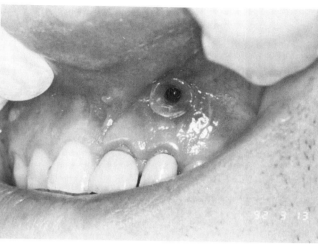

FIGURE 24-17

Decompression. Some cases require special procedures. **A,** A very large cyst fails to heal after root canal treatment. **B,** After surgical exposure and root-end surgery, a polyethylene tube is placed for several weeks to allow communication between the cyst cavity and the oral cavity. This allows collapse of the cyst wall. **C,** The lesion has resolved 1 year later, showing regeneration of bone. (Courtesy Dr. S. Gish.)

ment, prognostication, and follow-up evaluation. The general dentist should have knowledge in these areas but may prefer to refer the patient to or request input from an endodontist. The specialist is better able to accomplish these goals as well as to assess the short- and long-term outcome.[39]

REFERENCES

1. Hession RW: Long term evaluation of endodontic treatment, *Int Endod J* 14:179, 1981.
2. Morse DR, Esposito JV, Pike C, Furst ML: A radiographic evaluation of the periapical status of teeth treated by gutta-percha-eucapercha endodontic

method. Part III. A one-year follow-up study of 458 root canals, *Oral Surg Oral Med Oral Pathol* 56:190, 1983.

3. Van Nieuwenhuysen JP, et al: Re-treatment or radiographic monitoring in endodontics, *Int Endod J* 27:75, 1975.

4. Sundqvist G, Figdor D, Persson S, Sjogren U: Microbiologic analysis of teeth with failed endodontic treatment and the outcome of conservative re-treatment, *Oral Surg Oral Med Oral Pathol Radiol Endod* 85:86, 1998.

5. Chivian N: Surgical endodontics: a conservative approach, *J NJ Dent Soc* 40:1, 1969.

6. Siskin M: Surgical techniques applicable to endodontics, *Dent Clin North Am* 11:745, 1967.

7. Bellizzi R, Loushine R: *Clinical atlas of endodontic surgery,* Chicago, 1991, Quintessence Publishing.

8. Molven O, Halse A, Gruning B: Surgical management of endodontic failures: Indications and treatment results, *Int Dent J* 46:33, 1994.

9. Friedman S: Retrograde approaches in endodontic surgery, *Endod Dent Traumatol* 7:97, 1991.

10. Gutmann JL, Harrison JW: *Surgical endodontics,* Boston, 1991, Blackwell Scientific.

11. Arens DE, Torabinejad M, Chivian N, Rubenstein R: *Practical lessons in endodontic surgery,* Chicago, 1998, Quintessence Publishing.

12. Kramper BJ, Kaminski EJ, Osetek EM, Heuer MA: A comparative study of the wound healing of three types of flap design used in periapical surgery, *J Endod* 10:17, 1984.

13. Gilheany PA, Figdor D, Tyas MJ: Apical dentin permeability and microleakage associated with root end resection and retrograde filling, *J Endod* 20:22, 1994.

14. Grung B: Healing of gingival mucoperiosteal flaps after marginal incision in apicoectomy procedures, *Int J Oral Surg* 2:20, 1973.

15. Fister J, Gross BD: A histologic evaluation of bone response to bur cutting with and without water coolant, *Oral Surg Oral Med Oral Pathol* 49:105, 1980.

16. Morgan LA, Marshall JG: A scanning electron microscopic study of in vivo ultrasonic root-end preparations, *J Endod* 25:567, 1999.

17. Pileggi R, McDonald NJ: A qualitative scanning electron microscopic evaluation of ultrasonically cut retropreparations, *J Dent Res* 73:383, 1994.

18. Wuchenich G, Meadows D, Torabinejad M: A comparison between two root-end preparation techniques in human cadavers, *J Endod* 20:279, 1994.

19. Pantschev A, Carlsson A-P, Andersson L: Retrograde root filling with EBA cement or amalgam, a comparative clinical study, *Oral Surg Oral Med Oral Pathol* 78:101, 1994.

20. Marcotte LR, Dowson J, Rowe NH: Apical healing with retrofilling materials amalgam and gutta-percha, *J Endod* 2:63, 1975.

21. Flanders DH, James GA, Burch B, Dockum N: Comparative histopathologic study of zinc-free amalgam and Cavit in connective tissue of the rat, *J Endod* 1:56, 1975.

22. Witherspoon DE, Gutmann JL: Analysis of the healing response to gutta-percha and Diaket when used as root-end filling materials in periradicular surgery, *Int Endod J* 33:37, 2000.

23. Torabinejad M, Hong CU, Lee SJ, et al: Investigation of mineral trioxide aggregate for root-end filling in dogs, *J Endod* 21:603, 1995

24. Torabinejad M, Pitt Ford TR, McKendry DJ, et al: Histologic assessment of mineral trioxide aggregate as root-end filling in monkeys, *J Endod* 23:225, 1997.

25. Racey GL, Wallace WR, Cavalaris CJ, Marquard JV: Comparison of a polyglycolic acid suture to black silk and plain catgut in human oral tissues, *J Oral Surg* 36:766, 1978.

26. Lilly GE, Salem JE, Armstrong JH, Cutcher JL: Reaction of oral tissues to suture materials, *Oral Surg Oral Med Oral Pathol* 28:433, 1969.

27. Harrison JW, Jurosky KA Wound healing in the tissues of the periodontium following periradicular surgery. I. The incisional wound, *J Endod* 17:425, 1991.

28. Robbins SL, Kumar V: Inflammation and repair. In Robbins SL, Kumar V, editors: *Basic pathology*, ed 4, pp 28-61, Philadelphia, 1987, WB Saunders.

29. Hunt TK, Knighton DR, Thakral KK, et al: Studies on inflammation and wound healing: angiogenesis and collagen synthesis stimulated in vivo by resident and activated wound macrophages, *Surgery* 96:46, 1984.

30. Melcher AH, Chan J: Phagocytosis and digestion of collagen by gingival fibroblasts in vivo: a study of serial sections, *J Ultrastruct Res* 77:1, 1981.

31. Ross R: The fibroblast and wound repair, *Biol Rev* 43:51, 1968.

32. Harrison JW, Jurosky KA: Wound healing in the tissues of the periodontium following periradicular surgery. III. The osseous incisional wound, *J Endod* 18:76, 1992.

33. Ighaut J, Aukhill I, Simpson DM, et al: Progenitor cell kinetics during guided tissue regeneration in experimental periodontal wounds, *J Periodontal Res* 23:10, 1988.

34. Davis WL: *Oral histology: cell structure and function,* Philadelphia, 1986, WB Saunders.

35. Melcher AH, Irving JT: The healing mechanism in artificially created circumscribed defects in the femora of albino rats, *J Bone Joint Surg* 44:928, 1962.

36. American Association of Endodontists: *An annotated glossary of terms used in endodontics,* ed 6, Chicago, 1998, American Association of Endodontists.

37. Bergenholtz A: Radectomy of multirooted teeth, *J Am Dent Assoc* 85:870, 1972.

38. Langer B, Stein JD, Wagenberg B: An evaluation of root resections, *J Periodontol* 52:719, 1981.

39. Zuolo ML, Ferreira MOF, Gutmann JL. Prognosis in periradicular surgery: a clinical prospective study, *Int Endod J* 33:91, 2000.

Management of Traumatized Teeth

LEARNING OBJECTIVES

After reading this chapter, the student should be able to:

1 / Describe the clinical and radiographic features of the following: enamel fractures, crown fracture without pulp exposure, crown fracture with pulp exposure, crown-root fracture, root fracture, tooth luxation (concussion, subluxation, lateral luxation, extrusive luxation, intrusive luxation), avulsion, and alveolar fracture.

2 / Describe possible short- and long-term responses of pulp, periradicular tissues, and hard tissues to the injuries listed above.

3 / List pertinent information needed when examining patients with dental injuries (from health history, nature of injury, and symptoms).

4 / Describe the diagnostic tests and procedures used in examination of patients with dental injuries and interpret the findings.

5 / Describe appropriate treatment strategies (both at the time of injury and at follow-up) for various types of traumatic injuries.

6 / Identify the criteria for success or failure of various treatment modalities.

7 / Define pulp canal obliteration (calcific metamorphosis) and factors determining the appropriate treatment strategy.

8 / Differentiate between surface, inflammatory, and replacement resorption (ankylosis) and their respective treatment strategies.

9 / Describe the differences in treatment strategies for traumatic dental injuries in primary and permanent dentitions.

OUTLINE

Examination and Diagnosis
History
Clinical Examination
Specific Injuries
Enamel Fractures
Crown Fractures without Pulp Exposure
Crown Fractures with Pulp Exposure
Crown-Root Fractures
Root Fractures
Luxation Injuries
Avulsions
Alveolar Fractures

T rauma to teeth involves the dental pulp either directly or indirectly; consequently, endodontic considerations are important in evaluating and treating dental injuries. The purpose of this chapter is to describe examination procedures, emergency care, treatment options, and possible sequelae in traumatized teeth. Because injuries occur to primary teeth also, some of the topics discussed under "Specific Injuries" will include recommendations for these teeth.

Age is a significant factor in trauma to teeth. Injuries occur most often in the 7- to 12-year age group.[1] The significance of age is a "good news/bad news" situation. The good news is that pulps of teeth in children have a better blood supply than those in adults and better repair potential. The bad news is that growth may be interrupted in immature roots in teeth with damaged pulps, leaving the roots thin and weak (Figure 25-1). Spontaneous cervical fractures often occur because of thin dentin walls. Therefore when dental injuries occur in children, every effort is made to preserve pulp vitality.

Classification of traumatic injuries promotes better communication and dissemination of information. The system used in this chapter is based on Andreasen's modification of the World Health Organization's classification[1,2] (Box 25-1). It is preferable to other classification systems because it is internationally accepted and has a descriptive format based on anatomic and therapeutic considerations.

Examination and Diagnosis

Examination of a patient with dental injuries should include the following: chief complaint, history of present illness, pertinent medical history, and clinical examination. The emphasis in this chapter is on those aspects of the examination that specifically relate to dental trauma.[3]

HISTORY

Pertinent information regarding traumatic injuries should be obtained expeditiously by following a system.

Chief Complaint

The chief complaint is simply a statement in the patient's (or parent's) own words of the current problem, for example, "I broke my tooth," or "My tooth feels loose." It may also be unstated, as in a patient with obvious injuries.

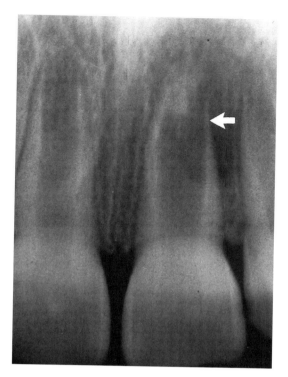

FIGURE 25-1
Trauma to an immature incisor resulted in pulp necrosis with interruption of tooth development, leaving the root with thin, weak walls *(arrow)*. Root canal treatment can be performed, but the tooth will be weak and prone to fracture.

> ### BOX 25-1
>
> ## Classification of Dental Injuries
>
> **Enamel fracture**: Involves the enamel only and includes enamel chipping and incomplete fractures or enamel cracks
> **Crown fracture without pulp involvement**: An uncomplicated fracture involving enamel and dentin with no pulp exposure
> **Crown fracture with pulp involvement**: A complicated fracture involving enamel and dentin and exposure of the pulp
> **Crown-root fracture**: Tooth fracture that includes enamel, dentin, and root cementum and may or may not include the pulp
> **Root fracture**: Fracture of root only involving cementum, dentin, and pulp; also referred to as horizontal root fracture
> **Luxation**: Tooth displacement, includes concussion, subluxation, extrusive luxation, lateral luxation, and intrusive luxation
> **Avulsion**: Complete displacement of a tooth out of its socket
> **Fracture of the alveolar process (mandible or maxilla)**: Fracture or comminution of the alveolar socket or of the alveolar process

History of Present Illness

To obtain the history of the present illness (injury), the dentist asks a few specific questions, such as the following:

When and how did the injury occur? The date and time of the accident are recorded. The record should include *how* it took place: car accident, playground, or other. Such information is useful in the search for avulsed teeth and embedded tooth fragments, assessment of possible contamination, determination of time factor with respect to choice of treatment and healing potential, and filling out accident reports.

Have you had any other injuries to your mouth or teeth in the past? Individuals may have repeated traumatic injuries if they are accident prone or participate in contact sports.[4] Crown or root fractures may have occurred as a result of an earlier injury but are observed at a later time.

What problems are you now having with your tooth or teeth? Pain, mobility, and occlusal interference are common symptoms. The patient's description of symptoms will help in diagnosis.

Medical History

The patient's medical history is often significant. For example, the patient may have an allergy to prescribed medication, may be taking medications that interact with proposed new medications, or may have a medical condition that affects treatment. Tetanus immunization status should be recorded; a booster may be indicated when there are contaminating injuries such as avulsions, intrusions, and penetrating lip and soft tissue lesions.[5]

CLINICAL EXAMINATION

The lips and oral soft tissues and facial skeleton should be examined as well as the teeth and supporting structures.

Soft Tissues

The purpose of the soft tissue evaluation is to determine the extent of tissue damage and to identify and remove foreign objects from wounds. In crown fractures with adjacent soft tissue lacerations, wounds are examined visually and radiographically for tooth fragments. Lips are likely areas for a foreign body impaction. Also, severe lacerations require suturing.

Facial Skeleton

The facial skeleton is evaluated for possible fractures of the jaw or alveolar process. Such fractures, when they involve tooth sockets, may produce pulpal necrosis in teeth associated with fracture lines.[6,7] Alveolar fractures are suspected when several teeth are displaced or move as a unit, when tooth displacement is extensive, or when occlusal misalignment is present.

Teeth and Supporting Tissues

Examination of teeth and supporting tissues should provide information about damage that may have occurred to dental hard tissues, pulps, periodontal ligaments, and bony sockets. The following guidelines provide a method of collecting information systematically.

Mobility. Teeth are examined (gently) for mobility, noting whether adjacent teeth also move when one tooth is moved (indicating alveolar fracture). The degree of horizontal mobility is recorded: 0 for no mobility; 1 for slight (<1 mm) mobility, 2 for marked (1 to 3 mm) mobility, and 3 for severe (>3 mm) mobility, both horizontally and vertically. If there is no mobility, the teeth are percussed for sounds of ankylosis (metallic sound). Absence of mobility may indicate normal status or "locking" of the tooth in bone, such as with intrusion.

Displacement. A displaced tooth has been moved from its normal position. If this occurs as a result of traumatic injury, it is referred to as "luxation." See the "Luxation Injuries" later in this chapter for descriptions of the various types of displacement.

Periradicular damage. Injury to the supporting structures of teeth may result in swelling and bleeding involving the periodontal ligament. Such teeth are sensitive to percussion, even light tapping. Apical displacement with injury to vessels entering the apical foramen may lead to pulp necrosis if the blood supply is compromised.[8]

Percussion identifies periradicular injury. Percussion must be done gently because traumatized teeth are often exquisitely painful to even light tapping. When examination or testing procedures are begun, uninjured teeth are examined first. This enhances the patient's confidence and understanding of the procedures. Importantly, in addition to testing the tooth or teeth involved

in the patient's complaint, several adjacent and opposing teeth are included also. This permits recognition of other dental injuries of which the patient may not be aware and that may not be obvious clinically. If later complications develop involving one of these adjacent or opposing teeth, early information will help in diagnosis.

Pulpal injury. Pulpal health is a very important consideration. Trauma may lead to resorption of dentin (internal) or calcific metamorphosis (radiographic obliteration) with tooth discoloration (yellowing effect). The trauma may induce pulp necrosis, which could result in external inflammatory root resorption.[9]

Pulpal status may be determined by symptoms, history, and clinical tests (see Chapter 4). Two clinical tests, however, deserve consideration here because of their applicability to traumatized teeth—the electrical pulp test (EPT) and carbon dioxide ice. These tests are generally reliable in evaluating and monitoring pulpal status except in teeth with incomplete root development.[8] A protocol for EPT and carbon dioxide ice is discussed later under "Luxation Injuries."

Radiographic examination. Radiographs are examined for fractures of bone or teeth and stage of development (Fig. 25-1). Horizontal root fractures and lateral luxations are often overlooked because the conventional angulation may miss irregularities that are not parallel with the x-ray beam. Therefore increased vertical occlusal exposure is a useful adjunct. Multiple exposures should be routine for examination of trauma to teeth to ensure complete disclosure and diagnosis of the injury.[10]

The film size should be such that it can accommodate two incisors without bending or distorting the image. It is also important to use a film holder to achieve standardized radiographic images, especially for subsequent comparisons.

A thorough examination combined with accurate records forms the basis of an appropriate treatment plan. The information gathered also provides information for accident reports that may be requested either immediately or later for legal or insurance purposes.

Specific Injuries

ENAMEL FRACTURES

Chips and cracks confined to enamel do not in themselves constitute a hazard to the pulp. The prognosis is good; however, the injury that produced the fracture may also have displaced (luxated) the tooth and damaged the blood vessels supplying the pulp. If the tooth is sensitive to

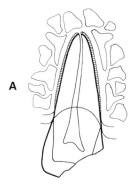
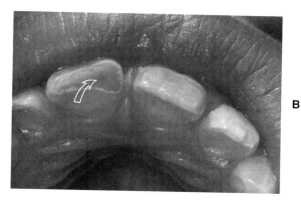

FIGURE 25-2
Crown fracture without pulp exposure. **A,** The injury results in loss of enamel and dentin without direct exposure to the pulp. **B,** Often a pink spot can be seen *(arrow)*, but if there is no direct exposure of pulp, the fracture is said to be "without pulp involvement."

percussion or if there are other signs of injury, the recommendations given under "Luxation Injuries" are followed. Grinding and smoothing the rough edges or restoring lost tooth structure may be all that is necessary.

CROWN FRACTURES WITHOUT PULP EXPOSURE
Description

These crown fractures involve enamel and dentin without pulp exposure (Figure 25-2). Such injuries are usually not associated with severe pain and generally do not require urgent care. The prognosis is good unless there is an accompanying luxation injury to periodontal ligament or to the apical vasculature supplying the pulp, in which case the tooth will be sensitive to percussion.[8] If so, the recommendations are followed as outlined under "Luxation Injuries" (as well as managing the crown fracture).

Treatment

Since the advent of the acid-etch technique, conservative restoration with composite resin of crown-fractured incisors has become possible without endangering the pulp (Figure 25-3). More conservative yet is reattachment of the separated enamel-dentin fragment (Figure 25-4). This requires a dentin bonding agent after acid-etching to improve fracture strength of the restored incisor. Clinical experiments as well as bonding studies have indicated that reattachment of dentin-enamel crown fragments is an acceptable restorative procedure and does not threaten pulp vitality.[11] Generally speaking, fracture bonding represents an ad-

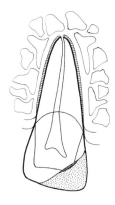

FIGURE 25-3
Restored crown fracture that does not involve the pulp directly. Exposed dentin is covered with a hard-setting liner followed by restoration of the missing tooth structure using acid-etched bonded resin.

vance in the treatment of anterior fractures. Dental anatomy is restored perfectly with normal tooth structure that abrades at a rate identical to that of the adjacent noninjured teeth. Also, pulpal status may be reliably monitored.

Chair time for the restorative procedure is minimal. The use of indirect veneering techniques at a later date to reinforce bonding or to restore the fractured incisor is a conservative approach to improving esthetics and function.[11]

Primary Teeth

Crown fractures are less common in primary than in permanent teeth. Ideally, treatment for primary teeth is the same as that for permanent teeth; however, patient cooperation may dictate the

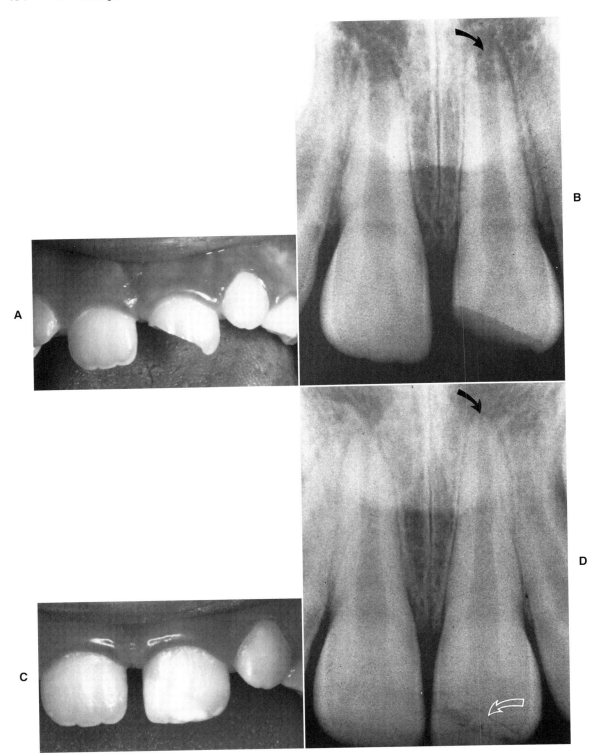

FIGURE 25-4
A, An 8-year-old patient with a fractured incisor without pulp exposure. **B,** Immature tooth with open apex *(arrow).* **C,** After the fractured segment was bonded into its original position. **D,** One-year evaluation showing continued root maturation and closing of apex *(black arrow).* Note the line where the fractured segment was bonded to the remaining tooth *(white arrow).* (From Bakland LK, Milledge T, Nation W: *Calif Dent Assoc J* 24:45, 1996.)

management approach. It is not as important to restore a primary crown fracture; thus the fracture site may be smoothed without restoring.

CROWN FRACTURES WITH PULP EXPOSURE
Description

This type of fracture involves enamel, dentin, and pulp (Figure 25-5). The pulp is exposed, and therefore the fracture becomes "complicated," a term often used for these types of injuries.[1] The extent of fracture, the stage of root development, and the length of time since injury are noted.

Extent of fracture helps to determine pulpal treatment as well as restorative needs; a small fracture may undergo vital pulp therapy and can be restored by an acid-etched composite restoration. An extensive fracture may require root canal treatment with a post and core-supported crown depending on the age of the patient.

The stage of root maturation is an important factor in choosing between pulpotomy and pulpectomy. Immature teeth have thin-walled roots (see Figure 25-1); an effort should be made to preserve the pulp to allow continued root development. That is best accomplished with a *shallow pulpotomy,* to be described in the next section. Vital pulp therapy followed by an acid-etched composite restoration or rebonding of the fractured segment is often feasible in mature teeth also. However, if the extent of tooth loss dictates restoration with a crown, root canal treatment is recommended.

The amount of time elapsed between injury and examination may directly affect pulpal health.[12] Generally, the sooner a tooth is treated, the better the prognosis for preserving the pulp. However, as a rule, pulps that have been exposed for less than a week can be treated by pulpotomy, if that is the treatment of choice. Successful pulpotomy procedures after pulp exposure of several weeks' duration have been reported,[13] but the prognosis becomes poorer the longer the pulp is exposed.[12]

Treatment of Crown Fractures

Teeth with crown fractures and exposed pulps can be treated either by pulpotomy or by root canal therapy before restoration of lost tooth structure. If vital pulp therapy is planned, it is important to perform treatment as soon after the injury as possible.

Pulpotomy. The main reason for recommending vital pulp therapy in a tooth with an exposed fracture is to preserve pulp tissue. This is particularly important in immature teeth in which continued root formation will result in a stronger tooth that is more resistant to fractures than one with thin root walls.

In the past, pulpotomy meant removal of pulp tissue to, or below, the cervical level. Loss of pulp tissue in that area means there is no additional dentin formation; this will result in a weakened tooth that is more prone to fracture. In recent years a more conservative and shallow pulpotomy has been popularized by Cvek and has sometimes been referred to as the *Cvek technique.*[13] This shallow pulpotomy preserves all the radicular and most of the coronal pulp tissue, allowing more hard tissue to develop in the root.

The pulp may need to be removed to or below the cervical level when the entire crown of an immature tooth fractures. Pulpotomy then is performed to encourage enough additional root development to allow subsequent post and core construction to support a crown. These situations are relatively uncommon. Recently a modification in the Cvek technique has been developed, using mineral trioxide aggregate (MTA), ProRoot MTA (Tulsa Dental Products, Tulsa, OK).[14,15]

Case selection. Both immature and mature teeth that can subsequently be restored with acid-etched composite are acceptable for shallow pulpotomies (Figure 25-6). Generally, immature teeth are more likely to be involved for the reasons stated previously.

Technique. The pulpotomy procedure (Figure 25-7) starts with anesthesia and rubber dam isolation. Exposed dentin is washed with saline or sodium hypochlorite solution. Extruding granulation tissue is removed with a spoon excavator from the pulp wound site. This provides an opportunity to determine more accurately the size and location of the exposure. Next, pulp tissue is removed to a depth of about 2 mm below the exposure. This relatively small amount of pulp removal is the reason for calling this procedure a shallow or partial pulpotomy.

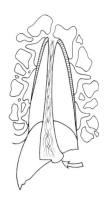

FIGURE 25-5
Crown fracture that results in exposure of the pulp. Granulation tissue *(arrow)* forms at the pulp wound within 24 hours and may actually proliferate and protrude with time.

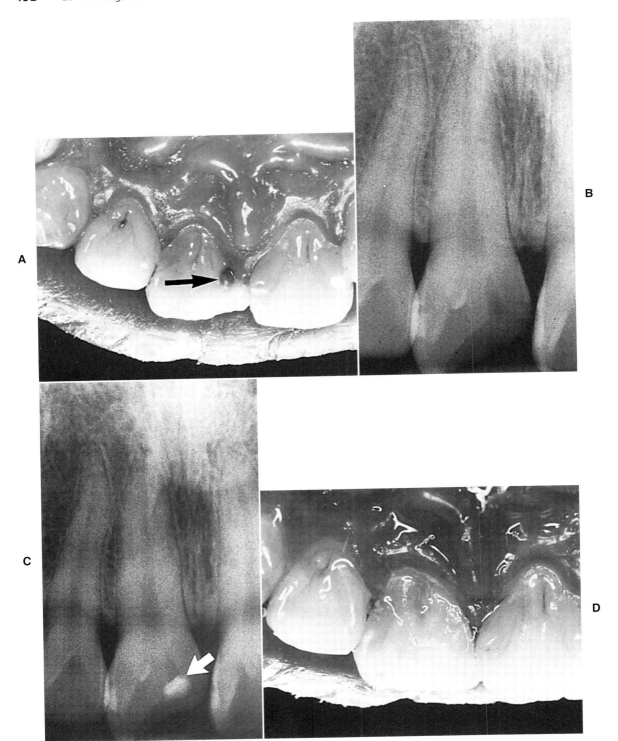

FIGURE 25-6
Shallow pulpotomy. **A,** A mesial-incisal-lingual chisel fracture occurred 3 days previously, exposing the pulp *(arrow).* **B,** Radiographic view. **C,** Preparation at exposure site is capped with calcium hydroxide liner and then sealed with ZnOE base *(arrow).* **D,** Fracture is immediately repaired with acid-etched composite resin. (Courtesy Dr. C. Noblett.)

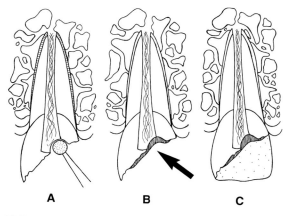

FIGURE 25-7

Shallow pulpotomy. **A,** Preparation of the pulp wound area with a round diamond stone cooled by a constant water spray. **B,** Protective dressing *(arrow)* of hard-setting calcium hydroxide covered with sealing cement (zinc oxide–eugenol, zinc phosphate, or glass ionomer). **C,** Missing tooth structure restored with acid-etched composite resin bonded to enamel.

Pulpotomy is accomplished with a water-cooled small round diamond (about the size of a No. 4 round bur) in the high-speed handpiece. Gently and gradually the surface layers of pulp tissue are wiped away, beginning at the exposure site and extending into the pulp to a depth of about 2 mm below the exposure site.

After the pulp is amputated to the desired level, a dentin shelf is created surrounding the pulp wound. The wound is gently washed with sterile saline and hemostasis is awaited. Then the wound is washed again to remove the clot (important!) and dressed with a hard-setting calcium hydroxide liner. Now the remainder of the cavity is carefully sealed with a hard-setting cement, such as IRM, or glass ionomer. When the cement has set, the tooth may be restored with acid-etched composite.

Considering the disintegration of calcium hydroxide liners with time, whenever possible the tooth is reentered after a period of 6 to 12 months to remove the initial calcium hydroxide layer and replace it with a dentin bonding material. This will prevent microleakage at the site where the initial calcium hydroxide has deteriorated and produced a space between the new dentin bridge and the covering restoration.

If MTA is used in place of calcium hydroxide, it is not necessary to wait for bleeding to stop completely. The material requires moisture for curing and can be placed directly onto the pulp tissue. Care should be followed to reduce the risk of forcing the material into the pulp proper; gently

dab small increments of the material onto the pulp using a moist cotton pellet. The pulpotomy space is filled with MTA so that it is completely flush with the fractured dentin surface. The material is then allowed to cure, which may take 6 to 12 hours. During the curing time, it is not necessary to protect the material with a restoration, but the patient must avoid using the tooth. After curing, the tooth may be restored, either with a composite resin or by bonding the fractured crown segment back onto the tooth.[15] It is not necessary to reenter the tooth after several months; MTA is stable.

Treatment evaluation. Treatment is evaluated after 6 months and then yearly. Successful shallow pulpotomy procedures (Box 25-2) may be considered definitive treatment[13] and have a very good long-term success rate.[13,16]

Root canal therapy. Teeth with mature roots may undergo either pulpotomy or root canal therapy; root canal therapy is usually necessary to accommodate prosthetic requirements. For example, if the crown has fractured in the gingival margin region, root canal treatment will allow post and core and crown placement.

Primary Teeth

Crown fractures with pulp exposures occur in primary teeth, although less often than in permanent teeth.[1] Treatment includes pulpotomy, root canal therapy, or extraction, depending on patient age and cooperation. If the root is more than half resorbed apically, the tooth is extracted. If root canal therapy is chosen, the canal is filled with a resorbable zinc oxide–eugenol based paste. Fractured crowns may be restored with acid-etched composite.

BOX 25-2

Criteria for a Successful Shallow Pulpotomy[1]

1. The tooth is asymptomatic and functions properly.
2. There is no radiographic evidence of periradicular periodontitis.
3. There is no indication of root resorption.
4. The tooth responds to pulp testing (if pulp testing is possible).
5. Continued root development and dentin formation are evident radiographically, if the root was immature at the time of treatment. If the pulp becomes necrotic or formation is arrested, apexification is then necessary.

CROWN-ROOT FRACTURES
Description

These fractures are usually oblique and involve both crown and root. Anterior teeth show the so-called chisel-type fracture, which splits the crown diagonally and extends subgingivally to a root surface (Figure 25-8). They resemble a crown fracture but are more extensive and more serious because they include the root. Another variation is the fracture that shatters the crown (Figure 25-9). The pieces are held in place only by the part of the fractured segment still attached to the periodontal ligament or gingival tissues. In all of these fractures, the pulp is usually exposed.

In contrast to other traumatic injuries in which posterior teeth are rarely involved, crown-root fractures often include the molars and premolars. Cusp fractures that extend subgingivally are common (Figure 25-10). Diagnostically they may, however, be difficult to identify in the early stages of development. Similarly, vertical fractures in the long axis of roots are difficult to detect and diagnose. Such crown-root fractures are discussed in more detail in Chapter 28.

Crown-root fractures in posterior teeth cannot always be associated with a single traumatic incident, although bicycle or automobile accidents at times may produce these results. The risk is increased with a sharp blow to the chin causing the jaws to slam together; skin abrasions under the chin may be a sign of such an impact. Also, all posterior teeth should be examined using a sharp explorer to detect movement of loose fragments.[1]

Examination

Crown-root fractures are complex injuries that are difficult both to evaluate and to treat. Until recently, it was recommended that all loose fragments had to be removed to evaluate the extent of injury. This may still be necessary in some instances, but with the availability of bonding agents it is now possible to bond loose fragments at least temporarily. The current recommendation is to attempt to bond loose fragments together, particularly if the tooth is immature and still developing. Clinical judgment must be used to decide when to follow one course of action or another.

It is not unusual, in a tooth in which the crown has broken into several pieces, to find that the same shattering effect has extended to the root as well. Additional radiographs at different angles

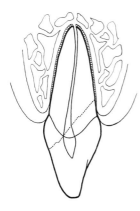

FIGURE 25-8
Crown-root fracture. Anterior teeth may develop "chisel-type" fractures, which extend below the cementoenamel junction. Because of the nature and location of these fractures, they are difficult to manage.

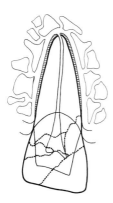

FIGURE 25-9
Crown-root fracture resulting in a shattered crown with subgingival extension.

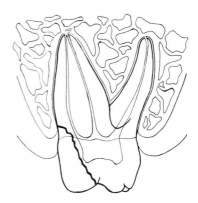

FIGURE 25-10
Pulp exposure may or may not be present with a crown-root fracture of a posterior tooth.

(as will be described under "Root Fractures") may help to identify radicular fracture lines.

Emergency Care

Teeth with crown-root fractures are often painful; such injuries often require urgent care. This may consist only of removing loose tooth fragments but often also includes pulp therapy (Figure 25-11). If the root is immature, pulpotomy (see "Crown Fractures with Pulp Exposure" in this chapter and also "Vital Pulp Therapy" in Chapter 22) is preferable to pulpectomy, whereas pulpectomy is the treatment of choice in patients with fully developed teeth. Definitive treatment should be postponed until an overall endodontic and restorative treatment plan is developed.

Treatment Planning

Crown-root fractures are often complicated by pulp exposures and extensive loss of tooth structure. In developing a treatment plan, many questions must be considered: Which is better for this tooth, pulpotomy or pulpectomy? After all loose fragments have been removed, will there be enough tooth structure to support a restoration? Is the subgingival fracture below a level at which a restorative margin can be placed, thus necessitating root extrusion or gingivoplasty or alveoplasty? Should the tooth be extracted and replaced with a bridge or implant? Or if extraction is chosen, can the space be closed orthodontically? These are but a few of the many questions. Because of such complexity, a team approach involving specialists in the areas of

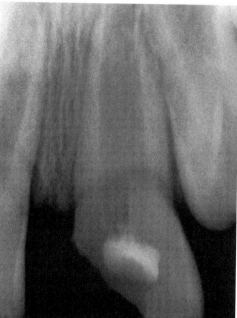

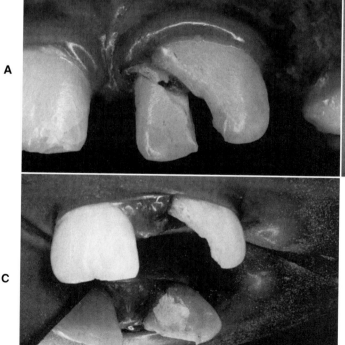

FIGURE 25-11
Urgent care of crown-root fracture. **A,** The mesial segments are mobile and must be removed. **B,** After removal of all loose fragments, the exposed pulp is managed by shallow pulpotomy. **C,** The crown can now be restored with acid-etched resin.

endodontics, periodontics, orthodontics, and prosthodontics is beneficial in developing the treatment plan.

Primary Teeth

A crown-root fracture in primary teeth usually dictates extraction. Occasionally, sufficient remaining tooth structure may be available for restoration or recontouring.

ROOT FRACTURES
Description

Fractures of roots (Figure 25-12) have been called intraalveolar root fractures, horizontal root fractures, and transverse root fractures. They do not occur often and may be difficult to detect.[17-21]

Radiographically, a root fracture is visualized if the x-ray beam passes through the fracture line. Because these fractures often are transverse-to-oblique (involving pulp, dentin, and cementum), they may be missed if the central beam's direction is not parallel or close to parallel to the fracture line. For this reason, a steep vertical angulation is included in addition to the normal parallel angulation whenever a root fracture is suspected. This additional angulation, i.e., foreshortened view (approximately 45 degrees), will detect many fractures, particularly in the apical regions (Figure 25-13).[1,20,21]

Clinically, root fractures may present as mobile or displaced teeth, with pain on biting. Symptoms are generally mild. If mobility and displacement of the coronal segment are absent or slight, the patient may have no chief complaint and may not seek treatment.[20] Generally, the more cervical the fracture, the more mobility and displacement of the coronal segment and a greater likelihood of pulp necrosis of this segment. Treatment (splinting) for root fractures is indicated if the coronal segment is mobile. Thus root fractures in the apical and middle thirds usually require no immediate treatment but must be observed long term.[20]

Emergency Care

If a root fracture is identified, initial treatment includes repositioning of the coronal segment (if displaced) and stabilization by splinting. Repositioning of the coronal segment may be as easy as applying finger pressure to the crown to align the segment, or it may be more complicated, requiring orthodontic approaches. When the coronal segment has been repositioned, it must be

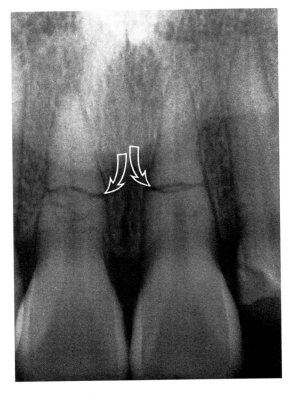

FIGURE 25-12
Horizontal root fractures. Central incisors are the teeth most often involved. Unless the coronal segments are displaced or mobile, no splinting or other treatment is necessary.

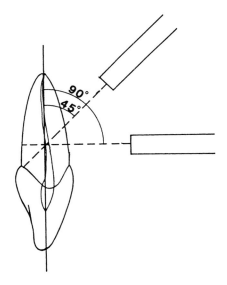

FIGURE 25-13
Radiographic technique used for suspected root fractures. At least two angulations are made: the conventional (90 degree) view and a steep vertical (45 degree) view. Additional angulations help to detect suspected root fractures by directing the x-ray beam through a diagonal fracture.

stabilized to allow repair of the periodontium (Figure 25-14).

Stabilization may be accomplished by the use of orthodontic wire and acid-etched resin. Splinting time must be sufficient to allow calcification to take place, probably both internally in the pulpal space and possibly externally across the fracture lines.[17] Up to 12 weeks' stabilization has been recommended.[20] If repair takes place with no evidence of pulp necrosis, root-fractured teeth do not require root canal treatment.[18]

Sequelae of Root Fractures

Root fractures are often characterized by development of calcific metamorphosis (radiographic obliteration) in one (usually coronal) or both segments; therefore EPT readings may be very high or absent. Lack of response to EPT by itself, however, in the absence of other evidence of pulp necrosis (bony lesions apically or laterally, adverse symptoms, and so on), does not indicate a need for root canal treatment. The majority of root fractures heal either spontaneously or following splint therapy.[18]

Root Canal Treatment

Root canal treatment is indicated when pathosis is evident, usually owing to development of pulp necrosis in the coronal portion, which subsequently leads to inflammatory lesions adjacent to the fracture lines (Figure 25-15).[19] The endodontic procedure, when necessary, usually is complex; referral to a specialist should be considered. The various treatment approaches are listed in Box 25-3. The current recommendation is to treat only the coronal segment canal (Figure 25-16). The pulp in the apical segment usually remains vital.

Primary Teeth

Root fractures are not common in primary teeth.[1] Those that occur with marked coronal displacement should be treated by removing the coronal segment and leaving the root apex in situ. Any attempt to remove the root apex may damage the subjacent permanent tooth bud. As in permanent teeth, root fractures not accompanied by mobility usually require no treatment unless problems develop subsequently.

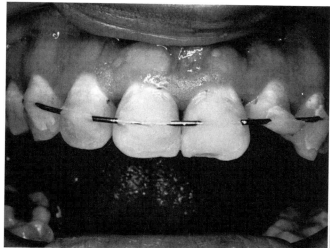
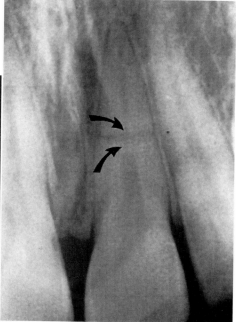

FIGURE 25-14

Stabilization of root fractures with a mobile coronal segment. **A,** Orthodontic wire is adapted to labial surfaces of anterior teeth and attached using the acid-etched resin technique. If possible, all six anterior teeth are included for better stabilization. **B,** At future evaluation, root formation has responded to treatment (stabilization). Internal calcification adjacent to the fracture *(arrows)* indicates repair.

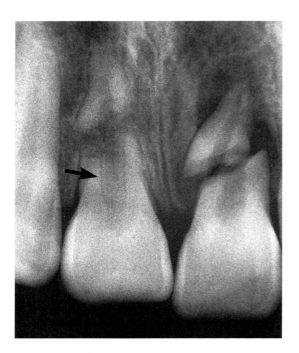

FIGURE 25-15
Two different long-term sequelae of horizontal root fractures. The incisor on the *left* shows bony interposition between the fractured segments, with bone growth into the coronal pulp space and formation of a lamina dura and periodontal ligament space *(arrow)*. The incisor on the *right* has undergone pulp necrosis of both segments; because of the location of the fracture and resulting damage, removal of both segments is indicated. (Courtesy Dr. M. Gomez.)

BOX 25-3

Treatment Procedures for Teeth with Root Fractures and Necrotic Pulps

1. Root canal therapy for both coronal and apical segments
2. Root canal therapy for coronal segment, no treatment for apical segment
3. Root canal therapy for coronal segment, surgical removal of apical segment
4. Coronal segment root canal therapy preceded by hard tissue induction at the fracture site ("apexification"-type procedure for the canal opening at the apical end of the coronal segment); no treatment for the apical segment*
5. Intraradicular splint, in which a post is used to brace the two segments internally
6. Endodontic implant, in which the apical part of the implant replaces the surgically removed apical root segment
7. Root extrusion, in which the coronal segment is removed and the apical segment is extruded to allow restoration of the missing coronal tooth structure; root canal therapy performed on the apical segment before its extrusion

*This procedure is the most common current recommendation and provides the most consistent results.

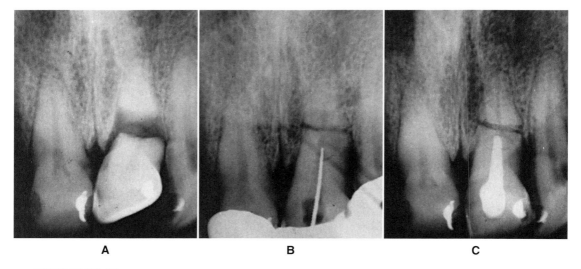

A	**B**	**C**

FIGURE 25-16
Successful treatment of pulp necrosis in a root-fractured incisor with root canal filling of coronal fragment. **A,** Condition after the injury. **B,** Segment is repositioned, stabilized, and treated. **C,** Five months after obturation; the segment is stable.

LUXATION INJURIES
Description

Luxation injuries (Figure 25-17) cause trauma to the supporting structures of teeth and often affect the neural and vascular supply to the pulp. The cause is usually a sudden impact, such as a blow or striking a hard object during a fall.[1,22] Generally, the more severe the luxation (involving more displacement), the greater the damage to the periodontium and to the dental pulp. Table 25-1 provides a summary of the typical clinical and radiographic findings associated with different types of luxation injuries.[1]

Concussion. The tooth is sensitive to percussion only. There is no increase in mobility, and the tooth has not been displaced. The pulp may respond normally to testing, and no radiographic changes are found.

Subluxation. Subluxation injuries include teeth that are sensitive to percussion and also have in-creased mobility. Often sulcular bleeding is present, indicating vessel damage and tearing of the periodontal ligament. No displacement is found, and the pulp may respond normally to testing. Radiographic findings are unremarkable.

Extrusive luxation. These teeth have been partially displaced from the socket along the long axis. Such extruded teeth have greatly increased mobility, and radiographs show displacement. The pulp usually does not respond to testing.

Lateral luxation. Trauma has displaced the tooth lingually, buccally, mesially, or distally, that is, out of its normal position away from its long axis. If the apex has been translocated during the displacement, the tooth may be quite firm. Percussion sensitivity may or may not be present with a metallic sound if the tooth is firm, indicating that the root has been forced into the alveolar bone.

Intrusive luxation. Teeth are forced into their sockets in an axial (apical) direction, at times to

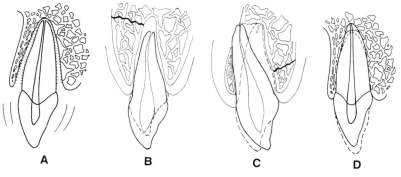

FIGURE 25-17
Luxation injuries. **A,** Subluxation: the tooth is loosened but not displaced. **B,** Extrusive luxation: the tooth is partially extruded from its socket. Occasionally this is accompanied by an alveolar fracture. **C,** Lateral luxation: the crown is displaced palatally and the root apex labially. **D,** Intrusive luxation: the tooth is displaced apically.

TABLE 25-1

Typical Clinical Findings with Different Types of Luxation Injuries

CLINICAL FINDINGS	CONCUSSION	SUBLUXATION	EXTRUSION	INTRUSION	LATERAL LUXATION
Abnormal mobility	−	+	+	− (+)*	− (+)
Tenderness to percussion	+	+ (−)	±	− (+)	− (+)
Percussion sound	Normal†	Dull	Dull	Metallic	Metallic
Positive response to pulp testing	±	±	− (+)	− (+)	− (+)
Clinical dislocation	−	−	+	+	+
Radiographic dislocation	−	−	+	+	+

From Andreasen JO, Andreasen FM: *Textbook and color atlas of traumatic injuries to the teeth*, ed. 3, St Louis, 1994, Mosby.
*(+), Less common occurrence.
†Teeth with incomplete root formation and teeth with marginal or periapical inflammatory lesions will also elicit a dull percussion sound.

the point of being buried and not visible. They have decreased mobility and resemble ankylosis.

Examination and Diagnosis

The clinical descriptions of the five types of luxation injuries should be sufficient to make the initial diagnosis. Pulpal status must be continually monitored until a definitive diagnosis can be made, which in some cases may require several months or years. Carbon dioxide ice and the EPT are used in monitoring pulpal status.[7]

Concussion injuries generally respond to pulp testing. Because the injury is less severe, pulpal blood supply is more likely to return to normal. Teeth in the *subluxation* injury group also tend to retain or recover pulpal responsiveness but less predictably than teeth with concussion injuries. In both cases, an immature tooth with an open apex has a better prognosis. *Extrusive, lateral,* and *intrusive* injuries involve more displacement and therefore more damage to apical vessels and nerves. Therefore pulp responses in teeth with extrusive, lateral, and intrusive luxations are often absent. These pulps often do not recover responsiveness even if the pulp is vital (has blood supply), because sensory nerves are permanently damaged. Exceptions are immature teeth with wide-open apices; these teeth often regain or retain pulp vitality (responsiveness) even after severe injuries.[8,23]

Monitoring pulp status requires a schedule of pulp testing and radiographic evaluation for a long enough time to permit determination of the outcome with some degree of certainty. That may require 2 or more years. Pulp status is best monitored with pulp testing, radiographs, developing symptoms, and observation for crown color changes.[7,8,23]

Pulp testing. Carbon dioxide ice or the EPT is used to test teeth that have been injured; several adjacent and opposing teeth are included in the test. An initial lack of response is neither unusual, nor is a high reading on the pulp tester. Retesting is done in 4 to 6 weeks; the results are recorded and compared with the initial responses. If the pulp responds in both instances, the prognosis for pulp survival is good. A pulp response that is absent initially and present at the second visit indicates a probable recovery of vitality, although cases of subsequent reversals have been noted.[1] If the pulp fails to respond both times, the prognosis is questionable and the pulp status uncertain. In the absence of other findings indicating pulp necrosis, the tooth is retested in 3 to 4 months. Continued lack of response may indicate pulp necrosis by infarct, but lack of response may not

be enough evidence to make a diagnosis of pulp necrosis. That is, the pulp may permanently lose sensory nerve supply but retain its blood supply. After a period of time, the pulp often responds to testing if it recovers.

Radiographic evaluation. The initial radiograph made after the injury will not disclose the pulp condition. However, it is very important for evaluation of the general injury to the tooth and alveolus and serves as a basis for comparison of subsequent radiographs. These radiographs are taken at the same intervals used for pulp testing. Evidence of resorption, both internal and external, and periradicular bony changes is sought. Resorptive changes, particularly external changes, may occur soon after injury; if no attempt is made to arrest the destructive process, much of the root may be rapidly lost. Inflammatory resorption can be intercepted by timely endodontic intervention.

Pulp space calcification or obliteration is a common finding after luxation injuries.[24] Also called *calcific metamorphosis,* this canal obliteration may be partial or nearly complete (after several years) and does not require root canal treatment, except when other signs and symptoms indicate pulp necrosis.

Crown color changes. Pulp injury may cause discoloration, even after only a few days. Initial changes tend to be pink. Subsequently, if the pulp does not recover and becomes necrotic, there may be a grayish darkening of the crown, often accompanied by a loss in translucency. Also, color changes may take place owing to increased calcific metamorphosis. Such color changes are likely to be yellow to brown and do not indicate pulp pathosis. Other signs, findings, or symptoms are necessary to diagnose pulp necrosis.

Finally, discoloration may be reversed. This usually happens relatively soon after the injury and indicates that the pulp is vital. Because of unpredictable changes associated with traumatized teeth, long-term evaluation is recommended.

Treatment of Luxation Injuries

Luxation injuries, regardless of type, often present diagnostic and treatment complexities that require consultation with specialists. For *concussion* injuries, no immediate treatment is necessary. The patient should allow the tooth to "rest" (avoid biting) until sensitivity has subsided. Pulp status is monitored as described. *Subluxations* may likewise require no treatment unless mobility is moderate; if mobility is graded 2, stabilization may be necessary.[1]

Extrusive and *lateral luxation* injuries require repositioning and splinting (see Figure 25-14). The length of time needed for splinting varies with the severity of injury. Extrusions may need only 2 to 3 weeks, whereas luxations that involve bony fractures need up to 8 weeks.[1] Root canal treatment is indicated for teeth with a diagnosis of irreversible pulpitis or pulp necrosis. Such a diagnosis often requires a combination of signs and symptoms such as discoloration of the crown, lack of pulp response to the EPT, and a periradicular lesion seen radiographically.[1] Severe pulp damage is more likely with greater degrees of displacement.

Treatment of *intrusive luxation* injuries depends on root maturity.[25] If the tooth is incompletely formed with an open apex, it may re-erupt. If it is fully developed, active extrusion will be necessary soon after the injury, usually by an orthodontic appliance. In extreme cases of intrusion, in which the tooth has been totally embedded into the alveolus, surgical repositioning may be necessary. Surgical repositioning should, however, be only partial and should be supplemented with orthodontic extrusion to reduce the risk of marginal bone loss and ankylosis. Root canal treatment is indicated for intruded teeth with the exception of those with immature roots, in which case the pulp may revascularize.[23]

A tooth with any luxation injury and also signs or symptoms of irreversible pulpitis requires root canal treatment; the procedure is conventional and may be completed in one appointment. If the pulp is necrotic, treatment may be accomplished in one or two visits with calcium hydroxide placed in the prepared canal for 1 to 2 weeks before obturation. If there is also evidence of external resorption in addition to pulp necrosis, calcium hydroxide should be left in the canal until evidence of root surface repair, such as reestablishment of periodontal ligament space, is evident.

Primary Teeth

Concussion and *subluxation* injuries require no treatment. Pulpal evaluation is limited to radiographic and clinical observation. Persistent crown discoloration usually indicates pulp necrosis, necessitating either root canal treatment or extraction.[26,27] Discolored primary teeth may return to normal color, probably indicating recovery of the pulp.[9] Calcific metamorphosis is common after luxation injuries. This changes the primary crown to a darker yellow color, which is not pathosis and so requires no treatment.

Teeth with lateral and extrusive luxations may be left untreated, or the tooth may be extracted, depending on the severity of injury. Teeth with intrusive luxations should be carefully evaluated to determine the direction of intrusion. Radiographs provide valuable information. If the in-

truded tooth appears foreshortened on the film, the apex is oriented toward the x-ray cone. Therefore these teeth should present no danger to the permanent successor and may be left to re-erupt. If the tooth appears elongated, the apex is oriented toward the permanent successor and may pose a risk to the permanent tooth bud. The tooth should be carefully extracted if it impinges on the permanent successor. Also evaluated is the symmetry of the permanent tooth buds.[1]

AVULSIONS
Description

An avulsed tooth is one that has been totally displaced out of its alveolar socket. If the tooth is replanted soon after avulsion (immediate replantation), the periodontal ligament has a good chance of healing. Time out of socket and the storage media used are the most critical factors in successful replantation. It is important to preserve the periodontal ligament cells and the fibers attached to the root surface by keeping the tooth moist and minimizing handling of the root.[1,28]

Treatment

Three situations involving avulsions may occur: (1) someone may telephone for advice about an avulsed tooth, presenting an opportunity for immediate replantation (within minutes); (2) the patient may be brought to the office with a tooth that has been out of the alveolus for *less* than 1 hour or kept in a suitable storage medium; or (3) the tooth has been out for *more* than 1 hour and not kept in a storage medium.

Immediate replantation. The prognosis is improved by replantation immediately after avulsion.[28] Many individuals—parents, athletic instructors, and others—are aware of this emergency procedure and can replant on site. Some may ask for advice by phone. The procedure used for immediate replantation is presented in Box 25-4.

BOX 25-4

First Aid for Avulsed Teeth

1. Rinse the tooth in cold, running tap water (10 seconds).
2. Do not scrub the tooth.
3. Replace the tooth in the socket using gentle finger pressure.
4. Hold (or have the patient hold) the tooth in position.
5. Seek dental care immediately.

When a patient who has had a tooth replanted at the accident site comes to the dental office, the replantation should be examined both clinically and radiographically. The dentist looks for additional injuries to adjacent or opposing teeth and evaluates the replanted tooth for stability and alignment. The procedure outlined in the next section (with the exception of the replantation step) is followed.

Replantation within 1 hour of avulsion. If immediate replantation is not feasible, the injured person should be brought to the dental office and the tooth transported in such a way as to keep it moist.[29] The best transport medium is a commercially available storage-transport medium or physiologic saline (usually neither is available); milk is an excellent alternative.[28,30] Saliva is acceptable, whereas water is not good for maintaining root-surface cell vitality.[1]

When the patient arrives:

1. The tooth is placed in a cup of physiologic saline.
2. The area of injury is radiographed, looking for evidence of alveolar fracture.
3. The avulsion site is examined carefully for any loose bone fragments that may be removed. If the alveolus is collapsed, it is spread open gently with an instrument.
4. The socket is gently irrigated with saline to remove contaminated coagulum.
5. In the cup of saline, the tooth is grasped with extraction forceps by the crown to avoid handling the root.
6. The tooth is examined for debris, which, if present, is gently removed with gauze moistened with saline.
7. The tooth is replaced into the socket; after partial insertion using the forceps, gentle finger pressure is used or the patient bites on gauze until the tooth is seated.
8. Proper alignment is checked, and hyperocclusion is corrected. Soft tissue lacerations are tightly sutured, particularly cervically.
9. The tooth is stabilized for 1 to 2 weeks with a splint (see Figure 25-14).
10. It has been suggested that antibiotics be prescribed in the same dosage as that used for mild to moderate oral infections.[31] A tetanus booster injection is recommended if the last one was administered more than 5 years previously.[4]
11. Supportive care is given; a soft diet and mild analgesics are suggested as needed.

Root canal treatment is indicated for mature teeth and should be done optimally after 1 week and before the splint is removed (the splint stabilizes the tooth during the procedure). The exception to routine root canal therapy is immature teeth with wide-open apices; they may revascularize but must be evaluated at regular intervals of 2, 6, and 12 months after replantation. If subsequent evaluations indicate pulp necrosis, root canal treatment, probably including apexification, is indicated.[32]

Replantation more than 1 hour after avulsion. If a tooth has been out of the alveolar socket for more than 1 hour (and not kept moist in a suitable medium), periodontal ligament cells and fibers will not survive regardless of the stage of root development. Replacement resorption (ankylosis) will probably be the eventual sequela after replantation. Therefore treatment efforts before replantation include treating the root surface with fluoride to reduce (slow) the resorptive process.[1]

When the patient arrives:

1. The area of tooth avulsion is examined and radiographs are examined for evidence of alveolar fractures.
2. Debris and pieces of soft tissue adhering to the root surface are removed.
3. The tooth is soaked in a 2.4% solution of sodium fluoride (acidulated to pH 5.5) for 5 to 20 minutes.

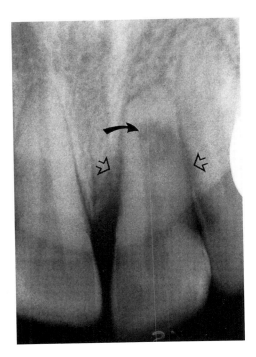

FIGURE 25-18
Replanted tooth with inflammatory resorption characterized by resorption of tooth structure *(curved arrow)* and a periodontal lesion in the periradicular bone *(open arrows)*. Although the inflammatory resorption appears internal, it is in fact superimposed and is external.

4. The pulp is extirpated, and the canal is cleaned, shaped, and filled while the tooth is held in a fluoride-soaked piece of gauze. Often the procedure can be accomplished from an apical direction if the root is immature.

5. The alveolar socket is carefully suctioned to remove the blood clot. The socket is irrigated with saline.[33] Anesthesia may be necessary first.

6. The tooth is gently replanted into the socket, checking for proper alignment and occlusal contact.

7. The tooth is splinted for 3 to 6 weeks (see Figure 25-14).

Sequelae to Replantation

Generally external resorption occurs. Three types have been identified: surface, inflammatory, and replacement.[1]

Surface resorption. Microscopic examination of replanted teeth reveals lacunae of resorption in the cementum. These are not usually visible on radiographs. They are repaired by deposition of new cementum, which represents healing.

Inflammatory resorption. Inflammatory resorption occurs as a response to the presence of infected necrotic pulp in conjunction with injury to the periodontal ligament. It occurs with replanted teeth (Figure 25-18) as well as with other types of luxation injuries. It is characterized by loss of tooth structure and adjacent alveolar bone. Resorption usually subsides after removal of the necrotic pulp, so the prognosis is good. Root canal treatment is therefore recommended routinely for replanted teeth with closed apexes.

Replacement resorption. In replacement resorption the tooth structure is resorbed and replaced by bone (Figure 25-19). This is the result of ankylosis; bone fuses directly to the root surface. The characteristics of ankylosis are lack of physiologic mobility, failure of the tooth to erupt along with adjacent teeth (leading to infraocclusion in young individuals), and a "solid" metallic sound when percussed. Currently, no known treatment is available for replacement resorption, which tends to be continuous until the root is replaced by bone. In teeth that have had long extraalveolar dry periods, the resorptive process is apparently slowed (but not halted) by immersing the tooth in fluoride before replantation.[1]

Primary Teeth

Replantation of avulsed primary teeth is not recommended because of the risk of damage to the permanent successor. Premature loss of a primary incisor is generally not serious.

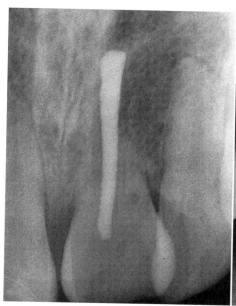
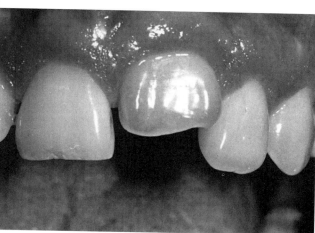

A

B

FIGURE 25-19
Replacement resorption (ankylosis). **A,** The root of this replanted root canal treated tooth has been almost totally resorbed and has been replaced by bone that fuses to the tooth structure, resulting in ankylosis and resorption. **B,** Tooth is in infraocclusion owing to ankylosis, which prevents normal eruption, as evidenced by continuous eruption of the adjacent teeth.

Root Canal Treatment

Mature avulsed teeth, when replanted, cannot be expected to reestablish pulpal blood supply.[32] Revascularization may occur in immature teeth with wide open apexes, but it is unpredictable. These teeth must be monitored radiographically over a period of time to watch for evidence of pulp necrosis.

In the mature replanted tooth, root canal treatment is definitely indicated and should be done about 1 to 2 weeks after replantation. The splint may remain during treatment for stability. The use of calcium hydroxide as an antimicrobial intracanal interappointment medicament may be helpful[34]; it is particularly beneficial if the root canal is infected, a condition that would be likely to occur when root canal treatment is delayed more than a few weeks after replantation.

The procedure consists of cleaning and shaping, followed by calcium hydroxide placement for a minimum of 1 to 2 weeks.[28] Obturation is then accomplished with gutta-percha and sealer. Long-term evaluation is necessary; complex problems may develop in the future.

Restoration, both temporary and permanent, is the key to success. Sealing of the access is critical between appointments and after obturation.

For long-term stability, a dentin bonding agent with acid-etched composite is indicated.[28]

ALVEOLAR FRACTURES

Pulp necrosis is often associated with alveolar fractures, which may in turn be associated with other major facial injuries.[5,6] The initial, urgent need is management of the fracture, which is splinting of the segment to the adjacent teeth and often is performed by oral and maxillofacial surgeons. When the patient is able to have the teeth examined, those in the line of fracture as well as adjacent teeth are evaluated. Lack of response to an EPT, if not reversed within 3 to 6 months, often, but not always, indicates pulp necrosis. Therefore the presence of other indicators (apical radiolucency or symptoms) is necessary before further treatment is given (Figure 25-20). Root canal treatment is indicated when pulp necrosis is diagnosed.[35]

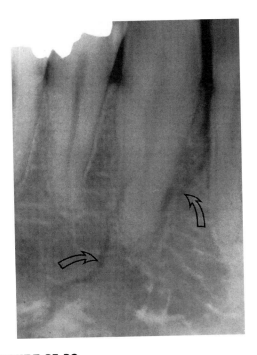

FIGURE 25-20
Alveolar fracture (arrows). Teeth involved in an alveolar fracture should have careful short- and long-term monitoring for pulp responsiveness or other signs of pathosis.

REFERENCES

1. Andreasen JO, Andreasen FM: *Textbook and color atlas of traumatic injuries to the teeth,* ed 3, St Louis, 1994, Mosby.
2. World Health Organization: *Application of the international classification of diseases to dentistry and stomatology,* ed 3, Geneva, 1993, ICD-DA.
3. Bakland LK, Andreasen JO: Examination of the dentally traumatized patient, *Calif Dent Assoc J* 24:35, 1996.
4. Glendor U, Koucheki B, Halling A: Risk evaluation and type of treatment of multiple dental trauma episodes to permanent teeth, *Endod Dent Traumatol* 16:205, 2000.
5. Arnon SS: Tetanus. In Behrman RE, Kleigman R, Arvin AM, editors: *Nelson's textbook of pediatrics,* ed 15, Philadelphia, 1995, WB Saunders.
6. Kamboozia AH, Punnia-Moorthy A: The fate of teeth in mandibular fracture lines. A clinical and radiographic follow-up study, *Int J Oral Maxillofac Surg* 22:97, 1993.
7. Oikarinen K, Lahti J, Raustia AM: Prognosis of permanent teeth in the line of mandibular fractures, *Endod Dent Traumatol* 6:177, 1990.
8. Andreasen FM, Andreasen JO: Diagnosis of luxation injuries: the importance of standardized clinical, radiographic and photographic techniques in clinical investigations, *Endod Dent Traumatol* 1:160, 1985.
9. Andreasen FM, Vestergaard Pedersen B: Prognosis of luxated permanent teeth the development of pulp necrosis, *Endod Dent Traumatol* 1:207, 1985.
10. Andreasen FM, Andreasen JO: Treatment of traumatic injuries: shift in strategy, *Int J Technol Assess Health Care* 6:588, 1990.
11. Andreasen FM, Flugge E, Daugaard-Jensen J, Munksgaard EC: Treatment of crown fractured incisors with laminate veneer restorations. An experimental study, *Endod Dent Traumatol* 8:30, 1992.

12. Heide S: Pulp reactions to exposure for 4, 48, or 168 hours, *J Dent Res* 59:1910, 1980 (abstract).
13. Cvek M: A clinical report on partial pulpotomy and capping with calcium hydroxide in permanent incisors with complicated crown fracture, *J Endod* 4:232, 1978.
14. Pitt Ford TR, Torabinejad M, Abedi HR, et al: Using mineral trioxide aggregate as a pulp-capping material, *J Am Dent Assoc* 127:1491, 1996.
15. Bakland LK: Management of traumatically injured pulps in immature teeth using MTA, *Calif Dent Assoc J* 28:855, 2000.
16. Fuks A, Chosack S: Long-term follow-up of traumatized incisors treated by partial pulpotomy, *Pediatr Dent* 15:334, 1993.
17. Herweijer JA, Torabinejad M, Bakland LK: Healing of horizontal root fractures, *J Endod* 18:118, 1992.
18. Zachrisson BV, Jacobsen I: Long-term prognosis of 66 permanent anterior teeth with root fracture, *Scand J Dent Res* 83:345, 1975.
19. Andreasen JO, Hjorting-Hansen E: Intraalveolar root fractures: radiographic and histologic study of 50 cases, *J Oral Surg* 25:414, 1967.
20. Andreasen FM, Andreasen JO, Bayer T: Prognosis of root-fractured permanent incisors: prediction of healing modalities, *Endod Dent Traumatol* 5:11, 1989.
21. Bender IB, Freedland JB: Clinical considerations in the diagnosis and treatment of intra-alveolar root fractures, *J Am Dent Assoc* 107:595, 1983.
22. Crona-Larson G, Noren JG: Luxation injuries to permanent teeth—a retrospective study of etiological factors, *Endod Dent Traumatol* 5:176, 1989.
23. Andreasen FM: Pulpal healing after luxation injuries and root fractures in the permanent dentition, *Endod Dent Traumatol* 5:111, 1989.
24. Andreasen FM, Zhijie Y, Thomsen BL, Andersen PK: Occurrence of pulp canal obliteration after luxation injuries in the permanent dentition, *Endod Dent Traumatol* 3:103, 1987.
25. Jacobsen I: Long term evaluation, prognosis and subsequent management of traumatic tooth injuries. In *Proceedings of the International Conference on Oral Trauma*, Chicago, 1986, American Association of Endodontists.
26. Holan G, Topf J, Fuks A: Effect of root canal infection and treatment of traumatized primary incisors on permanent successors, *Endod Dent Traumatol* 8:12, 1992.
27. Soxman JA, Nazif MM, Bouquot J: Pulpal pathology in relation to discoloration of primary anterior teeth, *J Dent Child* 51:282, 1984.
28. American Association of Endodontists: Treating the avulsed permanent tooth, *Endodontics: Colleagues for Excellence,* Winter/Spring, 1994.
29. Trope M: Protocol for treating the avulsed tooth, *Calif Dent Assoc J* 24:43, 1996.
30. Krasner P, Person P: Preserving avulsed teeth for replantation, *J Am Dent Assoc* 123:80, 1992.
31. Hammarström L, Blomlof L, Feiglin B, et al: Replantation of teeth and antibiotic treatment, *Endod Dent Traumatol* 2:51, 1986.
32. Kling M, Cvek M, Mejare I: Rate and predictability of pulp revascularization in therapeutically reimplanted permanent teeth, *Endod Dent Traumatol* 2:83, 1986.
33. Matsson L, Klinge B, Hallstrom H: Effect on periodontal healing of saline irrigation of the tooth socket before replantation, *Endod Dent Traumatol* 3:64, 1987.
34. Trope M, Yesilsoy C, Koren L, et al: Effect of different endodontic treatment protocols on periodontal repair and root resorption of replanted dog teeth, *J Endod* 18:492, 1992.
35. Andreasen JO: Fractures of the alveolar process of the jaw. A clinical and radiographic follow-up study, *Scand J Dent Res* 78:263, 1970.

Gerald W. Harrington and David R. Steiner

Periodontal-Endodontic Considerations

LEARNING OBJECTIVES

After reading this chapter, the student should be able to:

1 / State the anatomic pathways of communication between the dental pulp and the gingival sulcus or periodontal ligament.

2 / Describe the effects of pulpal disease and endodontic procedures on the periodontium.

3 / Describe the effects of periodontal disease and procedures on the pulp.

4 / Identify which clinical diagnostic procedures and findings are of importance in differentiating between those defects in the integrity of the gingival sulcus that will respond to root canal treatment and those that will require periodontal therapy for resolution.

5 / Establish treatment requirements and sequencing according to diagnostic findings.

6 / Identify which patients with complex problems should be considered for referral.

OUTLINE

Pathways of Communication between the Dental Pulp and the Periodontium
Dentinal Tubules
Lateral or Accessory Canals
Apical Foramen

Effects of Pulpal Disease and Endodontic Procedures on the Periodontium
Pulpal Disease
Endodontic Procedures

Effects of Endodontically Involved Teeth on Periodontal Health and Healing

Effects of Periodontal Disease and Procedures on the Pulp
Periodontal Disease
Periodontal Procedures

Clinical Diagnostic Procedures
Radiographic Findings
Pulp Testing Procedures
Periodontal Probing

Definition of a Perio-Endo Lesion*

Clinical Situations That Can Be Identified*
Acute or "Blow-Out" Lesions
Typical Periodontal Lesions
Radiolucent Lesions in Which the Gingival Sulcus Is Intact
Lesions with Narrow Sinus Tract Type Probing
Independent Periodontal and Periapical or Lateral Lesions That Do Not Communicate
True Combined Perio-Endo Lesions

Basis for Patient Referral

O ne of the more difficult dilemmas for a clinician is interpretation of the cause of a defect in the integrity of the gingival sulcus. Such a defect is identified by carefully probing all the way around a tooth with a periodontal probe. Either the gingival sulcus is intact or it is not. If the gingival sulcus is not intact (probing depth is greater than 2 to 3 mm), it is critical for the patient that the clinician choose appropriate treatment for resolution of the defect. The purpose of this chapter is to identify those clinical situations that will respond favorably to root canal treatment and those that will not.

Pathways of Communication Between the Dental Pulp and the Periodontium

Direct communication between the dental pulp and the periodontium may be through (1) patent dentinal tubules where the cementum is developmentally missing on the root surface or has been removed by periodontal root planing, (2) lateral and/or accessory canals, and (3) the apical foramen or foramina.

DENTINAL TUBULES

An understanding of the anatomy of patent dentinal tubules and changes brought about by age or periodontal treatment is essential to our understanding of the permeability of root dentin and dentin hypersensitivity. In the root, dentinal tubules extend from the intermediate dentin just inside the cementum-dentin junction to the pulp-predentin junction. Dentinal tubules in the root run a relatively straight course between the periphery and the pulp in contrast to the typical S-shaped contours of the tubules in the crown. Tubules range in size from about 1 to 3 μm in diameter.[1] They are approximately 1 μm in diameter near the cementum-dentin junction and approximately 2.5 μm near the pulp-predentin junction.[2] The diameter of tubules decreases with age by the laying down of highly mineralized peritubular dentin. It is possible for tubules to become completely calcified, particularly in the root. When the dentinal tubules in a section of root dentin become completely calcified, dentin is referred to as sclerotic or translucent.

The number of dentinal tubules per square millimeter varies from 8000 to 57,000.[1] At the periphery of the root at the cemento-enamel junction, the number has been estimated to be approximately 15,000/mm^2. The density, or number

*Adapted with permission from Harrington GW: The perio-endo question: differential diagnosis, *Dent Clin North Am* 23(4):673-690, 1979 and from Natkin E: *An introduction to endodontic diagnosis and treatment,* Seattle, 1989, University of Washington.

of tubules per square millimeter, increases from the cementum-dentin junction to the dentin-predentin junction. In periodontal disease the root surface becomes exposed to the oral cavity. Cementum acts as a protective barrier, but direct communication may be established between the contents of patent dentinal tubules and the oral environment if the cementum is congenitally missing at the cementum-dentin junction[3] or the cementum layer is removed by root planing. Therefore direct communication between the oral environment and the dental pulp may be established through patent dentinal tubules.

LATERAL OR ACCESSORY CANALS

Considerable speculation exists about the role lateral or accessory canals may play in the spread of inflammation from a periodontal pocket into the dental pulp or from the dental pulp into the periodontal ligament. Although there is little doubt that the spread of inflammation can and does occur in both directions, the clinical significance is open to question.

A lateral or accessory canal may be present anywhere on a root surface. The majority are found in the apical third of the root. The occurrence of lateral canals in the coronal third of the root is rare. The percentage of roots that may have a lateral canal or canals increases as the apex of the root is approached. Overall it is estimated that 30% to 40% of teeth have lateral or accessory canals. DeDeus[4] suggests that 1.6% of teeth have lateral canals in the coronal third of the root, 8.8% in the middle third, and 17% in the apical third. Obviously, the farther periodontal disease extends down the root surface, the greater the possibility that a lateral canal may become exposed by periodontal disease. In a study of 100 human teeth with extensive periodontal disease, however, only 2% had lateral canals located in an involved periodontal pocket.[5]

The incidence of lateral canals in the furcation region of molars is stated to be approximately 30% to 50%.[6,7] The clinical significance of lateral canals in the furcation, therefore, has been a subject of much speculation.

Clinical identification of the presence of a lateral canal is very difficult or impossible in most instances. An overall incidence of 30.6% has been identified when two-view radiographs of extracted teeth were examined.[8] In interpretation of standard intraoral radiographs, however, an incidence of only 7.6% was identified.[8] This disparity clearly demonstrates the difficulty encountered in the clinical identification of lateral canals. Moreover, the investigators were unable to identify any lateral canals in the furcation area of molar teeth. Therefore in the usual situations encountered in clinical practice, accurate positive identification of lateral canals on the basis of radiographic interpretation can be accomplished only in a very small percentage of cases.

Clinically, positive identification of the presence of a lateral canal can usually be made only when a discrete lateral lesion associated with a necrotic pulp can be identified radiographically or when some of the root canal filling material is forced into a lateral canal during the condensation procedure (Figure 26-1). In addition, the radiographic identification of a notch on the lateral root surface suggests the presence of an orifice into a lateral canal.

The clinical significance of the incidence of lateral canals at various levels on the root surface lies in the fact that the farther apical the lateral canal, the more extensive the periodontal destruction must be to involve the tissue in the lateral canal in the inflammatory process. If the incidence of lateral canals in the coronal third of the root is rare (with the exception of furcations), the incidence in the middle third is 12% or less,[8] and the preponderance of lateral canals occur in the apical third, then in most instances periodontal pathosis would have to be extensive for the inflammatory process to extend through a lateral canal to involve the dental pulp. In such instances, the overall prognosis for a tooth will then depend on the periodontal prognosis, i.e., how extensive the periodontal destruction is and the likelihood of resolving such periodontal pathosis with periodontal therapy.

If the dental pulp is necrotic and a patent lateral canal is exposed, periodontal reattachment to the root surface can be inhibited if definitive periodontal therapy is undertaken before root canal treatment. Therefore *if the pulp is necrotic and the periodontal prognosis is favorable, root canal treatment should always precede periodontal therapy.*

If the dental pulp is vital but there has been extension of the inflammatory process from a periodontal lesion into the tissue in a lateral canal, it is open to question whether or not the amount of tissue irritants present in the lateral canal would impede periodontal reattachment. *Because it is not possible to determine the exact histologic status of the dental pulp by the clinical testing procedures currently available and in most instances impossible to positively identify the presence or absence of a lateral canal, periodontal therapy alone should be undertaken to resolve a periodontal lesion if the tooth responds within normal limits to pulp testing procedures and there is no other evidence to indicate that the clinician should question the validity of the pulp test responses.*

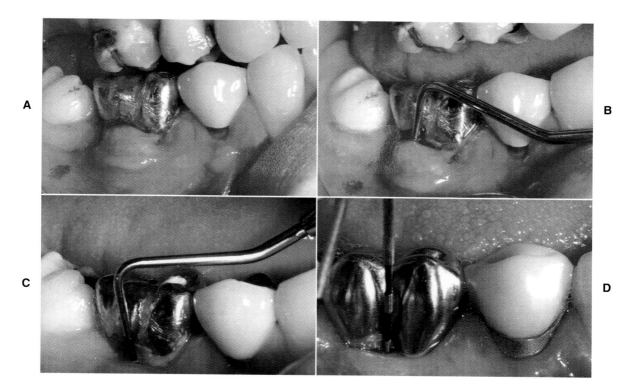

COLOR FIGURE 26-1
(Refer to Figure 26-5.) **A,** Typical swelling in a "blow out" type of lesion. **B,** A periodontal probe in the lesion at the time of initial examination. **C,** Probing is reduced to a narrow sinus tract type of probing after starting root canal treatment. **D,** Resolution of the lesion after completion of root canal treatment. (From Harrington GW: *Dent Clin North Am* 23:673, 1979.)

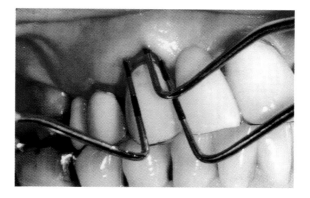

COLOR FIGURE 26-2
(Refer to Figure 26-8.) Clinical presentation of a narrow sinus tract type of probing. (From Harrington GW: *Dent Clin North Am* 23:673, 1979.)

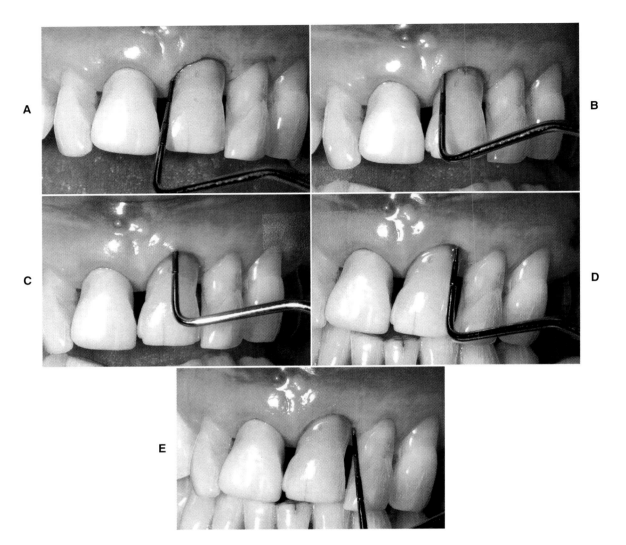

COLOR FIGURE 26-3
(Refer to Figure 26-6.) **A** to **E**, Typical probing of a lesion caused by periodontal disease. (From Harrington GW: *Dent Clin North Am* 23:673, 1979.)

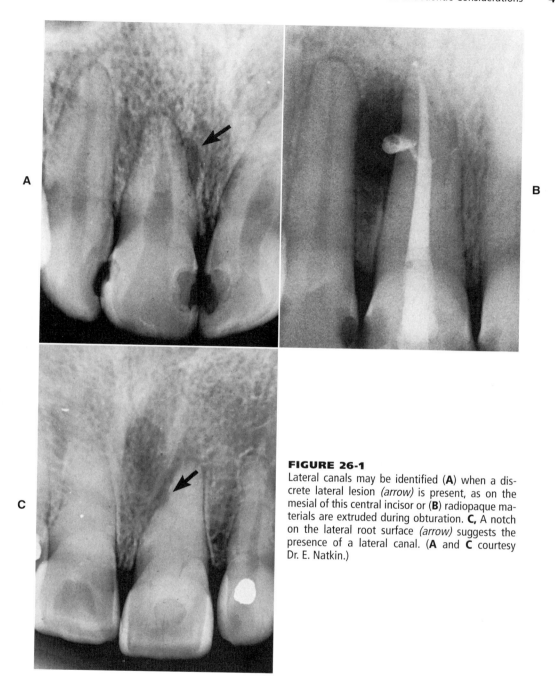

FIGURE 26-1
Lateral canals may be identified (**A**) when a discrete lateral lesion *(arrow)* is present, as on the mesial of this central incisor or (**B**) radiopaque materials are extruded during obturation. **C,** A notch on the lateral root surface *(arrow)* suggests the presence of a lateral canal. (**A** and **C** courtesy Dr. E. Natkin.)

APICAL FORAMEN

The major pathway of communication between the dental pulp and the periodontal ligament in all teeth is through the apical foramen or foramina. The effect of extensive pulp inflammation or necrosis is extension of the inflammatory process into the periodontal ligament contiguous with the pulp at the apical foramen.

Effects of Pulpal Disease and Endodontic Procedures on the Periodontium

PULPAL DISEASE

Pulp inflammation or necrosis may lead to an inflammatory response in the periodontal ligament at the apical foramen or foramina or at the site of a lateral or accessory canal. The resulting inflammatory lesion can range in extent from a minimal inflammatory process confined to the periodontal ligament to extensive destruction of the periodontal ligament, tooth socket, and surrounding bone. Such a lesion may result in a localized or diffuse swelling that occasionally may involve the gingival attachment. A lesion related to pulpal necrosis may also result in a draining sinus tract that drains through the alveolar mucosa or attached gingiva, but may occasionally drain through the gingival sulcus of the involved tooth or through the gingival sulcus of an adjacent tooth. After adequate root canal treatment, lesions resulting from pulpal necrosis resolve an exceptionally high percentage of the time.[9] The integrity of the periodontium will be reestablished if root canal treatment is done well. If a draining sinus tract through the periodontal ligament is present before root canal treatment, resolution of the defect that can be probed is expected.

ENDODONTIC PROCEDURES

Technical procedures involved in root canal treatment, irrigants, medicaments, dressings, sealers, and filling materials have the potential to cause an inflammatory response in the periodontium. An inflammatory response resulting from commonly used root canal treatment methods and materials, however, is usually transient in nature and resolves quickly if filling materials are confined within the canal space.

In young patients there is evidence that a caustic agent such as 30% hydrogen peroxide may move through large patent dentinal tubules from the pulp chamber and canal to cause an inflammatory response in the periodontal ligament.[10-12] As a tooth matures, however, and the diameter of dentinal tubules is reduced significantly, there is little clinical evidence that any of the materials used in root canal treatment cause an inflammatory response in periodontal tissues other than through a lateral canal or the apical foramen.

Procedural errors during root canal treatment can, and often do, cause major destructive inflammatory processes in the periodontium. Breakdown of the attachment resulting in a periodontal defect that can be probed may occur after procedural errors such as access perforations in the floor of a pulp chamber or on the root surface apical to the gingival attachment, strip perforations or root perforations related to cleaning and shaping procedures, and vertical root fractures. Reattachment after a periodontal defect has been established because of a procedural error is usually difficult to attain.

Effects of Endodontically Involved Teeth on Periodontal Health and Healing

Current literature suggests that a pulpless tooth may be one of several site characteristics that may influence treatment outcomes for periodontal lesions.[13] In this chapter, a pulpless tooth is defined as a tooth without a vital pulp; i.e., a tooth with a necrotic pulp or a tooth that has previously had root canal treatment. Recent retrospective statistical studies suggest that pulpless teeth with periapical lesions promote the initiation of periodontal pocket formation, promote the progression of periodontal disease, and interfere with healing of periodontal lesions after periodontal treatment.[14-18] The presumed pathways include patent dentinal tubules as well as accessory or lateral canals.[14] The extrapolated difference in periodontal pocket depth related to teeth with no periapical lesions compared with teeth with periapical lesions, however, is stated to be 0.5 to 1.0 mm. On a clinical basis detection of small changes in probing depth with any degree of accuracy is difficult. The standard deviations in clinical probing results are stated to be 0.5 to 1.3 mm.[19]

The reported statistical differences between teeth with and without periapical lesions are also somewhat inconsistent with differing periodontal responses to different treatment modalities. The data suggest that periodontally involved teeth managed by periodontal surgery and osteoplasty are not influenced by pulp pathosis.[15] In addition, nonsurgical treatment of vertical marginal defects showed no correlation between periapical pathosis and mean pocket depth reduction.[15] In summary, the data presented by these studies are equivocal at best, appear to present trifling distinctions, and appear to have little clinical significance.

In an attempt to relate disease etiology and progression with the assignment of prognosis, McGuire and Nunn[20-23] found that some commonly accepted clinical parameters did not accurately predict a tooth's survival. Their statistical model[20] had predicted that endodontic involvement would be associated with the probability that the prognosis for such a tooth would worsen over time. In their clinical study,[22] however, the actual outcome was that none of the 131 teeth lost out of a total 2509 teeth had endodontic involvement. Initial endodontic involvement was determined not to be a significant clinical factor associated with tooth loss.

Because the alternative to maintenance of a pulpless tooth is extraction, long-term prognosis studies are significant. A recent retrospective clinical study of patients with advanced periodontal disease 5 to 14 years after completion of active periodontal and endodontic treatment showed that the risk of endodontic failure is very low and that there is little risk of tooth loss for periodontal reasons.[24] Of 911 periodontally involved teeth, overall tooth loss was 2%. Of the 571 teeth that did not have root canal treatment before the recall period, only one tooth needed root canal treatment over the 5- to 14-year follow-up period. None of the teeth were lost for endodontic reasons, and the overall failure rate of the 340 endodontically treated teeth was 1.2%.

The prognosis is quite good even for molars with extensive periodontal disease that requires root amputation.[25,26] It has been suggested that survival rates of teeth with root resections are not substantially different from those for osseointegrated implants.[27] In fact, a current periodontics textbook suggests that substituting an osseointegrated implant for a tooth with furcation involvement should be considered with extreme caution and only if the implant will improve the success of the overall treatment plan.[28] In the benchmark research study on prognosis for osseointegrated implants, Adell et al.[29] reported an overall success rate of 91% for mandibular implants and 81% for maxillary implants for a follow-up period of 5 years or more.

In summary, *although it has been suggested that a pulpless tooth may represent an etiologic risk factor related to periodontal disease, the comparative risk must be considered negligible based on clinical outcomes.*

Effects of Periodontal Disease and Procedures on the Pulp

PERIODONTAL DISEASE

Over the years there has been considerable speculation on the effect of periodontal disease on the health of the pulp. The accumulated evidence suggests that there is little or no effect on human pulps.[30-35] In some of these studies, the pulps of intact, caries-free, periodontally involved teeth were all histologically within normal limits regardless of the severity of periodontal disease.[32,35] Indeed, there is some evidence that periodontal disease must extend all the way to the apical foramen before the accumulation of plaque can cause significant pulp involvement.[36]

PERIODONTAL PROCEDURES

Periodontal root planing removes cementum and dentin from the root surface, exposing patent dentinal tubules to the oral environment. Dentin hypersensitivity often results, but it can usually be managed by desensitization procedures.

The pulp response to cementum and dentin removal and exposure of patent dentinal tubules by periodontal root planing will vary with the remaining dentin thickness. Unless dentin removal is excessive, pulp response will be negligible. Although the pulp is exposed to a bacterial challenge through patent dentinal tubules, it is quite capable of repair and healing. Production of reparative dentin and reduced canal diameter may result, but pulp tissue remains relatively unaffected.

In a study of patients with maxillary molar furcation involvement in which a high percentage of the teeth had lost at least 50% percent or more bone support around one root before periodontal treatment, only 4% required root canal treatment from 5 to 24 years after completion of periodontal treatment.[32] In no case was the cause for root canal treatment ascribed to the effects of periodontal disease or periodontal treatment. In a 4- to 13-year recall study of nonabutment teeth with advanced periodontal disease in which the crestal bone level of over half of the teeth was in the apical two-thirds of the root, only 3% developed pulp necrosis.[35] With the exception of several teeth that subsequently had progression of periodontal disease to involve the root apices, neither the cumulative effects of periodontal treatment nor periodontal disease itself were reasons cited for pulp necrosis.

If periodontal treatment is to be considered for managing periodontal disease that extends around the apical foramen, curetting the periodontal lesion as part of the treatment will sever the blood supply to the pulp and will require prophylactic endodontic treatment. Root canal treatment should be completed before periodontal treatment because the necrotic pulp will prevent healing of the periodontal tissues.

In summary, *unless periodontal disease has progressed to involve the tooth apex, the effect of periodontal disease on the pulp appears to be negligible. Prognosis for a tooth involved with periodontal disease is determined by the outcome expected from periodontal therapy.*

Clinical Diagnostic Procedures

Appropriate diagnosis is critical. The clinician must be able to identify the clinical characteristics of a lesion, determine whether or not root canal treatment has the potential to resolve the lesion, and establish a reasoned prognosis.

RADIOGRAPHIC FINDINGS

Interpretation of radiographs of good quality is a very important part of diagnosis. Identification of the proximal crestal bone and its position in relation to the cementum-enamel junction and the coronal level of superimposition of the trabecular pattern over the root of a tooth requires careful examination. Crestal bone level can be identified by the clear-cut image of the root itself and clarity of the canal space contrasted with superimposition of the trabecular pattern over the root (Figure 26-2). If there is crestal bone loss, the more apical margin of the superimposed trabecular pattern identifies the level of bone loss on one side of the tooth. In some cases the superimposition of the trabecular pattern will appear to have two distinct levels on the root. There is no way to interpret from a single radiograph whether the apically positioned bone level is on the buccal or the lingual side. This discrimination can only be made by clinical examination of the area.

Interpretation of discrete periapical or lateral lesions and discrete periodontal lesions is of clinical importance in suggesting the cause of the lesion and the proper diagnostic procedures to follow to confirm the cause. However, when there is radiographic evidence that bone loss extends from the level of crestal bone to or near the apex of the tooth, the radiograph is of little value in determining the cause (Figure 26-3).

PULP TESTING PROCEDURES

The presence or absence of vital tissue in a tooth with a single canal can be determined with confidence with current pulp testing procedures. The exact histologic status cannot be determined. In teeth with multiple canals there may be vital tissue in one or more canals while pulp necrosis may have occurred in the remaining canal or canals. Therefore the same degree of confidence cannot be ascribed to positive pulp test responses in a tooth with multiple canals as can be attributed to positive tests in a tooth with a single canal. Limitations related to the interpretation of pulp test responses complicate diagnosis of the cause of a defect in the integrity of the gingival sulcus. Chapter 4 of this text presents an in-depth discussion of the interpretation of pulp test responses.

PERIODONTAL PROBING

Considering the limitations in the diagnostic armamentarium, discrimination of "perio-endo"

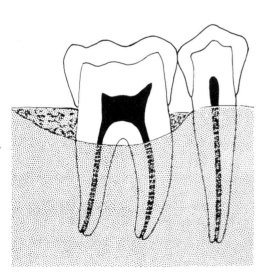

A

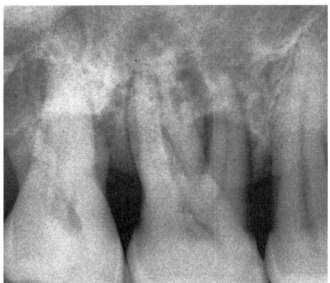

B

FIGURE 26-2
A, Clear definition of the root and root canal space indicates bone loss on one side of the tooth down to the level of the superimposed trabecular pattern. **B,** The image of the mesiobuccal root of the first molar demonstrates the clarity of definition of the root outline and of the root canal space up to the level of the superimposed trabecular pattern. (**A** from Harrington GW: *Dent Clin North Am* 23:673, 1979.)

lesions must be made primarily on the basis of the critical examination of the area by means of a periodontal probe. By development of acute tactile discriminations the nature and cause of the lesion can be determined. This determination is made by identifying the physical characteristics of the lesion itself. Careful, accurate probing all the way around the external root surface of the tooth is required. A fine periodontal probe must be used (Marquis periodontal probe, Marquis Dental Manufacturing Co., Denver, CO). Differentiation must also be made between "probing" and "sounding." As used in this chapter, *probing* is defined as the tactile discrimination of the level of the epithelial attachment through use of the periodontal probe. In contrast, *sounding* implies penetrating through the attachment to define the most coronal level of the alveolar bone. As there may be considerable differences between the two, the clinician must understand and appreciate this clear distinction to develop the quality of tactile discrimination required. In the descriptions to follow, probing is the procedure referred to in all instances.

Definition of a Perio-Endo Lesion

A perio-endo lesion is defined as follows:
1. The tooth involved must be pulpless.
2. There must be destruction of the periodontal attachment apparatus from the gingival sulcus to either the apex of the tooth or to the area of an involved lateral canal; i.e., there must be a defect in the attachment that can be probed.

3. Both root canal treatment and periodontal therapy are required to resolve the entirety of the lesion.

The second and third criteria will be extensively described in the following clinical examples, but the first criterion requires some clarification. Clinical experience shows that if a tooth has an advanced irreversible pulpitis, there is often minimal disruption of the lamina dura and periodontal ligament space at the apex of the tooth. With some teeth there may be radiographic evidence of a very small periapical lesion, particularly in young patients. However, it is not common to find irreversible pulpitis associated with a large radiolucent periapical lesion. In fact, if vital tissue is found in the pulp chamber of a tooth with a single canal and there is a large radiolucent lesion associated with the apex, it is incumbent to positively identify the cause of the lesion. In a tooth with multiple canals at least one canal will have pulpal necrosis if there is a large lesion associated with the apex or apices. In summary, *at least one necrotic, not simply irreversibly inflamed, canal is to be expected when a moderate-to-large periapical lesion is present.*

Similarly, when a large lesion is associated with the lateral surface of the root, the pulp of the tooth must be necrotic if there is an actual endodontic component to the lesion. The role, if any, of inflammatory tissue in a lateral canal in development of a lesion that can be probed along the lateral surface of the root must be questioned. Hence, it is inferred that some pulpal necrosis must be present for a lateral or apical lesion to develop. In the discussion to follow there must be evidence of pulpal necrosis for the lesion to be considered a true perio-endo lesion.

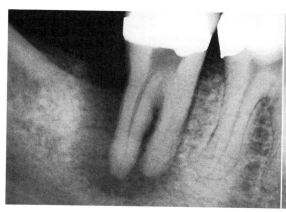 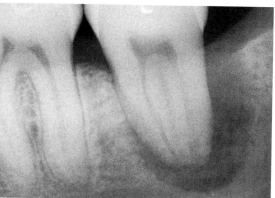

A   B

FIGURE 26-3
These lesions have similar radiographic characteristics. **A,** Lesion is due solely to pulpal necrosis. **B,** Lesion is strictly a periodontal lesion.

Clinical Situations That Can Be Identified

A periodontal-endodontic decision tree is presented in Figure 26-4.

ACUTE OR "BLOW-OUT" LESIONS

When a patient presents with a localized swelling that involves the gingival sulcus, it may be difficult to determine if the swelling is due to a periodontal abscess or an abscess of endodontic origin. The tooth must be pulpless. The swelling is usually on the labial or buccal side of the tooth but may be on the lingual side. As the sulcus is probed there is usually normal sulcus depth all the way around the tooth until the area of the swelling is probed. At the edge of the swelling the probe drops precipitously to a level near the apex of the tooth, and the probing depth remains the full width of the swelling (Figure 26-5 and Color Figure 26-1). At the opposite edge of the swelling, probing is once again within normal limits. The width of the detached gingiva can be as broad as the entire buccal or lingual surface of the tooth. This swelling can be characterized as having "blown out" the entire attachment on that side.

When probing carefully around the neck of the tooth in the area of swelling, intact crestal bone may sometimes be felt. This would indicate that there has been a pathologic perforation of the cortical plate farther apically and that the periosteum has been lifted off the coronal cortical plate by the swelling. If intact crestal bone is present, rapid reattachment can be expected after resolution of the swelling. In some instances, on the other hand, careful probing will reveal the absence of the buccal cortical plate to the depth of approximately the apical extent of the swelling. With this blow out type of probing, indicating loss of bone along a broad front, rapid reattachment can also be expected. In furcations, however, healing may first proceed to what will be described later in this chapter as a "sinus tract type of probing," but eventually complete reattachment can be expected.

Treatment for a blow out lesion involves customary endodontic emergency procedures that would be used if there were a similar swelling but the entire sulcus were intact. The root surface need not be curetted, nor the area surgically flapped. Endodontic treatment only is indicated. As the result of endodontic management of the swelling, complete periodontal reattachment occurs within 1 week in most cases. As mentioned earlier, however, the broad, precipitous probing may resolve to a narrow, deep sinus tract type of probing, which may remain until after completion of root canal treatment.

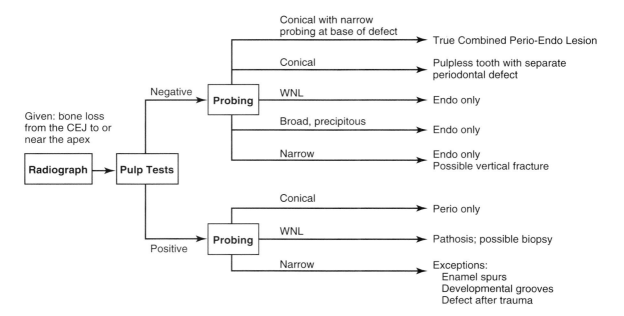

FIGURE 26-4
Periodontal-endodontic decision tree. Appropriate tests and findings indicate both the diagnosis and etiology of the pathosis. *CEJ,* Cementum-enamel junction; *WNL,* within normal limits. (Courtesy Dr. D. Steiner, from Natkin E: *An introduction to endodontic diagnosis and treatment,* Seattle, 1989, University of Washington Press.)

It should also be apparent that probing in other areas around the root surface of a tooth may vary from what is considered to be within normal limits, but the blow out probing in the area of the swelling will be distinctive.

TYPICAL PERIODONTAL LESIONS

In periodontal disease bone loss always begins at crestal bone level and progresses apically. The typical lesion is conical in contour. The probing may start from a sulcus depth that is within normal limits, then gradually step down a slope to the apical extent of the lesion, and then step up again on the other side to a sulcus depth within normal limits (Figure 26-6). The slope of the lesion will vary and may depend on the coronal width of the lesion. Regardless of the degree of the slope, a distinctive conical shape will be distinguished by carefully feeling the increasing and then decreasing depth of the attachment as the periodontal probe is stepped down into and then up out of the lesion.

Occasionally the clinical presentation of a periodontal lesion will have the sloping contour of a conical lesion on one side but a more precipitous, sharp drop-off on the other. Such probing should be considered to be of the "periodontal type" of probing.

A periodontal lesion will not resolve in response to root canal treatment even if the associated tooth is pulpless. The prognosis for a tooth with conical shaped probing must be based on the prognosis for resolving the periodontal lesion. If it can be demonstrated that a tooth is pulpless and if the periodontal prognosis is favorable, root canal treatment should be completed before periodontal therapy. In summary, *conical shaped probing indicates periodontal pathosis.*

RADIOLUCENT LESIONS IN WHICH THE GINGIVAL SULCUS IS INTACT

Because bone loss from periodontal disease always begins at crestal bone level and progresses apically, an intact gingival sulcus demonstrated by careful probing eliminates periodontal disease as the cause of a lesion. If a patient presents with a tooth with a necrotic pulp and the gingival sulcus is intact, adequate nonsurgical root canal treatment will resolve either a radiolucent lesion that extends up the lateral root surface of the

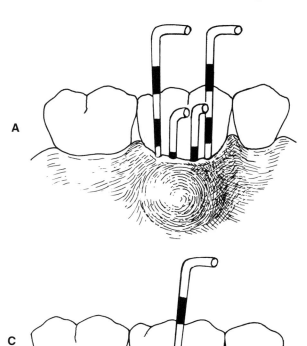

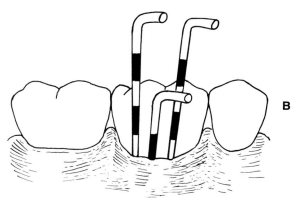

FIGURE 26-5
(Refer to Color Figure 26-1.) **A,** Periodontal probing in a typical "blow-out" type of lesion. Probings are within normal limits on either side of the swelling. The lesion can be probed to a level near the apices for the width of the swelling. **B,** After initiation of root canal treatment the swelling has resolved and the probing is reduced to a narrow sinus tract type probing in the furcation. **C,** After completion of root canal treatment the sulcus is intact. (From Harrington GW: *Dent Clin North Am* 23:673, 1979.)

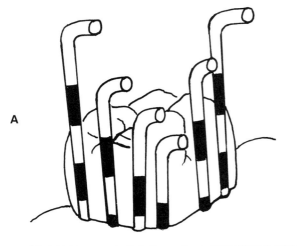

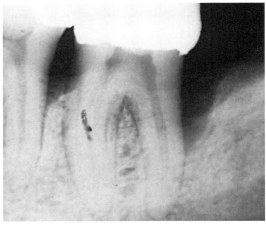

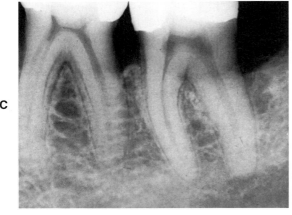

FIGURE 26-6

(Refer to Color Figure 26-3.) **A,** Probing in a typical periodontal lesion demonstrates the conical characteristics of the lesion. **B,** Pretreatment radiograph of a periodontal lesion. All teeth respond within normal limits to pulp tests. **C,** Two-year recall radiograph of successful periodontal treatment. (**A** from Harrington GW: *Dent Clin North Am* 23:673, 1979.)

tooth to involve crestal bone or a radiolucent lesion in the furcation (Figure 26-7).

If there is radiographic evidence of a radiolucent lesion as described, but there is no evidence of pulp necrosis in at least one canal, then a biopsy should be performed to determine the nature of the lesion (see Chapter 3).

LESIONS WITH NARROW SINUS TRACT TYPE PROBING

An apparent periodontal lesion may or may not be detectable radiographically. Clinically, a lesion may be probed for some distance down the root surface of the involved tooth, but the defect is in fact a sinus tract. Typically, probing reveals a sulcus depth within normal limits with the exception of one very narrow area that can be probed some distance down the root surface of the tooth and in many cases all the way to the apex of the tooth (Figure 26-8 and Color Figure 26-2). Usually the break in the attachment is only about 1 mm wide, and probing 1 mm to either side of the le-

sion will be within normal limits. A lesion that probes in this manner is in fact a sinus tract, and the probing represents a typical sinus tract type of probing.

The tooth is pulpless. Customary root canal procedures are indicated. The lesion need not be curetted or surgically flapped. It is strictly a sinus tract similar to a sinus tract exiting in the alveolar mucosa or attached gingiva. Simply passing a periodontal probe down through the sulcus along the lateral root surface of the tooth does not mean that a lesion is the result of periodontal disease. When a sinus tract occurs over the lateral root surface of a tooth, it will respond to root canal treatment like any other sinus tract. Typically the orifice into such a sinus tract will close within 1 week after the cleaning and shaping appointment.

Occasionally this lesion will have the same type of probing except that the sinus tract is much wider than usual (Figure 26-9). In some instances the disruption in the gingival sulcus may be up to 5 or 6 mm wide. There is no swelling in the area.

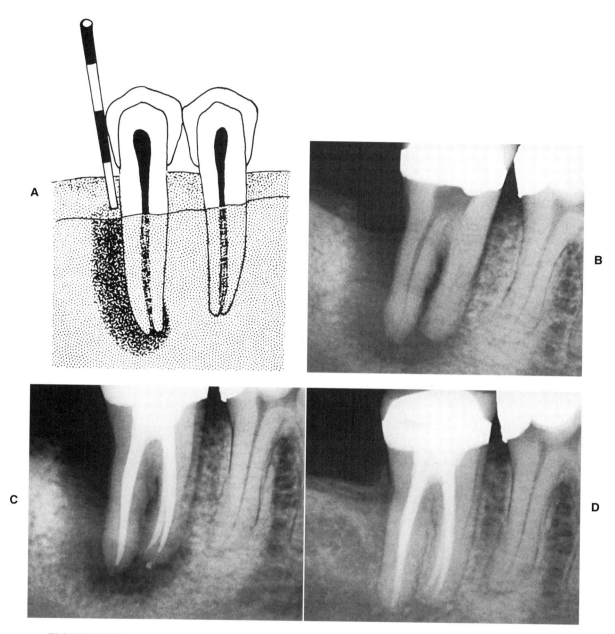

FIGURE 26-7
A, This radiolucent lesion has the radiographic appearance of a periodontal lesion. Careful periodontal probing demonstrates that the gingival sulcus is intact. **B,** The initial radiograph indicates bone loss from the crest of the ridge around the apices of the tooth. Periodontal probing demonstrates that the gingival sulcus is intact. There is no response to pulpal tests. **C,** Root canal treatment completed. **D,** Four-year recall shows resolution of the radiolucency. (**A** from Harrington GW: *Dent Clin North Am* 23:673, 1979.)

Typically the sulcus probes within normal limits to the very edge of the sinus tract, then falls off precipitously to approach the apex of the tooth. Approximately the same depth is probed across the entire 3 to 6 mm width of the sinus tract, and then sharply at the demarcation of the sinus tract the probing is again within normal limits.

There are some indications that the increased width is associated with chronicity, although this has not been documented. In any case, the treat-

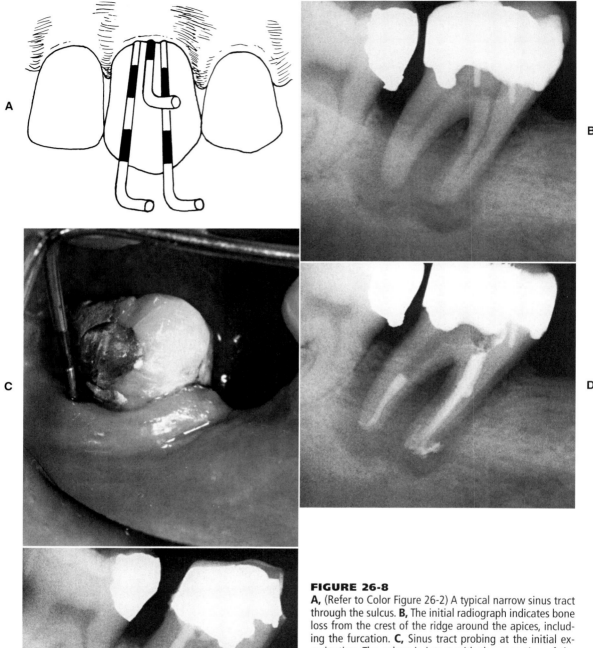

FIGURE 26-8

A, (Refer to Color Figure 26-2) A typical narrow sinus tract through the sulcus. **B,** The initial radiograph indicates bone loss from the crest of the ridge around the apices, including the furcation. **C,** Sinus tract probing at the initial examination. The sulcus is intact with the exception of the sinus tract. **D,** Root canal treatment completed. **E,** A 1-year recall shows resolution of the radiolucency. Probing is within normal limits. (**A** from Harrington GW: *Dent Clin North Am* 23:673, 1979.)

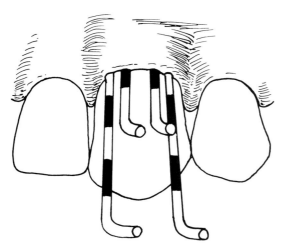

FIGURE 26-9
Periodontal probing of a typical wide sinus tract through the sulcus. There is no swelling in the area. (From Harrington GW: *Dent Clin North Am* 23:673, 1979.)

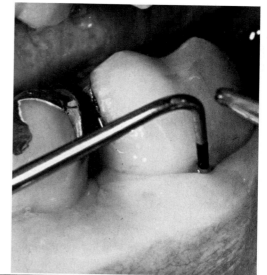

A

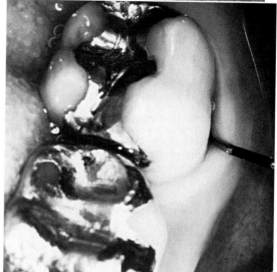

B

FIGURE 26-10
A, Vertical sinus tract type probing down the distal side of the mesial root in the furcation. **B,** Horizontal probing into the furcation.

ment is once again nonsurgical root canal treatment. The lesion need not be curetted, and a surgical flap is not necessary for resolution. However, closure of the orifice into the sinus tract may require somewhat more time than closure of a similar sinus tract of smaller width.

An exception to the above is a wide sinus tract type of probing on the direct palatal surface of maxillary teeth. Experience has shown that this type of probing does not resolve by root canal treatment. In such instances, prognosis is determined by the prognosis for the periodontal procedure required to resolve such a defect.

Special consideration must be given to probing the furcations of multirooted teeth. A vertical sinus tract type of probing in the furcation down the distal aspect of the mesial root or the mesial aspect of the distal root of a pulpless mandibular molar will respond to adequate root canal treatment by closure of the sinus tract. However, closure may be somewhat slower in the furcation area than on a lateral root surface of a tooth, and complete closure of the sinus tract may not occur until 2 to 3 months after obturation of the canals. Again, neither curettage nor a surgical procedure will be required for resolution of a lesion with a typical sinus tract type of vertical probing in the furcation. Although the example refers to a mandibular molar specifically, the same holds true for each furcation area of a maxillary molar.

Careful attention must also be given to probing the furcation areas in a *horizontal direction* (Figure 26-10). Because of the height of the soft tissue

and the contour of the furcation, this procedure may not be adequately carried out with a periodontal probe in many cases. A special curved probe or a thin periodontal curette may be required to follow the contour of the furcation to adequately explore the horizontal component of a furcation involvement. In many instances in which there is furcation involvement, there will be a horizontal as well as a vertical component to the lesion.

In younger patients, a lesion with a horizontal type of sinus tract probing in the furcation resolves with no complications after root canal treatment. In older patients, if a lesion with a horizontal component in the furcation is associated with a pulpless tooth, resolution is unlikely. Although such lesions may occasionally fill in slowly after adequate root canal treatment, resolution of the horizontal component by means of endodontic treatment alone occurs rarely in older patients. Therefore resolution of a lesion with a horizontal probing into a furcation associated with a pulpless tooth must be viewed with skepticism in an older patient. The prognosis in such cases should be determined by consideration of the typical periodontal criteria for determining prognosis of a furcation involvement.

There are several other clinical situations in which a sinus tract type of probing may occur but do not indicate a typical sinus tract. These exceptions include the presence of enamel spurs, developmental grooves, vertical root fractures, and periodontal defects after trauma.

Enamel Spurs

Enamel spurs or extensions into the furcation area of multirooted teeth usually are identified by visual examination of the furcation during flap reflection.

Developmental Grooves

Developmental grooves occur most often on the lingual surface of maxillary lateral incisors but may involve central incisors and less often other teeth. Developmental grooves are identified by careful evaluation of radiographs, visual examination, and tactile discrimination. The pulp of a tooth with a deep developmental groove may become necrotic and develop a periapical lesion. Adequate root canal treatment will resolve the periapical lesion but will not resolve the periodontal defect associated with the developmental groove. Prognosis should be determined by the extent of the periodontal defect.

Vertical Root Fracture

A sinus tract type of probing is not pathognomonic of a vertical root fracture in a tooth that has previously had root canal treatment, but a sinus tract type of probing is very often associated with such fractures. Visual confirmation of a fracture is required to make the diagnosis. If a sinus tract type of probing occurs on both the buccal and lingual aspects of such a root, it is highly suggestive of a vertical root fracture. The prognosis for teeth with confirmed vertical root fractures that extend to the level of crestal bone is poor.

Similarly, a sinus tract type of probing may be found in the proximal areas of posterior teeth that have incomplete coronal fractures that extend into the roots. More information on these longitudinal fractures is in Chapter 28.

Periodontal Defect After Trauma

Occasionally a sinus tract type of probing may be associated with a tooth that has been involved in a traumatic incident. This defect usually occurs on the lingual surface of anterior teeth. The tooth involved will usually respond within normal limits to pulp testing procedures, although occasionally such traumatized teeth may not respond to pulp tests for a period of time after trauma. The defect will gradually resolve but may be present for as long as several months after the impact injury. No treatment is required for resolution of this lesion.

With the exception of the above four circumstances, a sinus tract type of probing indicates a lesion associated with a pulpless tooth. The sinus tract may be coming from either a periapical or lateral lesion. Although it is rare, a sinus tract may develop through the periodontal ligament of a tooth other than the tooth that is pulpless. Careful pulp testing reveals this situation. In such a case, adequate root canal treatment for the pulpless tooth will resolve the sinus tract associated with the adjacent tooth.

In many instances, a sinus tract type of probing will be associated with a lateral lesion involving a pulpless tooth that has a root perforation or a resorptive lesion. Such lesions on the lateral surface of the root seem predisposed to development of sinus tracts through the periodontal ligament. A sinus tract type of probing itself is not diagnostic of such defects but should alert the clinician toward careful evaluation for the cause of the sinus tract.

In all cases, a sinus tract should be considered a sign associated with the problem and should not be considered to be a pathologic entity in itself. If adequate endodontic treatment can be accomplished, a sinus tract will resolve without any further definitive therapy directed toward its elimination. In summary, then, *pulpal necrosis does not cause periodontal disease. It may cause the formation of a sinus tract through the periodontal ligament. Bone loss resulting from pulpal necrosis is reversible. The periodontal attachment apparatus will regenerate completely after adequate root canal treatment.*

INDEPENDENT PERIODONTAL AND PERIAPICAL OR LATERAL LESIONS THAT DO NOT COMMUNICATE

A tooth with periodontal disease may also be pulpless and present with radiographic evidence of a discrete periapical or lateral lesion (Figure 26-11).

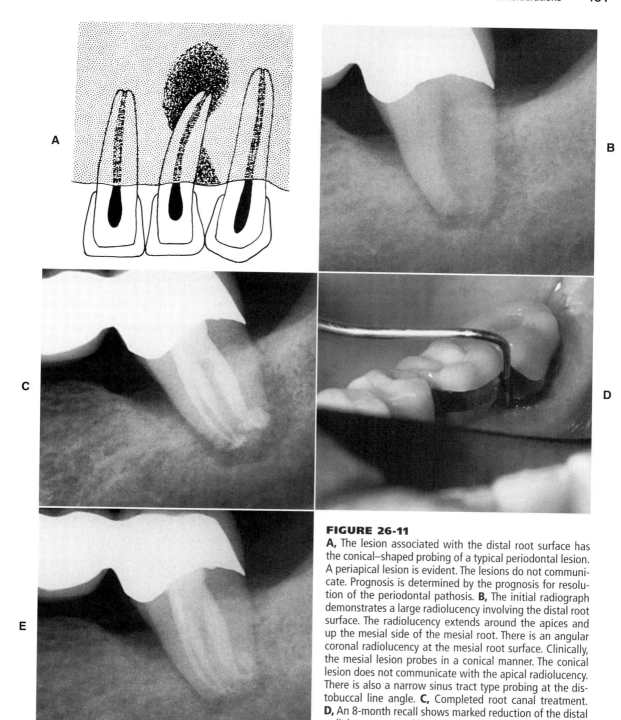

FIGURE 26-11
A, The lesion associated with the distal root surface has the conical–shaped probing of a typical periodontal lesion. A periapical lesion is evident. The lesions do not communicate. Prognosis is determined by the prognosis for resolution of the periodontal pathosis. **B,** The initial radiograph demonstrates a large radiolucency involving the distal root surface. The radiolucency extends around the apices and up the mesial side of the mesial root. There is an angular coronal radiolucency at the mesial root surface. Clinically, the mesial lesion probes in a conical manner. The conical lesion does not communicate with the apical radiolucency. There is also a narrow sinus tract type probing at the distobuccal line angle. **C,** Completed root canal treatment. **D,** An 8-month recall shows marked reduction of the distal radiolucency caused by the necrotic pulp. Probing is within normal limits around the distal sulcus. **E,** The mesial lesion probes in the same conical manner and to the same depth as before root canal treatment, indicating a periodontal lesion. (**A** from Harrington GW: *Dent Clin North Am* 23:673, 1979.)

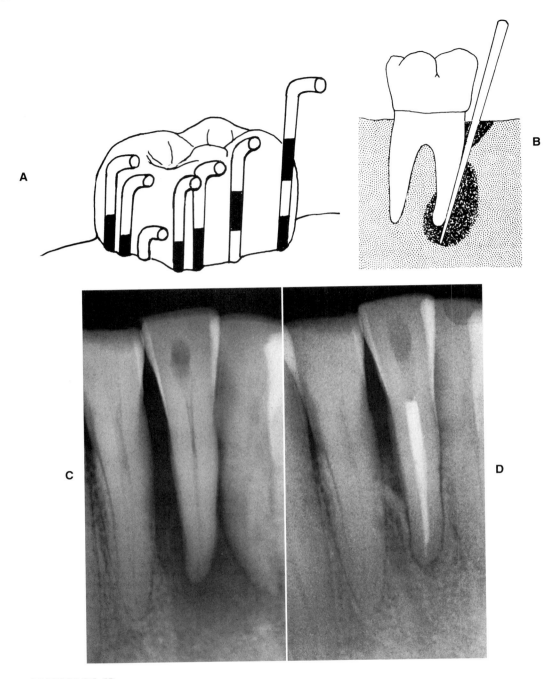

FIGURE 26-12
A, Periodontal probing in a true combined perio-endo lesion. **B,** Communication between a periodontal lesion and a lesion caused by a necrotic pulp in a combined perio-endo lesion. **C,** Mandibular incisor with a large lesion at the distal. The lesion probed with a conical contour. Within the conical lesion there was a defect that probed to the apex, demonstrating communication. **D,** An 11-year recall demonstrates resolution of the lesion around the apex. An angular defect remains at the distal. (**A** and **B** from Harrington GW: *Dent Clin North Am* 23:673, 1979.)

The periodontal lesion probes in a manner consistent with the typical conical periodontal type of probing. The tooth is pulpless. The prognosis for the tooth depends upon the periodontal prognosis. Adequate root canal treatment will resolve the discrete periapical or lateral lesion. Although both periodontal and periapical lesions are present, the findings are not consistent with a true combined perio-endo lesion as there is no demonstrable communication between the two lesions.

TRUE COMBINED PERIO-ENDO LESIONS

True combined perio-endo lesions occur when independent periodontal and periapical or lateral lesions are present and do communicate. Either such combined lesions are extremely rare, or the criteria to make the discrimination have not been fully elaborated. The typical combined perio-endo lesion that can be identified presents radiographic evidence of bone loss, which appears to extend some distance down the lateral root surface from crestal bone. Probing reveals the typical conical periodontal type of probing with the exception that at the base of the periodontal lesion the probe will abruptly drop farther down the lateral root surface and may even extend to the apex of the tooth (Figure 26-12). The lesion can be characterized as a typical sinus tract type of probing at the base of a periodontal lesion.

Adequate root canal treatment will resolve the periapical lesion up to the extent of the periodontal lesion either with or without periodontal therapy. The overall prognosis for the tooth, therefore, depends on the likelihood of resolution of the periodontal aspects of the lesion. In all such instances, if the periodontal prognosis is satisfactory, root canal treatment should be completed before initiation of definitive periodontal therapy. Otherwise, drainage from the periapical lesion through the sinus tract into the periodontal aspect of the lesion will interfere with periodontal repair if definitive periodontal therapy is initiated before root canal treatment.

Basis for Patient Referral

When clinical diagnostic criteria as defined in this chapter are applied to dental patients, distinguishing between lesions of periodontal origin and those resulting from pulpal necrosis is very often straightforward. In many cases, however, discriminations are difficult and appropriate treatment planning may prove to be quite complex. Required treatment procedures and sequencing may also be complicated. The interest of the patient is paramount. If the etiology of a defect is unclear, a consultation with or referral to a specialist for appropriate diagnosis and treatment is indicated.

REFERENCES

1. Mjör IA, Nordahl I: The density and branching of dentinal tubules in human teeth, *Arch Oral Biol* 41:401, 1996.
2. Garberoglio R, Brannström M: Scanning electron microscopic investigation of human dentinal tubules, *Arch Oral Biol* 21:355, 1976.
3. Furseth R, Mjör IA: Cementum. In Mjör I, Pindborg JJ, editors: *Histology of the human tooth,* Copenhagen, 1973, Munksgaard, Scandinavian University Books.
4. DeDeus DD: Frequency, location, and direction of the lateral secondary and accessory canals, *J Endod* 1:361, 1975.
5. Kirkham DB: The location and incidence of accessory pulpal canals in periodontal pockets, *J Am Dent Assoc* 91:353, 1975.
6. Vertucci FJ, Williams RG: Furcation canals in the human mandibular first molar, *Oral Surg Oral Med Oral Pathol* 38:308, 1974.
7. Gutmann JL: Prevalence, location, and patency of accessory canals in the furcation region of permanent molars, *J Periodontol* 49:21, 1978.
8. Pineda F, Kuttler Y: Mesiodistal and buccolingual roentgenographic investigation of 7,275 root canals, *Oral Surg Oral Med Oral Pathol* 33:101, 1972.
9. Sjögren U, Hägglund B, Sundqvist G, Wing K: Factors affecting the long-term results of endodontic treatment, *J Endod* 16:498, 1990.
10. Harrington GW, Natkin E: External resorption associated with bleaching of pulpless teeth, *J Endod* 5:344, 1979.
11. Madison S, Walton RE: Cervical root resorption following bleaching of endodontically treated teeth, *J Endod* 16:570, 1990.
12. Rotstein I, Friedman S, Mor C, et al: Histological characterization of bleaching-induced external root resorption in dogs, *J Endod* 17:436, 1991.
13. Kornman KS, Robertson PB: Fundamental principles affecting the outcomes of therapy for osseous lesions, *Periodontol 2000* 22:22, 2000.
14. Jansson L, Ehnevid H, Lindskog S, Blomlof L: Relationship between periapical and periodontal status. A clinical retrospective study, *J Clin Periodontol* 20:117, 1993.
15. Ehnevid H, Jansson L, Lindskog S, Blomlof LB: Periodontal healing in teeth with periapical lesions. A clinical retrospective study, *J Clin Periodontol* 20:254, 1993.
16. Jansson LE, Ehnevid H, Lindskog SF, Blomlof LB: Radiographic attachment in periodontitis-prone teeth with endodontic infection, *J Periodontol* 64:947, 1993.
17. Ehnevid H, Jansson LE, Lindskog SF, Blomlof LB: Periodontal healing in relation to radiographic attachment and endodontic infection, *J Periodontol* 64:1199, 1993.

18. Jansson L, Ehnevid H, Lindskog S, Blomlof L: The influence of endodontic infection on progression of marginal bone loss in periodontitis, *J Clin Periodontol* 22:729, 1995.

19. Newman MG, Sanz M: Advanced diagnostic techniques. In Carranza FA, Newman MG, editors: *Clinical periodontology*, ed 8, Philadelphia, 1996, WB Saunders.

20. McGuire MK: Prognosis versus actual outcome: a long-term survey of 100 treated periodontal patients under maintenance care, *J Periodontol* 62:51, 1991.

21. McGuire MK, Nunn ME: Prognosis versus actual outcome. II. The effectiveness of clinical parameters in developing an accurate prognosis, *J Periodontal* 67:658, 1996.

22. McGuire MK, Nunn ME: Prognosis versus actual outcome. III. The effectiveness of clinical parameters in accurately predicting tooth survival, *J Periodontol* 67:666, 1996.

23. McGuire MK: Prognosis vs outcome: predicting tooth survival, *Compend Contin Educ Dent* 21:217, 2000.

24. Jaoui L, Machtou P, Ouhayoun JP: Long-term evaluation of endodontic and periodontal treatment, *Int Endod J* 28:249, 1995.

25. Carnevale G, Di Febo G, Tonelli MP, et al: A retrospective analysis of the periodontal-prosthetic treatment of molars with interradicular lesions, *Int J Periodontics Restorative Dent* 11:188, 1991.

26. Basten CH-J, Ammons WF, Persson R: Long-term evaluation of root resected molars: a retrospective study, *Int J Periodontics Restorative Dent* 16:207, 1996.

27. Buhler H: Survival rates of hemisected teeth: an attempt to compare them with survival rates of alloplastic implants, *Int J Periodontics Restorative Dent* 14:537, 1994.

28. Carnevale G, Pontoriero R, Lindhe J: Treatment of furcation-involved teeth. In Lindhe J, Karring T, Lang NP, editors: *Clinical periodontology and implant dentistry*, ed 3, Copenhagen, 1997, Munksgaard.

29. Adell R, Lekholm U, Rockler B, Brånemark P-I: A 15-year study of osseointegrated implants in the treatment of the edentulous jaw, *Int J Oral Surg* 10:387, 1981.

30. Tagger M, Smukler H: Microscopic study of the pulps of human teeth following vital root resection, *Oral Surg Oral Med Oral Pathol* 44:96, 1977.

31. Ross IF, Thompson RH: A long term study of root retention in the treatment of maxillary molars with furcation involvement, *J Periodontol* 49:238, 1978.

32. Czarnecki RT, Schilder H: A histological evaluation of the human pulp in teeth with varying degrees of periodontal disease, *J Endod* 5:242, 1979.

33. Haskell EW, Stanley H, Goldman S: A new approach to vital root resection, *J Periodontol* 51:217, 1980.

34. Bergenholtz G, Nyman S: Endodontic complications following periodontal and prosthetic treatment of patients with advanced periodontal disease, *J Periodontol* 55:63, 1984.

35. Torabinejad M, Kiger RD: A histologic evaluation of dental pulp tissue of a patient with periodontal disease, *Oral Surg Oral Med Oral Pathol* 59:198, 1985.

36. Langeland K, Rodrigues H, Dowden W: Periodontal disease, bacteria and pulpal histopathology, *Oral Surg Oral Med Oral Pathol* 37:257, 1974.

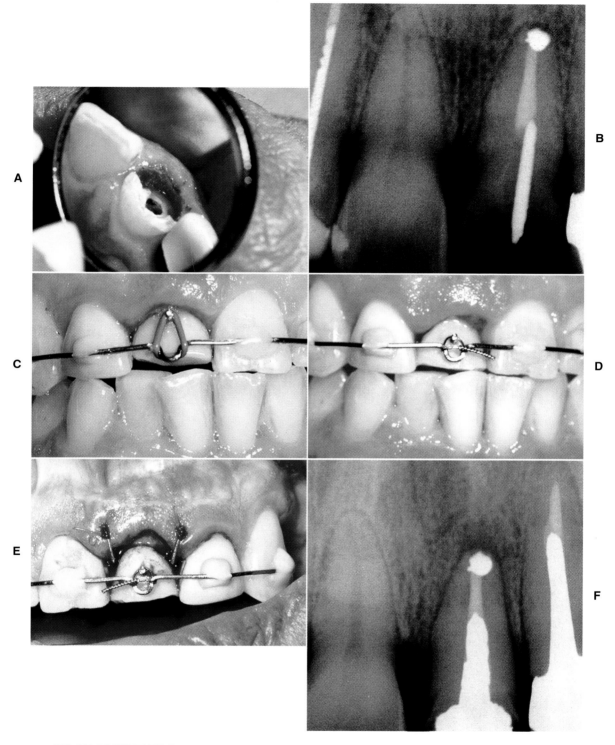

COLOR FIGURE 27-1
Orthodontic extrusion. **A,** Tooth with prior endodontic procedures experienced trauma, resulting in a deep shearing fracture. **B,** Post space has been prepared, and a temporary post is cemented. **C,** A temporary crown is placed. An omega-shaped loop with elastic bands is attached to the TMS pin in the temporary crown. **D,** Extrusion is near completion; occlusion of the temporary restoration is relieved as the tooth erupts. Extrusion is complete because the gingival margin of the TMS pin is level with interdental gingival margin of the anchorage wire. Note the level of gingival margin on the facial surface. **E,** After several weeks of stabilization, periodontal surgery is necessary to modify alveolar bone height and gingival contour. **F,** New position permits restoration with a permanent post, core, and crown. (Courtesy Dr. M. Messersmith.)

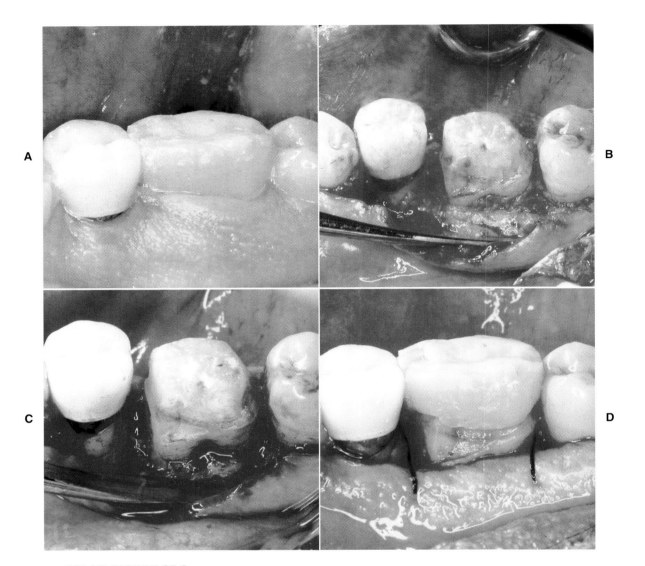

COLOR FIGURE 27-2

Crown lengthening. **A,** Acrylic temporary crown on the first molar is encroaching on the lingual gingiva and biologic width by extending to 0.5 mm from alveolar bone. **B,** After crown removal, full-thickness flaps were elevated, exposing a collar of excess tissue. **C,** Ostectomy and osteoplasty remove bone at the lingual and mesial surfaces to a distance of at least 3 mm from the future crown margins. **D,** An apically positioned flap sutured; sufficient biologic width is now established. (From Freeman K, Bebermeyer R, Moretti A, Koh S: *J Gt Houst Dent Soc* 71:14, 2000.)

Gerald N. Glickman and James A. Wallace

27

Endodontic Adjuncts

LEARNING OBJECTIVES

After reading this chapter, the student should be able to:

1 / Define the endodontic adjunct treatments described herein.

2 / Describe indications and contraindications for these treatments.

3 / Describe briefly the clinical technique, step-by-step, for each adjunct procedure.

4 / Discuss the prognosis for each adjunct procedure, both short-term and long-term.

5 / Identify findings that would indicate failure both short-term and long-term.

6 / Identify the appropriate general treatment options if the adjunct treatment fails.

7 / Briefly describe what the treatment entails for the patient (time, orthodontic appliances, surgical trauma, and so forth).

8 / Determine when consultation is indicated to devise a treatment plan.

9 / Determine when a patient should be referred to the appropriate specialist for treatment.

OUTLINE

Intentional Replantation
  Definitions
  Case Selection
  Clinical Technique
  Evaluation
  Prognosis

Transplantation
  Definitions
  Case Selection
  Clinical Technique
  Evaluation
  Prognosis

Orthodontic Extrusion
  Definition
  Case Selection
  Clinical Technique
  Evaluation
  Prognosis

Crown Lengthening
  Definition
  Case Selection
  Clinical Technique

Root Submersion
  Definition
  Case Selection
  Clinical Technique
  Evaluation
  Prognosis

Endodontic Implants
  Definition
  Prognosis

ypes of therapy not performed routinely but considered an integral part of endodontics include intentional replantation, transplantation, orthodontic extrusion, crown lengthening, root submersion, and endodontic implants. Patients have changing profiles and expectations. Their dental needs and demands necessitate familiarity with treatments that have been considered radical or last-resort options. This chapter discusses those options. Also included are case selection, a summary of techniques, evaluation of success or failure, and prognosis.

The general practitioner may or may not perform the procedures described in this chapter; however, the generalist should know the indications and contraindications for such treatments, understand the techniques, and know how to apply this knowledge in case selection. Referral to an endodontist may then be considered, or the general practitioner may choose to treat the patient in accordance with his or her level of training and experience. Most important, the generalist needs to understand these procedures sufficiently to be able to explain them to the patient, regardless of who performs the actual treatment.

Intentional Replantation

DEFINITIONS

Replantation is the return of a tooth to its alveolus. *Intentional replantation* is the insertion of a tooth into its alveolus after the tooth has been extracted for the purpose of performing root-end surgery.[1] Replantation is not a new procedure; it was first reported in 1593, when Paré replanted three avulsed teeth.[2]

CASE SELECTION
Indications

These root canal treatments cannot be performed conventionally because of calcifications or other blockages or because the patient cannot open his or her mouth sufficiently. Also included are treatment failures that cannot be retreated by conventional means because of unusual anatomy (Figure 27-1); canals that are blocked with broken instruments, crowns, ledges, or restorative materials such as posts; areas that are inaccessible; or roots that have unmanageable perforations. Ordinarily, surgery would be indicated but cannot be performed owing to anatomic restraints such as the external oblique ridge or nerve bundle proximity (inferior alveolar, lingual, or mental nerves).

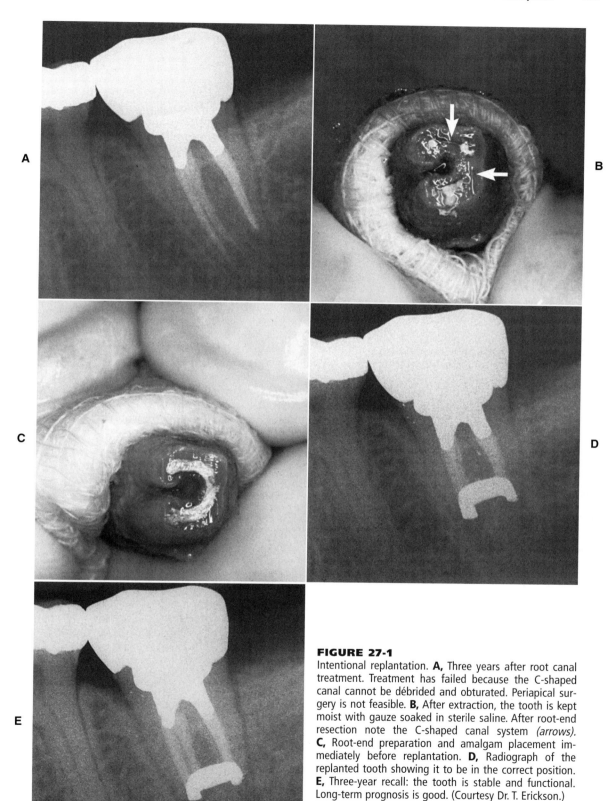

FIGURE 27-1
Intentional replantation. **A,** Three years after root canal treatment. Treatment has failed because the C-shaped canal cannot be débrided and obturated. Periapical surgery is not feasible. **B,** After extraction, the tooth is kept moist with gauze soaked in sterile saline. After root-end resection note the C-shaped canal system *(arrows)*. **C,** Root-end preparation and amalgam placement immediately before replantation. **D,** Radiograph of the replanted tooth showing it to be in the correct position. **E,** Three-year recall: the tooth is stable and functional. Long-term prognosis is good. (Courtesy Dr. T. Erickson.)

In essence, intentional replantation is indicated when there is no other treatment alternative to maintain a strategic tooth (Figure 27-1, *A*).

Contraindications

Intentional replantation is not a substitute for endodontic surgery if that procedure can be successfully performed. Replantation is contraindicated in patients who have a major comminution or fracture of the jaws or alveolus or an extensive medical history resulting in poor healing capacity. Replantation is not indicated for a tooth with advanced periodontal disease with mobility or furcation involvement. Caution is the rule for extractions of teeth if there is a strong possibility of fracturing the tooth or supporting bone.

CLINICAL TECHNIQUE

Important for success of this procedure are minimizing the out-of-socket time for the extracted tooth and minimizing damage to the root surface while the tooth is held. Adherence to these principles will decrease periodontal ligament cell death and decrease future ankylosis/resorption. The procedure of replantation involves first anesthesia, then luxation, and then gentle extraction with forceps that do not damage the root surface cervically. The tooth is held carefully by the crown in saline-soaked gauze and inspected closely for fractures, perforations, or other damage. Three to 4 mm of the apex is resected with a high-speed fissure bur using copious saline irrigation (Figure 27-1, *B*). An apical root-end preparation is made with small burs or an endodontic ultrasonic handpiece. This is followed by condensation of a root-end filling material (Figure 27-1, *C*). It is important not to damage the root and to keep the tooth moist, thus maintaining viable cells on the root surface. Apical pathosis may be curetted, taking care not to damage the socket walls; however, this procedure is probably unnecessary. The tooth is then carefully replanted, usually with finger or with forceps.

A perforation, resorptive defect, or other problem also may be repaired after extraction and before replantation using similar techniques.

Stabilization (if needed) after replantation may be done with sutures and/or a periodontal packing or with an acid-etch composite and orthodontic wire splinted to adjacent teeth; the splint is removed within 7 to 14 days. A radiograph is made immediately after replantation (Figure 27-1, *D*).

A very effective and simple stabilization approach is to have the patient close in centric occlusion and hold this position for the remainder of the day. He or she may release for short periods to ingest soft foods; fluids are taken through a straw.

EVALUATION

Recall evaluations are performed to search for signs of mobility, periodontal defects, root resorption, persistent periradicular pathosis, and evidence of healing (Figure 27-1, *E*).

PROGNOSIS

Intentional replants tend to be more successful short-term than long-term. Usually connective tissue and epithelial reattachment and stabilization occur initially. Problems may appear later, sometimes after several years.

However, intentional replants often are successful long-term. Some authors,[3,4] including Grossman,[5] have reported good success rates for 5 years or more. Factors affecting prognosis include the time the tooth is out of the socket, damage to the socket wall or roots, or problems during extraction.

Serious complications include periodontal defects or, most often, ankylosis with severe replacement resorption. Thus long-term follow-up is necessary.[6,7] If these problems develop, extraction is indicated.

Transplantation

DEFINITIONS

Transplantation is the transfer of a tooth from one alveolar socket to another either in the same or in another person.[1] An *autogenous* transplant is the transfer of a tooth from one alveolar socket to another in the same patient.[8,9] *Homogeneous* (allogeneic) transplantation is the transfer of a tooth from one patient to another. This can be performed immediately or after storage of the tooth in physiologic media or with cryopreservation.[10] *Heterogeneous* transplantation is a transfer from one species to another (for example, from monkey to human)[11]; this process is not feasible clinically.

CASE SELECTION
Indications

Usually autogenous tooth transplants involve third molars or premolars. Canine or incisor locations that were congenitally missing or lost owing to caries, trauma, juvenile periodontitis, or impaction are often the recipient sites for transplanted premolars. Posterior teeth may be replaced after extraction because of severe caries or a procedural accident (Figure 27-2).

A transplanted tooth should possess an intact crown. Ideally, there is partial root formation approximately equal to crown length, although teeth with more developed roots may also be candidates to transplant. Donor dimensions should be similar to those of the recipient site. An immature root often has an epithelial root sheath; pulp survival and root formation may then continue. Transplants of donor teeth with partial root development generally are easier and have a better prognosis; usually the pulps survive.

Contraindications

The same systemic contraindications apply as with intentional replantation. Local considerations are anatomic and may prevent transplan-tation. For example, a relatively narrow alveolar ridge may not accommodate a molar with divergent roots.

CLINICAL TECHNIQUE

Transplantation involves four steps: (1) at the recipient site, extraction and/or surgical preparation of the socket to receive the transplant; (2) extraction and placement of the transplant; (3) stabilization; and then (4) root canal treatment (if needed).

Socket Preparation

Preparation of the recipient socket is related to transplant shape as well as to time. If root morphology and length are similar and the extraction is performed at the same visit, the recipient socket often requires minimal preparation (Figure 27-3).

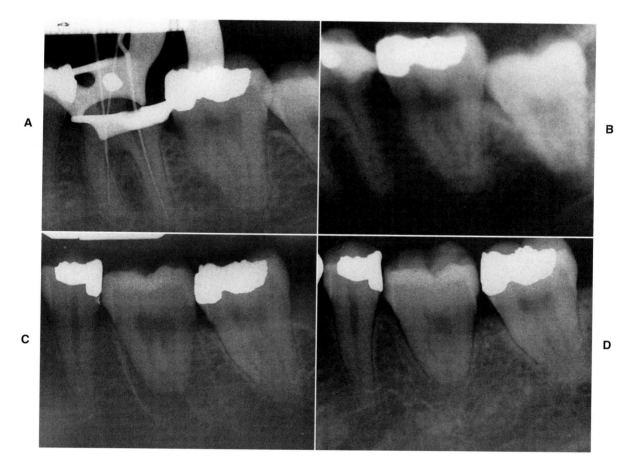

A

B

C

D

FIGURE 27-2
Transplantation. **A,** First molar requires extraction because of a large furcation perforation. **B,** Earlier panelipse radiograph shows a partially erupted third molar with root formation almost complete—a suitable donor. The third molar is transplanted to the first molar site after extraction. **C,** Two years post-transplantation. The donor is in occlusion and the pulp responds to pulp testing. (Courtesy Dr. H. Perinpanayagam.)

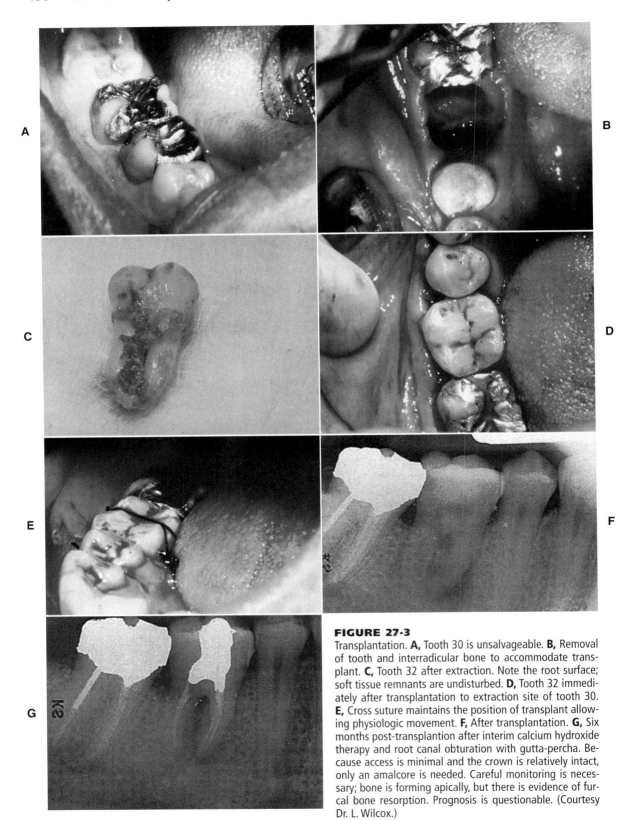

FIGURE 27-3
Transplantation. **A,** Tooth 30 is unsalvageable. **B,** Removal of tooth and interradicular bone to accommodate transplant. **C,** Tooth 32 after extraction. Note the root surface; soft tissue remnants are undisturbed. **D,** Tooth 32 immediately after transplantation to extraction site of tooth 30. **E,** Cross suture maintains the position of transplant allowing physiologic movement. **F,** After transplantation. **G,** Six months post-transplantion after interim calcium hydroxide therapy and root canal obturation with gutta-percha. Because access is minimal and the crown is relatively intact, only an amalcore is needed. Careful monitoring is necessary; bone is forming apically, but there is evidence of furcal bone resorption. Prognosis is questionable. (Courtesy Dr. L. Wilcox.)

If transplantation is done at a separate appointment from socket preparation, or if socket size and transplant size do not match, the socket requires shaping. This is best accomplished with an electric slow-speed handpiece and copious saline irrigation. Socket size is measured and compared to transplant size with a periodontal probe, and the socket is surgically adjusted until a fit is obtained. The tooth is placed gently in the socket and stabilized (see under "Intentional Replantation") if necessary.

If the area to receive the transplant is edentulous, preparation of both soft and hard tissue is necessary. A full-thickness flap is elevated from the alveolar crest buccally and lingually. Osseous tissue is removed (as in socket preparation) to allow the transplant to fit passively but snugly in the socket.

Extraction

Extraction should be performed as atraumatically as possible to maintain periodontal ligament fibers and cells. After extraction the donor site is managed carefully. The transplanted tooth is kept moist by wrapping and holding it in saline-soaked gauze.

Transplantation

The prepared socket is rinsed with sterile saline. The tooth is gently positioned in the socket and the flap is sutured snugly.

Stabilization

If the transplant exhibits mobility (usually) or if continued hemorrhage causes supraeruption, stabilization should be used to maintain the tooth in position, as with replantation. An alternative method is to suture over the occlusal surface and place periodontal packing. Certain situations may require more elaborate long-term splints, such as wire and bonded composite.

Follow-up

Conventional postsurgical instructions are given. The patient should return in 7 to 10 days for evaluation of healing and splint removal. If the transplant has roots that are incompletely developed, periodic radiographic evaluation is performed at 3- to 6-month intervals to monitor development. Arrested development and appearance of a resorptive lesion is a sign of pulp necrosis, requiring root canal treatment.

Teeth with fully developed roots require root canal treatment soon after transplantation. The protocol is similar to that used for traumatically avulsed and replanted teeth (see Chapter 25). After stabilization, the canals should be cleaned, shaped, and obturated, and the tooth is restored. Calcium hydroxide placement is probably unnecessary. This agent was once believed to inhibit root resorption, but evidence indicates that this is not true.[12]

EVALUATION

Transplants may not manifest signs of failure (periodontitis or resorption) for several years. Therefore, they should be evaluated clinically and radiographically for a *minimum* of 5 years for evidence of pathosis. The criteria for success are absence of pathosis, no adverse signs and symptoms, and no evidence of severe progressive external resorption (which is common in transplants).

Pulps that become necrotic in a transplant donor with immature roots require root-end closure (see Chapter 22) followed by root canal treatment.

PROGNOSIS

The prognosis for autogenous transplants varies widely.[13,14] Factors identified as most important for success are preservation of the periodontium on the roots and socket walls, developmental root stage (immature roots are best), and location of the donor tooth in the arch. The ipsilateral or contralateral third molar is the donor tooth of choice for replacement of molars.[15] Premolars can replace premolars or anterior teeth.[16] Failure of transplantation (replacement resorption, periodontal lesions, or adverse signs and symptoms) requires extraction.

Orthodontic Extrusion
DEFINITION

Orthodontic extrusion is defined as forced-controlled vertical tooth movement occlusally in the socket.[17] Vertical orthodontic repositioning after root canal treatment has been suggested in situations in which loss of tooth structure cervically makes restoration and periodontal maintenance impossible.[18] Through extrusion the area in question becomes accessible for restoration; thus surgery (which often creates a periodontal defect) is avoided. However, because gingival tissues and alveolar bone of the extruding tooth move coronally, a surgical periodontal procedure is often needed to reestablish biologic width and to restore the tooth's normal bony and gingival contour.[19,20] These procedures tend to be complex and may require cooperative treatment by the generalist, endodontist, periodontist, prosthodontist, and orthodontist.

CASE SELECTION
Indications

Indications are subgingival pathoses that are untreatable by standard restorative techniques, including coronal or root fractures in the cervical area, caries, deep marginal preparations, periodontal defects, resorptive lesions, and perforations.[19,20] Some of these lesions may be corrected by crown lengthening; however, the resultant periodontal defect may be impossible to treat or may be unattractive or unmaintainable. In these situations, extrusion provides a more desirable treatment and restorative environment. Orthodontic extrusion is also a common indication prior to implant placement. Forced occlusal movement results in an increase in vertical bone height, thereby providing more implant support. The tooth is first extruded, then extracted.

Contraindications

Orthodontic extrusion should not be considered if (1) there is such extensive loss of structure that vertical extrusion would result in a poor crown-root ratio or (2) the new tooth position would expose and create unmanageable furcation problems.

Other Considerations

An additional factor is patient acceptance of the procedure, because orthodontic appliances are involved. Time and expense may also be factors; the tooth has to be orthodontically repositioned and then stabilized before it is restored. Finally, a restoration may be somewhat difficult to design because the available root surface is smaller and may have proximal concavities.

Alternative treatment options include surgical crown lengthening, surgical repositioning of the tooth, and extraction with prosthetic replacement.

CLINICAL TECHNIQUE

The technique involves several phases: (1) root canal treatment, (2) post space preparation, (3) post and core fabrication with a hook on the occlusal surface (or a pin or bracket on the facial surface), (4) extrusion, (5) crown lengthening, (6) stabilization, and (7) restoration. Adjacent teeth function as anchors during extrusion or, in some cases, a removable appliance is used. After root canal treatment various approaches can be used depending on the situation.

One technique is a modification of the T-loop to prevent tipping (Figure 27-4).[21] A more common approach is to fabricate a hook to accommodate an orthodontic appliance or elastic. A large-gauge wire with an occlusal hook may be used as a temporary post. Brackets are placed on the facial surfaces of adjacent teeth. A horizontal wire engages the brackets, and the hook is activated to exert a vertical extrusive force. Alternatively, an orthodontic wire is bonded to the facial surfaces and an elastic force is used (see Color Figure 27-1 immediately following page 484). If the facial surface of the tooth to be extruded is intact, a post and hook may not be necessary. A bracket is bonded to the enamel and abutments, and the horizontal wire is attached to all brackets.

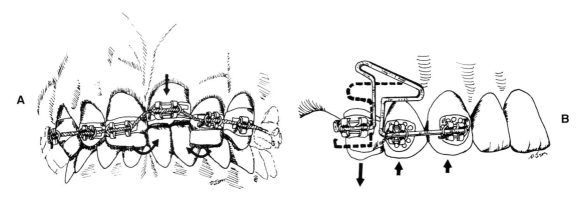

FIGURE 27-4
A, Orthodontic appliance used for extrusion; this is not a good design because it tends to tip adjacent teeth into the extrusion site. **B,** T-loop appliance used for extruding a terminal tooth. This design prevents tipping of anchors. (From Tuncay O, Cunningham C: *J Endod* 8:368, 1982.)

The patient should be evaluated often (every 1 to 2 weeks) during eruption. The tooth usually moves quickly; the occlusion usually requires adjusting, or the wire may have to be reactivated. The forced eruption period lasts approximately 4 to 6 weeks. Alveolar crestal bone and gingiva usually move coronally with the tooth. Periodontal procedures (bony recontouring or gingivectomy) may be required during or after orthodontic extrusion to correct gingival contours. These procedures may be unnecessary or minimized if, during extrusion, an intrasulcular incision (gingival fiberotomy) of the supracrestal attachment is performed every 2 weeks.[22]

Stabilization with a passive arch wire is required for 6 to 8 weeks to prevent intrusion. This allows time for the periodontal tissues to establish new attachments.[23]

The area involved is often of cosmetic concern. The following techniques improve appearance during movement and stabilization. Hollow-ground acrylic or a natural crown may be positioned facially to the root. Also, removable appliances may replace the missing tooth structure without interfering with movement.[24] When extrusion is complete and gingival appearance is satisfactory, the tooth is permanently restored. Importantly, the patient must be trained to follow special oral hygiene procedures both during and after movement and restoration.

EVALUATION

The patient should be recalled periodically. A minimal follow-up period is 1 year; however, long-term evaluation is recommended. Both radiographic and clinical examinations are necessary to assess periodontal status and mobility and check for the presence of caries as well as for periradicular pathoses.

PROGNOSIS

The outcome of orthodontic extrusion is good, provided periodontal attachment remains intact and the crown-root ratio is acceptable.[25] Because periodontal ligament fibers are reorganized (but not destroyed) during extrusion and alveolar bone moves with the tooth, root resorption is rarely a problem.[25] Developing periradicular and periodontal pathoses usually are correctable. Again, meticulous oral hygiene is critical.

Crown Lengthening
DEFINITION

Crown lengthening is a surgical procedure used to increase the extent of supragingival tooth structure for restorative or esthetic purposes. The basic procedure is apical positioning of the gingival margin and/or reducing cervical bone.[26]

CASE SELECTION
Indications

Crown lengthening is generally used for restoring teeth with subgingival defects such as caries, perforations, or resorptions. Other indications are cosmetic factors or short clinical crowns that may be lengthened to improve retention and appearance. To repeat, with orthodontic extrusion, the periodontium usually accompanies the tooth; surgical crown lengthening is necessary for appearance and function.

Impingement by restoration margins on the attachment apparatus may result in inflammation, pain, and loss of periodontal attachment (see Color Figure 27-2 immediately following page 484).[27] Margins should not be placed near or at the alveolar crest. Preferably, the relationship should allow at least 2 mm of root surface between the alveolar crest and the restoration; such is the concept of the "biologic width."[28] Biologic width (Figure 27-5) has two components cervical to the margin of the alveolar crest, each averaging 1 mm in width: (1) the connective tissue attachment and (2) the epithelial attachment.[29] Sulcus depth varies.

Many factors are considered in planning treatment. These include extent and location of fractures, perforations, caries, root length, periodontal support, periodontal status of adjacent teeth, tooth position, and esthetics.

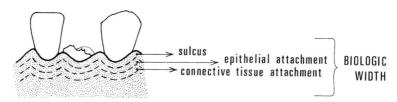

FIGURE 27-5
Levels of factors related to biologic width. Each anatomic division is approximately 1 mm.

Contraindications

Usually adverse factors can be determined before the procedure is undertaken. However, occasionally some situations are encountered during surgery, including creation of an unattractive gingival deformity, production of an unfavorable root-to-crown ratio, compromise of bone support for adjacent teeth, and exposure of the furcation.

CLINICAL TECHNIQUE

Studies have shown no correlation between the width of the attached gingiva and periodontal health except in association with restorations; however, the attached gingiva should not be indiscriminately removed.[30-32] In patients with subgingival restorations it is recommended that at least 2 mm of attached keratinized gingiva be left to maintain periodontal health and protect the restoration.[33] This requires an internal bevel incision with elevation of a full-thickness flap. Then crestal bone is removed to at least 2.5 to 3.0 mm below the level of the free gingival margin desired (Figure 27-6). Thorough root planing follows the osteotomy. Then the flap is sutured at this level (apical to its original height).

On anterior teeth, for esthetic purposes, crown preparation should be delayed for approximately 14 weeks after surgery. The best method of determining preparation time is to measure from the provisional crown margin to the free gingival margin; final restoration is done when the area within this measurement has stabilized for at least 1 month.[34] Posterior crown preparation may be done 2 to 4 weeks after crown lengthening because appearance is not a factor, and crown margins are supragingival.

Root Submersion

DEFINITION

Root submersion is a surgical procedure in which the tooth roots are resected approximately 3 mm below the alveolar crest and then covered with a mucoperiosteal flap. Eventually the area is shaped by hard tissue. Root submersions are generally not complex; the more straightforward procedures may be managed by the general practitioner.

CASE SELECTION
Indications

After tooth extraction the alveolar ridges resorb, approximately 0.1 mm/yr for the maxilla and 0.4 mm/yr for the mandible.[35,36] Alveolar bone resorption is prevented by maintaining the roots. Proprioception is also retained.[37] Three considerations related to root submersion are (1) roots with vital pulps,[38] (2) root canal treatment in situ,[39] and (3) root canal treatment after extraction and replantation to encourage ankylosis.[40] The first method has been most successful because it results in a blending of healthy pulpal tissue with overlying connective tissue followed by osteodentin covering the root face and eventual bone formation. The second technique has shown similar results in some patients. The third method shows little promise because no bone forms coronally and many roots are resorbed.

Conditions that indicate root submersion include rampant caries, poor periodontal conditions, poor oral hygiene, and repeated prosthetic failures. These types of conditions tend to be seen in aged, medically compromised or handicapped, or financially compromised patients who require

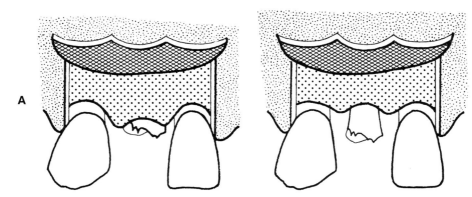

FIGURE 27-6
Crown lengthening after orthodontic extrusion. **A,** Full-thickness flap exposes bony margin. **B,** Reduction and recontouring of crestal bone reestablishes biologic width. Often some removal of bone from adjacent teeth is necessary.

denture support and have a need for proprioception. Roots are occasionally retained when extraction would produce surgical or esthetic defects (Figure 27-7).

Contraindications

Root resorption, unresolved endodontic pathosis, and inadequate bone support are contraindications. Loss of vestibular depth may result from surgery (which may interfere with prosthetic retention and use); this may be treated with vestibuloplasty or a free gingival graft. An anatomic problem occurs when the facial gingiva is thin, the root is prominent, and a bony dehiscence or fenestration is likely. These patients often develop a soft tissue fenestration with root exposure (failure) at varying times after root submersion, which requires resubmergence or extraction.

CLINICAL TECHNIQUE

Preferably, healthy pulp should not be removed before submersion. However, in patients with pulp or periradicular pathosis, root canal treatment is first necessary. Both situations require a similar surgical approach. An inverse beveled intrasulcular incision is made to remove the sulcular (or pocket) epithelium. A mucoperiosteal flap, extending both buccally and lingually, is elevated

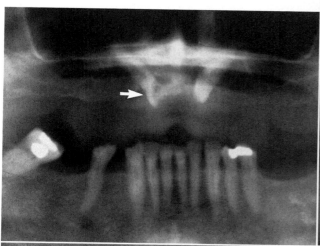

A

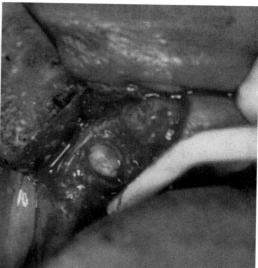

B

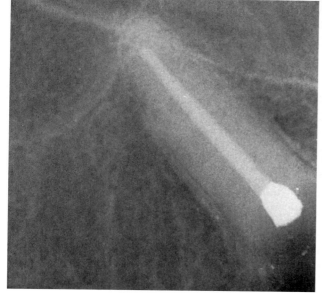

C

FIGURE 27-7
Root submergence. **A,** Carious, partially impacted maxillary canine tooth *(arrow)*. **B,** Flap is reflected, and then root canal treatment is performed because of pulp pathosis. The root is submerged by bur reduction 3 mm below the alveolar crest and the flap is sutured for primary closure. **C,** Postendodontic treatment, submersion, and amalgam seal.

far enough apically to allow reapproximation (primary closure) of the flap margins. The root is resected at least 3 mm below the alveolar crest. If the pulp is to be retained, the resection is done with copious water spray and gentle reduction. If root canal treatment was performed, an amalgam seal may be placed in the canal, although this is generally unnecessary.

Flap margins are apposed (primary closure) with mattress sutures. Postoperative instructions are the same as those given for surgical extractions (Figure 27-7). Sutures are removed in 5 to 7 days.

EVALUATION

Postoperative evaluation is critical and is recommended initially every 3 months for 1 year; thereafter, recall is performed yearly. Failures generally result from four factors: (1) flap breakdown immediately after the procedure; (2) denture impingement with ulceration and fenestration (root exposure) through overlying tissue; (3) passive

eruption or crestal bone resorption, also resulting in soft tissue fenestration; and (4) obliteration of the vestibule. This decrease in vestibular depth is a major disadvantage of this technique because it limits prosthesis retention.

PROGNOSIS

Short-term success tends to be much better than long-term success. Good results continue for an average of about 2 years, after which the rate of failure increases.[41] Success with vital pulp root submersion is higher than when the roots have root canal treatment; the latter have an overall moderate success rate.[42] Presently, root submersion cannot be recommended as a routine procedure, but for selected patients it is a practical means of retaining alveolar bone.[43]

The major reasons for failure are soft tissue fenestration with exposure of roots or loss of vestibular depth. Endodontic failure with apical or coronal pathosis may occur as well. Failures generally require surgical removal of the tooth or reoperation to submerge the root further into bone.

Endodontic Implants
DEFINITION

Endodontic implants are metallic extensions of a tooth root using a post prepared for that purpose. The tooth first has root canal treatment, then a metallic post is placed into the canal and out the apex, extending beyond the root apex and inserted into a previously prepared channel in bone. The purpose is to increase the root-crown ratio, thus stabilizing the tooth. A potential advantage over osseous integrated implants is the absence of communication (direct contact) of a material with the tissues of the oral cavity; epithelium and connective tissue remain attached to the tooth surface.[44] Offsetting major disadvantages are the difficulty of achieving anatomic adaptability and creating and maintaining an apical seal of the implant.

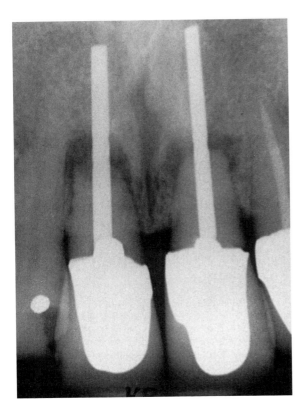

FIGURE 27-8
Seventeen years after implant placement. Note the apical radiolucencies. There is a sinus tract associated with tooth 9, and deep probing defects. Despite eventual failure, the implants served the patient for many years. (Courtesy Dr. S. Madison.)

PROGNOSIS

Under good conditions, the success rate for endodontic implants is reasonable for several years, but they usually show problems with time.[44,45] Usually the initial evaluation is very good; the tooth feels solid, and periradicular findings are favorable. These positive findings generally do not persist and with time periodontal lesions, increasing mobility, or periradicular pathosis (often) may be seen (Figure 27-8). Long-term failure is often related to coronal or apical leakage[46,47] or periodontal communication with the apex.[48] The poor long-term prognosis for endodontic implants has discouraged their use. Most patients are now treated with extraction and immediate insertion of a single-tooth osseous integrated implant.

REFERENCES

1. American Association of Endodontists: *An annotated glossary of terms used in endodontics,* ed 6, Chicago, 1998, American Association of Endodontists.
2. Kupfer IJ, Sidney R, Kupfer BS: Tooth replantation following avulsion, *NY State Dent J* 19:80, 1952.
3. Kingsbury BC, Wiesenbaugh JM: Intentional replantation of mandibular premolars and molars, *J Am Dent Assoc* 83:1053, 1971.
4. Bender I, Rossman L: Intentional replantation of endodontically treated teeth, *Oral Surg Oral Med Oral Pathol* 76:623, 1993.
5. Grossman L: Intentional reimplantation of teeth, *J Am Dent Assoc* 72:1111, 1966.
6. Holland G, Robinson P: Pulp reinnervation in reimplanted canine teeth of the cat, *Arch Oral Biol* 32:593, 1987.
7. Andreasen J: *Atlas of replantation and transplantation of teeth,* Philadelphia, 1992, WB Saunders.
8. Apfel H: Autoplasty of enucleated perfunctional third molars, *J Oral Surg* 8:289, 1950.
9. Miller HM: Transplantation: a case report, *J Am Dent Assoc* 40:237, 1950.
10. Andreasen J, Schwartz O: *Atlas of replantation and transplantation of teeth,* Philadelphia, 1992, WB Saunders.
11. Natiella J, Armitage J, Green G: The replantation and transplantation of teeth: a review, *Oral Surg Oral Med Oral Pathol* 23:397, 1970.
12. Dumsha T, Hovland E: Evaluation of long-term calcium hydroxide treatment in avulsed teeth, *Int Endod J* 28:7, 1995.
13. Tsukibashi M: Autogenous tooth transplantation: a reevaluation, *Int J Periodontics Restorative Dent* 13:121, 1993.
14. Akiyama Y, Fukuda H, Hashimoto K: A clinical and radiographic study of 25 autotransplanted molars, *J Oral Rehabil* 25:640, 1998.
15. Andreasen J: Third molar autotransplantation relation between successful healing and stage of root development at time of grafting. Presented at the annual meeting of the Scandinavian Association of Oral and Maxillofacial Surgeons, Nyborg, Denmark, August 15-19, 1990.
16. Andreasen J, Paulsen H, Yu Z, et al: A long-term study of 370 autotransplanted premolars. Part II. Tooth survival and pulp healing subsequent to transplantation, *Eur J Orthod* 12:14, 1990.
17. Berglundhl T, Marinello CP, Lindhe J, et al: Periodontal tissue reactions to orthodontic extrusion: an experimental study in the dog, *J Clin Periodontol* 18:330, 1991.
18. Heathersay G: Combined endodontic orthodontic treatment of transverse root fractures in the region of the alveolar crest, *Oral Surg Oral Med Oral Pathol* 36:408, 1973.
19. Stevens H, Levine R: Forced eruption: a multidisciplinary approach for form, function, and biologic predictability, *Compend Contin Educ Dent* 19:994, 1998.
20. Ingber J: Forced eruption. Part I. A method of treating isolated one and two walled infrabony osseous defects rationale and case report, *J Periodontol* 45:199, 1974.
21. Tuncay O, Cunningham C: T-loop appliance in endodontic-orthodontic interactions, *J Endod* 8:367, 1982.
22. Kozlorsky A, Tal H, Lieberman M: Forced eruption combined with gingival fiberotomy: a technique for clinical crown lengthening, *J Clin Periodontol* 15:534, 1988.
23. Simon J, Lythgoe J, Torabinejad M: Clinical and histological evaluation of extruded endodontically treated teeth, *Oral Surg Oral Med Oral Pathol* 50:361, 1980.
24. Delivanis P, Delivanis H: Esthetic solutions in orthodontic extrusion of compromised teeth, *J Endod* 10:221, 1984.
25. Hamilton R, Gutmann J: Endodontic-orthodontic relationships: a review of integrated treatment planning challenges, *Int Endod J* 32:343, 1999.
26. American Academy of Periodontology: *Glossary of periodontal terms,* ed 3, Chicago, 1992, American Academy of Periodontology.
27. Freeman K, Bebermeyer R, Moretti A, Koh S: Single-tooth crown lengthening by the restorative dentist: a case report, *J Gt Houst Dent Soc* 71:14, 2000.
28. Eissman H, Radke A, Noble W: Physiologic design criteria for fixed dental restoration, *Dent Clin North Am* 15:543, 1971.
29. Gargiulo A, Wentz F, Orban B: Dimensions and relations of the dentogingival junction in humans, *J Periodontol* 32:261, 1961.
30. Hangorsky W, Bissada N: Clinical assessment of free gingival grafts' effectiveness on the maintenance of periodontal health, *J Periodontol* 51:274, 1980.
31. Dorfman H, Kennedy J, Bird W: Longitudinal evaluation of free autogenous gingival grafts, *J Clin Periodontol* 7:316, 1980.
32. Wennstrom J, Lindhe J, Myman S: Role of keratinized gingiva for gingival health, *J Clin Periodontol* 8:311, 1981.
33. Statler K, Bisada N: Significance of the width of keratinized gingiva in the periodontal status of teeth with submarginal restorations, *J Periodontol* 58:698, 1987.
34. Wise MD: Stability of gingival crest after surgery and before anterior crown placement, *J Prosthet Dent* 53:20, 1985.
35. Tallgren A: The continuing reduction of the residual alveolar ridges in complete denture wearers: a mixed longitudinal study covering 245 years, *J Prosthet Dent* 27:120, 1972.
36. Atwood D, Clay KW: Clinical cephalometric and densitometric study of reduction of residual ridges, *J Prosthet Dent* 26:280, 1971.
37. Simpson HE: Histologic changes in retained roots, *J Can Dent Assoc* 25:287, 1989.

38. Poe GS, Johnson DL, Hillenbrand DJ: Vital root retention in dogs, Technical report 019, Bethesda, MD, 1971, Naval Dental School.

39. Bjorn H, Hollender L, Lindhe J: Tissue regeneration in patients with periodontal disease, *Odontol Rev* 16:317, 1965.

40. Simon JH, Kimura JT: Maintenance of alveolar bone by the intentional replantation of roots, *Oral Surg Oral Med Oral Pathol* 37:963, 1974.

41. Goska FA, Vandrak RK: Roots submerged to preserve alveolar bone: a case report, *Milit Med* 137:446, 1972.

42. Whitaker DD, Shankle RJ: A study of the histologic reaction of submerged root segments, *Oral Surg Oral Med Oral Pathol* 37:819, 1974.

43. Wallace J, Carman J, Jimenez J: Endodontic therapy and root submergence of an impacted maxillary canine, *Oral Surg Oral Med Oral Pathol* 77:519, 1994.

44. Madison S, Bjorndal A: Clinical application of endodontic implants, *J Prosthet Dent* 5:603, 1988.

45. Cranin AN, Robin MF: A statistical evaluation of 952 endosteal implants in humans, *J Am Dent Assoc* 94:315, 1977.

46. Frank AL, Abrams MF: Histologic evaluation of endodontic implants, *J Am Dent Assoc* 78:520, 1969.

47. Simon JH, Frank AL: The endodontic stabilizer: additional histologic evaluation, *J Endod* 6:450, 1980.

48. Perel ML: *Dental implantology and prosthesis,* Philadelphia, 1977, JB Lippincott.

Longitudinal Tooth Fractures

LEARNING OBJECTIVES

After reading this chapter, the student should be able to:

1 / Define and differentiate craze line, cusp fracture, cracked tooth, split tooth, and vertical root fracture.

2 / Describe the causes of these fractures of tooth structure.

3 / List and describe the five considerations (characteristics) of fractures in dentin.

4 / Describe in general each of the five categories of fracture in regard to
  a. Incidence
  b. Pathogenesis
  c. Clinical features
  d. Etiologies
  e. Diagnosis
  f. Treatment
  g. Prognosis
  h. Prevention

5 / Identify patients with difficult situations who should be considered for referral.

OUTLINE

Incidence

Categories

Craze Lines

Fractured Cusp
Incidence
Pathogenesis
Clinical Features
Etiologies
Diagnosis
Treatment
Prognosis
Prevention

Cracked Tooth
Incidence
Pathogenesis
Clinical Features
Etiologies
Diagnosis
Treatment
Prognosis
Prevention

Split Tooth
Incidence
Pathogenesis
Clinical Features
Etiologies
Diagnosis
Treatment
Prognosis
Prevention

Vertical Root Fracture
Incidence
Pathogenesis
Clinical Features
Etiologies
Diagnosis
Treatment
Prognosis
Prevention

Cracked teeth and their related entities as well as vertical root fractures are longitudinal fractures of the crown and/or root. These contrast with horizontal fractures, which predominate in anterior teeth and result from impact trauma. Longitudinal (vertical) fractures occur in all tooth groups and are caused by occlusal forces and by dental procedures.

There is relatively little research on longitudinal tooth fractures, particularly on clinical outcomes related to diagnosis and treatment. Most treatment modalities are based on opinion and anecdotal information.[1] Therefore many recommendations have not been substantiated in controlled clinical trials but are based on experience. This chapter deals with longitudinal fractures in the vertical plane, that is, the long axis of the crown or root.

Treating longitudinal fractures is usually challenging. Sometimes they are not difficult to diagnose or manage, whereas at other times they are so devastating that the involved tooth must be extracted. Notwithstanding, many situations present problems with both diagnosis and treatment and these patients should be considered for referral.

Incidence

The incidence of longitudinal fractures is apparently increasing. There are several reasons for this unfortunate occurrence. One is the increasing age of patients with decreased numbers of tooth extractions. Therefore more teeth undergo complex procedures and are present for longer periods of time. These procedures include restorative and endodontic treatments that remove dentin, thereby compromising internal strength. Also, the teeth absorb external forces, usually occlusal, that exceed the strength of dentin and gradually alter tooth structure. When the destructive force is beyond the elastic limit of dentin or enamel, a fracture occurs.[2,3] Therefore the longer a tooth is present and the more forces it undergoes, the greater the chances of an eventual fracture. Another reason for the increased incidence is more awareness and better diagnosis and identification of the problem. Importantly, such fractures are not confined to elderly patients and do not occur only in restored teeth.[4-6]

Categories

There are five categories of longitudinal fractures. From least to most severe they are (1) craze lines, (2) fractured cusp, (3) cracked tooth, (4) split tooth, and (5) vertical root fracture. These types of fracture differ but they are often confused or combined in clinical articles.[7-10] This leads to misunderstanding, with incorrect diagnosis and inappropriate treatment. Table 28-1 identifies four of the five entities by findings, diagnostic methods, and treatment. The reader is referred to this table throughout the chapter.

Fractures occur primarily in two areas, crown and root. Either area may be the site of initiation as well as the region of principal damage. In the crown (usually extending to the root), these lesions take the form of a craze line, fractured cusp, cracked tooth, or split tooth (Figure 28-1); the latter three usually extend to the root. Roots show vertical root fracture (Figure 28-2). The remainder of the chapter is subdivided into these five categories.

Craze Lines

Craze lines are common, particularly in permanent teeth in adults. They usually extend over

---

Considerations for Cracked Teeth

Five important considerations of which patients must be informed are the following:
1. Longitudinal fractures result from excessive forces, usually (but not always) long-term forces.
2. Visualization of the presence or extent of the fracture may be difficult to identify clinically; they are often tiny and are not demonstrable until growth or expansion occurs. Also, they may be hidden under restorations or bone and gingiva and thus not be visible even after flap reflection.
3. With time, fracture spaces tend to acquire stains and become more visible.
4. Fractures have a tendency to grow, although initially they are very small. This propagation may be very slow. An analogy is a small crack in a windshield that may lengthen over months or years.
5. Signs and symptoms often are not present early but become manifest months, years, or decades after fracture initiation.

TABLE 28-1

Categories of Fractures

	FRACTURED CUSP	CRACKED TOOTH	SPLIT TOOTH	VERTICAL ROOT FRACTURE
Location	Crown and cervical margin of root	Crown to root extension (depth varies)	Crown and root; extension to all surfaces	Root only
Direction	Mesiodistal and faciolingual	Mesiodistal	Mesiodistal	Facioligual
Origination	Occlusal surface	Occlusal surface	Occlusal surface	Root (any level)
Etiologies	Undermined cusp, damaging habits	Damaging habits, weakened tooth structure	Damaging habits, weakened tooth structure	Wedging posts, obturation forces, excessive root-dentin removal
Symptoms	Sharp pain with mastication and with cold	Cracked tooth syndrome, or highly variable	Pain with mastication	None to slight
Signs	None of significance	Variable	Separable segments, periodontal abscess	Variable
Identification	Visualize, remove restoration	Biting, remove restoration	Remove restoration	Reflect flap and transilluminate
Diagnostic tests	Visible fractures of cusps, biting, transillumination	Transillumination, staining, wedge segments (unseparable)	Wedge segments (separable)	Reflect flap and transilluminate
Treatment	Remove cusp and/or restore	Root canal treatment usually, restore with full crown	Variable, must remove one segment, restore, or extract	Remove tooth or fractured root
Prognosis	Very good	Always questionable to poor	Maintain intact (hopeless) Remove segment (variable)	Hopeless for fractured root
Prevention	Place conservative class-II restorations, coronal protection (onlay undermined cusps)	Eliminate damaging habits (ice chewing, etc.), coronal protection (onlay undermined cusps)	Eliminate damaging habits, coronal protection (onlay cusps)	Minimize root dentin removal, avoid wedging posts, reduce condensation forces

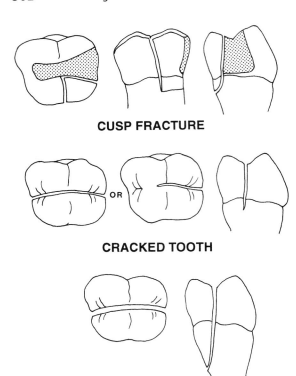

CUSP FRACTURE

CRACKED TOOTH

SPLIT TOOTH

FIGURE 28-1
The three fracture types that originate occlusally and then extend toward the root.

marginal ridges and along buccal and lingual surfaces in posterior teeth but also appear as long vertical defects from incisal to cervical aspect on anterior teeth (Figure 28-3). Craze lines are confined to enamel.[1,7]

Craze lines occur naturally but their incidence increases in patients who have had restorations or impact injuries. It is unknown (but unlikely) whether they are precursors to dentin fractures. Craze lines are unimportant other than as a common source of misidentification and confusion with cracked teeth. Because of their insignificance, they are not included in Table 28-1.

Fractured Cusp

Fractured cusps are usually relatively easy to diagnose and treat and generally have a good prognosis (see Table 28-1).

INCIDENCE

Fractured cusps are more common than the other major entities discussed in this chapter, which is fortunate because these are the least devastating and are the most manageable.[1] This fracture occurs often in teeth with extensive caries or large restorations that do not protect undermined cusps.[11]

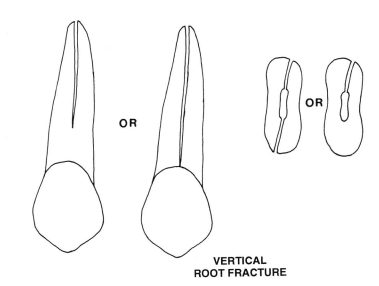

VERTICAL ROOT FRACTURE

FIGURE 28-2
This fracture begins and ends on the root. Usually the fracture extends facially and lingually, but may not extend to both surfaces or from apical to cervical.

PATHOGENESIS

These fractures are related to lack of cusp support. A second, but uncommon, cause is a traumatic upward blow to the mandible, resulting in a sharp impact between the maxillary and mandibular teeth. Fortunately, this mishap does not happen often; a single injury may cause fracture or loss of several cusps.

CLINICAL FEATURES

Cusp fractures are usually associated with a weakened marginal ridge in conjunction with an undermined cusp. These compromise dentin support for the cusp, which is supplied primarily by the marginal ridge.[12] Either a single cusp or two cusps (in molars) are involved. The fracture includes a mesial-distal and a facial-lingual component (Figure 28-4). Therefore the crack lines (see Figure 28-1) cross the marginal ridge and then extend, down a facial or lingual groove and often into the cervical region parallel to the gingival margin (or somewhat subgingivally, which is more common). If two cusps are involved, the fracture lines will be mesial and distal, without a facial or lingual component. *Very rarely* are two mesial or two distal cusps fractured together.

These are oblique shearing fractures extending from the occlusal, often at the base of a cavity (Figure 28-5). The defect often includes the region of epithelial attachment and does not extend beyond the cervical third of the root.[13] There usually is no pulp exposure, particularly in older teeth with smaller pulp chambers.

ETIOLOGIES

Typically there is a history of extensive deep interproximal caries or a subsequent class II restoration. Occasionally these cusp fractures occur in nonrestored teeth with extensive undermining caries.

DIAGNOSIS
Subjective Symptoms

Often the patient reports brief, sharp pain on mastication or with temperature changes, particularly cold. Often the pain is more distinct with masticatory release (not with closure but with separation of teeth after biting). Pain is neither severe nor spontaneous and occurs only on stimulus. Interestingly, the symptoms are often relieved when the cusp finally breaks off.

Objective Tests

The most indicative test is biting. The patient may close onto a cotton swab applicator, a rubber

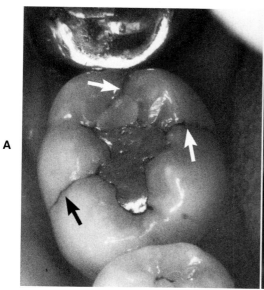
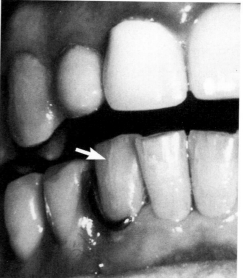

A **B**

FIGURE 28-3
Craze lines are common. These are fractures that are limited to the enamel and do not extend to dentin. **A,** This molar shows craze lines over marginal ridges and through buccal and lingual grooves *(arrows)*. **B,** Vertical craze lines are common in anterior teeth *(arrow),* particularly in older patients.

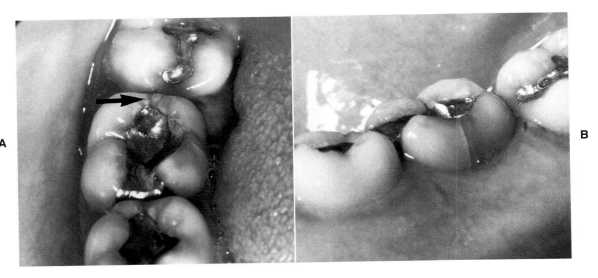

FIGURE 28-4
Cusp fracture. **A,** This fracture is usually associated with a class II restoration, extending across at least one marginal ridge *(arrow)* and often **(B)** down a lingual or buccal surface. These fractures tend to acquire stain with time, are usually symptomatic, and will stop light with transillumination.

polishing (burlew) wheel, or a specially designed bite-testing instrument (Figure 28-6). An occlusal, gnashing force on the involved cusp elicits pain. Ordinarily, pulp tests indicate vitality.

Radiographic Findings

Radiographs are not useful because cusp fractures are not visible radiographically.

Other Findings

The restoration may have to be removed to observe the underlying dentin. The fracture may then be readily visible, or it may be disclosed by either staining or transillumination. Older fractures may have already acquired stain (see Figure 28-4). The cusp fracture line usually originates at the cavity floor at a line angle.

TREATMENT

Retaining the fractured cusp is often not indicated. The cusp is removed, and the tooth is restored as appropriate. The restoration will probably be a three-fourths or full crown extending below or to the fracture margin. Root canal treatment is often not required, because the pulp is not exposed. Occasionally, restoration is unnecessary.

If the cusp is not mobile, the fracture line probably does not extend to a root surface sub-

gingivally. In these cases, the cusp need not be removed; a crown should be placed to hold the segments.

PROGNOSIS

Long-term success is good because fractures tend to be shallow. Cusp fractures occasionally extend deeper, below the gingival attachment; treatment of these is more challenging. An approach to restoring deep-extending cusp fractures is described later in this chapter.

PREVENTION

Extensive removal of dentin support should be avoided. The width and particularly the depth of restorations should be minimized.[14] Those that wedge, such as inlays, require adequate dentin support. Cusps should be reduced and onlayed if undermined; both amalgam and gold onlays provide fracture resistance.[15] Composite resins that are bonded to enamel or dentin and improperly placed may shrink excessively upon polymerization; this contraction may displace and weaken cusps, rendering them susceptible to occlusal forces and fracture.

In terms of bonding, adhesive resins, if placed with special techniques, may reinforce weakened cusps.[16-18] However, studies are still short-term and "bench-top" and do not include long-term evaluations made under clinical conditions. In

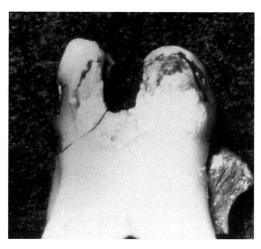

FIGURE 28-5
Cusp fracture. Typically, the separation occurs from the line angle of the cavity to the cervical surface.

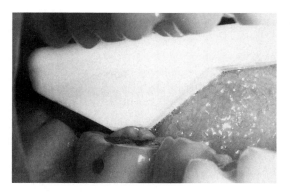

FIGURE 28-6
Special diagnostic "biting" instruments (Tooth Slooth) are placed on one cusp at a time while the patient grinds with opposing teeth. Sharp pain on pressure or release may indicate a cusp fracture or cracked tooth.

other words, such bonded restorations may provide only temporary reinforcement.

Cracked Tooth

Cracked teeth are also described as "incomplete (greenstick) fractures," which describes their form.[19] Cracked tooth is a variation of the cusp fracture, but the associated fracture is centered more occlusally (see Figure 28-1). The effects of cracked teeth tend to be more devastating because their extent and direction are more centered and more apical (see Table 28-1).

INCIDENCE

The occurrence of cracked tooth is unknown but is apparently increasing.[5,8] Cracked teeth are predominantly seen in older patients, although they may occur at any age in adults.[4,6] The longevity and complexity of restorations are related factors, although cracked teeth often are minimally restored or not restored at all.[8] Mastication for many years, particularly of hard objects, is also a factor. Continued and repeated forces finally cause fatigue of tooth structure resulting in fracture followed by continued growth of that fracture.

The teeth usually involved are mandibular molars (both restored and nonrestored) followed by maxillary premolars and then by maxillary first molars.[6] Anterior teeth do not develop true cracks, and true cracks are seen rarely on mandibular premolars. Furthermore, class I restored teeth fracture as often as do class II restored teeth, particularly molars. Therefore the phenomenon is not always dependent on violation of tooth structure by access preparations, caries, or restorations. There has been speculation that teeth treated by root canals are more brittle and weakened and therefore are more susceptible to fracture. Evidence does not support this assumption.[12,20-22]

PATHOGENESIS

As stated previously, cracks in teeth tend to depend on time and patient habits. Obviously, forces in excess of dentin strength are responsible; these forces are greater in the posterior region, i.e., close to the fulcrum of the mandible, invoking the "nutcracker" effect.[6,23]

Although occlusal anatomy (deep fissures or prominent or functional cusps) and occlusal dysfunction might render a tooth more susceptible to cracking, these factors are only speculative; no relationship with cracked teeth has been demonstrated.

CLINICAL FEATURES

Cracks in teeth are almost invariably mesiodistal fractures (Figure 28-7), although mandibular molars occasionally (rarely) fracture toward the facial-lingual surface. The diagnosis of a facial-lingual cracked molar is a common misinterpretation because of visualization of facial and lingual fractures (see Figure 28-3, *A*). These are actually craze lines, which follow the buccal and

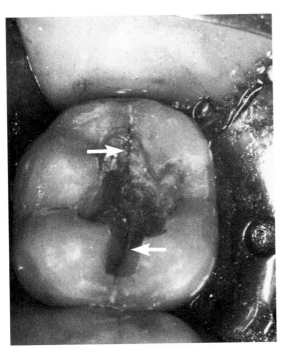

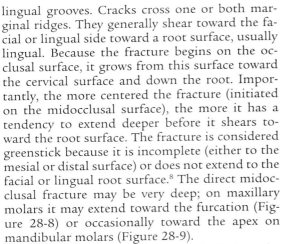

FIGURE 28-7
Cracked tooth. The fracture extends across both marginal ridges and across the cavity floor *(arrows)*. Fractures in the mesial-distal direction are by far the most common.

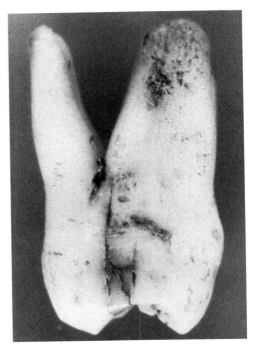

FIGURE 28-8
Cracked tooth. The fracture extends across the marginal ridge and down the proximal close to the furcation (greenstick fracture).

lingual grooves. Cracks cross one or both marginal ridges. They generally shear toward the facial or lingual side toward a root surface, usually lingual. Because the fracture begins on the occlusal surface, it grows from this surface toward the cervical surface and down the root. Importantly, the more centered the fracture (initiated on the midocclusal surface), the more it has a tendency to extend deeper before it shears toward the root surface. The fracture is considered greenstick because it is incomplete (either to the mesial or distal surface) or does not extend to the facial or lingual root surface.[8] The direct midocclusal fracture may be very deep; on maxillary molars it may extend toward the furcation (Figure 28-8) or occasionally toward the apex on mandibular molars (Figure 28-9).

The fracture may or may not include the pulp. The more centered the fracture is, the greater is the chance of pulp exposure now or later. Occasionally, fractures oriented toward the facial-lingual surface shear away from the pulp, although this is not likely and is difficult to determine clinically. Therefore many cracked teeth require root canal treatment, preferably before restoration for coronal protection. Wedging forces must be minimized during both root canal treatment and restoration to avoid aggravating the fracture.

ETIOLOGIES

Cracked teeth are often found in patients who chew hard, brittle substances (ice, unpopped popcorn kernels, hard candy, and so on). These patients may have prominent masticatory muscles and show excessive occlusal wear as a result of heavy occlusal forces.[23] If these teeth are restored, the restorations may be class I or a deep class II. Interestingly, cracks associated with wide class II restorations are more likely to be cusp fractures and their effects are not as devastating.[24]

Thermal stresses are also thought to be a cause of fractures, although the evidence of this is inconclusive. Supposedly, differences in expansion and contraction of restorations versus tooth structure may weaken and crack dentin.[25,26]

DIAGNOSIS

Cracked teeth show a variety of test results, radiographic findings, and signs and symptoms, depending on many factors.[7] This variety and un-

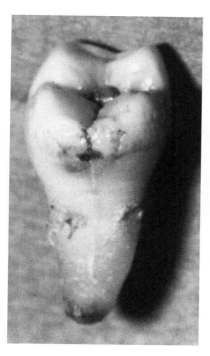

FIGURE 28-9
Centered fracture on this lightly restored second molar extends toward the apex. Treatment of these fractures is hopeless.

predictability often make the cracked tooth a perplexing diagnostic and treatment entity.

Subjective Findings

Often cracked teeth manifest as the so-called cracked tooth syndrome.[27] This syndrome is characterized by acute pain on mastication (pressure or release) of grainy, tough foods and sharp, brief pain with cold.[24] These findings are also related to cusp fracture. However, there may be a variety of symptoms ranging from slight to very severe spontaneous pain consistent with irreversible pulpitis, pulp necrosis, or apical periodontitis. Even an acute apical abscess may be present if the pulp has undergone necrosis. There may be apical pathosis related to acute apical abscess (with or without swelling) or a draining sinus tract. In other words, once the fracture has extended to and exposed the pulp, severe pulp or periradicular pathosis will be present. This explains the variation in signs and symptoms.

Objective Tests

Pulp and periradicular tests also have variable results. The pulp is usually responsive (vital) but may be nonresponsive (necrosis). Periapical tests also vary, but usually pain is not elicited with percussion or palpation if the pulp is vital. Directional percussion is also advocated. Percussion that separates the crack may cause pain. Opposite-direction percussion usually is asymptomatic. This pain is probably related to stimulation of the periodontal ligament proprioceptors.

Radiographic Findings

Because of the mesiodistal direction of the fracture, it is not visible. Radiographs are to help determine the pulp-periradicular status. Usually there are no significant findings, although occasionally different entities also occur. At times, loss of proximal (horizontal, vertical, or furcal) bone is related to the fracture; bone loss increases as the severity of the crack increases.

Other Findings

Craze lines in posterior teeth that cross marginal ridges or buccal and lingual surfaces must be differentiated with transillumination.

With craze lines, transilluminated light from the facial or lingual surface is not blocked or reflected; the entire tooth in a facial-lingual orientation is illuminated.

When a crack is suspected, it is important to try to visualize the length and location of the fracture. Occlusal and proximal restorations are first removed. Then transillumination (Figure 28-10), which often shows a characteristic abrupt blockage of transmitted light, is performed. With transillumination the portion of the tooth where the light originates illuminates to the fracture. A fracture contains a thin air space, which does not readily transmit light. Therefore the crack (or fracture) blocks or reflects the light, causing the other portion to appear dark.

Staining with methylene blue or iodine may also disclose the fracture, although not predictably. A cotton pledget soaked with methylene blue or other dye is placed against the cavity floor; the dye is held in by a sealing temporary such as IRM. The temporary restoration and pledget are removed after a few days. The dye may have contacted the crack long enough to disclose it clearly (Figure 28-11). Patients should be advised that the tooth will temporarily turn blue; they may wish to forgo this test.

If a fracture is detected, an instrument is placed in the cavity with moderate pressure exerted on opposing walls to try to separate the segments. If no movement is detected, the classification is a cracked tooth; when the segments

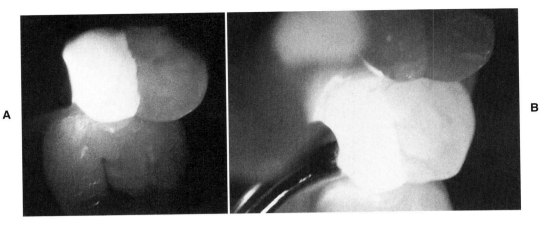

FIGURE 28-10
Cracked tooth. **A,** Fracture through dentin reflects transilluminated light showing abrupt change in brightness.
B, For comparison, an adjacent noncracked premolar transmits light readily.

separate it is a split tooth (discussed later). It is debatable whether wedging should be performed; wedging may split the tooth iatrogenically. However, if controlled force exacerbates the crack, certainly the tooth is predisposed to a later split anyway.

Occasionally (particularly if the crack is centered), an access preparation is necessary to disclose the extent (Figure 28-12) of the crack. After the chamber roof and coronal pulp have been removed, the floor is transilluminated as for a fracture (not to be confused with anatomic grooves). Sealing in a disclosing dye for a few days may be helpful.

Periodontal probing is important and may disclose the approximate depth and severity of the fracture. Removal of interproximal restorations is helpful because it allows improved access for placement of the periodontal probe. However, subgingival fractures often do not create a probing defect. Therefore the absence of deep probing does not preclude a cracked tooth. The presence of deep probing is serious and indicates an adverse prognosis.

Selective biting on objects (as described earlier under "Fractured Cusp") is helpful (see Figure 28-6), particularly when pain is reported on mastication.

TREATMENT
Prognosis

The five important considerations listed in the box on p. 501 should be reviewed. When both clinician and patient are aware of the complications and questionable outcomes, a treatment plan is formulated. Extraction is a reasonable solution in many situations. Much depends on the nature (depth and location) of the fracture. Again, the segments must not separate on wedging. If they do not separate, there are many treatment alternatives to retain the tooth intact. If the occlusal-proximal fracture is centered in the facial-lingual aspect and involves the floor of the cavity preparation, there are treatment options. If there are no symptoms of irreversible pulpitis, a crown may be placed, although some of these teeth will eventually manifest irreversible pulpitis or pulp necrosis. They will then require treatment through the crown.[28]

Further Examination

After access has been gained, the chamber floor is examined. If the fracture extends through the chamber floor, generally further treatment is hopeless and extraction is preferred (Figure 28-12).[29] An exception is the maxillary molar, which may be hemisected along the fracture, saving half (or both halves) of the crown and supporting roots. Many of these treatments are complex, and the patient should be considered for referral to an endodontist. If a partial fracture of the chamber floor is detected, the crown is bound with a well-fitting cemented orthodontic band (Figure 28-12) or temporary crown to protect the cusps until final restoration is performed.[30] This also helps to determine whether symptoms decrease during root canal treatment. The rationale (unsupported) is that if pain symptoms are not relieved, the prognosis is significantly poorer and extraction may be necessary.

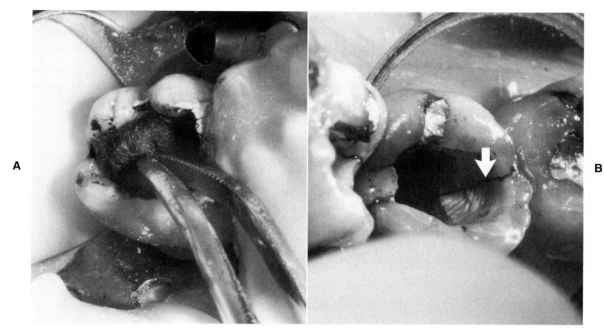

FIGURE 28-11
A, Disclosing solution on a cotton pellet (in this case, methylene blue) is placed in the cavity for a few minutes or sealed in for a week. **B,** This technique may clearly disclose the fracture *(arrow)* and its extent.

Restoration

If the fracture appears to be incomplete (not terminating on a root surface), the tooth is restored to bind the fractured segments (barrel-stave effect) and also to protect the cusps. For a permanent restoration, a full crown is preferred, although an onlay with bevels may suffice. Posts and internally wedging foundations are to be avoided. Acid-etch dentin bonding resins or bonded amalgams may help to provide a foundation for the crown to prevent crack propagation, although this approach is unproven.[31]

One suggested approach has been to remove dentin with burs until the crack disappears in an effort to eliminate or determine the extent of the crack. This is not rational; the fracture is small and invisible at the furthest extent (even after staining). Therefore the crack probably continues deeper into dentin than can be visualized. This procedure removes sound tooth structure unnecessarily, thereby further decreasing tooth strength.

PROGNOSIS

The overall prognosis depends on the situation but is always questionable at best. The patient is informed about the possible outcomes and the unpredictability of duration of treatment. The

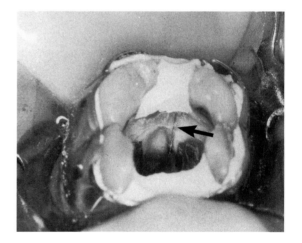

FIGURE 28-12
Managing a cracked tooth. To minimize movement of segments, an orthodontic band has been placed. The access is now completed to determine the depth of the fracture. The fracture *(arrow)* extends across the floor; the prognosis is poor.

fracture may continue to grow with eventually devastating consequences, requiring tooth extraction or additional treatments (Figure 28-13). Furthermore, the patient should be informed that cracks may be present in other teeth as well and could manifest in the future.

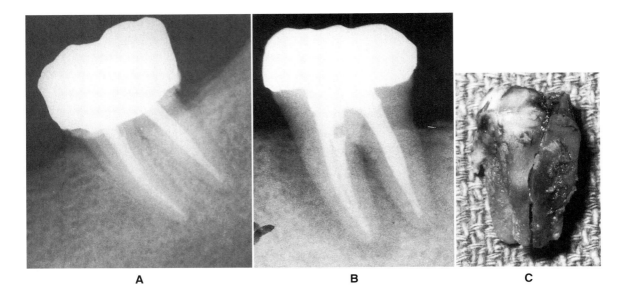

A   **B**   **C**

FIGURE 28-13
Cracked tooth resulting in eventual split tooth. **A,** A cracked tooth was identified, root canal treatment was completed, and a full crown was placed. **B,** After 3½ years the fracture became manifest with extensive bony destruction. **C,** The fracture had grown over time to become a split tooth.

In general, the more centered the origin of the fracture is on the occlusal surface, the poorer the long-term prognosis; these fractures tend to *remain* centered and grow deeper. The result is major damage to the tooth and periodontium. In other words, the cracked tooth may ultimately evolve to a split tooth or develop severe periodontal defects.

PREVENTION

Generally, patients are encouraged to forego destructive habits such as ice chewing. In addition, most suggestions made earlier for prevention of cusp fractures apply here. The use of deep class I or class II restorations should be minimized, particularly on maxillary premolars (cusp protection may be helpful).[32] Altering the occlusal anatomy or changing occlusal relationships is not useful.

Split Tooth

A split tooth is the evolution of a cracked tooth. The fracture is now complete and extends to a surface in all areas.[5] The root surface involved is probably in the middle or apical third. There are no dentin connections; tooth segments are entirely separate (Figure 28-13, C). The split may occur suddenly, but it more likely results from long-term growth of an incomplete fracture (see Table 28-1).

INCIDENCE

As with cracked tooth, the occurrence of split tooth is apparently increasing.[19] Obviously, many factors related to cracked tooth are endemic to split tooth. An assumption is that root canal treatment weakens dentin and renders teeth more susceptible to severe fractures; this is unlikely.[21,33]

PATHOGENESIS

Causative factors related to cracked tooth also apply to split tooth. Why some cracked tooth fractures continue to grow to a complete split is unknown. Two major causes are probably persistent destructive wedging or displacing forces on existing restorations and new traumatic forces that exceed the elastic limits of the remaining intact dentin.

CLINICAL FEATURES

These are primarily mesiodistal fractures that cross both marginal ridges and extend deep to shear onto the root surfaces. The more centered the fracture is occlusally, the greater the tendency to extend apically. These fractures are more devastating. Mobility (or separation) of one or both segments is present.

These fractures usually include the pulp. The more centered the fracture is, the greater the probability of exposure.

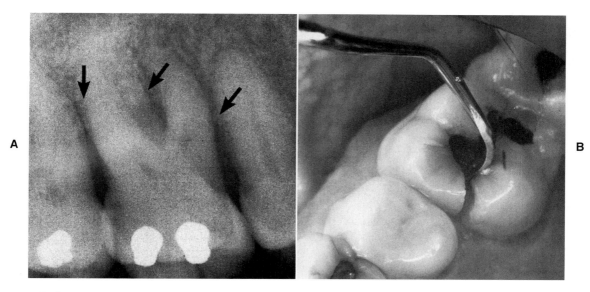

FIGURE 28-14
Split tooth. **A,** Often split teeth demonstrate marked horizontal and vertical bone loss *(arrows)* interproximally and in the furcation. **B,** This molar shows the definitive sign: separation of the segments on wedging.

ETIOLOGIES

Split tooth has the same causes as cracked tooth. Split tooth may be more common in root canal treated teeth. However, this is not because the treatment per se weakens the tooth by dehydrating or altering dentin.[33] Rather, the strength of these teeth has already been compromised by caries, restorations, or overextended access preparations.

DIAGNOSIS

Split tooth does not have the same variety of confusing signs, symptoms, and test results as cracked tooth. Generally, split teeth are easier to identify.[19] Damage to periodontium is usually significant and is detected by both patient and dentist.

Subjective Findings

Commonly, the patient reports marked pain on mastication. These teeth tend to be less painful with occlusal centric contacts than with mastication. A periodontal abscess may be present, often resulting in mistaken diagnosis.

Objective Findings

Objective findings are not particularly helpful but should include both pulp and periradicular tests.

Radiographic Findings

Findings on radiographs depend partially on pulp status but are more likely to reflect damage to the periodontium. Often there is marked horizontal loss of interproximal or interradicular bone (Figures 28-13, *B,* and 28-14, *A*).

Other Findings

The most important consideration is to identify the extent and severity of the fracture, which often requires removal of a restoration. With split tooth the fracture line is usually readily visible under or adjacent to the restoration; it includes the occlusal surface and both marginal ridges.

Separability of the segments is also important. As with cracked tooth, an instrument is placed in the cavity. Wedging against the walls is done with moderate pressure; the walls are then visualized for separation (Figure 28-14, *B*). A separating movement indicates a through-and-through fracture.

Periodontal probing generally shows deep defects; probings tend to be adjacent to the fracture. Here again, removal of existing restorations is helpful in visualizing interproximal areas.

TREATMENT

Maintaining an intact tooth is impossible. If the fracture is severe (that is, deep apically), the tooth must be extracted. If the fracture shears to a root

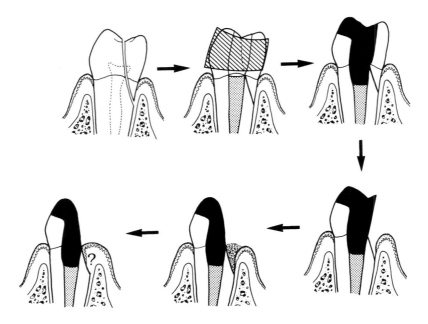

FIGURE 28-15
A technique for managing certain split teeth and cusp fractures. From *upper left* to *lower left*. Separable segment is held with a matrix or band. Root canal treatment is followed by an amalcore onlay. The fractured segment is removed and the amalgam is contoured. The tissue will heal and usually reattach; the nature of the attachment (connective or epithelial tissue) is unknown. Usually, normal sulcus depth is reestablished.

surface that is not too far apical (middle to cervical ⅓ of the root), the smaller segment will be very mobile. Then there is a good possibility that the small segment can be removed and the remainder of the tooth salvaged.

Different approaches to maintenance are used, depending on conditions. Some choices are the following.

Remove the fractured segment. Then the type of treatment and restoration are determined. However, the following choice (retention of fractured segment temporarily) is preferred and is generally less complicated.

Retain the fractured segment temporarily (Figure 28-15). First, a rubber dam is applied with a strong rubber dam clamp to isolate and hold the segments together. Root canal treatment is completed (if not already performed), and restoration with a retentive amalcore (onlaying the undermined cusps) is performed. Then the fractured segment is removed. Granulation tissue proliferates to occupy the space and reattach the periodontium to the root dentin surface. The final restoration usually is the amalcore but may be a full crown with a margin related to the new attachment.

Remove the fractured segment and perform crown lengthening. The mobile segment is removed first,

and root canal treatment is performed next followed by crown lengthening and appropriate restoration. This is not feasible in most situations because the fracture is too deep on the root surface.

Remove the fractured segment and perform no further treatment. This choice is appropriate when root canal treatment has been completed previously and the tooth already restored. All pulp space areas *must* be filled to the margins with permanent restorative material (for example, amalgam) with no obturating material (e.g., gutta-percha) exposed (Figure 28-16). The defect often granulates in, and reattachment to the fractured dentin surface occurs.

In summary, treatment may be complex or relatively simple depending on the situation. Because of the complexity of their situations, these patients should be considered for referral to a specialist for diagnosis or treatment.

PROGNOSIS

As expected, prognosis is variable. Some treatments of split tooth are successful, whereas others are doomed to failure if attempted. When the fracture surfaces in the middle to cervical third of the root, there is a reasonable chance of successful

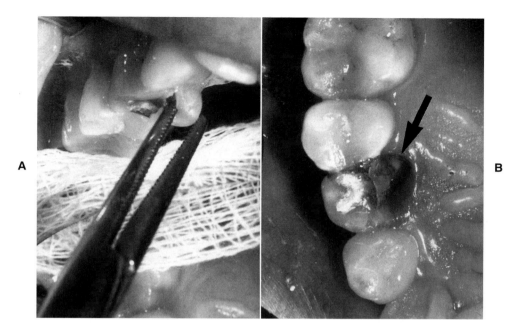

FIGURE 28-16
A technique for managing fractures. Root canal treatment and amalcore onlay had been done earlier; the fracture occurred after treatment. **A,** The mobile segment is removed. **B,** A space is created with raw root dentin exposed *(arrow).* Tissue usually granulates in and is reattached to the dentin (but not to the amalgam). No further treatment is needed.

treatment and restoration. If the fracture surfaces in the middle to apical third, the prognosis is poor. With these deep fractures, usually too much of the pulp space is exposed to the periodontium; root canal treatment with restoration of this space would result in deep periodontal defects.

Sometimes prediction of success or failure cannot be determined before treatment is completed if the more conservative approach is taken, that is, if the segment is temporarily held in place during root canal treatment and restoration. After root canal treatment has been completed and the segment has been removed, the dentist may discover that, unfortunately, the fracture is indeed very deep and the tooth is unsalvageable. The patient must be informed of all these possibilities before treatment is begun.

PREVENTION

Generally, preventive measures are similar to those recommended for cracked tooth, that is, eliminating oral habits that damage tooth structure and impose wedging forces. Teeth requiring large, deep access preparations should be protected by an onlay or full crown. Large access preparations also require appropriate cusp protection.[12]

Vertical Root Fracture

Vertical root fracture (VRF) differs from the entities (see Table 28-1) described previously in this chapter because the treatment plan is easy, but diagnosis often is tricky and elusive because the VRF mimics other conditions.[34,35] Because treatment invariably consists of tooth extraction or removal of the fractured root, an error in diagnosis has serious consequences.

INCIDENCE

The overall occurrence is unknown, but VRF is common.[36] These defects occur more often in teeth that have undergone complex restorative procedures, that is, root canal treatment and intraradicular post retention.

PATHOGENESIS

This fracture results from wedging forces within the canal. These excessive forces exceed the binding strength of existing dentin, causing fatigue and fracture. Irritants that induce severe inflammation in the adjacent periodontium result from the fracture.[37] Generally, this periodontal destruction and the accompanying findings, signs,

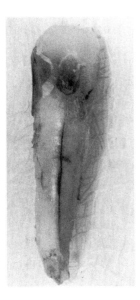

FIGURE 28-17
Vertical root fracture extends facially and lingually and, in this case, in an apical to cervical direction.

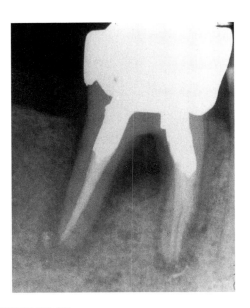

FIGURE 28-18
Vertical root fracture of the distal root. A common radiographic pattern of bone resorption is seen. The defect extends along the fractured root and into the furcation.

and symptoms bring the fracture to the attention of the patient or dentist.

CLINICAL FEATURES

These fractures occur primarily in the facial-lingual plane (see Figure 28-2). They are longitudinal and may either be short or extend the length of the root, that is, from apical to cervical (Figure 28-17). The fracture probably begins internally (canal wall) and grows outward to the root surface. In addition, the fracture may begin at the apex or at midroot.[38] Therefore it may be incomplete (see Figure 28-2), extending neither to both facial and lingual root surfaces nor from apical to cervical root surfaces.

Although VRFs usually show only mild clinical signs and symptoms, the effects on the periodontium are eventually devastating and irresolvable.

ETIOLOGIES

There are two major causes (the only demonstrated ones) of VRFs. These are (1) post placement (cementation) and (2) condensation during obturation.[39] The only reported cases of VRF occurring in nonendodontically treated teeth are in Chinese patients.[40,41] Other causes, such as occlusal forces, wedging of restorations, corrosion and expansion of metallic posts, and expansion of postsurgical retrograde restorations, have been mentioned but not convincingly shown.[42]

Condensation, both lateral and vertical, may cause excessive wedging forces, creating a VRF.[43,44] Intraradicular retentive posts have also been implicated.[34,39,45] Two aspects of posts cause wedging forces. Wedging occurs during cementation of posts and also during the seating of tapered posts or with posts that depend on frictional retention.[39,46] Occlusal forces exerted on the post after cementation and restoration may also be a factor but probably a minor one. Post placement has been shown to exert a greater wedging force than lateral condensation.[46]

Certain root shapes and sizes are more susceptible to VRF. Roots that are deep facially and lingually but narrow mesially and distally are particularly prone to fracture.[38] Examples are mandibular incisors and premolars, maxillary second premolars, mesiobuccal roots of maxillary molars, and mesial and distal roots of mandibular molars. Round, oval, or bulky roots are resistant to fracture; examples are maxillary central incisors, lingual roots of maxillary molars, and maxillary canines.

Susceptibility of any root to fracture is markedly increased by excessive dentin removal during canal instrumentation or post preparation.[47,48] An additional factor occurring during condensation is the placement of excessive numbers of accessory cones requiring multiple spreader insertions.[38,49] Also, the insertion of tapered, inflexible condensing instruments into curved canals creates root distortion and the potential for fracture.[50]

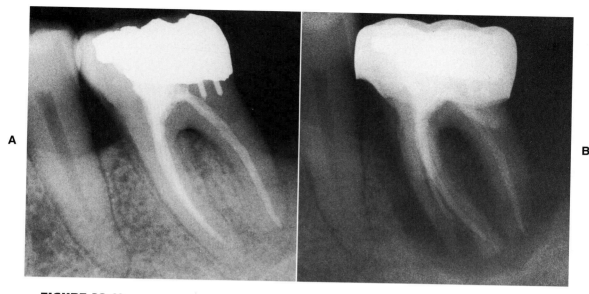

FIGURE 28-19
Vertical root fracture. **A,** At the time of root canal treatment and restoration. **B,** Several years later the fracture manifests devastating results. Visualizing the fracture on a radiograph is unusual.

DIAGNOSIS

Vertical root fractures become manifest by a variety of signs, symptoms, and other clinical findings. They may mimic other entities such as periodontal disease or failed root canal treatment. This variety of findings often makes VRF a perplexing diagnosis.[51,52] Interestingly, because VRFs are often mistaken for periodontal lesions or for failed root canal treatment, the dentist may refer these difficult diagnosis patients to the periodontist or endodontist, presumably for periodontal therapy or endodontic retreatment.

Diagnostic findings of VRF were reported in a series of 42 clinical cases in a study performed by Michelich et al.[35] Much of the information that follows is derived from the findings in that study in conjunction with other reports.

Subjective Findings

Symptoms tend to be minimal. Seldom is the VRF painful, and it is often asymptomatic or shows mild, insignificant signs and symptoms. Often, some mobility is detectable, but many teeth are stable. Periradicular symptoms (pain on pressure or mastication) are common but mild.

Because many VRFs resemble periodontal lesions, a periodontal-type abscess (either as a presenting sign or in the history) is a common occurrence.[37,45] In fact, this localized swelling is often what brings the patient to the dentist's office.

Objective Tests

Periradicular tests of palpation and percussion are not particularly helpful. Periodontal probing patterns are more diagnostic. Significantly, some teeth with VRFs have normal probing patterns.[35] Most show significant probing depths with narrow or rectangular patterns, which are more typical of endodontic-type lesions.[45,53] These deep probing depths are not necessarily evident on both the facial and lingual aspects. Overall, probing patterns are not in themselves totally diagnostic, but they are helpful.

Radiographic Findings

Radiographs also show a variety of patterns. At times there are no significant changes.[35] However, when present, bone resorptive patterns tend to be marked, extending from the apex along the lateral surface of the root and often include angular resorption at the cervical root (Figure 28-18).[54] However, many of the resorptive patterns related to VRF mimic other entities. Lesions may resemble failed root canal treatment; that is, they have an apical "hanging drop" appearance. In only a small percentage of teeth is there a visible separation of fractured root segments (Figure 28-19). Interestingly, VRFs may be more readily identified using computed tomography rather than conventional radiography.[55]

The idea that a radiolucent line separating the filling (i.e., gutta-percha) from the canal wall is diagnostic has been advocated. However, this radiolucent line may be a radiographic artifact, incomplete obturation, an overlying bony pattern, or other radiographic structure that is confused with a fracture. Therefore radiographs are helpful but are not solely diagnostic except in those few instances in which the fracture is obvious.

Dental History

Virtually all teeth with a VRF have had root canal treatment[9]; many have been restored with cast or prefabricated posts. Potentially greater destructive forces exist with tapered, wedging posts.[56,57]

Interestingly, endodontic and restorative treatment may have been done months or years before the fracture. Forces (without fracture) are established at the time of treatment or restoration.[41,45,46] These forces are stored in root dentin but may not result in an actual fracture until later; neither patient nor dentist may relate the fracture to earlier procedures.

Other Findings

Signs, symptoms, and radiographs all give variable findings. *Flap reflection* is the only reliable diagnostic approach. Surgical exposure of bone overlying the root surface is the best method of identification.[34,35] VRFs have consistent patterns (Figure 28-20). There is usually a "punched-out" bony defect that tends to be oblong and overlies the root surface. This defect may take the form of a dehiscence or fenestration at various root levels. The defect is filled with granulomatous tissue.

After inflammatory tissue has been removed, the fracture is usually (but not always) visible on the root (Figure 28-21). If it is not obvious, the fracture line may be hidden or very small and undeveloped. However, the characteristic punched-out, granulomatous tissue filled defect is fairly diagnostic of VRF, which should be strongly suspected.[35] Transillumination or staining with dyes are helpful. Also, the root-end could be resected and examined under magnification to detect the fracture.

PATTERNS OF BONE RESORPTION

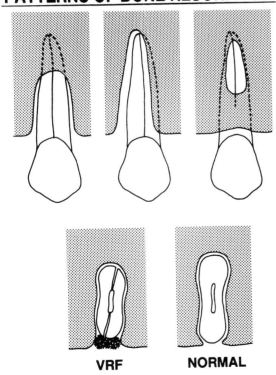

VRF   **NORMAL**

FIGURE 28-20
Vertical root fracture. After flap reflection and visualization, the pattern of bony changes tends to be consistent with oval or oblong "punched-out" defects filled with granulomatous tissue (VRF). This is differentiated from the normal bony fenestration.

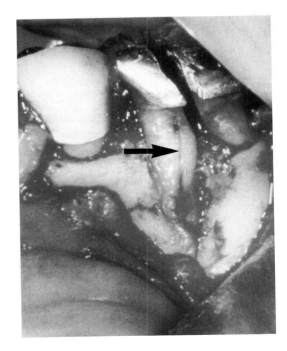

FIGURE 28-21
Vertical root fracture is usually but not always identified *(arrow)* after flap reflection. Usually (as in this case), the bone has been resorbed, showing a long defect. This molar has been hemisected; the fractured mesial segment will now be removed.

Fracture Characteristics

Histologic fracture characteristics have been described with VRF after removal.[37] All fractures extended from the canal to at least one root surface but not necessarily to both (Figure 28-22). Similarly, fractures often extended only the partial length of the root, usually to the apex but not always to the cervix.

Many irritants occupy the fracture space and adjacent canal.[37] Fractures usually harbor bacteria, sealer particles, and amorphous material. Canals adjacent to the fracture often contain necrotic tissue as well as concentrations of bacteria. Periodontal tissues adjacent to the fracture are chronically inflamed. Occasionally, connective tissue grows into the fracture toward the canal; this is often associated with resorption at the root surface (Figure 28-23).

Thus profound irritants related to the fracture with resulting inflammation at the surface were identified in the study.[37] VRFs resemble a very long apical foramen that communicates with necrotic pulp containing bacteria—thus the hopeless prognosis.

TREATMENT

As stated earlier, the only treatment is removal of the fractured root. In multirooted teeth, this could be done by root amputation or hemisection (see Figure 28-21).

Other modalities have been suggested in attempts to reduce the fracture or retain the root, such as placement of calcium hydroxide, ligation of the fractured segments, or cementation of the fractured segments, trying to bind them by adhesive resins, epoxies, or glass ionomer.[58] A unique approach is to extract the tooth, repair the fracture with a laser or with a cement, and then replant the tooth. Many of these suggested methods are impractical and have not been shown to be effective long-term. Surgical repairs such as removal of one of the fractured segments or repair with amalgam or resin after surgical exposure and

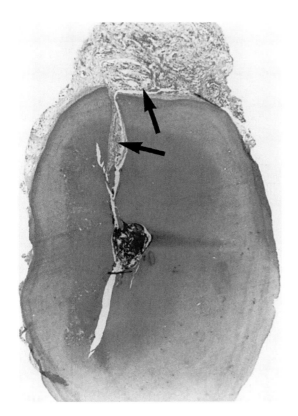

FIGURE 28-22
Vertical root fracture. This histologic cross section shows a fracture extending to only one surface and to the canal. The fracture space and root surface show inflammatory tissue *(arrows)*.

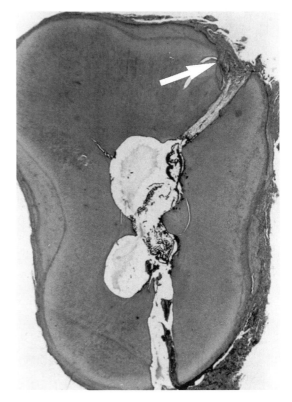

FIGURE 28-23
Vertical root fracture extends to both surfaces (facial and lingual). The facial surface shows resorption *(arrows)* and ingrowth of connective tissue. The lingual component contains necrotic debris and bacteria.

preparation have also been suggested, but no successful results have been documented.

PROGNOSIS

At present, prognosis is virtually hopeless for tooth with a vertically fractured root.

PREVENTION

Because the causes of VRF are well known, prevention should not be difficult. The cardinal rules for safety are to (1) *avoid excessive removal of intraradicular dentin* and (2) *minimize internal wedging forces.* The binding strength of root dentin is considerable but it is easily compromised. Treatment and restorative procedures that require minimal dentin preparation should be selected. Condensation of obturating materials should be carefully controlled. More flexible and less tapered finger pluggers or spreaders are preferred because they are safer than stiff, conventional hand-type spreaders.[49,50]

Posts weaken roots and should not be used unless they are necessary to retain a foundation (see Chapter 15). The post design least likely to cause stress and fracture dentin is the flexible (including carbon-fiber carbon) or cylindrical (parallel-sided) preformed post,[39,56] although these designs are not suitable in all restorative situations. Cast posts or some of the tapered preformed posts may be necessary. Their shape may exert wedging forces that readily split roots or cause dentin strain, particularly if they lack a stop or ferrule on the root seat.[59,60] Any post used should be as small as possible, have a passive fit, and not lock or grip the root internally with threads.[39] Cementation should be done carefully and slowly; an escape vent for the cement is probably helpful.

REFERENCES

1. American Association of Endodontists: Cracking the cracked tooth code, *Endodontics: Colleagues for Excellence,* Nov 1997.
2. Renson CE, Braden M: The experimental determination of the rigidity modulus, Poisson's ratio and the elastic limit in shear of human dentin, *Arch Oral Biol* 20:43, 1975.
3. Carter J, Sorenson S, Johnson R, et al: Punch shear testing of extracted vital and endodontically treated teeth, *J Biomech* 16:841, 1983.
4. Eakle W, Maxwell E, Braley B: Fractures of posterior teeth in adults, *J Am Dent Assoc* 112:215, 1986.
5. Ehrmann E, Tyas M: Cracked tooth syndrome: diagnosis, treatment and correlation between symptoms and post-extraction findings, *Aust Dent J* 35:105, 1990.
6. Hiatt W: Incomplete crown-root fracture in pulpal-periodontal disease, *J Periodontol* 44:369, 1973.
7. Rosen H: Cracked tooth syndrome, *J Prosthet Dent* 47:36, 1982.
8. Abou-Rass M: Crack lines: precursors of tooth fractures—their diagnosis and treatment, *Quintessence Int* 4:437, 1983.
9. Gehr M, Denlap R, Anderson M, Kuhl L: Clinical survey of fractured teeth, *J Am Dent Assoc* 114:174, 1987.
10. Schweitzer J, Gutmann J, Bliss R: Odonto-iatrogenic tooth fracture, *Int Endod J* 22:64, 1989.
11. Silvestri A, Singh I: Treatment rationale of fractured posterior teeth, *J Am Dent Assoc* 97:806, 1978.
12. Reeh E, Messer H, Douglas W: Reduction in tooth stiffness as a result of endodontic and restorative procedures, *J Endod* 15:512, 1989.
13. Cavel W, Kelsey W, Blankenau R: An in vivo study of cuspal fracture, *J Prosthet Dent* 53:38, 1985.
14. Re G, Norling B, Draheim R: Fracture resistance of lower molars with varying facio-occlusolingual amalgam restorations, *J Prosthet Dent* 47:518, 1982.
15. Salis S, Hood J, Kirk E: Impact-fracture energy of human premolar teeth, *J Prosthet Dent* 58:43, 1987.
16. Trope M, Langer I, Maltz D, Tronstad L: Resistance to fracture of restored endodontically treated premolars, *Endod Dent Traumatol* 2:35, 1986.
17. Reeh E, Douglas W, Messer H: Stiffness of endodontically-treated teeth related to restoration technique, *J Dent Res* 68:1540, 1989.
18. Trope M, Tronstad L: Resistance to fracture of endodontically treated premolars restored with glass ionomer or acid-etched composite resins, *J Endod* 17:257, 1991.
19. Burke F: Tooth fracture in vivo and in vitro, *J Dent* 20:131, 1992.
20. Howe C, McKendry D: Effect of endodontic access preparation on resistance to crown-root fracture, *J Am Dent Assoc* 121:712, 1990.
21. Rivera E, Yamauchi M: Site comparisons of dentine collagen cross-links from extracted human teeth, *Arch Oral Biol* 38:541,1993.
22. Huang T-J, Schilder H, Nathanson D: Effect of moisture content and endodontic treatment on some mechanical properties of human dentin, *J Endod* 18:209, 1992.
23. Cameron C: The cracked tooth syndrome: additional findings, *J Am Dent Assoc* 93:971, 1976.
24. Homewood C: Cracked tooth syndrome—incidence, clinical findings, and treatment, *Aust Dent J* 43:217, 1998.
25. Brown W, Jacobs H, Thompson R: Thermal fatigue in teeth, *J Dent Res* 51:461, 1972.
26. Harper R, et al: In vivo measurement of thermal diffusion through restorative material, *J Prosthet Dent* 42:180, 1980.
27. Christensen G: The cracked tooth syndrome: a pragmatic treatment approach, *J Am Dent Assoc* 124:107, 1993.
28. Krell K, Rivera E: Six-year evaluation of cracked teeth diagnosed with reversible pulpitis, *J Endod* 26:540, 2000 (abstract).

29. Turp J, Gobetti J: The cracked tooth syndrome: an elusive diagnosis, *J Am Dent Assoc* 127:1502, 1996.
30. Ailor J: Managing incomplete tooth fractures, *J Am Dent Assoc* 131:1168, 2000.
31. Franchi M, Breschi L, Ruggeri O: Cusp fracture resistance in composite-amalgam combined restorations, *J Dent* 27:47, 1999.
32. Blaser P, Lund M, Cochran M, et al: Effects of designs of class II preparations on resistance of teeth to fracture, *Oper Dent* 8:11, 1983.
33. Sedgley C, Messer H: Are endodontically treated teeth more brittle? *J Endod* 18:332, 1992.
34. Pitts D, Natkin E: Diagnosis and treatment of vertical root fractures, *J Endod* 9:338, 1983.
35. Michelich R, Smith G, Walton R: Vertical root fracture: clinical features (unpublished).
36. Fuss A, Lustig J, Tamse A: Prevalence of vertical root fractures in extracted endodontically treated teeth, *Int Endod J* 32:283, 1999.
37. Walton R, Michelich R, Smith G: The histopathogenesis of vertical root fractures, *J Endod* 10:48, 1984.
38. Holcomb Q, Pitts D, Nicholls J: Further investigation of spreader loads required to cause vertical root fracture during lateral condensation, *J Endod* 13:277, 1987.
39. Ross R, Nicholls J, Harrington G: A comparison of strains generated during placement of five endodontic posts, *J Endod* 17:9, 1991.
40. Yang S, Rivera E, Walton R: Vertical root fractures in non-endodontically treated teeth, *J Endod* 21:337, 1995.
41. Chan C, Lin C, Tseng S, et al: Vertical root fracture in endodontically versus nonendodontically treated teeth: a survey of 315 cases in Chinese patients, *Oral Surg Oral Med Oral Pathol Oral Radiol Endod* 87:504, 1999.
42. Rud J, Onmell D: Root fractures due to corrosion: diagnostic aspects, *Scand J Dent Res* 78:397, 1970.
43. Ricks-Williamson L, Fotos P, Goel V, et al: A three-dimensional finite-element stress analysis of an endodontically prepared maxillary central incisor, *J Endod* 21:362, 1995.
44. Harvey T, White J, Leeb I: Lateral condensation stress in root canals, *J Endod* 7:151, 1981.
45. Meister F, Lommel T, Gerstein H: Diagnosis and possible causes of vertical root fractures, *Oral Surg Oral Med Oral Pathol* 49:243, 1980.
46. Obermayr G, Walton R, Leary M, Krell K: Vertical root fracture and relative deformation during obturation and post-cementation, *J Prosthet Dent* 66:181, 1991.
47. Sornkul E, Stannas J: Strength of roots before and after endodontic treatment and restoration, *J Endod* 18:440, 1992.
48. Trope M, Ray H: Resistance to fracture of endodontically treated roots, *Oral Surg Oral Med Oral Pathol* 73:99, 1992.
49. Dang D, Walton R: Vertical root fracture and root distortion: effect of spreader design, *J Endod* 15:294, 1989.
50. Murgel C, Walton R: Vertical root fracture and dentin deformation in curved roots: the influence of spreader design, *Endod Traumatol* 6:273, 1990.
51. Moule A, Kahler B: Diagnosis and management of teeth with vertical root fractures, *Aust Dent J* 44:75, 1999.
52. Tamse A, Fuss, Z, Lustig J, Kaplavi J: An evaluation of endodontically treated vertically fractured teeth, *J Endod* 7:506, 1999.
53. Harrington G: The perio-endo question: differential diagnosis, *Dent Clin North Am* 23:673, 1979.
54. Tamse A, Fuss Z, Lustig J, et al: Radiographic features of vertically fractured, endodontically treated maxillary premolars, *Oral Surg Oral Med Oral Pathol Oral Radiol Endod* 88:348, 1999.
55. Youssefzadeh S, Gahleitner A, Dorffner R, et al: Dental vertical root fractures: value of CT in detection, *Radiology* 210:545, 1999.
56. Standlee J, Caputo A, Collard E, Pollack M: Analysis of stress distribution by endodontic posts, *Oral Surg Oral Med Oral Pathol* 33:952, 1972.
57. Johnson J, Schwartz H, Blackwell R: Evaluation and restoration of endodontically treated posterior teeth, *J Am Dent Assoc* 93:597, 1976.
58. Trope M, Rosenberg E: Multidisciplinary approach to repair of vertically fractured teeth, *J Endod* 18:460, 1992.
59. Sorenson J, Englemen M: Ferrule design and fracture resistance of endodontically treated teeth, *J Prosthet Dent* 63:529, 1990.
60. Milot P, Stein R: Root fracture in endodontically treated teeth related to post selection and crown design, *J Prosthet Dent* 68:428, 1992.

Differential Diagnosis of Orofacial Pain

LEARNING OBJECTIVES

After reading this chapter, the student should be able to:

1 / Describe the basic components of pain mechanisms while recognizing that current knowledge is incomplete.

2 / Explain why an understanding of physiology, psychology, and pathology of pain is important to dental practice.

3 / Explain the mechanisms of referred and spreading pain and how these may lead to misdiagnosis.

4 / Describe the difference between acute and chronic pain.

5 / Recognize the bases for migraine, neuritis, and neuralgia and explain how these syndromes may mimic tooth pain.

6 / Understand that pain may be largely or entirely of psychogenic origin.

7 / Differentiate between deep and superficial pain, and relate this to the difference between pain of pulpal or periradicular origin and that of periodontal origin.

8 / List the main characteristics of pulpal, periradicular, periodontal, and mucosal pain.

9 / Describe how history and diagnostic tests help clarify difficult diagnoses.

10 / Describe procedures to be followed when a definitive diagnosis and localization of pain are not possible.

OUTLINE

Significance of Pain Diagnosis

Pain Mechanisms
Specificity
Gating

Pain as an Experience

The Versatility of Pain

Superficial Versus Deep Pain
Periodontal Pain
Pulpal Pain

Phenomena Complicating the Diagnosis of Dental Pain
Referred Pain
Spreading Pain
Psychogenic pain
Headaches
Neuritis
Trigeminal Neuralgia
Atypical Oral and Facial Pain

Diagnostic Procedures
Recognition of Difficult Diagnoses
Approach to Difficult Diagnoses
Important Clues

Significance of Pain Diagnosis

Many dental patients are in pain when they are seen. The most common cause of pain in the orofacial region is inflammatory disease of either the pulp or the tooth's supporting structures. Effective treatment is based on careful, accurate diagnosis. However, diagnosis and identification of the source of pain are not simple. Pain originating from the teeth may be referred to or spread to other structures; conversely, pain from nondental sites can be referred to teeth. Because rational treatment involves removal of the cause or causes of pain rather than merely addressing the symptoms, it is imperative to establish first whether pain is of dental origin. When pain is dental, determination of which tooth or teeth are involved is the most important consideration. Difficulties in the localization of pain may result in extraction or endodontic treatment of the wrong tooth. The pain may originate from other sources such as the muscles of mastication or mucosa of the nose and sinuses; again, neither tooth extraction or root canal therapy will resolve the symptoms. Unfortunately, such inappropriate treatments in attempts to relieve pain are all too common. Not only are such misadventures ineffective in resolving pain, they may also lead to litigation.

Thus before a practitioner treats a patient in pain, a correct diagnosis is essential. When diagnosis is difficult, two measures are recommended. One is to provide symptomatic relief and to observe the patient. When pain intensifies, identification is easier; an example is when pulpal inflammation invades the periradicular tissues. The second option is to seek an expert opinion. Pain is a versatile phenomenon; many forms of chronic pain and myofascial pain elude simple diagnosis and may be beyond the expertise of a general dentist. For example, temporomandibular joint and muscle disorders are often found in conjunction with other, more generalized conditions such as fibromyalgia. Complete diagnosis of orofacial pain may necessitate input from specialists from several disciplines.

This chapter does not provide a complete or comprehensive discussion of the complexities of diagnosis of orofacial pain. This warrants an entire text.[1,2] It does provide a guide to (1) determining whether a pain is of dental origin and (2) locating the site and nature of the origin of the pain (Box 29-1). Importantly, although most dental pain results from inflammatory changes, such inflammation of pulp and periradicular tissues is often not painful. In fact, pain severe enough for the patient to seek dental treatment may occur only a small proportion of the time.

BOX 29-1

Definitions

Acute pain: The unpleasant experience arising from the excitation of pain pathways by stimuli that cause or threaten tissue damage. Acute pain is of great survival value.

Allodynia: Lowering of the pain threshold such that stimuli that were previously innocuous now evoke pain.

Anesthesia: Absence of all sensation.

Atypical orofacial pain: A poorly defined category that includes a variety of syndromes such as phantom tooth pain, atypical odontalgia, atypical facial neuralgia, and burning mouth.

Chronic pain: This arises in the absence of overt stimuli and tissue damage, is an experience of no value, and may be regarded as a disease of the pain warning system.

Convergence: Many primary afferent axons end on the same second-order neuron (*convergence*). If the sensory terminals of these axons are active and are close together in terms of time or position, they then interact.

Deep pain: Dull, depressing, poorly localized pain arising from nerve fibers supplying blood vessels, gut, and other deep structures. It often induces nausea.

Dysesthesia, Paresthesia: Disturbed unpleasant sensation of variable presentation; often described as a combination of tingling, burning, and numbness accompanied by a lowered pain threshold. It may be spontaneous or evoked.

Hyperalgesia: An exaggerated response to a stimulus that is normally less painful.

Hyperesthesia: Increased sensitivity to all stimuli.

Hypoalgesia: A reduced response to a stimulus that is normally painful.

Neuralgia: Chronic pain syndromes characterized by severe, unremitting, or paroxysmal pain. Although in many conditions (e.g., trigeminal neuralgia) the cause is unclear, neuralgia is often associated with peripheral nerve damage (e.g., postherpetic neuralgia).

Neuritis: Inflammation of a nerve that, if it involves pain-conducting fibers, results in pain. The pain will be experienced in the anatomic distribution of the affected nerve.

Neuroplasticity: The ability of the central nervous system to modify the processing of afferent information.

Nociceptors: Receptors that respond at high threshold to stimuli normally interpreted as painful. Several types have been identified responding to mechanical, thermal, or chemical stimuli. A noxious stimulus is of sufficient intensity (mechanical or thermal) or specificity (chemical) to initiate activity in nociceptors.

Noxious stimulus: A stimulus capable of causing tissue injury.

Pain system: Components of the nervous system involved in the input and processing of noxious information.

Pathologic pain: Pain produced by a disease process rather than by laboratory stimulation.

Psychologic pain: A pain syndrome in which the psychologic factors predominate; there may be little or no evidence of noxious stimulation of peripheral nerves.

Referred pain: Pain experienced from a site other than the site of the stimulus or tissue damage. Afferent fibers from several sites (possibly some distance from each other) converge on second-order neurons; then central cognitive processes mistake the true site.

Spreading pain: Inflammatory mediators spread from a site of tissue damage into adjacent tissues, inducing hyperalgesia and painful muscle spasms.

Superficial pain: A bright, sharp, well-localized pain produced by noxious stimulation of receptors on the body surface.

Temporomandibular myofascial pain dysfunction syndrome: Pain related to the jaw musculature and joint that may arise from the joint itself, from bone, from soft connective tissue, or, most commonly, from muscle.

Vascular pain: Deep pains thought to arise from noxious stimulation of sensory fibers supplying blood vessels.

Many inflammatory pulpal or periradicular lesions are detected by chance in a patient with no history of previous pain.

Pain Mechanisms

Differential diagnosis must be based on an understanding of pain mechanisms. This is still an area of discovery; a comprehensive account is not currently possible. Only a very brief summary of contemporary knowledge is possible here. More details may be sought elsewhere.[3-7]

Many hypotheses have been developed in attempts to explain the mechanics of pain. The most distinct and distinguished of these are the "specificity theory" and the "gate control theory." Although originally developed as alternatives, the key elements of "specificity"[3,5] and "gating"[3,6,8] are compatible.

SPECIFICITY

A longstanding belief is that a specific part of the nervous system is responsible for carrying pain from pain receptors to a pain center in the central nervous system. There are, in fact, some nerve fibers that respond only (or maximally) to stimuli in the noxious range. However, the existence of such a dedicated "pain system" is not sufficient, in itself, to explain all experimental and clinical features of pain. Referred pain (in which the sensation

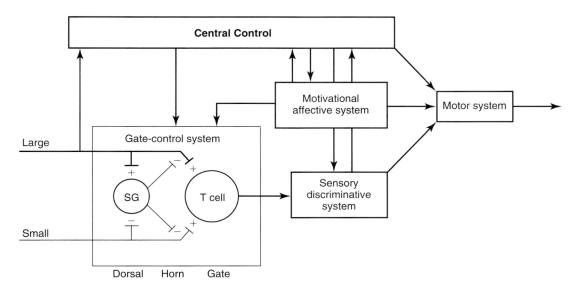

FIGURE 29-1
Gating in the central nervous system. Large and small afferent fibers interact through a gating mechanism in the dorsal horn of the spinal cord and trigeminal nucleus (dorsal horn gate). Branches of the afferent fibers act on specialized interneurons, the spinal gating cells *(SG)*, which, by presynaptic inhibition, control input to the transmission cells *(T cell)*. These cells are the second-order sensory neurons responsible for passing on sensory input to higher nerve centers where motivational/affective factors and the sensory discriminative components interact, which may result in perception of a pain experience and lead to motor activity. The dorsal horn gate is also influenced by descending central control. (Adapted from Melzack R, Wall PD: *Science* 150:971-979, 1965.)

is incorrectly localized) and pathologic pain (such as trigeminal neuralgia, which is initiated by mild nonnoxious stimuli) as well as the clearly documented effects of emotional and motivational factors require an explanation. The best explanation includes mechanisms such as summation and inhibition acting on a "gate' which controls the progress of potentially painful input.[3,8]

GATING

All incoming afferent activity from the peripheral nervous system is subject to modulating effects upon entering the central nervous system (Figure 29-1). The central nervous system actually filters and integrates a vast amount of sensory information, only a very small proportion of which will reach the level of consciousness. Much of the information is discarded and much is used in unnoticed autonomic reflex activities. Incoming noxious information is a part of this overall pattern. The integrating process has been described as analogous to a gate. When the gate is open, incoming sensory activity passes through and goes on to the next level.

The anatomic substrate of the gating mechanism for pain is in the dorsal horn of the gray matter of the spinal cord and brainstem. The gate either *inhibits* or *facilitates* the activity of transmission cells that carry activity further along the nervous pathway. A number of factors determine whether the gate is open or not. One important factor is the relative degree of activity in large diameter $A\beta$ fibers and small diameter $A\delta$ and C fibers. The large diameter $A\beta$ fibers are activated by nonnoxious stimuli, and the small $A\delta$ and C fibers by noxious stimuli. Large fiber activity tends to *close* the gate, whereas small fiber activity *opens* the gate. Descending control mechanisms from higher levels in the central nervous system are influenced by cognitive, motivational, and affective processes. These higher level mechanisms also modulate the gate. Activity in large afferent fibers not only tends to close the gate directly but also activates the central control mechanisms, which may also close the gate.

When the gate is open and activity in the incoming afferents is sufficient to activate the transmission system, two main ascending pathways are activated. One is the sensory-discriminative pathway, which connects to the somatosensory cortex by way of the ventroposterior thalamus. This pathway allows the localization of pain. The second ascending pathway involves the reticular information through the medial thalamic and limbic system, which deals with the unpleasant, aversive, and emotional aspects of pain. Descending pathways, as well as acting on the dorsal horn gate, may also interact with these two ascending systems. One of the principal descending pathways uses endogenously secreted opioid-like peptides (e.g., endorphin) to suppress or reduce transmission in pain pathways.

Pain as an Experience

This overall description of the processing of noxious information integrates the presence of receptors and pathways specialized to conduct pain. It also explains how this noxious information may be suppressed, amplified, or altered by other afferent input as well as by the influence of higher centers. Hence pain is not a simple sensation such as touch, heat, or taste but an "experience," resulting from extensive integration.[3]

This outline explains the versatility of pain. Why, for example, do similar tissue injuries produce different degrees of pain either in different individuals or in the same individual on different occasions? This difference occurs because of variations in the magnitude and effect of other inputs and higher nerve centers. The involvement of higher centers can also explain why the pain experience can vary with age[9,10], gender,[10] and cultural background.[11-13] The flexible pain "system" also allows recognition of the difference between acute and chronic pain. Acute pain provides a warning of actual or impending tissue damage and is essential to survival. Significantly, subjects who show congenital insensitivity to pain have a short life expectancy. Chronic pain such as trigeminal neuralgia has no survival value but is interpreted as a disease of the pain system.

The Versatility of Pain

Many elements contribute to the experience of pain. Therefore the presentation of pain may be highly variable and the identification of the source and cause may be difficult.

Some pain characteristics arising from and around the teeth (for example, the hyperalgesia that occurs with inflammation) may be explained by the sensitization of nociceptors. Many inflammatory mediators, neuropeptides, growth factors, and other cytokines are involved in tissue injury and the body's response. This array of factors gives wide variability in the response to tissue injury. Many of the peptides present in the dental pulp[14] (e.g., substance P, calcitonin gene-related peptide, neuropeptide Y) primarily regulate blood flow.[15] Many peptides are released from sensory terminals by axon reflexes in neurogenic inflammation. The principal role of the afferent innervation of the dental pulp may not be sensory but vasomotor and possibly trophic.

Other mechanisms such as referred and psychogenic pain require the inclusion of central interactions. In general, the differential diagnosis of dental pain requires *identifying* pain from other sources (real or imagined), such as psychogenic and chronic pain, as well as from other sites, such as pain from the muscles of mastication.

Social, cultural, and sex- and age-related factors all affect the pain experience through the emotional-motivational component. For example, the pain threshold is similar in different racial groups but pain perception may differ between different groups.[9,11] Social and cultural factors determine the symptoms that patients emphasize.[12]

The characteristics of pain can change with time because of the adaptation of peripheral receptors, facilitation or fatigue among central connections, or a number of other causes. The central nervous system exhibits considerable plasticity. Persisting noxious input, particularly from C fibers, can produce changes in the dorsal horn neurons, especially in the presence and distribution of membrane receptors.[16] The changes in these altered neurons can persist long after the original stimulus, a phenomenon known as central sensitization or "wind-up."[17] These long-term changes in excitability can lead to spontaneous pain or decreased pain thresholds and may be a component of some chronic pain syndromes. It is also possible that the so-called "hot tooth" syndrome in which a tooth with longstanding, intense pulpitis is difficult to anesthetize may be the result of this effect.

Superficial Versus Deep Pain

Pain arising from damage to deep visceral tissue differs from that arising from superficial tissues. Viscera are insensitive to procedures such as cutting or burning but are highly sensitive to distension, pressure, and inflammation. Pain from deep tissues is poorly localized. In contrast, larger, faster nerve fibers in superficial tissues and less central convergence allow more precise localization of superficial pain. Pulpal pain may be considered deep (visceral). Periradicular pain is superficial (peripheral). Thus extension of inflammation from a deep site (pulp) to a superficial one (periradicular tissues) often allows localization of the tooth that is the culprit.

PERIODONTAL PAIN

Periodontal disease is widespread primarily because it is largely painless. It may occasionally manifest with acute pain such as that associated with a lateral periodontal abscess. Periradicular inflammation extending from a necrotic or inflamed pulp may be painful when acute but not when chronic. Mild inflammation arising from the early stages of the extension of pulpal disease or from a high restoration may result in tenderness without spontaneous pain. Locating a tooth with periodontal pain is usually straightforward due to the presence of proprioceptors whose position the nervous system is able to identify.[1]

PULPAL PAIN

Pulpal inflammation is often not painful. Many patients with pulpal necrosis and periradicular pathosis relate no history of endodontic pain. However, at times, an inflamed pulp may be exquisitely painful, causing spontaneous, throbbing, and intense pain that is worsened by hot and cold stimuli.[1] When pain is not spontaneous but evoked by a stimulus, it may outlast the stimulus. It is unclear why pulpal inflammation is, on some occasions, painful and, on other occasions, not painful. If evoked pain from pulpitis significantly outlasts the stimulus, the pulpitis is deemed "irreversible." If the pain subsides quickly, the inflammation is more likely "reversible."

Unfortunately the correlation between symptoms and the histologic condition of the pulp is not consistent. Patients describe pain from pulpitis in a variety of ways. It may increase and throb when they are lying down. It may present as a continuous dull ache that is increased by a stimulus. The pain is intermittent and may abate suddenly for no apparent cause or, conversely, awaken the patient.

Pulpal pain tends to be diffuse and to be referred. As the pain increases in intensity it may spread to the ear, temple, cheek, or other teeth, although never across the midline.[18] If the inflammation extends into the periradicular tissues, localization is usually easier, presumably because of proprioceptors.

Phenomena Complicating the Diagnosis of Dental Pain

REFERRED PAIN

Referred pain in the oral and perioral region is common and important.[18] By definition, *referred pain* comprises input from a site of tissue damage

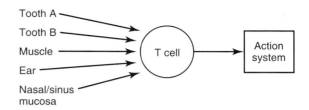

FIGURE 29-2
Referred pain mechanism. Afferent nerves from a variety of tissues converge on the cell body of the second-order neuron (the transmission T cell) in the brainstem, which stimulates the action system. Once the T cell is activated, it may be difficult for higher centers to determine the exact location of the initiating pain, which may be wrongly assigned. A higher center may assume that the painful input comes from a recently activated pathway, resulting in the assignment of painful input to a recently restored tooth.

combined with input from another site where there is no tissue damage; therefore the pain is referred and is perceived to originate from the site of no damage. The convergent neurons are the cells in the dorsal horn gate. When the transmission system is activated and nerve impulses pass along the sensory discriminative pathway, the higher centers in the brain are unable to distinguish the source of the noxious stimuli (Figure 29-2). Therefore the brain may interpret the source wrongly, particularly when previous non-noxious stimuli have been received from the same (referred) site.

This pattern explains the not uncommon phenomenon of pain being referred to a recently restored tooth. Pain from a tooth may then seem to originate from a different tooth. Tooth pain may also appear to originate from a nondental site or, conversely, a tooth may be identified as the source of pain when the origin is nondental. A good example (and a common occurrence) is pain from sinusitis being referred to a maxillary molar.

Odontogenic pain is more likely to be referred when it is more intense, but duration and quality do not seem to be related to referral. The association of intensity to referral is attributed to central nervous system hyperexcitability (central sensitization), causing the expansion of receptive fields. Pain is never referred across the midline but readily from arch to arch.

Some referral patterns are more common than others; it is important to be aware of these possibilities. When the offending tooth is not obvious and cannot be stimulated to reproduce the patient's symptoms, examination should be extended to include these other possibilities. For example, muscles of mastication, the ear, sinuses, the heart, and other teeth may be the source of the referred pain.

Muscles of Mastication

Many patients with myofascial pain dysfunction syndrome describe toothache among their symptoms. Some may describe a toothache but be unaware that the problem is a joint/muscle disorder. This pattern of referral is common and may result in unnecessary extraction or root canal therapy. It is important to examine the temporomandibular joint and muscles of mastication in the diagnosis of all but the most obvious toothaches.[19-22]

CASE

PAIN REFERRED TO A TOOTH FROM MUSCLES OF MASTICATION

Complaint: Moderately severe but continuous dull ache in left lower jaw.

History: The pain has lasted several weeks, being most severe in the morning. It is not intensified by hot and cold stimuli and is relieved temporarily by mild analgesics. A three-unit mandibular-posterior bridge had been placed a few days earlier. There was neither recent acute infection nor trauma. The referring dentist had completed root canal treatment on the premolar abutment with no change in symptoms.

Examination: No visible or palpable intraoral soft tissue abnormalities are present. All teeth on the left side respond within normal limits to vitality tests and percussion. Radiographs show no hard tissue lesions. Discomfort is not relieved by an inferior alveolar nerve block. Palpation of the left masseter muscle shows it to be acutely tender, particularly on the anterior border. Occlusal examination shows imbalances and premature contacts on the left side. Injecting a local anesthetic into the tender region of the muscle relieves the pain.

Diagnosis: Acute myofascial pain in the left masseter muscle after dental treatment.

Etiology: Afferents from the muscle (probably in tendons or fascia) converge on the same second-order neuron in the brainstem trigeminal nucleus as periodontal afferents from the mandibular abutment teeth. The higher centers to which the second-order neuron projects are unable to differentiate between the two inputs. The higher nerve centers "assume" that the new input (from the muscle) originates from the same site as the original input (the teeth).

Treatment: A night guard was worn for 1 week followed by occlusal adjustment. Short-term splint therapy was necessary to ensure that occlusal changes did not occur while the muscle was in spasm.

Ear, Nasal, and Sinus Mucosa

Referred pain from respiratory mucosa to teeth has been demonstrated by stimulating the mucosa 1 week after cavity preparation. Clinically, posterior maxillary teeth are tender to mastication and hypersensitive to cold. The patient often gives a history of an upper respiratory tract infection or recent pollen allergies. The inflamed, fluid-filled sinus may be tender to pressure anterior to the zygomatic buttress. Pain increases when the patient lowers his or her head or jumps and lands on the heels with a jarring motion. Pain of dental origin can also be referred to the ear and preauricular region and may present as tinnitus.[23-25]

CASE

PAIN REFERRED FROM NASAL AND ANTRAL MUCOSA

Complaint: Continuous, dull, widespread toothache from the maxillary molars bilaterally.

History: Symptoms have recurred on several occasions over a period of years; the discomfort at times spreads over the cheek. Teeth are tender to mastication and somewhat sensitive to cold. Symptoms seem to resolve spontaneously. The patient has frequent colds and often feels "stuffed up."

Examination: Nasal and oropharyngeal discharge and inflamed mucosa are seen. Tenderness is reported with strong pressure to the cheek. Soft tissues around the teeth are normal. The molars respond briefly and sharply to a cold stimulus but not with lingering pain. Other teeth test within normal limits. Maxillary molars on both sides are slightly tender to pressure. Radiographs reveal no caries, deep restorations, nor periradicular pathosis.

Diagnosis: Acute upper respiratory tract infection with involvement of the maxillary sinuses.

Etiology: Afferents from both mucosa and teeth converge on the same second-order neurons in the brainstem. Possibly, some afferents supplying the teeth that travel along the wall of the sinus are also stimulated "en passant" by sinus pressure.

Treatment: No dental treatment was indicated. The patient was referred to her medical practitioner to treat the respiratory complaint. On recall, the "toothaches" had resolved; all molars responded within normal limits to vitality and percussion tests.

Cardiac Origin

Cardiac disease may refer pain to the teeth. Pain arising from both narrowing of the coronary artery (angina pectoris) and myocardial infarction may refer to either arch but most commonly to the left mandible.[26-28] Occasionally the oral symptoms are not accompanied by chest pains; cardiac pain is felt only in the face and jaws.

CASE

REFERRED PAIN OF CARDIAC ORIGIN

Complaint: Dull toothache in tooth No. 20, usually after physical exertion.
History: The patient has a long history of cardiac disease with previous infarctions and two bypass operations. The hospital cardiac unit referred him for dental evaluation and treatment before performing a third surgical procedure. Radiographs reveal a periradicular lesion on tooth No. 20, although the tooth is asymptomatic. Neither aspirin nor acetaminophen relieves the pain, but amyl nitrite does.
Diagnosis: Angina pectoris referred to a tooth with an otherwise asymptomatic lesion.
Etiology: Cardiac pain is a "deep" pain and as such is poorly localized. Oral and cardiac afferents are likely to converge above the brainstem level.
Treatment: Tooth No. 20 was treated endodontically with appropriate medical precautions. The patient was warned that the discomfort might continue with referred pain until his cardiac problems were resolved.

Other Teeth

Toothache may refer not only to nondental sites but to other teeth as well.[29]

CASE

TOOTH-TO-TOOTH REFERRAL

Complaint: Intermittent, poorly localized, dull pain in the upper right quadrant.
History: The pain has lasted several weeks, following no fixed pattern. Root canal treatment of tooth No. 4 was completed 1 year ago and treatment of tooth No. 3 was done 2 months ago. The referring dentist suspected that tooth No. 3 was the problem and retreated the tooth, but symptoms did not resolve.
Examination: No soft tissue abnormalities are visible or palpable in the area. None of the teeth are tender to percussion and palpation. Teeth without root canal treatment respond within normal limits to vitality tests, although a response in tooth No. 2 is slow to develop. Radiographs reveal

apparently successful root canal treatment on tooth No. 3 and tooth No. 2 has a crown with three pins visible.

The patient was treated symptomatically with analgesics and advised that a definitive diagnosis was not possible until symptoms were focused. The discomfort level increased 2 weeks later. On examination tooth No. 2 is very tender to pressure and responds to electrical and thermal stimuli, although now with lingering pain. All other teeth remain asymptomatic.
Diagnosis: Irreversible pulpitis and acute apical periodontitis in tooth No. 2 that became localized as inflammation spread from the pulp to periradicular tissues.
Etiology: Afferents from teeth Nos. 2, 3, and 4 converge on the same brainstem neuron. Possibly when the origin and site of referral are close together, afferent fibers branch and supply two teeth.
Treatment: Pulpectomy of tooth No. 2 resolved the symptoms. This was followed by full root canal treatment. Symptoms have not returned.

SPREADING PAIN

As inflammation increases and mediators spread through the adjacent tissues, pain may diffuse in an increasingly wider area.[1,30,31] The pain may not be localizable because the origin is somewhere within that area. This is *primary spreading pain*. The term *secondary spreading pain* describes pain from muscle spasms. These may result from masticatory function disturbed by a painful tooth.

CASE

SPREADING PAIN

Complaint: Soreness of the temporomandibular joint and stiffness in the jaw musculature resulting in trismus.
History: Two months earlier a periradicular abscess on tooth No. 14 had spread through soft tissues, causing extensive swelling. Incision and drainage followed by root canal treatment resulted in resolution of tooth symptoms, although joint soreness and stiffness persisted.
Examination: Tooth No. 14 is asymptomatic after apparently successful root canal treatment. Opening of the jaw is limited with tenderness of the anterior border of the right masseter muscle.
Diagnosis: Spasms in the right masseter muscle.
Etiology: The spread of inflammatory mediators from the periradicular abscess induced spasms in

the masseter muscle. These spasms often persist after resolution of the inflammation.

Treatment: Therapy is focused on the muscle spasm. Heat, exercise, and possibly muscle relaxants should be effective.

PSYCHOGENIC PAIN

Pain has strong emotional and affective components.[32] The gate control theory helps to explain this by incorporating the role of higher nerve centers in the overall description of pain mechanisms. Support comes from the finding that antidepressant drugs, particularly tricyclic antidepressants are often effective for treating chronic pain syndromes. Importantly (and confusingly), pain may originate in higher centers even without input from peripheral nerves. A patient suffering from psychogenic pain often indicates a painful site. Because the mouth and face have unusual emotional significance, these sites are commonly indicated as major sources of pain. The complex psychology of psychogenic pain is beyond the scope of this chapter. Accurate diagnosis and treatment are difficult. Importantly, psychogenic pain is common and should be included in a differential diagnosis. A psychologic component is suspected when the pain does not fit known physiologic patterns:

- No identifiable origin
- Multiple (particularly when bilateral) pain sites
- No predictable response to therapy (especially analgesics)
- Unusual, inconsistent, nonanatomically logical pain patterns
- No demonstrable etiology for the pain

As a clue, patients suffering from psychogenic pain often focus on social and emotional problems when giving their history. Although all pain has an emotional component, with psychogenic pain it is the predominant component. Psychogenic pain is a tentative diagnosis of last resort and an indication for referral. Often there is a true cause for the pain, but the dentist is unable to make a definitive diagnosis and mistakenly dismisses the problem as being of emotional or psychogenic origin.

CASE

PSYCHOGENIC PAIN

Complaint: A 45-year-old woman was seen with a continuous, moderate, dull, but occasionally severe ache from bilateral temporomandibular joints and molars. Discomfort began with the onset of marital problems and financial hardship. Root canal treatment of tooth No. 3 provided temporary relief, as did occlusal splint therapy and pharmacologic treatment for depression. However, the discomfort returned.

Examination: Clinical and radiographic examinations of teeth show no abnormalities. Treatment of tooth No. 3 appears successful. Palpation of the temporomandibular joint reveals no abnormality. Further questioning reveals extended emotional stress after marital break-up.

Diagnosis: Orofacial pain of psychogenic origin (tentative).

Etiology: Pain originates from higher nerve centers and is probably entirely affective. Various forms of treatment are transiently effective because they affect higher central nervous system centers.

Treatment: Long-term relief depends on the emotional problems sustaining the central nervous system changes being removed or on the patient adopting suppressive strategies. A careful nonjudgmental explanation of psychogenic pain was given to the patient. In particular, the contribution of both organic and psychologic components to the pain experience was described. Clearly the patient was experiencing pain, but, because no organic cause was evident, interventional dental treatment would not bring long-term relief. Addressing the emotional component of the pain with the help of a physician, family, and other support services may eliminate it. The prescription of antidepressants by the physician is virtually always a component of treatment.

HEADACHES

Headaches are the most common painful entities of the head and neck.[33] The pain is often referred to teeth and may be confused with toothache. Headache presents in many forms. There are many classifications but two primary groups of headaches: functional and organic.

Functional

Functional headaches are caused by vascular (migraine, cluster, toxic vascular, and hypertensive), musculoskeletal, and emotional disturbances.

Migraine headaches. These may be referred to the teeth (commonly the maxillary canine teeth and premolars), although the principal experience is headache.[34] Classic migraine is readily diagnosed (unilateral throbbing associated with photophobia and nausea); patients usually have a history of recurrent episodes. Atypical variants may confuse diagnosis.

Cluster headaches. These are severe. The patient experiences several (sometimes daily) within a 2- or 3-month period, each lasting up to an hour.[35] The pain is usually limited to the distribution of the first and second divisions of the trigeminal nerve and may be manifest in the maxillary and occasionally the mandibular teeth.

Tension headache. This is the most common form of headache. Involved are muscle spasms that induce pain, which may be referred over a wide area, including the forehead, temples, and back of the neck.[1]

Organic

These headaches are caused by mass lesions (tumors, hematomas, and so on), infection, arteritis, phlebitis, vascular occlusion, cranial neuralgias, and diseases of the eye, ear, nose, throat, and teeth.

Brain tumors may produce a range of no to severe headache. When present, the headache is most often a deep, aching, steady, dull pain. The most severe head pains are associated with neuralgias and vascular headaches. Headaches caused by intracranial hematomas usually are seen after injury.

NEURITIS

Neuritic pains from nerves supplying teeth often cause or mimic toothache.[1] A neuritis may arise from trauma or spread of disease (inflammatory or neoplastic) from adjacent structures. Neuritis is best distinguished from pain originating from the teeth by the history, which usually includes trauma, other disease processes, or other neurologic symptoms such as anesthesia, paresthesia, or occasional muscle weakness and paralysis.

TRIGEMINAL NEURALGIA

Trigeminal neuralgia is is initiated by innocuous stimuli from a trigger zone and causes severe pain.[1,36-38] More common in older patients, it has a neuroanatomic pattern, usually being limited to one division of the trigeminal nerve, most often the mandibular branch. Most trigger sites are extraoral but may be intraoral and therefore confused with tooth pain. The cause of trigeminal neuralgia is controversial.

ATYPICAL ORAL AND FACIAL PAIN

This poorly defined group includes conditions such as atypical facial neuralgia, atypical odontal-gia, phantom tooth pain, and burning mouth.[6,39-41] Their most consistent characteristic is chronic pain of a steady intensity (usually burning but sometimes throbbing) that is poorly localized. The pain often changes location and may cross the midline. Most patients are female. Because these conditions may include tooth pain in their presentation, they are a source of possible misdiagnosis. Multiple dental procedures have often been conducted on patients with these conditions. The etiology is unknown but a psychiatric basis is strongly suspected. Treatment with antidepressants, commonly tricyclics, has been reported to be successful though topical capsaicin may also be effective.

Failure to recognize chronic pain may lead to inappropriate and ineffective treatment. In a rather extreme example,[41] a 22-year-old woman underwent 38 separate root canal treatments, 22 apicoectomies, and 12 extractions, all in a futile attempt to relieve perceived oral pain. Her problem was probably psychogenic.

Diagnostic Procedures

Thorough diagnosis of orofacial pain in some patients may be difficult and time-consuming[1,42] and is beyond the scope of this chapter. The discussion here is limited to determining whether the presenting pain is of dental or other origin and, if dental, to locating its origin. The procedures and tests used in endodontic diagnosis were described in Chapter 4. There is a definite tendency to attribute orofacial pain to a pulpal or periradicular cause. Root canal treatment is not initiated until indicated by a definitive diagnosis.

RECOGNITION OF DIFFICULT DIAGNOSES

In most cases the diagnosis of dental pain is relatively straightforward. The history identifies a consistent, logical pattern of symptoms. The patient indicates a particular tooth, which, when examined, reveals a diseased pulp or periradicular tissues and when stimulated, appropriately reproduces the significant symptoms described in the history. Any departure from this pattern should alert the dentist (Table 29-1, Box 29-2 and Box 29-3).

APPROACH TO DIFFICULT DIAGNOSES

The major weapons are knowledge, an understanding of the mechanisms of pain, and, in particular an appreciation of the phenomena of

TABLE 29-1

Characteristics of Oral Pain

SOURCE OF PAIN	HISTORY					PHYSICAL EXAMINATION		RADIOGRAPHY	
	ABILITY TO LOCALIZE PERIRADICULAR	CHARACTER OF PAIN	PAIN INTENSIFIED BY	PAIN INTENSITY	ASSOCIATED SIGNS	PAIN DUPLICATED BY	BITEWING	PERIRADICULAR
Dentinal	Poor	Evoked does not outlast stimulus; brief	Hot, cold, sweet, sour	Mild to moderate	Caries, defective restoration, exposed dentin	Hot or cold, scratching	Caries, defective restoration	N/A
Pulpal	Very poor	Explosive, intermittent, throbbing, boring	Hot, cold, sometimes chewing	Usually severe; may be mild to moderate	Deep caries, extensive restoration	Hot, cold, probing, sometimes percussion	Deep caries and deep restoration with no secondary dentin	None, or early periradicular changes
Periradicular	Good	For hours at same level, deep, boring	Chewing	Moderate to severe	Periradicular swelling and redness, tooth mobility	Percussion, palpation of periradicular area	Sometimes deep caries, deep restoration	Sometimes periradicular changes, sometimes gutta-percha point in sinus
Periodontal	Good	For hours at same level, boring	Chewing	Moderate to severe	Periodontal swelling, deep pockets with pus, tooth mobility	Percussion, palpation of periodontal area	Sometimes alveolar bone loss	Useful with probe in pocket
Gingival	Good	Pressing, annoying	Food impaction, brushing	Mild to severe	Acute gingival inflammation	Touch, percussion	N/A	N/A
Mucosal	Usually good	Burning, sharp	Sour, sharp, and hot food	Mild to moderate	Erosive or ulcerative lesions, redness	Palpation of lesion	N/A	N/A

Adapted from Sharav Y: Orofacial pain. In Wall PD, Melzack R, editors: *Textbook of pain*, ed 4, New York, 1999, Churchill Livingstone.
N/A, Not applicable

BOX 29-2

Signs of a Difficult Diagnosis

- The patient cannot localize the pain, or it appears in different locations at different times.
- The pain is spontaneous and intermittent and is not necessarily associated with precipitating factors such as thermal stimuli or mastication.
- Stimulation of the suspected tooth or teeth does not reproduce the symptoms.
- The indicated tooth lacks any defect (etiology) that may lead to pulpal damage (pulps do not become inflamed or necrotic spontaneously).
- More than one tooth appears to be involved, or the symptoms are bilateral.

BOX 29-3

Suspicions That Pain Is Not of Tooth Origin

Suspicions that pain is not of tooth origin should be raised when there is (are):[6,42]
- Unidentified local dental cause for pain
- Stimulating, burning, nonpulsatile toothaches
- Constant, unremitting, nonvariable toothaches
- Spontaneous multiple toothaches
- Nonelimination of pain from the suspected tooth after a local anesthetic block
- Failure to respond to reasonable dental therapy of the tooth

---

referred and spreading pain and their patterns. *Dental pains are extremely versatile and have the propensity to simulate nearly any pain syndrome.*

IMPORTANT CLUES

The following items are important clues in the differential diagnosis of orofacial pain:

- *Recent medical history* may include colds or flu with suspected sinusitis and ear infections. The symptoms may become worse when the head is lowered. *Examination should include the oropharynx, sinuses, and ears for signs of inflammation.*
- *Stress and insomnia* are correlated with bruxism and myofascial pain syndromes. *The patient should be questioned about these conditions and habits; include an examination of the muscles of mastication and temporomandibular joint.*
- *Recent dental treatment* suggests that a compromised pulp has succumbed to the final insult of cavity preparation and restoration. Pain is commonly referred to the most recently treated tooth or teeth. *Pain in recently treated teeth should always be approached with suspicion.*
- The *true origin of pain* is sometimes silent, but pain may be initiated by direct stimulation. *Stimulating the site of perceived pain neither initiates nor worsens pain that has been referred from another source.*
- *Anesthetizing the site* to which pain is referred may reduce but not eliminate the pain. *Anesthetizing the true origin of the pain eliminates the pain. Selective infiltration anesthesia should be conducted on maxillary teeth beginning with the anterior teeth because these are more easily anesthetized individually.*

- *More than one source of pain* is possible; the sources may be related. For example, a tender tooth may cause an occlusal imbalance. Avoiding this tooth could lead to a secondary, painful muscle spasm. *Pulpitis in more than one tooth is uncommon, but in occlusal derangements several teeth may become tender.*
- *Pain from the pulp is poorly localized* because it is a deep tissue. When the inflammation spreads to the superficial periodontium it becomes well localized. *If pain is poorly localized and pulpitis is suspected, allow for inflammation to spread to the periodontal tissues, at which time localization will be clear.*

REFERENCES

1. Okeson J: *Bell's orofacial pains,* Chicago, 1995, Quintessence Publishing.
2. Dubner R, Sessle B, Lavigne G: *Physiology, diagnosis and management of oro-facial pain,* Chicago, 2000, Quintessence Publishing.
3. Melzack R, Wall P: *The challenge of pain,* ed 2, New York, 1988, Penguin Viking.
4. Dubner R, Sessle B, Storey A: *The neural basis of oral and facial function,* New York, 1978, Plenum.
5. Willis W: *The pain system,* Basel, 1988, Karger.
6. Wall P, Melzack R: *Textbook of pain,* ed 4, Edinburgh, 1999, Churchill Livingstone.
7. Sessle B: Acute and chronic craniofacial pain: brainstem mechanisms of nociceptive transmission and neuroplasticity, and their clinical correlates, *Crit Rev Oral Biol Med* 11:57, 2000.
8. Melzack R, Wall P: Pain mechanisms: a new theory, *Science* 150:971, 1965.
9. Isberg A, Hagglund M, Paesani D: The effect of age and gender on the onset of symptomatic temporomandibular joint disk displacement, *Oral Surg Oral Med Oral Pathol Oral Radiol Endod* 85:252, 1998.

10. Riley J, Gilbert G, Heft M: Orofacial pain symptom prevalence: selective sex differences in the elderly? *Pain* 76:97,1988.

11. Zola I: Culture and symptoms—an analysis of patients' presenting complaints, *Am Soc Rev* 31:615, 1966.

12. Craig K, Wycoff M: Cultural factors in chronic pain management. In Burrows GD, Elton D, Stanley G, editors, *Handbook of chronic pain management,* Amsterdam, 1987, Elsevier.

13. Moore R, Miller M, Weinstein P, et al: Cultural perceptions of pain and pain coping among patients and dentists, *Community Dent Oral Epidemiol* 14:327, 1986.

14. Casasco A, Calligaro A, Casasco M, et al: Peptidergic nerves in human dental pulp: an immunocytochemical study, *Histochemistry* 95:115, 1990.

15. Olgart L: Neural control of pulpal blood flow, *Crit Rev Oral Biol Med* 7:159, 1996.

16. Bennett G: Update on the neurophysiology of pain transmission and modulation: focus on the NMDA-receptor, *Pain* 19:S2, 2000.

17. Mannion R, Costigan M, Decosterd I, et al: Neurotrophins: peripherally and centrally acting modulators of tactile stimulus-induced inflammatory pain hypersensitivity, *Proc Natl Acad Sci USA* 96:9385, 1999.

18. Falace D, Reid K, Rayens MK: The influence of deep (odontogenic) pain intensity, quality, and duration on the incidence and characteristics of referred orofacial pain, *J Orofac Pain* 10:232, 1996.

19. Travell J: Temporomandibular joint pain referred from muscles of the head and neck, *J Prosthet Dent* 10:745, 1960.

20. Fricton J, Kroenig R, Haley D, Siegert R: Myofascial pain syndrome of the head and neck: A review of clinical characteristics of 164 patients, *Oral Surg Oral Med Oral Pathol* 60:615, 1985.

21. Reeh E, El Deeb M: Referred pain of muscular origin resembling endodontic involvement, *Oral Surg Oral Med Oral Pathol* 71:223, 1991.

22. Raphael K, Marbach J, Klausner J: Myofascial pain: clinical characteristics of those with regional vs. widespread pain, *J Am Dent Assoc* 131:161, 2000.

23. Wright E, Gullickson D: Dental pulpalgia contributing to bilateral preauricular pain and tinnitus, *J Orofac Pain* 10:166, 1996.

24. Hutchins H, Reynolds O: Experimental investigation of the referred pain of aerodontalgia, *J Dent Res* 26:3, 1947.

25. Silverglade D: Dental pain without dental etiology: a manifestation of referred pain from otitis media, *J Dent Child* 47:358, 1980.

26. Matson M: Pain in the orofacial region associated with coronary insufficiency, *Oral Surg Oral Med Oral Pathol* 16:284, 1963.

27. Natkin E, Harrington G, Mandel M: Anginal pain referred to the teeth, *Oral Surg Oral Med Oral Pathol* 40:678, 1975.

28. Kreiner M, Okeson J: Toothache of cardiac origin, *J Orofac Pain* 13, 201, 1999.

29. Glick D: Locating referred pulpal pains, *Oral Surg Oral Med Oral Pathol* 15:613, 1962.

30. Okeson J: *Orofacial pain: guidelines for assessment, diagnosis, and management,* Chicago, 1996, Quintessence Publishing.

31. Sharav Y, Leviner E, Tzukert A, McGrath P: The spatial distribution, intensity and unpleasantness of acute dental pain, *Pain* 20:363, 1984.

32. Baron R, Logan H, Hoppe S: Emotional and sensor focus as mediator of dental pain among patients differing in desired and felt control, *Health Psychol* 12:381, 1993.

33. Dalessio D: *Wolff's headache and other head pain,* ed 4, New York, 1980, Oxford University Press.

34. Brooke R: Periodic migranous neuralgia: a cause of dental pain, *Oral Surg Oral Med Oral Pathol* 46:511, 1978.

35. Bittar G, Graff-Radford S: A retrospective study of patients with cluster headaches, *Oral Surg Oral Med Oral Pathol* 73:519, 1992.

36. Loser J: Tic douloureux and atypical facial pain, *J Can Dent Assoc* 12:917, 1985.

37. Law A, Lilly J: Trigeminal neuralgia mimicking odontogenic pain: a report of two cases, *Oral Surg Oral Med Oral Pathol* 80:96, 1995.

38. Turp J, Gobetti J: Trigeminal neuralgia—an update, *Compend Contin Educ Dent* 21:279, 2000.

39. Brooke R: Atypical odontalgia, *Oral Surg Oral Med Oral Pathol* 49:196, 1980.

40. Bates R, Stewart C: Atypical odontalgia: phantom tooth pain, *Oral Surg Oral Med Oral Pathol* 72:479, 1991.

41. Marbach J, Hulbrook J, Hohn C, Segal A: Incidence of phantom tooth pain: an atypical facial neuralgia, *Oral Surg Oral Med Oral Pathol* 53:190, 1982.

42. Okeson JP, Falace DA: Nonodontogenic toothache, *Dent Clin North Am* 41:367 1997.

Endodontic Therapeutics

LEARNING OBJECTIVES

After reading this chapter, the student should be able to:

1 / Identify patients with a higher risk for experiencing pain after endodontic procedures.

2 / Understand the indications and contraindications for prescribing analgesics, antibiotics, antiinflammatory agents and anxiolytics.

3 / Develop a treatment plan consisting of appropriate endodontic and pharmacologic strategies for managing pain, anxiety, and infection.

4 / Diagnose and treat odontogenic infections.

5 / Monitor patient response to treatment.

6 / Make alternative therapeutic selections when required.

OUTLINE

Odontalgia

Predictors of Post-Treatment Endodontic Pain

    Risk Factors for Post-Treatment Endodontic Pain

    Flare-up

Pain Management Strategies: the "3D's"

    Diagnosis

    Definitive Treatment

    Drugs

Antibiotics

    Prophylactic Antibiotics for Medically Compromised Patients

    Antibiotics Used in Treatment

    Selection of an Antibiotic Regimen

    Role of Bacteria and Their Control

Anxiolytics

    Oral

    Inhalation

T his chapter is not a complete review of the pharmacology of certain drug classes. Instead, it reviews therapeutic strategies for combining both pharmacologic and endodontic treatments for managing pain, infection, and anxiety.

Odontalgia

The management of the endodontic patient does not end at the completion of the appointment. Continuing treatment includes strategies to control pain and/or infection both before and after treatment. Thus endodontic therapeutics includes clinical procedures as well as appropriate adjunctive pharmacotherapy. Indeed the most common form of orofacial pain is toothache (odontalgia), yearly affecting 12% of the population or about 22 million citizens in the United States.[1] Thus strategies for managing odontalgia are important components of root canal treatment.

Predictors of Post-Treatment Endodontic Pain

Fortunately not all endodontic patients experience pain after treatment. Studies have shown that more than one-half of endodontic patients do not report post-treatment pain.[2-4] However, this also means that approximately 40% of patients experience some pain after endodontic procedures, with about 20 percent of all patients reporting moderate-to-severe pain.[2,4] Therefore patients who are at increased risk for post-treatment pain should be identified and receive additional pharmacotherapy for pain management.

RISK FACTORS FOR POST-TREATMENT ENDODONTIC PAIN

Unfortunately, there are no tests that reliably predict which patients will experience pain; however, certain risk factors have been identified. One major risk factor is the presence of preoperative pain or percussion sensitivity.[5] This may be due to hyperalgesia or allodynia initiated by pulpal and/or periradicular inflammation. *Hyperalgesia* (exaggerated pain response) is due to both peripheral and central mechanisms and, significantly, can persist with little-to-no peripheral input.[6-8] *Allodynia* (a reduction in pain threshold) is identified by the symptom of painful chewing or a positive percussion test, in which a normally innocuous stimulus (e.g., gentle tapping of a tooth with a mirror handle) is now perceived as painful. As summarized in Box 30-1, patients with preoperative hyperalgesia or allodynia have an increased risk for developing post-treatment endodontic pain.[9-11]

FLARE-UP

A small proportion of patients (2% to 4%) experience a post-treatment flare-up.[12-14] A *flare-up* is the development of severe post-treatment pain and/or swelling that requires an emergency dental visit. Risk factors include apprehension, retreatment, female sex and age older than 40, a history of allergy, and a diagnosis of pulpal necrosis.[10,11,14] Patients with an apical periodontitis who have endodontic treatment completed in one visit have an almost 10-fold increase in the risk of developing a flare-up.[12] Patients with risk factors should be informed of this possibility; this may increase their compliance in taking analgesics and may decrease the tendency to blame the clinician.

Pain Management Strategies: the "3D's"

A simple effective algorithm for managing the patient with odontalgia is the "3D's": *D*iagnosis, *D*efinitive treatment, and *D*rugs. First, the 3D's provides an easy mnemonic to summarize an integrated approach. Second, this algorithm combines pharmacologic and nonpharmacologic approaches to obtain maximal clinical benefit. And third, the order of the 3D's is a logical sequence for developing a plan for management of post-treatment pain.

DIAGNOSIS

Diagnosis is the first "D" and is a critical initial step in managing pain. Diagnosis of the cause and localization of the pain are critical in effective pain management. Two general issues should be considered in examining a patient with pain. First, can the chief complaint be reproduced? If the chief complaint cannot be reproduced, then possibly the pain is originating from another location, including another tooth (see Chapter 29). This possibility can be evaluated by using a local anesthetic block to rule out pain referred from distant sites, although there are limitations in interpreting diagnostic local anesthetic injections (see Chapters 7 and 29).

The second general issue is identification of a cause for the odontalgia. If the patient points to a certain tooth as the source of the pain, then clinical examination should reveal an etiologic factor.

BOX 30-1	
Diagnostic Features of Hyperalgesia Caused by Odontalgia	
Characteristic of Hyperalgesia	**Diagnostic Sign or Symptom**
Spontaneous pain	Spontaneous pain
Increased pain response	Increased pain to vitality testing
Reduced pain threshold (= allodynia)	Positive percussion or palpation test

In most cases odontalgia is due either to acute stimulation (i.e., dentinal hypersensitivity), to trauma, or to pulp inflammation. Thus clinical examination should reveal corresponding etiologic factors such as exposed dentin, traumatic occlusion (or a history of trauma, bruxism, etc), caries, or a leaking restoration. If the suspected tooth has no apparent etiologic factors that could contribute to the pain, then the differential diagnosis should be expanded. It is appropriate and ethical to consider referring the patient to a specialist for more detailed clinical examination if either the chief complaint cannot be reproduced or etiologic factors are not apparent. Ignoring these factors may increase the risk of misdiagnosis and mistreatment.

DEFINITIVE TREATMENT

The second "D" refers to definitive dental treatment. Examples include pulpotomy, pulpectomy, incision for drainage, and even immediate extraction for teeth with a hopeless prognosis. Definitive treatment reduces or eliminates the peripheral causative factors contributing to hyperalgesia, resulting in a significant reduction in pain levels. Figure 30-1 compiles data from studies of more than 1000 patients with pain after endodontic procedures. Whenever possible, data from the control groups are shown (e.g., patients taking placebo tablets instead of active analgesics); thus the major source for the pain reduction presumably was the definitive dental treatment. Both pulpotomy and pulpectomy substantially reduce post-treatment pain by 50% to 75%, compared with pretreatment pain values.

Figure 30-1 illustrates and reinforces an important therapeutic concept. The optimal method to control post-treatment pain is to combine both definitive treatment and appropriate drugs. Effective treatment, such as canal débridement and

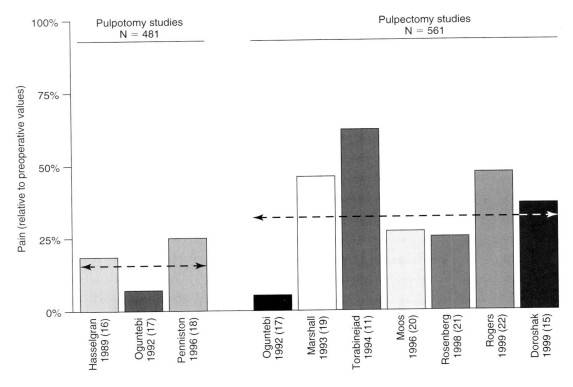

FIGURE 30-1
Evaluation of the effects of pulpotomy or pulpectomy on post-treatment pain in patients experiencing pain *before* treatment. Data are presented relative to the mean pre-treatment pain values reported for each study. Pre-treatment pain values *(solid lines at 100%)* and mean post-treatment pain values *(dashed arrows)* are normalized by sample size for each study. The first author, year, and reference number (in parentheses) are noted for each study.

irrigation, will reduce or eliminate many of the peripheral factors that lead to activation of nociceptors innervating pulpal or periradicular tissue, thus altering the peripheral component of hyperalgesia. Prescribing drugs without dental treatment is unlikely to provide the same level of pain relief as compared to the combination of both techniques.

After definitive treatment, pain is often reduced fairly quickly. An average time course of post-treatment endodontic pain is illustrated in Figure 30-2, as shown in a multicenter clinical trial.[11] Two important concepts emerge from this figure. First, the best predictor of post-treatment pain appears to be the magnitude of pretreatment pain. Figure 30-2 shows that patients with moderate-to-severe pretreatment pain report greater pain after endodontic treatment compared with those who report no or mild pretreatment pain. Second, on average, maximal pain is experienced in the first 24 hours of treatment with levels diminishing thereafter.[3,15-22]

These pain predictors have important implications for dispensing of analgesics. Patients who

are at increased risk (e.g., presenting with more pain) for post-treatment pain should take analgesics "by the clock" (e.g., every 6 hours) for the first 2 to 3 days. This maintains a more predictable blood level of analgesics compared with the traditional "take as needed" (prn) instruction. After 2 to 3 days, patients may then take analgesics as needed.

DRUGS

The third "D" refers to drugs. The three major areas covered in this section on drugs are a flexible prescription plan, the use of long-acting local anesthetics, and indications for steroids.

Analgesics

A flexible analgesic prescription strategy, based on research, has been developed.[5,23] The overall objective of a flexible analgesic prescription strategy is to obtain maximal analgesia and minimal side effects. Thus a flexible pain management plan selects the optimal analgesic based upon the pa-

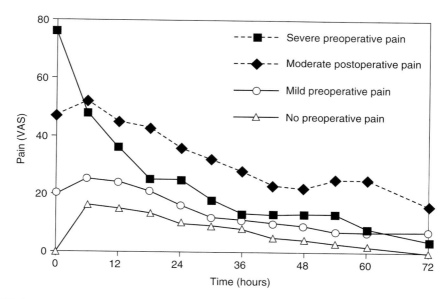

FIGURE 30-2

Time course of post-treatment pain in 53 patients. This was a multicenter clinical trial evaluating the effects of various analgesics on post-treatment pain after anesthesia, isolation, and complete cleaning and shaping of the root canal systems. Only patients given a placebo are presented in this figure. The patients are subdivided into four groups depending on the magnitude of pre-treatment pain they reported before treatment. (Modifed from Torabinejad M, Cymerman JJ, Frankson M, et al: *J Endod* 20:345, 1994.)

tient's medical history, level of pain, and presence of risk factors for post-treatment pain.

The selection of the appropriate analgesic is based in part upon the observation that the non-narcotic component of a combination drug often provides greater analgesia with fewer side effects than the opioid component. This is based on re-sults of studies evaluating both acetaminophen-codeine combinations (e.g., the equivalent of two tablets of Tylenol III and ibuprofen [200 mg]-hydrocodone [7.5 mg] combinations [i.e., the equivalent of Vicoprofen]).[24,25] Thus analgesia can be maximized with fewer side-effects by using the strategy of first prescribing the most effective dose of a nonnarcotic analgesic.

There are important dose-response considera-tions for the nonnarcotic drugs such as ibuprofen or acetaminophen, because they have a ceiling in their dose-response curve. Thus after a maximally effective dose is ingested, additional amounts of the same drug will not provide a proportionate analgesic benefit. This last point has important clinical implications. Patients with endodontic pain should always be asked about how much pain they have (i.e., estimated on a scale of 1 to 10) and about their recent history of analgesic use (type of analgesic, total dose, and time of last dose). These factors will guide the selection of an appropriate analgesic treatment plan.

Figure 30-3 presents a simplified model of a flexible analgesic prescription plan. This plan is di-vided into two columns, for patients who can take nonsteroidal antiinflammatory drugs (NSAIDs) and for patients who cannot (e.g., those with active ulcers, ulcerative colitis, or asthma, or those with a potential interaction with certain concomitant drugs). Each column is then divided into three general categories of analgesic recommendations based on the level of pain or the clinician's assess-ment of risk factors for post-treatment pain. The overall strategy is to first obtain the best analgesia as a result of the use of the nonnarcotic drug and then to add narcotic drugs when needed for ad-ditional pain control. This approach maximizes analgesia benefit while minimizing the potential for side effects.

NSAIDs alone are usually sufficient for patients who can tolerate them because of the relatively low incidence of post-treatment pain (most patients have no to slight pain).[3,4] Thus a prescription for an NSAID, such as ibuprofen 600 mg every 6 hours, is optimal for the majority of patients. If patients cannot tolerate an NSAID, a 1000 mg dose of acetaminophen is often suitable for man-aging post-treatment pain.

Some patients have moderate-to-severe post-treatment pain[4]; these patients may not obtain adequate pain relief by a single drug approach.

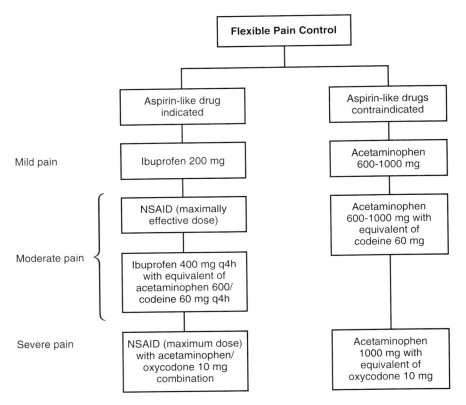

FIGURE 30-3
A simplified analgesic prescription plan to guide drug selection based upon patient history and level of present pain or anticipated post-treatment pain. *NSAID,* Nonsteroidal antiinflammatory drug.

For these patients, there are two general analgesic approaches. A first approach is to coprescribe the alternating schedule of NSAID described earlier with an acetaminophen-opioid combination (Figure 30-3). This provides predictable control for severe pain and can be used to modify a standard NSAID-only regimen if pain control is inadequate.[26,27] Moreover, all three drugs (the NSAID, acetaminophen, and the opioid) are active analgesics that can have additive effects when combined.[25,27,28] A second general approach would be to switch to a fixed drug combination of ibuprofen 200 mg with hydrocodone 7.5 mg (e.g., Vicoprofen); this combination is effective for pain of inflammatory origin.[25] In general, a flexible analgesic prescription strategy offers the best combination of pain relief with minimal side effects, in addition to providing the clinician with a rational approach for customizing an analgesic plan suitable for the patient's needs.

Local Anesthetics

Another important element in a review of the third "D" of pain control (drugs) is local anes-

thetics. Chapter 7 provides a detailed description of the use of local anesthetics. Local anesthetics offer the benefit of prolonged pain control after completion of the endodontic appointment. Long-acting local anesthetics, etidocaine or bupivacaine, offer prolonged pain control for up to 6 to 8 or more hours after injection.[29,30]

However, recent basic research on pain mechanisms have revealed the existence of a central component to hyperalgesia, which can be established by an intense barrage of activity from peripheral nociceptors.[6,8] The *preemptive analgesia hypothesis* states that clinical pain is reduced if the peripheral barrage of nociceptors is reduced.[31] Subsequent studies on orofacial pain have provided support for this concept. For example, patients given a bupivacaine injection for an inferior alveolar nerve block before an oral surgical procedure reported less pain at *2 days* after the procedure compared with placebo-injected patients.[32] This result is not restricted to extraction procedures because infiltration with bupivacaine before tonsillectomy reduced postoperative pain for 7 days compared with placebo injections.[33] Collectively, these studies indicate that long-acting local anesthetics should be considered for treating endodontic pain patients.

Steroids

Steroids represent another example of the third "D" of pain control (drugs). In general, the decision to use a drug depends on the risks, benefits, patient factors, and pharmacologic alternatives. The decision to prescribe steroids is not always simple because potential risks include suppression of immune function and wound healing. Single-dose administration of a steroid produces a reduction in circulating lymphocytes and monocytes for 24 hours with no reduction in circulating neutrophils or antibody response.[34]

Controlled clinical trials for mild-to-moderate pain indicated that steroids provide analgesia in patients with endodontic pain after oral, intramuscular, or intracanal routes of administration.[22,35,36] Short-term administration of steroids may have a place in management of endodontic pain for patients in whom the benefits outweigh the potential modulation of infection, wound healing, or other adverse effects. However, this benefit must be balanced against the known efficacy of alternative drugs (e.g., NSAIDs) and the particular factors of each case. No evidence supports the prophylactic use of steroids for prevention of more severe levels of endodontic pain.

Antibiotics

As described above, odontogenic pain is best managed by a combined approach using both local treatment and pharmacotherapeutic measures. The same philosophy holds for odontogenic infections—optimal management includes both definitive treatment (e.g., canal débridement and, often, incision for drainage) and pharmacologic adjuncts (e.g., antibiotics) when indicated. Systemic antibiotics are not a substitute for proper local treatment. Indeed, the vast majority of endodontic infections can be treated without antibiotics. Pain and swelling are managed by débridement of the pulp space and drainage of the soft and hard tissues. Healthy patients without systemic signs and symptoms of infection but with symptomatic pulpitis, symptomatic apical periodontitis, a draining sinus tract, or localized swelling do not require antibiotics.[37,38]

Likewise, the use of "prophylactic antibiotics" to prevent post-treatment pain or flare-ups after root canal treatment is neither effective, rational nor justified.[39,40] Even if antibiotics were helpful, because only a small percentage of endodontic patients experience a flare-up, the risk-benefit ratio would not support their routine use.[12,14,41,42] The use of prophylactic antibiotics places patients at risk for side effects. In addition, these patients are subjected to the possibility of selection of resistant microorganisms and "superinfections." Also, antibiotics may be very costly.

PROPHYLACTIC ANTIBIOTICS FOR MEDICALLY COMPROMISED PATIENTS

Medically compromised patients who have an increased risk of a secondary infection at a distant site (metastatic) after a bacteremia include those with rheumatic or congenital heart disease, prosthetic cardiac valves, mitral valve prolapse with regurgitation, previous infective endocarditis, systemic pulmonary shunts, indwelling arteriovenous shunts, uncontrolled diabetes, and an immunosuppressed or immunologically deficient status. These dental patients who are at risk of metastatic infection after a bacteremia must receive a regimen of antibiotics that either follows the recommendations of the American Heart Association (AHA) or is determined in consultation with the patient's physician. A team approach by the patient, dentist, and physician helps to ensure compliance and adequate therapy.[43,44] The regimens recommended by the AHA are given in Table 30-1.

The AHA recommends the use of antibiotics to protect against endocarditis for canal instrumentation beyond the apex, for endodontic surgery, and for anesthesia delivered via the periodontal ligament.[43,44] Although the incidence of bacteremia is low with root canal procedures, a transient bacteremia can result from instrumentation confined to the root canal[45,46] Care must be taken when positioning rubber dam clamps and performing other procedures that may produce bleeding with an accompanying bacteremia. The use of chlorhexidine, povidone-iodine, or iodine-glycerin on isolated and dried gingiva for 5 minutes along with irrigation of the gingival sulcus before surgical procedures are performed has been recommended.[43,47]

Antibiotic prophylaxis guidelines for patients with total joint replacements have recently been updated.[48] Patients considered to be at risk include immunocompromised/immunosuppressed patients, insulin-dependent (type I) diabetic patients, patients who have had joint replacements in the past 2 years, and those with previous joint infections, malnourishment, and hemophilia.[48,49]

TABLE 30-1

American Heart Association Guidelines for Antibiotic Prophylaxis for Bacterial Endocarditis: Prophylactic Regimens for Dental, Oral, Respiratory Tract, or Esophageal Procedures

SITUATION	AGENT	REGIMEN*
Standard general prophylaxis	Amoxicillin	Adults: 2.0 g Children: 50 mg/kg orally 1 hour before procedure
Unable to take oral medications	Ampicillin	Adults: 2.0 g IM or IV Children: 50 mg/kg IM or IV 30 min before procedure
Allergic to penicillin	Clindamycin	Adults:600 mg Children: 20 mg/kg orally 1 hour before procedure
	OR Cephalexin† or cefadroxil† OR Azithromycin or clarithromycin	Adults: 2.0 g Children: 50 mg/kg orally 1 hour before procedure Adults: 500 mg Children: 15 mg/kg orally 1 hour before procedure
Allergic to penicillin and unable to take oral medications	Clindamycin	Adults: 600 mg Children: 20 mg/kg IV within 30 minutes before procedure
	OR Cefazolin†	Adults: 1.0 g Children: 25 mg/kg IM or IV within 30 minutes before procedure

Adapted from Dajani A, Taubert K, Wilson W, et al: Prevention of bacterial endocarditis: recommendations by the American Heart Association, *JADA* 128:1142-1151, August 1997. Copyright © 1997 American Dental Association. Reprinted by permission of ADA Publishing, a Division of ADA Business Enterprises, Inc.
IV, Intravenous; *IM,* intramuscular.
*Total children's dose should not exceed adult dose.
†Cephalosporins should not be used in individuals with immediate-type hypersensitivity reactions (urticaria, angioedema, or anaphylaxis) to penicillins.

ANTIBIOTICS USED IN TREATMENT

An antibiotic regimen should be prescribed in conjunction with the appropriate endodontic procedure when there is systemic involvement, a persistent infection, or a spreading infection. The signs and symptoms of systemic involvement and spread of infection include fever ($>100°$ F or $>38°$ C), malaise, cellulitis, progressive abscess, and unexplained trismus, alone or in combination. Under these circumstances, an antibiotic should be given only as an adjunct to débridement and drainage or extraction when indicated. Patients with these signs and symptoms must be closely followed on a daily basis, in person or by telephone. After the source of infection has been treated, improvement is usually rapid. Systemically administered antibiotics will not be effective against a reservoir of microorganisms in an infected root canal system or a periradicular abscess because of absence of normal circulation.

Initial empirical selection of an antibiotic (antimicrobial agent) is based on the microorganisms commonly associated with endodontic infections.[50,51] The clinician must be thoroughly familiar with the drug and inform the patient of benefits, side effects, and possible sequelae of not taking the proper dosage. If the patient's condition does not rapidly improve, consultation or referral to a specialist should be done immediately.

SELECTION OF AN ANTIBIOTIC REGIMEN

Under ideal circumstances, susceptibility testing would be undertaken before the prescription of antimicrobial drugs. Unfortunately with the polymicrobial nature of endodontic infections, it may take from several days to weeks to obtain a complete susceptibility profile of the bacteria. Therefore by necessity, the initial antibiotic prescribed is empiric. Penicillin VK remains the first antibiotic (antimicrobial) of choice because it has remained effective against most of the facultative and strict anaerobes commonly found in polymicrobial endodontic infections.[50-53] Bacteria sensitive to penicillin include anaerobes (*Porphyromonas, Prevotella, Peptostreptococcus, Fusobacterium,* and *Actinomyces*), and Gram-positive facultative bacteria (e.g., streptococci and enterococci).[50-53]

Penicillin is inexpensive and has low toxicity, but importantly, approximately 10% of the population may be allergic to this medication. Most allergic reactions occur in patients with no reported history of penicillin allergy.[54] However, obtaining a careful history of the patient's drug reactions is mandatory. If a decision is made to prescribe penicillin, an adequate blood level must be obtained. An initial oral loading dose of 1000 mg of penicillin VK is followed by 500 mg every 6 hours for 7 days. A loading dose provides an adequate therapeutic level and helps prevent development of resistant strains. Antibiotics should be continued for 2 to 3 days after resolution of the signs and symptoms of the infection. When an antibiotic is prescribed in conjunction with débridement of the root canal system and soft tissue drainage, significant improvement should be seen within 2 to 3 days. If the infection is not resolving, referral to a specialist is indicated.

Amoxicillin has a broader spectrum than penicillin VK that includes bacteria not usually found in endodontic infections. Thus it selects for resistant organisms commonly found in the gastrointestinal tract. For patients with severe infections or if immunocompromised, the prescription of the broader spectrum amoxicillin may be warranted. An oral loading dose of 1000 mg is followed by 500 mg every 8 hours for 7 days. The combination of amoxicillin and clavulanate (Augmentin) may be indicated if tests demonstrate the presence of β-lactamase-producing bacteria or if the infection is life-threatening.

Metronidazole is bactericidal against strict anaerobes but does not have activity against aerobes or facultative anaerobes. The addition of metronidazole to penicillin for combined therapy is indicated if the patient's condition is not improving after 72 hours. The patient should continue to take the prescribed penicillin for its efficacy against aerobes or facultative anaerobes. When the patient's condition is not improving, the initial diagnosis and treatment must be reviewed and further treatment rendered if indicated. The recommended dose of metronidazole is 500 mg every 6 hours for 7 days. Patients taking metronidazole have an intolerance to alcohol.

Clindamycin is effective against many Gram-positive and Gram-negative microorganisms including both facultative and strict anaerobes. Clindamycin is a good (but expensive) alternative to penicillin and is recommended for patients allergic to penicillin. It is well distributed throughout the body and reaches bone concentrations similar to those in plasma. Clindamycin therapy has been associated (very seldom) with pseudomembranous colitis. However, antibiotic-associated colitis is now known to be caused by all antibiotics except the aminoglycosides. Clindamycin, ampicillin/amoxicillin, and the cephalosporins each cause about one-third of cases of antibiotic-associated colitis. The usual adult dose of clindamycin is a 300 mg loading dose followed by 150 to 300 mg every 6 hours for 7 days.

Clarithromycin and azithromycin are macrolides like erythromycin with some advantages over erythromycin.[55] They may be prescribed for patients allergic to penicillin with relatively mild indications for systemic antibiotic therapy. They produce less gastrointestinal upset and have a spectrum of antimicrobial activity that includes some of the anaerobic bacteria associated with endodontic infections. Clarithromycin may be given with or without meals in a dose of 250 to 500 mg every 12 hours for 7 days. Azithromycin should be taken 1 hour before meals or 1 hour after meals. A loading dose of 500 mg is followed by 250 mg daily for 5 to 7 days. These antimicrobials block the metabolism of warfarin and anisindione, which can lead to serious bleeding in patients taking anticoagulant medication.[56]

Patients using oral contraception should be warned to use alternative methods of contraception after the prescription of antibiotics. Although rifampin seems to be the only antimicrobial proven to be associated with reduced effectiveness of oral contraceptives, case reports have implicated others.[56]

ROLE OF BACTERIA AND THEIR CONTROL

Antimicrobials in the form of irrigants, intracanal medicaments, and antibiotics have been an integral part of endodontic practice. With the advent of improved microbiologic techniques, scientific data suggest that diseases of endodontic origin are either primarily or secondarily caused by microorganisms. Clinicians must understand the role of microorganisms in the pathogenesis of these pathoses. Important treatment modalities are complete root canal débridement and incision for drainage in conjunction with appropriate use of antimicrobials.

Anxiolytics

A third realm of endodontic pharmacotherapy is the control of anxiety. Surveys of dental patients indicate that both endodontic and oral surgical procedures rank as the most fearful for patients, with many patients reporting that they are "nervous" when facing an impending endodontic appointment.[57,58] Similar to the control of pain and infection, an integrated approach for the control of anxiety includes both nonpharmacologic and pharmacologic techniques.

Several nonpharmacologic techniques for the control of anxiety, ranging from behavioral management techniques to distraction to hypnosis have been evaluated in endodontic patients.[59,60] These techniques reduce reports of pain or anxiety during endodontic treatment.[61,62] Nonpharmacologic techniques are often combined with pharmacologic techniques for control of anxiety.[63]

Pharmacologic routes for control of anxiety include oral, inhalation, and intravenous techniques; because of the scope of this topic, only the first two methods will be reviewed. Advantages of oral routes of drug administration for control of anxiety include demonstrated efficacy, reduced monitoring, and decreased likelihood of serious morbidity.[64,65]

ORAL

Commonly and conveniently used oral benzodiazepines include diazepam and triazolam. Diazepam (Valium), at an adult dose of 5 to 15 mg, can be administered to reduce anxiety in endodontic patients.[66] Triazolam (Halcion), at a 0.25 mg oral dose, is also effective. It has rapid onset and reduces anxiety comparable to an intravenous dose of 19 mg of diazepam.[66,67] Unlike diazepam, triazolam does not have an active metabolite and provides faster recovery; however, patients cannot drive because they may experience transient reductions in psychomotor impairment.[67] Sublingual administration of the triazolam tablet bypasses first-pass hepatic clearance of the drug and increases the peak anxiolytic effect; an indication for this approach may be patients requiring a faster onset of anxiolytic activity.[68] Diazepam is available in tablet form, or for a more rapid onset, may be prepared as a liquid at 5 mg/ml and administered approximately one hour before the appointment.

INHALATIONAL

The primary inhalational anxiolytic drug is nitrous oxide (N_2O). Although 40% N_2O appears to have marginal effects on anxiety, the delivery of 50% N_2O has been reported to be effective.[67,69] N_2O does not appear to have additive effects when combined with either triazolam or diazepam.[67,70] Intraoperative scavenging of N_2O is important because chronic exposure to the gas has medical implications.[71,72] Although patient acceptance is often high with N_2O, the clinician should consider the potential for effective gas scavenging as well as the effectiveness of alternative drugs. Also there is some difficulty in completing endodontic procedures and radiographic examination because of interference from the inhalation apparatus.

REFERENCES

1. Lipton J, Ship J, Larach-Robinson D: Estimated prevalence and distribution of reported orofacial pain in the United States, *J Am Dent Assoc* 124:115, 1993.
2. Seltzer S, Bender I, Ehrenreich J: Incidence and duration of pain following endodontic therapy, *Oral Surg Oral Med Oral Pathol* 14:74, 1961.
3. Harrison JW, Baumgartner CJ, Zielke DR: Analysis of interappointment pain associated with the combined use of endodontic irrigants and medicaments, *J Endod* 7:272, 1981.
4. Georgopoulou M, Anastassiadis P, Sykaras S: Pain after chemomechanical preparation, *Int Endod J* 19: 309, 1996.
5. Hargreaves KM, Hutter J: Endodontic pharmacology. In Cohen S, Burns R., editors: *Pathways of the pulp,* ed 8, St Louis, 2001, Mosby.
6. Hargreaves KM, Roszkowski M, Jackson D, et al: Neuroendocrine and immune responses to injury, degeneration and repair. In Sessle B, Dionne R, Bryant P, editors: *Temporomandibular disorders and related pain conditions,* Seattle, 1995, IASP Press.
7. Hargreaves K: Neurochemical factors in injury and inflammation in orofacial tissues. In Lund J, Lavigne G, Dubner R, Sessle B, editors: *Orofacial pain: basic sciences to clinical management,* Chicago, 2001, Quintessence Publishing.
8. Dickenson A, Stanfa L, Chapman V, Yaksh T: Response properties of dorsal horn neurons: pharmacology of the dorsal horn. In Yaksh T, Lynch C, Zapol W, et al, editors: *Anesthesia: biological foundations,* Philadelphia, 1998, Lippincott.
9. Imura N, Zuolo ML: Factors associated with endodontic flare-ups: a prospective study, *Int Endod J* 28:261, 1995.
10. Torabinejad M, Kettering JD, McGraw JC, et al: Factors associated with endodontic interappointment emergencies of teeth with necrotic pulps, *J Endod* 14:261, 1988.
11. Torabinejad M, Cymerman JJ, Frankson M, et al: Effectiveness of various medications on postoperative pain following complete instrumentation, *J Endod* 20:345, 1994.
12. Trope M. Flare-up rate of single-visit endodontics, *Int Endod J* 24:24, 1991.
13. Mor C, Rotstein I, Friedman S: Incidence of interappointment emergency associated with endodontic therapy, *J Endod* 18:509, 1992.
14. Walton R, Fouad A: Endodontic interappointment flare-ups: a prospective study of incidence and related factors, *J Endod* 18:172, 1992.
15. Doroshak A, Bowles W, Hargreaves K: Evaluation of the combination of flurbiprofen and tramadol for management of endodontic pain, *J Endod* 25:660, 1999.

16. Hasselgren G, Reit C: Emergency pulpotomy: pain relieving effect with and without the use of sedative dressings, *J Endod* 15:254, 1989.

17. Oguntebi BR, DeSchepper EJ, Taylor TS, et al: Postoperative pain incidence related to the type of emergency treatment of symptomatic pulpitis, *Oral Surg Oral Med Oral Pathol* 73:479, 1992.

18. Penniston SG, Hargreaves KM: Evaluation of periapical injection of Ketorolac for management of endodontic pain, *J Endod* 22:55, 1996.

19. Marshall JG, Liesinger AW: Factors associated with endodontic posttreatment pain, *J Endod* 19:573, 1993.

20. Moos HL, Bramwell JD, Roahen JO: A comparison of pulpectomy alone versus pulpectomy with trephination for the relief of pain, *J Endod* 22:422, 1996.

21. Rosenberg PA, Babick PJ, Schertzer L, Leung A: The effect of occlusal reduction on pain after endodontic instrumentation, *J Endod* 24:492, 1998.

22. Rogers M, Johnson B, Remeikis N, BeGole E: Comparison of effect of intracanal use of ketorolac tromethamine and dexamethasone with oral ibuprofen on post treatment endodontic pain, *J Endod* 25:381, 1999.

23. Hargreaves KM, Troullos E, Dionne R: Pharmacologic rationale for the treatment of acute pain, *Dent Clin North Am.* 31:675, 1987.

24. Cooper S: New peripherally acting oral analgesics, *Annu Rev Pharmacol Toxicol* 23:617, 1983.

25. Wideman G, Keffer. M, Morris E, et al: Analgesic efficacy of a combination of hydrocodone with ibuprofen in postoperative pain, *Clin Pharmacol Ther* 65:667, 1999.

26. Cooper S: The relative efficacy of ibuprofen in dental pain, *Compend Contin Educ Dent* 7:578, 1986.

27. Breivik E, Barkvoll P, Skovlund E: Combining diclofenac with acetaminophen or acetaminophen-codeine after oral surgery: a randomized, double-blind, single oral dose study, *Clin Pharmacol Ther* 66:625, 1999.

28. Sunshine A, Olson N, ONeill E, et al: Analgesic efficacy of a hydrocodone with ibuprofen combination compared with ibuprofen alone for the treatment of acute postoperative pain, *J Clin Pharmacol* 37:908, 1997.

29. Dionne R: Suppression of dental pain by the preoperative administration of flurbiprofen, *Am J Med* 80:41, 1986.

30. Dunsky JL, Moore PA: Long-acting local anesthetics: a comparison of bupivacaine and etidocaine in endodontics, *J Endod* 10:457, 1984.

31. Woolf C: Transcriptional and posttranslational plasticity and the generation of inflammatory pain, *Proc Natl Acad Sci USA* 96:7723, 1999.

32. Gordon S, Dionne R, Brahim J, et al: Blockade of peripheral neuronal barrage reduces postoperative pain, *Pain* 70:209, 1997.

33. Jebeles J, Reilly J, Gutierrez J, et al: Tonsillectomy and adenoidectomy pain reduction by local bupivacaine infiltration in children, *Int J Pediatr Otorhinolaryngol* 25:149, 1993.

34. Haynes R: Adrenocorticotrophic hormone: adrenocortical steroids and their synthetic analogs; inhibitors of the synthesis and actions of adrenocortical hormones. In Gilman A, Rall T, Nies A, Taylor P, editors: *Goodman and Gilman's the pharmacological basis of therapeutics,* ed 8, New York, 1990, Pergamon.

35. Marshall JG, Walton RE: The effect of intramuscular injection of steroid on posttreatment endodontic pain, *J Endod* 10:584, 1984.

36. Liesinger A, Marshall FJ, Marshall JG: Effect of variable doses of dexamethasone on posttreatment endodontic pain, *J Endod* 19:35, 1993.

37. Fouad AF, Rivera EM, Walton RE: Penicillin as a supplement in resolving the localized acute apical abscess, *Oral Surg Oral Med Oral Pathol* 81:590, 1996.

38. Henry M, Reader A, Beck M: Effect of penicillin on postoperative endodontic pain and swelling in symptomatic necrotic teeth, *J Endod* 27:117, 2001.

39. Walton RE, Chiappinelli J: Prophylactic penicillin: effect on posttreatment symptoms following root canal treatment of asymptomatic periapical pathosis, *J Endod* 19:466, 1993.

40. Pickenpaugh L, Reader A, Beck M et al: Effect of prophylactic amoxicillin on endodontic flare-up in asymptomatic, necrotic teeth, *J Endod* 27:53, 2001.

41. Pallasch T: Infectious disease at the millennium, *J Calif Dent Assoc* 27:367, 1999.

42. Pallasch T: Pharmacokinetic principles of antimicrobial therapy, *Periodontol 2000* 10:5, 1996.

43. Dajani A, Taubert K, Wilson W, et al: Prevention of bacterial endocarditis, *JAMA* 277:1794, 1997.

44. Tong D, Rothwell BR: Antibiotic prophylaxis in dentistry: a review and practice recommendations, *J Am Dent Assoc* 131:366, 2000.

45. Debelian GJ, Olsen I, Tronstad L: Bacteremia in conjunction with endodontic therapy, *Endod Dent Traumatol* 11:142, 1995.

46. Baumgartner JC, Heggers JP, Harrison JW: The incidence of bacteremias related to endodontic procedures. I. Nonsurgical endodontics, *J Endod* 2:135, 1976.

47. Bender I, Barkan M: Dental bacteremia and its relationship to bacterial endocarditis: preventive measures, *Compend Contin Educ Dent* 10:472, 1989.

48. American Dental Association and American Academy of Orthopaedic Surgeons: Advisory statement: Antibiotic prophylaxis for dental patients with total joint replacements, *J Am Dent Assoc* 128:1004, 1997.

49. ADA Council on Scientific Affairs: Antibiotic use in dentistry, *J Am Dent Assoc* 128:648, 1997.

50. Yamamoto K, Fukushima H, Tsuchiya H, Sagawa H: Antimicrobial susceptibilities of *Eubacterium, Peptostreptococcus,* and *Bacteroides* isolated from root canals of teeth with periapical pathosis, *J Endod* 15:112, 1989.

51. Baker P, Evans R, Slots J, Genco R: Antibiotic susceptibility of anaerobic bacteria from the human oral cavity, *J Dent Res* 64:1233, 1985.

52. Ranta H: Bacteriology of odontogenic apical periodontitis and effect of penicillin treatment, *Scand J Infect Dis* 20:187, 1988.

53. Vigil GV, Wayman BE, Dazey SE, et al: Identification and antibiotic sensitivity of bacteria isolated from periapical lesions, *J Endod* 23:110, 1997.

54. Erffmeyer J, Blaiss M: Proving penicillin allergy, *Postgrad Med* 87:33, 1990.

55. Moore P: Dental therapeutic indications for the newer long-acting macrolide antibiotics, *J Am Dent Assoc* 130:1341, 1999.

56. Hersh E: Adverse drug interactions in dental practice, *J Am Dent Assoc* 130:236, 1999.

57. Wong M, Lytle WR: A comparison of anxiety levels associated with root canal therapy and oral surgery treatment, *J Endod* 17:461, 1991.

58. Dionne RA, Gordon SM, McCullagh LM, Phero JC: Assessing the need for anesthesia and sedation in the general population, *J Am Dent Assoc* 129:167, 1998.

59. Aartman IH, de Jongh A, Makkes PC, Hoogstraten J: Treatment modalities in a dental fear clinic and the relation with general psychopathology and oral health variables, *Br Dent J* 186:467, 1999.

60. Selden HS: Patient empowerment—a strategy for pain management in endodontics, *J Endod* 19:521, 1993.

61. Morse DR: Use of meditative state for hypnotic induction in the practice of endodontics, *Oral Surg Oral Med Oral Pathol* 41:664, 1976.

62. Peretz B, Katz J, Zilburg I, Shemer J: Treating dental phobic patients in the Israeli Defense Force, *Int Dent J* 46:108, 1996.

63. Morse DR, Schacterle GR, Furst ML, Bose K: Stress, relaxation, and saliva: a pilot study involving endodontic patients, *Oral Surg Oral Med Oral Pathol* 52:308, 1981.

64. Dionne R: Oral sedation, *Compend Contin Educ Dent* 19:868, 1998.

65. Haas DA: Oral and inhalation conscious sedation, *Dent Clin North Am* 43:341, 1999.

66. Ehrich DG, Lundgren JP, Dionne RA, et al: Comparison of triazolam, diazepam, and placebo as outpatient oral premedication for endodontic patients, *J Endod* 23:181, 1997.

67. Kaufman E, Hargreaves K, Dionne R: Comparison of oral triazolam and nitrous oxide with placebo and intravenous diazepam for outpatient medication, *Oral Surg Oral Med Oral Pathol* 75:156, 1993.

68. Berthold CW, Dionne RA, Corey SE: Comparison of sublingually and orally administered triazolam for premedication before oral surgery, *Oral Surg Oral Med Oral Pathol* 84:119, 1997.

69. Berge TI: Acceptance and side effects of nitrous oxide oxygen sedation for oral surgical procedures, *Acta Odontol Scand* 57:201, 1999.

70. Houpt MI, Kupietzky A, Tofsky NS, Koenigsberg SR: Effects of nitrous oxide on diazepam sedation of young children, *Pediatr Dent* 18:236, 1996.

71. Girdler NM, Sterling PA: Investigation of nitrous oxide pollution arising from inhalational sedation for the extraction of teeth in child patients, *Int J Paediatr Dent* 8:93, 1998.

72. Howard WR: Nitrous oxide in the dental environment: assessing the risk, reducing the exposure, *J Am Dent Assoc* 128:356, 1997 [published erratum appears in *J Am Dent Assoc* 128:700, 1997].

Richard E. Walton

31

Geriatric Endodontics

LEARNING OBJECTIVES

After reading this chapter, the student should be able to:

1 / Identify those biologic aspects in the elderly patient that are similar to and different from those in the younger patient.

2 / Discuss age changes in the older dental pulp, both physiologic and anatomic.

3 / Discuss differences in healing patterns in the older patient.

4 / Describe complications presented by the medically compromised older patient.

5 / Describe, step by step, the process of diagnosis and treatment planning in the elderly patient.

6 / Identify factors that complicate case selection.

7 / Discuss why there are differences and what those differences are when root canal treatment is performed in the older patient.

8 / Recognize the complications of endodontic surgery.

9 / Select the appropriate restoration after root canal treatment.

10 / Identify those elderly patients who should be considered for referral.

OUTLINE

Biologic Considerations

Pulp Response
Changes with Age
Nature of Response to Injury

Periradicular Response

Healing

Medically Compromised Patients

Diagnosis
Diagnostic Procedure
Radiographic Findings

Differential Diagnosis
Endodontic Pathosis
Other Pathoses

Treatment Planning and Case Selection
Procedure
Prognosis
Number of Appointments
Additional Considerations

Root Canal Treatment
Treatment Considerations

Impact of Restoration

Retreatment

Endodontic Surgery
Medical Considerations
Biologic and Anatomic Factors
Healing After Surgery

Bleaching
External Stains
Internal Stains

Restorative Considerations
Overdenture Abutments
Coronal Seal

Trauma

Endodontic considerations in the elderly patient are similar in many ways to those in the younger patient, but with differences. This chapter will discuss those similarities as well as concentrating on the differences. The topics will include the biologic aspects of pulpal and periradicular tissues, healing patterns, diagnosis, and treatment aspects in the geriatric patient.

The number of persons aged 65 and over in the United States exceeds 35 million. Not only is this age group expanding in numbers, but their dental needs continue to increase.[1,2] More elderly patients will not accept tooth extraction unless there are no alternatives.[3,4] Their expectations for dental health parallel their demands for quality medical care. An even more important consideration is that their dentitions will have experienced decades of dental disease as well as restorative[5] and periodontal procedures (Figure 31-1). These all have compound adverse effects on the pulp, periradicular, and surrounding tissues (Figure 31-2). In other words, the more injuries that are inflicted, the greater the likelihood of irreversible disease and thus the greater the need for treatment.

The combination of an increase in pathosis and dental needs, coupled with greater expectations, has resulted in more endodontic procedures among these aging patients (Figure 31-3). Furthermore, expanded dental insurance benefits for retirees as well as more disposable income has made complex treatment more affordable.[2]

Endodontic considerations in elderly patients include biologic, medical, and some psychologic differences from younger patients as well as treatment complications. These considerations will be further discussed in the chapter.

Biologic Considerations

Biologic considerations are both systemic and local. The wide variety of systemic changes related to the patient's medical status are covered in other textbooks. In the older patient, there are no systemic or local changes particularly unique to endodontics that are different from those for other dental procedures. Similarly, pulp and periradicular tissues do not respond markedly differently.

Pulp Response

CHANGES WITH AGE

There are two considerations: (1) structural (histologic) changes that take place as a function of time; and (2) tissue changes that occur in response

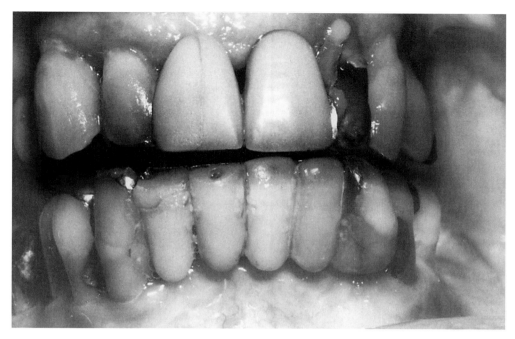

FIGURE 31-1
Dentitions in older individuals often have multiple appearances and diverse problems caused by many years of disease, restorations, and oral and systemic changes. These dentitions often are a challenge to restore to acceptable function and esthetics.

to irritation from injury. These tend to have similar appearances in the pulp. In other words, injury may prematurely "age" a pulp. Therefore an "old" pulp may be found in a tooth of a younger person, i.e., a tooth that has experienced caries, restorations, etc. Whatever the etiology, these older (or injured) pulps react somewhat differently than do younger (or noninjured) pulps.

Chronologic Versus Physiologic

Does a pulp in an older individual react differently than an injured pulp in a younger individual? This question has not been answered. Probably a previously injured pulp (from caries, restoration, etc.) in a younger person has *less* resistance to injury than an undamaged pulp in an older individual. At a histologic level, there are some consistent changes in these older pulps as well as in irritated pulps.

Structural

The pulp is a dynamic connective tissue. It has been well documented that, with age, there are changes in both cellular, extracellular, and supportive elements (see Chapter 2). There is a decrease in cells, including both odontoblasts and fibroblasts. There is also a decrease in the supportive elements, i.e.,

blood vessels and nerves.[6,7] There is presumably an increase in the percentage of space occupied by collagen, but less ground substance; these changes in proportions have not been measured, but only have been observed histologically.[8]

Calcifications

These include denticles (pulp stones) and diffuse (linear) calcifications. These increase in the aged pulp[9] as well as in the irritated pulp.[10] Pulp stones tend to be found in the coronal pulp, and diffuse calcifications are in the radicular pulp. It has been speculated that the indices of calcification arise from degenerated nerves or blood vessels, but this has not been proven. Another common speculation is that pulp stones may cause odontogenic pain; this is not true.

Dimensional

Pulp spaces generally progressively decrease in size and often become very small.[11,12] Dentin formation is not necessarily continuous throughout life, but it often does occur and may be accelerated by irritation from caries, restorations, and periodontal disease. Dentin formation with time or irritation is not uniform. For example, in molar

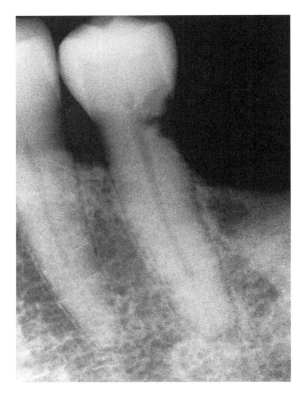

FIGURE 31-2
Cervical external resorption exposing the pulp. A free-end removable partial denture has settled posteriorly, exerting pressure on the gingiva and inducing inflammation and root resorption. (From Walton RE: *Dent Clin North Am* 41:795, 1997.)

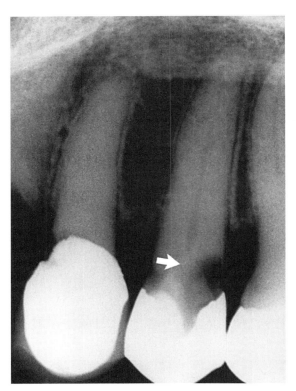

FIGURE 31-3
Restorations, caries, and time have all combined to result in dentin formation. The first premolar shows calcific metamorphosis (a very small pulp space is present). The second premolar has dentin formation *(arrow)* in response to recurrent caries. Both will be difficult to treat and restore. (From Walton RE: *Dent Clin North Am* 41:795, 1997.)

pulp chambers there is more dentin formation on the roof and floor than on the walls.[6] The result is a flattened (disc-like) chamber (Figure 31-4).

NATURE OF RESPONSE TO INJURY

The older patient does tend to have more adverse pulpal reactions to irritation than those that occur in the younger patient. The reason for these differences is debatable and not fully understood, but they are probably the result of a lifetime of cumulative injuries.

From Irritation

There are reasons for pulp pathosis after restorative procedures. First, the tooth may have experienced several injuries in the past. Second, there are likely to be more extensive procedures that involve considerable tooth structure, such as crown preparation. There are multiple potential injuries associated with a full crown: foundation place-

ment, bur preparation, impressions, temporary crown placement (often these leak), cementation, and unsealed crown margins. The coup de grace of a pulp that is already stumbling along may be that final restoration.

Age

Although it would seem that a pulp with fewer cells, blood vessels, and nerves would be less resistant to injury, this has not been proven. Pulp responses to various procedures in different age groups have not shown differences, although the large number of variables in these types of clinical studies make it difficult to isolate age as a factor. This is not necessarily the case with the immature tooth (open apex), in which pulps have indeed been shown to be more resistant to injury. There are some who theorize that pulps in older teeth may, in fact, be *more* resistant because of de-

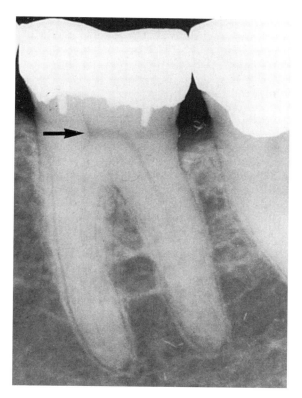

FIGURE 31-4
Disc-like chamber (arrow). The chamber is flattened because of dentin formation on the roof and floor. These chambers and canals are a challenge to locate. (From Walton RE: Dent Clin North Am 41:795, 1997.)

creased permeability of dentin.[13] Again this resistance to injury in old teeth has not been proven.[14] The bottom line is that older pulps in older patients do require more care in preparation and restoration; this is probably due to a history of previous insults rather than age per se.

Systemic Conditions

There is no conclusive evidence that systemic or medical conditions directly affect (decrease) pulp resistance to injury. One proposed condition is atherosclerosis, which has been presumed to directly affect pulp vessels[15]; however the phenomenon of pulpal atherosclerosis could not be demonstrated.[16]

Periradicular Response

Little information is available on changes of bone and soft tissues with age, and how these might affect the response to irritants or to subsequent healing after removal of those irritants. The indicators are that there is relatively little change in periradicular cellularity, vascularity, or nerve supply with aging.[17] Therefore it is unlikely that there are significantly different periapical responses in older compared with younger individuals.

Healing

There is a popular concept that healing in older individuals is impaired, compromised, or delayed compared with that in younger patients. This is not necessarily true. Studies in animals have shown remarkably similar patterns of repair of oral tissues in young versus old, but with a slight delay in healing response.[18] Radiographic evidence of healing of younger versus older patients after root canal treatment demonstrated no apparent difference in success and failure.[19] There is no evidence that vascular or connective tissue changes in older individuals result in significantly slower or in impaired healing. Overall, there is little difference in the speed or nature of healing between the different age groups; this includes both bone and soft tissue. Critical to healing is vascularity. In healthy individuals, blood flow is not impaired with age.[20]

Medically Compromised Patients

Certainly, systemic problems in the older patient tend to occur more often and with greater severity. In general, medical conditions are no more significant for endodontic procedures in the older patient than for other types of dental treatment. In fact, there is little information on the relationship of medical conditions or medically compromised patients as to adverse reactions during or after endodontic procedures.

It has been presumed that systemic conditions such as diabetes or immunosuppressant therapy would predispose an endodontic patient to infection or to delayed healing. There is no evidence that this presumption is true nor that these conditions will have more of an adverse effect in elderly patients. There is concern, however, about the person with severe, uncontrolled diabetes, who may require additional precautions and careful monitoring.[21]

Of interest is osteoporosis, a rather common condition of older women. There is evidence that osteoporosis is associated with a decrease in trabecular bone density in the jaws, particularly in the anterior maxilla and the posterior mandible.[22,23] However, it is not known whether patients with osteoporosis have impaired bony healing after root canal treatment or surgery. As related to diagnosis of periapical pathosis, osteoporotic changes are probably not of sufficient magnitude[24] to confuse pre- or post-treatment evaluation.

In summary, elderly medically compromised patients are at no more risk for complications than are other age groups. In fact, for any medically compromised patient, root canal treatment or other endodontic procedures are far less traumatic and damaging than extraction. However, one important consideration is that older patients are more likely to be taking more and stronger medications.[25] Caution is required, particularly when prescribing additional medications.

Diagnosis

Again, the same basic principles apply with older as with younger patients.

DIAGNOSTIC PROCEDURE

It is important that a routine sequence be applied to diagnosis, particularly with elderly patients. The most important findings are from the subjective examination to determine symptoms and history. Careful questioning and then allowing sufficient time for the older patient to recall and answer often yields valuable information.

Chief Complaint

Allow the patient to express the problem(s) in his or her own words. Not only will this divulge symptoms, but also it provides an opportunity to determine the patient's dental knowledge and ability to communicate; this ability may be impaired because of problems with sight, hearing, or mental status.

Medical History

The prudent diagnostician not only discusses positive responses marked on the medical history form but repeats important items that may not have been marked or were overlooked by the patient. Systemic conditions, medications, and related considerations should be discussed in depth. It is now appropriate to explain how the patient's condition might affect diagnosis, treatment planning, treatment, and outcomes.

Dental History

In general, elderly patients have a lot of history to review and recall. There may have been important dental occurrences that are only a dim memory, which require prompting by the examiner. Examples include a history of traumatic injury, fractures, caries, or pain and/or swelling.

Subjective Findings

By definition, subjective findings include information obtained by questioning the patient's description of current signs and symptoms. Many older patients are stoic. They do not readily express adverse symptoms and may consider them to be minor relative to other systemic problems or pains. A careful, concerned discussion about these seemingly minor problems also helps establish rapport and confidence.

Overall, symptoms of pulpitis do not seem to be as acute in the older patient. One reason may be that there is a reduced pulp volume and a decrease in sensory nerves,[26] particularly in dentin.

The *absence* of significant signs and symptoms is also very common, more so than the *presence*. Of course, the absence does not indicate the lack of significant pathosis; most irreversible pulpal and apical pathoses are asymptomatic at any age. Thus when pathosis is suspected, objec-

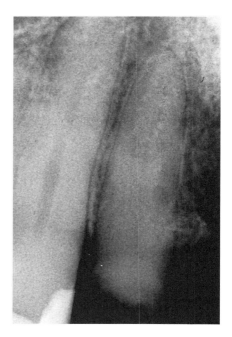

FIGURE 31-5
Calcific metamorphosis. Although there usually is vital pulp tissue, these teeth in older adults often do not respond to pulp testing because of decreased nerve supply and an increase in insulating dentin. (From Walton RE: *Dent Clin North Am* 41:795, 1997.)

tive tests are required whether or not there are significant signs and symptoms.

Objective Tests

These are primarily related to pulpal and periapical tests. Oral examination and transillumination are also commonly required.

1. *Pulp testing:* Although similar in older and younger patients, there are some differences. The pulp becomes less responsive to stimuli with age (Figure 31-5). Thus testing in older patients should be done slowly and carefully, with the use of different stimuli. It is common for a tooth with a vital pulp to be nonresponsive to one form of testing (e.g., electrical) but respond to another stimulus (e.g., cold). These results must be correlated with other tests and findings as well as with radiographs.

   There is a question of whether electric pulp tests should be used in patients with pacemakers.[27] Although it is unlikely that these tests could cause a pacemaker to malfunction, there usually are other tests that can be used safely to give information on pulp status.

   A test cavity is often indicated but may not be as useful in the older patient because of reduced dentin innervation. A false-negative (no response/vital pulp) response is not unusual, even with a test cavity.

2. *Periapical testing:* Percussion (biting and tapping) and palpation tests indicate periapical inflammation but are not particularly useful unless the patient reports significant pain. These are most useful to confirm that such symptoms are indeed from a particular tooth and determine the severity of response.

RADIOGRAPHIC FINDINGS

Current, good quality periapical films are always necessary; the same principles apply as in the younger patient. The techniques of making radiographs are similar but with some differences. Bony growths such as tori and muscle attachments (frena) may affect film positioning. Also, the older patient may have difficulty in placing the film; holders should be used. Generally, a parallel film is preferred for diagnosis with occasional supplementation of mesially or distally angled cone positioning or a Panelipse or occlusal view. Often bitewing projections are helpful in showing chamber size and location and relative depths of caries and restorations.

Apically, there may be some differences in the older patient. The incidence of nonendodontic pathosis of the jaws tends to increase with age; careful determination of pulp status is even more important in these situations when the nature of the pathosis is uncertain. If the pulp is vital, a lesion in the apical region is not endodontic.

Radiographs are studied for pulp size and for root and pulp anatomy. Again, pulps tend to be smaller and may disappear radiographically (Figure 31-6). Importantly, nonvisualization of a pulp space does not mean that a pulp is not present. In

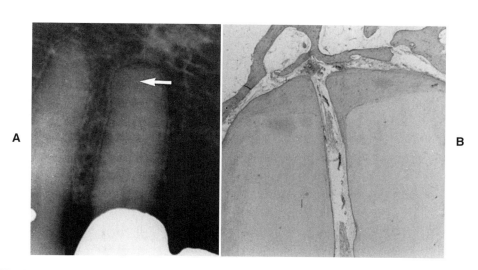

FIGURE 31-6
A, Although the pulp is barely visible apically *(arrow)*, a corresponding histologic section of this region (**B**) shows a sizable pulp space containing vital tissue. (From Walton RE: *Dent Clin North Am* 41:795, 1997.)

fact, it has been demonstrated[28] that there is always a pulp space, even when it is not visible radiographically. Apical root and canal anatomy tends to be somewhat different in elderly patients because of continued cementum formation.[29,30] This may be further complicated by apical root resorption from pathosis.[31]

Differential Diagnosis

This is the ultimate determination of whether there is an endodontic or another type of pathosis and, if endodontic, the specific details of the pulp or periapical lesion.

ENDODONTIC PATHOSIS

Signs and symptoms, test results, and other observations in the older patient should follow a fairly consistent pattern. There may be the complications of mind-altering medications as well as occasional perceptive problems in elderly patients. Vague symptoms that cannot be localized or do not follow an identifiable pattern probably are not endodontic in origin. Other pathosis or nonpathologic entities must then be considered.

OTHER PATHOSES

These include numerous entities, many of which are more common in elderly patients. The lesion

that commonly mimics endodontic pathosis is periodontal. Nonendodontic symptomatic disorders that may mimic endodontic pathosis include headaches, temporomandibular joint dysfunction, and neuritis and neuralgia. The incidence of these tends to increase somewhat with age, particularly in patients who have specific disorders such as arthritis that may affect the joints.

Differentiating periodontal from endodontic pathosis is a common problem because of the increasing incidence of both endodontic and periodontal disease. Usually the underlying problem is either periodontic or endodontic, with few true combined lesions (see Chapter 26). Radiographic changes, swellings, sinus tracts, and deep probing defects may be either endodontic or periodontal in origin. Although all findings should be considered, the ultimate indicator is pulp testing. If the pulp is indeed vital, the problem is periodontal. If the pulp is necrotic, the likelihood is that the problem is endodontic. Pulp tests are critical; a test cavity may be helpful.

Treatment Planning and Case Selection

After differential diagnosis, a definitive treatment plan is determined—usually root canal treatment, but including additional procedures. Everything should be considered (restorability, periodontal status, and overall treatment plan). This would be

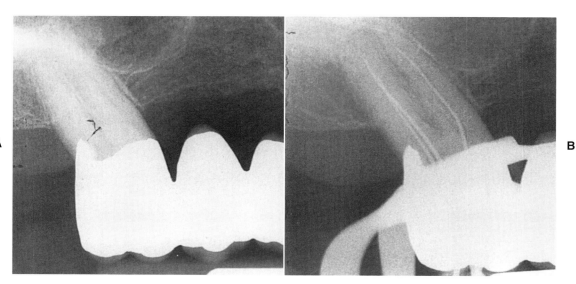

FIGURE 31-7
A, Castings are frequently misoriented due to tipping and rotation. **B,** Access is more challenging; observation before and caution during access are critical to avoid perforation. (From Walton RE: *Dent Clin North Am* 41:795, 1997.)

the time to consider referral of the patient to an endodontist if the situation is deemed too complex.

PROCEDURE

Whatever the treatment, procedures are generally more technically complex in older patients. Extensive restorations, a history of multiple carious insults, periodontal involvement, decreasing pulp size, tipping (Figure 31-7) and rotation are all factors. An original treatment plan often has to be modified during the procedure because of unexpected findings. For example, root canal treatment may be initiated only to find that a canal cannot be located or negotiated; periradicular surgery then becomes a necessity (Figure 31-8). These possibilities should be explained to the patient, preferably before treatment is begun.

PROGNOSIS

Although periradicular tissues will heal as readily in elderly as in young patients,[32,33] there are many factors that reduce the rate of success. The same factors that complicate treatment also may compromise ultimate success. An extensively restored tooth is more prone to coronal leakage. Canals that cannot be negotiated to length may contain persistent irritants. Tipped or rotated teeth restored with castings that are misaligned are more difficult to access and therefore to clean, shape, and obturate.

Each patient should have a pretreatment and post-treatment assessment of prognosis. The pretreatment assessment is the anticipated outcome; the post-treatment assessment reviews what should happen according to modifiers determined during treatment. Many teeth are severely compromised and would be a problem to retain (Figure 31-9). Extraction is often the preferred approach; a recent study[34] on the outcome of not replacing a missing tooth showed that the consequences generally were not significant. Thus when extraction is discussed as an option, the patient is informed that "filling the space" may be unnecessary.

NUMBER OF APPOINTMENTS

Whether to treat in a single visit or in multiple visits has always been a subject of debate and conjecture. Studies have shown that, overall, there are no advantages to multiple appointments relating to post-treatment pain or prognosis. However, with pulp necrosis, treatment in multiple appointments and the use of calcium hydroxide as an intracanal medicament may speed healing,[35] and longer term better outcomes were conclusively demonstrated.[36]

There are benefits to single appointment procedures in elderly patients. Longer appointments may be less of a problem than several shorter appointments if the patient must rely on others for transportation or requires assistance to reach

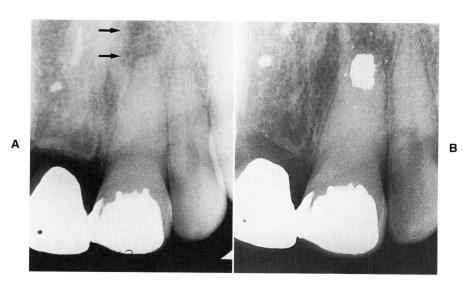

FIGURE 31-8
A, Calcific metamorphosis and apical pathosis *(arrows)* after trauma. In this tooth, conventional access would be difficult and would jeopardize retention of the bridge. **B,** A surgical approach was used with the hope of sealing in irritants apically. (From Walton RE: *Dent Clin North Am* 41:795, 1997.)

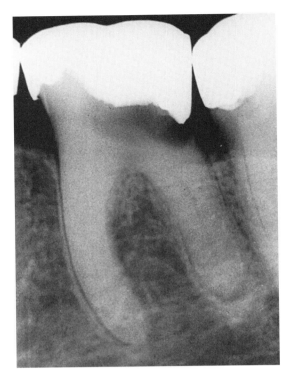

FIGURE 31-9
Recurrent caries have created challenges in retaining this molar. Crown lengthening would be necessary both for restoration and isolation during root canal treatment. Crown lengthening may infringe upon the furcation. Canals would be difficult to locate and negotiate. The tooth probably should be extracted. (From Walton RE: *Dent Clin North Am* 41:795, 1997.)

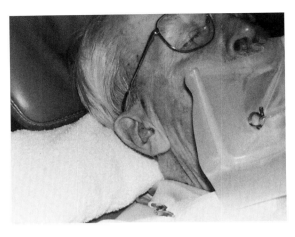

FIGURE 31-10
Elderly patients often have postural problems. This patient is made comfortable with a rolled-up towel, forming a brace under his neck.

the office or to get in the chair. At times, the elderly patient may require special positioning of the chair, support of the back or neck or limbs, or other such considerations (Figure 31-10). These problems may require shorter, multiple appointments.

ADDITIONAL CONSIDERATIONS

In treatment planning for elderly patients there is a tendency to plan according to anticipated longevity.[37] It is natural to assume that procedures need not be as permanent because the patient may not live for very long. The concept that treatment should not outlast the patient is not accepted by most elderly patients, who desire health care equivalent to that rendered to younger patients. Esthetic and functional concerns may be no different.

Root Canal Treatment

TREATMENT CONSIDERATIONS
Time Required

On average, longer appointments are necessary to accomplish the same procedures in elderly patients for the reasons discussed earlier.

Anesthesia

Primary injections. The need for anesthesia is somewhat less in the older patient. It is necessary for vital pulps but is often unnecessary for pulp necrosis, obturation appointments, and retreatments. Older patients tend to be less sensitive and are more likely to prefer procedures without anesthetic. Also, they tend to be less anxious and therefore have a higher threshold of pain. Although there are no differences in effectiveness of anesthetic solutions, various systemic problems or medications may preclude the use of vasoconstrictors.

Supplemental injections. Intraosseous, periodontal ligament (PDL), and intrapulpal anesthesia are effective adjuncts if the primary anesthesia is not give adequate. Again, certain cardiac conditions may preclude the use of epinephrine, particularly with the intraosseous and PDL techniques. Duration of anesthesia is considerably decreased without a vasoconstrictor; reinjection during the procedure may be required.

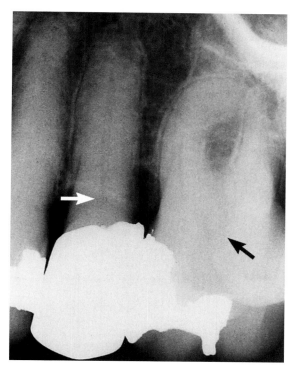

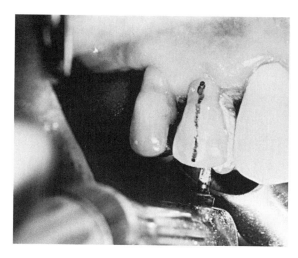

FIGURE 31-12
Aids in orientation during access. The preparation is initiated without the rubber dam in place. A mark to guide the bur is placed on the crown in the long axis of the root. (From Walton RE: *Dent Clin North Am* 41:795, 1997.)

FIGURE 31-11
Age, caries, and restorations have resulted in small chambers *(arrows)*; either would be a challenge to access.

Procedures

Isolation. Isolation is often difficult because of subgingival caries and/or defective restorations. However, placement of a rubber dam is imperative, often requiring ingenuity (see Chapter 8). A fluid-tight isolation reduces salivary contamination of the pulp space and prevents introduction of irrigants into the mouth. If there are questions about the integrity of a restoration, it should be removed before rubber dam placement. Also, temporary crowns, orthodontic bands, or temporary restorations should be removed in their entirety; improved visibility and good isolation are more predictable.

Access preparation. Achieving good access to enable locating and then negotiating canal orifices is challenging in old teeth because of internal anatomy (Figure 31-11). Radiographs are helpful. A slightly larger rather than a too small access opening is preferred, particularly through large restorations such as crowns. Magnification is also helpful, either from a microscope or other vision aids.

A supra-erupted tooth, as a result of caries or restoration, has a short clinical crown, requiring a less deep access preparation. The distance from the reference cusp to the chamber roof should be measured on the bur radiographically. A very small or nonvisible chamber may be an indication for beginning the access without the rubber dam; this aids in staying in the long axis of the tooth (Figure 31-12). Once the canal is located, the rubber dam is immediately placed before working length radiographs are made.

Locating canal orifices is often fatiguing and frustrating to both clinician and patient. Although a reasonable period of time should be allocated, there is a limit. It may be best to stop and have the patient return for another appointment. Often, the canals are readily located at a subsequent visit. This also is a time to consider a referral; another procedure, such as surgery, may be indicated.

Working length. There are some differences in the older patient.[38] Because the apical foramen varies more widely (Figure 31-13) than in the younger tooth and because of decreased diameter of the canal apically, it is more difficult to determine the preferred length.[29] In teeth of any age, materials and instruments are best confined to the canal space. One to 2 mm short of the radiographic apex is the preferred working and obturation length[39]; this should be decreased if an apical stop is not detected.

Cleaning and shaping. A common challenge is a much smaller canal that requires more time

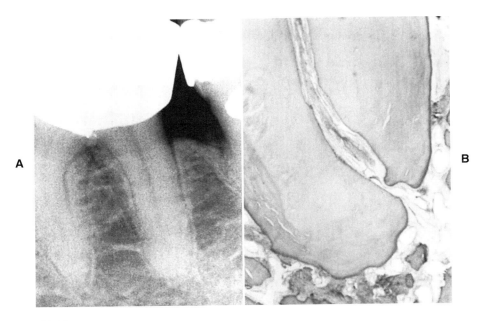

FIGURE 31-13
Variability in apical foramen location. **A,** The foramen is not visible radiographically. **B,** Histologically, the distal root shows the foramen to be well short of the apex. (From Walton RE: *Dent Clin North Am* 41:795, 1997.)

and effort to enlarge. A very small canal may be more easily negotiated and initially prepared with a lubricant, such as glycerin. This may be used through two or three smaller sizes of files to facilitate enlarging as well as to reduce the risk of binding and separation. The same principles of débridement and adequate shaping are followed.

Intracanal medicaments. These are contraindicated, with the exception of calcium hydroxide. This chemical is antimicrobial, inhibits bacterial growth between appointments, and may reduce periradicular inflammation.[40] It is indicated if the pulp is necrotic and the canal preparation is essentially complete.

Obturation. There is no demonstrated preferred approach, although cold-lateral and warm-vertical gutta-percha obturations are the most commonly used and the best documented.

Impact of Restoration

Generally the larger and deeper the restoration, the more complicated the root canal treatment. The old tooth is more likely to have a full crown. There are two concerns: (1) potential damage to retention or components of the crown and (2) blockage of access and poor internal visibility.

The porcelain-fused-to-metal crown is more common than a full metal crown and creates additional problems. Porcelain may fracture or craze. This problem is minimized by using burs specifically designed to prepare through porcelain[41] combined with slow cutting and copious use of water spray. Occlusal access is wide (Figure 31-14). Metal should not be removed after the chamber is opened to prevent metal shavings from entering and blocking canals. An access through a PFM or a gold crown (either anterior or posterior) that is to be retained, is best permanently repaired with amalgam. Anterior nonmetallic crowns may be repaired with composite.

Retreatment

Factors that lead to failure tend to increase with age; thus retreatment is more common in older patients. Retreatment at any age is often complicated and should be approached with caution; these patients should be considered for referral. Retreatment procedures and outcomes are similar in both older and younger teeth.

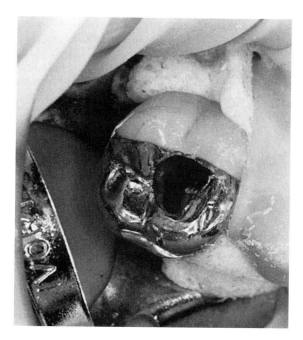

FIGURE 31-14
Access through a porcelain-fused-to-metal crown. The outline is large for visibility. Also, the preparation does not extend to the porcelain to avoid fracturing it. (From Walton RE: *Dent Clin North Am* 41:795, 1997.)

Endodontic Surgery

Considerations and indications for surgery are similar in elderly and younger patients. These include incision for drainage, periradicular procedures, corrective surgery, root removal, and intentional replantation. Overall, the incidence of most of these will increase with age. Small non-negotiable canals, resorptions, and canal blockages occur more often with age. Perforation during access or preparation, ledging, and instrument separation are related to restorative and anatomic problems.

MEDICAL CONSIDERATIONS

These may require consultation and are of concern but generally do not contraindicate a surgical approach.[42] This is particularly true when extraction is the alternative; surgery is often less traumatic.[43]

Excessive hemorrhage during or after surgery is of concern; many elderly patients are receiving anticoagulant therapy. Interestingly, recent studies examined bleeding patterns in oral surgery patients taking low-dose aspirin[44] and prescribed anticoagulants.[45,46] The findings were that anticoagulant therapy should preferably not be altered and that hemorrhage was controllable by local hemostatic agents.

BIOLOGIC AND ANATOMIC FACTORS

Bony and soft tissues are similar and respond the same in older and younger patients. There may be somewhat less thickness of overlying soft tissue; however, alveolar mucosa and gingiva seem to be structurally similar. Anatomic structures such as the sinuses, floor of the nose, and location of neurovascular bundles are essentially unchanged. Often, periodontal and endodontic surgery must be combined. Also, crown-to-root ratios may be compromised because of periodontal disease or root resorption.

HEALING AFTER SURGERY

Hard and soft tissues will heal as predictably although somewhat more slowly.[47-49] Postsurgical instructions should be given both verbally and in writing to minimize complications. If the patient has cognitive problems, instructions are repeated to the person accompanying the patient. Even very elderly patients will have good healing, provided they follow post-treatment protocols. Ice and pressure (in particular) applied over the surgical area reduces bleeding and edema and minimizes swelling. Overall, older patients experience no more significant adverse affects from surgery than do younger patients; outcomes are more dependent on oral hygiene than on age per se, as has been shown in periodontal surgery patients.[50]

One problem that seems to be more prevalent in older patients is ecchymosis after surgery. This is hemorrhage that often spreads widely through underlying tissue and commonly presents as discoloration (Figure 31-15). Patients are informed that this may occur and that it is not of concern. Normal color may take 1 to 2 weeks or longer to return. In addition, the discoloration may go through different color phases (purple, red, yellow, green) before disappearing.

Bleaching

Both internal and external tooth discoloration occurs in older patients.[13] Internal discoloration is related to dental (restorative or endodontic) procedures or to an increase in dentin formation with a loss of translucency. External discoloration occurs from stains and restorative procedures as well (see Figure 31-1). Overall, teeth tend to discolor with time and with age. Both external and

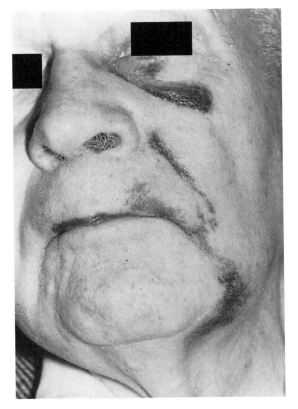

FIGURE 31-15
Postsurgical ecchymosis. Root-end surgery of a maxillary lateral incisor resulted in widespread migration of hemorrhage into the tissues, with resultant discoloration. This is not an uncommon occurrence in elderly patients. No treatment is indicated, and the problem resolves in 1 to 2 weeks.

internal bleaching procedures can be successful in these patients.

EXTERNAL STAINS

These are on, or close to, the enamel surface and are best managed by conventional night guard/oxidizing gel techniques.

INTERNAL STAINS

Stains that are most amenable to internal bleaching are related to discoloration after root canal treatment or pulp necrosis. The considerations related to diagnosis, etiology, treatment planning, and prognosis for successful short-term and long-term internal bleaching are detailed in Chapter 23. Often discolorations in these teeth can be significantly resolved, much to the satisfaction of the older patient.

Teeth that are discolored because of increased amounts of dentin formation and loss of translucency generally should not be considered for internal bleaching, which would require root canal treatment first. External bleaching may lighten the teeth somewhat.

Restorative Considerations

OVERDENTURE ABUTMENTS

This involves the reduction of a root to permit the resting of a removable partial or complete denture on a restored or natural root face.

An important consideration is that, although a pulp space may not be evident on a radiograph (Figure 31-16), usually small components of the pulp chamber extend into the crown.[28] Reduction would create an clinically undetectable exposure. If untreated, this will result in pulp necrosis. Teeth to be reduced for overdenture abutments should have root canal treatment followed by an appropriate restoration to seal the access. Amalgam, composite resin, and glass ionomer are adequate materials.[51]

CORONAL SEAL

In the elderly (as in the younger) patient, the coronal surface must be sealed from oral fluids forever to prevent failure. A concern for elderly patients is that the dentist will be less careful with the design and placement of a restoration or select less durable materials. In addition, the older patient is likely to be more susceptible to recurrent caries or abrasion, particularly on cervical root surfaces. These lesions do not have to penetrate as deeply to expose the obturating material. Subsequent to this exposure will be contamination of the obturating material by saliva and bacteria with resultant periapical pathosis. Again, this is probably the number one cause of treatment failure and reason for retreatment.

Trauma

Traumatic injuries occur in elderly patients more commonly with recreational activity and because of postural instability and loss of coordination. Generally, the older patient who experiences facial trauma will have different concerns and require some differing approaches than the younger patient.[52]

A major issue is that there may be cranial injuries that are masked by the obvious superficial facial trauma. Evidence of such injuries, as shown

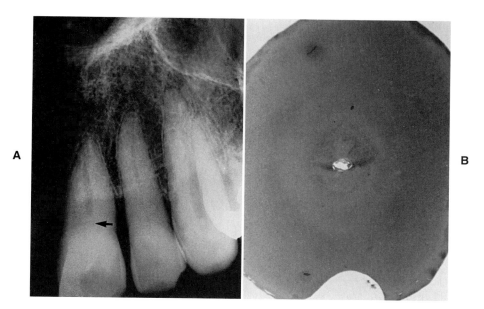

FIGURE 31-16
A, This central incisor was cross-sectioned at the level of the *arrow,* where no pulp space is visible. **B,** Histologically, a small pulp space is apparent. Reducing such a tooth for overdentures would result in pulp exposure. (From Walton RE: *Dent Clin North Am* 41:795, 1997.)

by in-office tests (see Chapter 25), would require an immediate hospital emergency room visit. Other concerns would be similar to those discussed earlier in this chapter: medical status, cognitive factors, and patient expectations. In conjunction with these considerations, the actual management of the hard and soft tissues would be similar to and have an expected outcome much like that of a younger patient.

Many of these elderly trauma patients may have initial injury management by a generalist and then be referred to an oral surgeon for facial injury assessment. Follow-up, long-term dentition care may then be best managed by the endodontist.

REFERENCES

1. Meskin L, Berg R: Impact of older adults on private dental practices, 1988-1998, *J Am Dent Assoc* 131:1188, 2000.
2. Berkey D, Berg R, Ettinger R, et al: The old-old dental patient, *J Am Dent Assoc* 127:321, 1996.
3. Marcus S, Drury T, Brown L, Zion G: Tooth retention and tooth loss in the permanent dentition of adults: United States, 1988-1991, *J Dent Res* 75 (special issue): 684, 1996.
4. Lloyd P: Oral and dental problems. In Yoshikawa T, Coobbs E, Brummel-Smith K, editors: *Practical ambulatory geriatrics,* ed 2, St Louis, 1998, Mosby.
5. Lloyd P: Fixed prosthodontics and esthetic considerations for the older adult, *J Prosthet Dent* 72:525, 1994.
6. Bernick S, Nedelman C: Effect of aging on the human pulp, *J Endod* 3:88, 1975.
7. Fried K: Changes in innervation of dentine and pulp with age. In Ferguson DB, editor: *The aging mouth,* New York, 1987, Karger.
8. Stanley H, Ranney R: Age changes in the human dental pulp: the quantity of collagen, *Oral Surg* 15:1396, 1962.
9. Barkhorder R, Linder D, Bui D: Pulp stones and aging [Abstract 669], *J Dent Res* 69 (special issue):192, 1990.
10. Sayegh F, Reed A: Calcification in the dental pulp, *Oral Surg Oral Med Oral Pathol* 25:873, 1968.
11. Philippas GG, Applebaum E: Age changes in the permanent upper canine teeth, *J Dent Res* 47:411, 1968.
12. Morse D, Esposito J, Schoor R, et al: A review of aging of dental components and a retrospective radiographic study of aging of the dental pulp and dentin in normal teeth, *Quintessence Int* 22:711, 1991.
13. Ketterl W: Age-induced changes in the teeth and their attachment apparatus, *Int Dent J* 33:262, 1983.
14. Stanley H: The factors of age and tooth size in human pulpal reactions, *Oral Surg Oral Med Oral Pathol* 14:498, 1961.
15. Bernick S: Age changes in the blood supply to human teeth, *J Dent Res* 46:544, 1967.
16. Krell K, McMurtrey L, Walton R: Vasculature of the dental pulp of atherosclerotic monkeys: light and electron microscopic findings, *J Endod* 20:469, 1994.
17. VanDerVelden V: Effect of age on the periodontium, *J Clin Periodontol* 11:281, 1984.

18. Hill H: Influence of age on the response of oral mucosa to injury. In Squier C, Hill M, editors: *Effect of aging in oral mucosa and skin,* Boca Raton, Fla, 1994, CRC Press.

19. Swift M, Wilcox L: Age and endodontic prognoses, *J Dent Res* 68 (special issue):142, 1989.

20. Johnson G: Effects of aging on microvasculature and microcirculation in skin and oral mucosa. In Squier C, Hill M, editors: *Effect of aging in oral mucosa and skin,* Boca Raton, Fla, 1994, CRC Press.

21. Murrah V: Diabetes mellitus and associated oral manifestations: a review, *J Oral Pathol* 14:271, 1985.

22. Jeffcoat M: Osteoporosis: a possible modifying factor in oral bone loss, *Ann Periodontol* 3:312, 1998.

23. White S, Rudolph D: Alterations of the trabecular pattern of the jaws in patients with osteoporosis, *Oral Surg Oral Med Oral Pathol Oral Radiol Endod* 88:628, 1999.

24. Mohajery M, Brooks S: Oral radiographs in the detection of early signs of osteoporosis, *Oral Surg Oral Med Oral Pathol Oral Radiol Endod* 73:112, 1992.

25. Miller C: Documenting medication use in adult dental patients: 1987-1991, *J Am Dent Assoc* 123:41, 1992.

26. Bernick S: Effect of aging on the nerve supply to human teeth, *J Dent Res* 46:694, 1967.

27. Woodly L, Woodworth J, Dobbs J: A preliminary evaluation of the effect of electric pulp testers on dogs with artificial pacemakers, *J Am Dent Assoc* 89:1099, 1974.

28. Kuyk J, Walton R: Comparison of the radiographic appearance of root canal size to its actual diameter, *J Endod* 16:528, 1990.

29. Zander H, Hurzeler B: Continuous cementum apposition, *J Dent Res* 37:1035, 1958.

30. Nitzan D, Michaeli Y, Weinreb M, et al: The effect of aging on tooth morphology: A study on impacted teeth, *Oral Surg Oral Med Oral Pathol Oral Radiol Endod* 61:54,1986.

31. Malueg L, Wilcox L, Johnson W: Examination of external apical root resorption with scanning electron microscopy, *Oral Surg Oral Med Oral Pathol Oral Radiol Endod* 82:89, 1996.

32. Barbakow F, Cleaton-Jones P, Friedman D: An evaluation of 566 cases of root canal therapy in general dental practice: postoperative observations, *J Endod* 6:485, 1980.

33. Swartz D, Skidmore A, Griffin J: Twenty years of endodontic success and failure, *J Endod* 9:198, 1983.

34. Shugars D, Bader J, Phillips W, et al: The consequences of not replacing a missing posterior tooth, *J Am Dent Assoc* 131:1317, 2000.

35. Trope M, Delano E, Ørstavik D: Endodontic treatment of teeth with apical periodontitis: single- vs multi-visit treatment, *J Endod* 25:245, 1999.

36. Weiger R, Rosendahl R, Lost C: Influence of calcium hydroxide intracanal dressings on the prognosis of

37. teeth with endodontically induced periapical lesions, *Int Endod J* 33:219, 2000.

37. Braun R, Marcus M: Comparing treatment decisions for elderly and young dental patients, *Gerodontics* 1:138, 1985.

38. Stein T, Corcoran J: Anatomy of the root apex and its histologic changes with age, *Oral Surg Oral Med Oral Pathol Oral Radiol Endod* 69:238, 1990.

39. Wu M-K, Wesselink P, Walton R: Apical terminus of root canal treatment procedures, *Oral Surg Oral Med Oral Pathol Oral Radiol Endod* 89:99, 2000.

40. Katebzadeh N, Sigurdsson A, Trope M: Radiographic evaluation of periapical healing after obturation of infected root canals: an in vivo study, *Int Endod J* 33:60, 2000.

41. Haselton D, Lloyd P, Johnson W: An in-vitro comparison of the effect of two burs used for endodontic access on all-ceramic high lucite crowns, *Oral Surg Oral Med Oral Pathol Oral Radiol Endod* 89:486, 2000.

42. Campbell J, Huizinga P, Das S, et al: Incidence and significance of cardiac arrhythmia in geriatric oral surgery patients, *Oral Surg Oral Med Oral Pathol Oral Radiol Endod* 82:42,1996.

43. Ingle J: Geriatric endodontics, *Alpha Omegan* 79:47, 1986.

44. Ardekian L, Gaspar R, Peled M, et al: Does low-dose aspirin therapy complicate oral surgical procedures? *J Am Dent Assoc* 131:331, 2000.

45. Blinder D, Manor Y, Martinowitz U, Taicher S: Dental extractions in patients maintained on continued oral anticoagulant: comparison of local hemostatic modalities, *Oral Surg Oral Med Oral Pathol Oral Radiol Endod* 88:137, 1999.

46. Wahl M: Myths of dental surgery in patients receiving anticoagulant therapy, *J Am Dent Assoc* 131:77, 2000.

47. Stahl S, Witkin G, Cantor N, et al: Gingival healing: II. Clinical and histological repair sequences following gingivectomy, *J Periodontol* 39:109, 1968.

48. Holm-Pedersen P, Löe H: Wound healing in the gingiva of young and old individuals, *Scand J Dent Res* 79:40, 1971.

49. Rapp E, Brown C Jr, Newton C: An analysis of success and failure of apicoectomies, *J Endod* 17:10, 1991.

50. Lindhe J, Socransky S, Nyman S, et al: Effect of age on healing following periodontal therapy, *J Clin Periodontol* 12:774, 1985.

51. Keltjens H, Creugers T, van't Hof M, Creugers N: A 4-year clinical study on amalgam, resin composite and resin-modified glass ionomer cement restorations in overdenture abutments, *J Dent* 27:551, 1999.

52. Marciani R: Critical systemic and psychosocial considerations in management of trauma in the elderly, *Oral Surg Oral Med Oral Pathol Oral Radiol Endod* 87:272, 1999.

Lisa R. Wilcox

Pulpal Anatomy and Access Preparations

The illustrations in this section depict the size, shape, and location of the pulp space within each tooth, as well as the more common morphologic variations. Based on this knowledge of the shape of the pulp and its spatial relationship to the crown and root, the correct outline form for access preparation is presented from both the occlusal-lingual and proximal views. From these illustrations, the following features can be observed:

1. The *location* of access on posterior teeth relative to occlusal landmarks such as marginal ridges and cusp tips.

2. The *size* and *appearance* of the access on anterior teeth as viewed from the incisal surface.
3. The *approximate size* of the access opening.
4. The *location of canal orifices* and their positions relative to occlusal landmarks and to each other.
5. The *canal curvatures* and the location of the apical formamens.
6. The *configuration of the chamber* and cervical portion of the canals following straight-line access preparation.
7. The *root curvatures* that are most common.

Each illustration gives the following information:

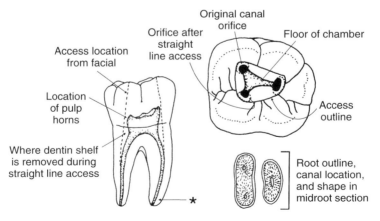

Original canal orifice
Orifice after straight line access
Floor of chamber
Access location from facial
Location of pulp horns
Access outline
Where dentin shelf is removed during straight line access
Root outline, canal location, and shape in midroot section
*

*Most common root curvatures

In addition, the percentages of the more common morphologic variations of the roots and canals are given. With many of the tooth groups, the percentages do not total 100 percent. The remaining percentage represents the less common variations not illustrated. Percentages are approx-imate to give general information, primarily to demonstrate relative occurrences. The more common root and canal curvatures are included. These are curvatures not readily identified on radiographs, that is, toward the facial and lingual aspects.

Maxillary Right Central Incisor

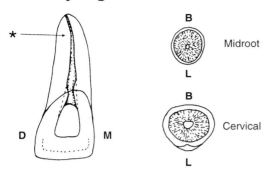

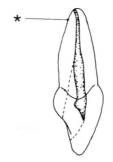

B

Midroot

L

B

Cervical

L

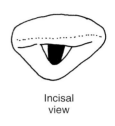

*

Incisal
view

1 canal: 100%

*Most common root curvatures

Maxillary Right Lateral Incisor

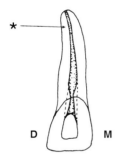

B

Midroot

L

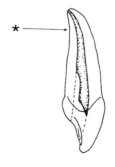

*

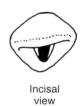

Incisal
view

1 canal: 100%

*Most common root curvatures

Maxillary Right Canine

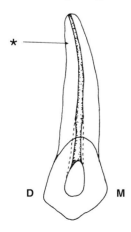

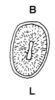

B

Midroot

L

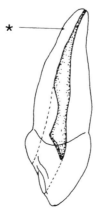

*

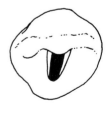

Incisal
view

1 canal: 100%

*Most common root curvatures

Maxillary Right First Premolar

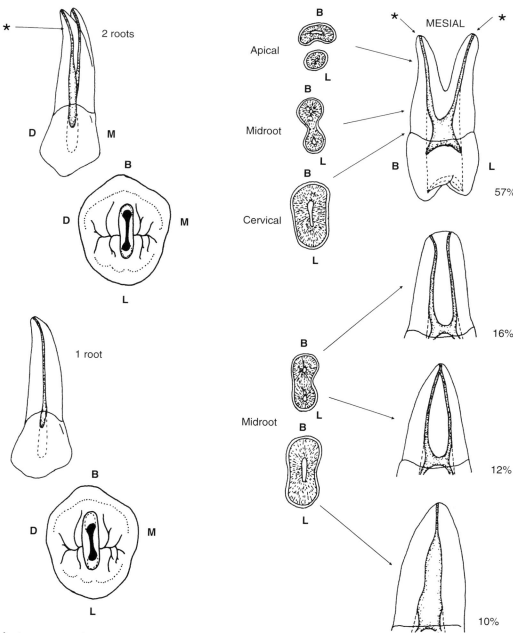

2 roots

1 root

*Most common root curvatures

Maxillary Right Second Premolar

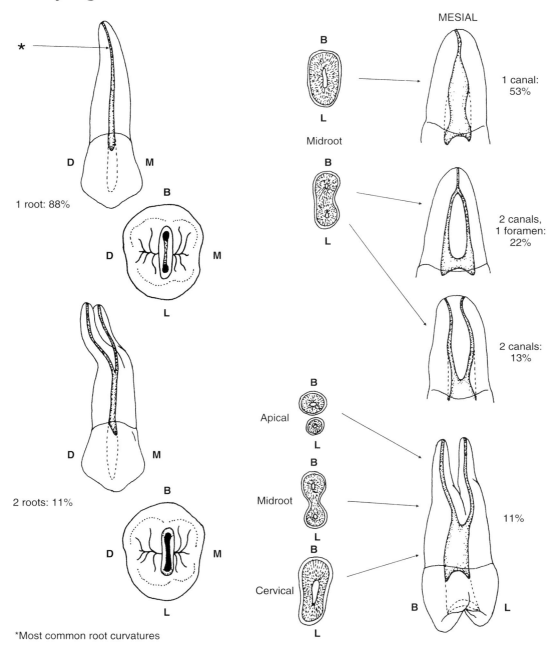

MESIAL

B

L

Midroot

1 canal:
53%

2 canals,
1 foramen:
22%

2 canals:
13%

Apical

Midroot

Cervical

11%

*

D   M

1 root: 88%

B

D   M

L

D   M

2 roots: 11%

B

D   M

L

*Most common root curvatures

Maxillary Right First Molar

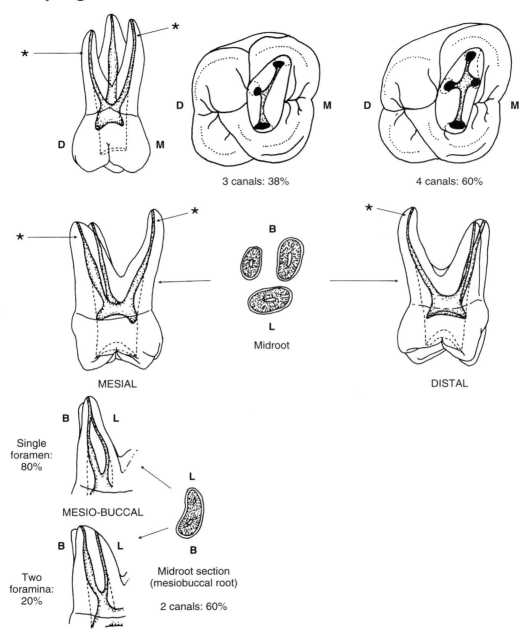

3 canals: 38%

4 canals: 60%

B

L

Midroot

MESIAL

DISTAL

Single
foramen:
80%

B   L

MESIO-BUCCAL

L

Two
foramina:
20%

B   L

Midroot section
(mesiobuccal root)

2 canals: 60%

B

*Most common root curvatures

Maxillary Right Second Molar

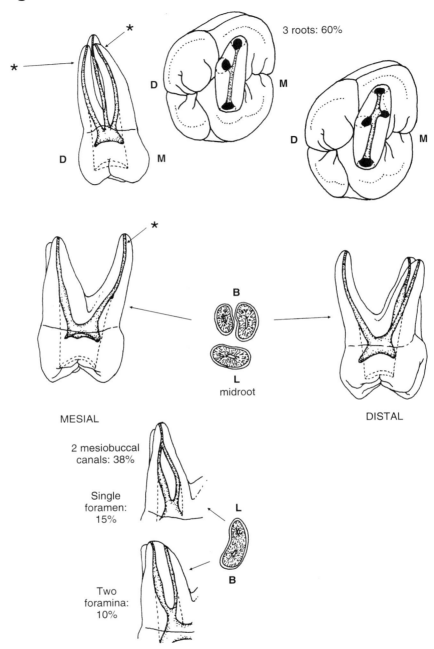

3 roots: 60%

D M

D M

D

B

L
midroot

M

MESIAL

DISTAL

2 mesiobuccal
canals: 38%

Single
foramen:
15%

L

Two
foramina:
10%

B

*Most common root curvatures

Maxillary Right Second Molar

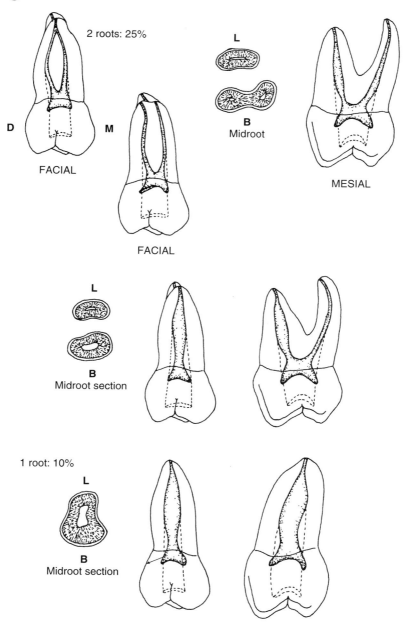

2 roots: 25%

D   M

FACIAL

L

B
Midroot

MESIAL

FACIAL

L

B
Midroot section

1 root: 10%

L

B
Midroot section

*Most common root curvatures

Mandibular Right Central and Lateral Incisor

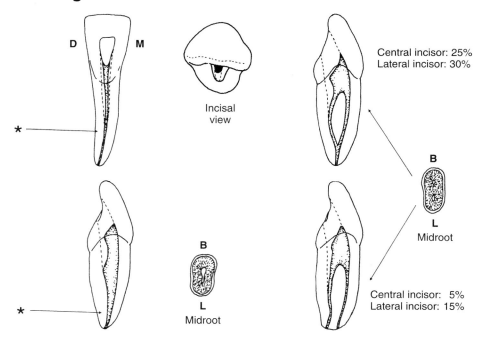

Incisal view

B
L
Midroot

Central incisor: 25%
Lateral incisor: 30%

B
L
Midroot

Central incisor: 5%
Lateral incisor: 15%

*Most common root curvatures

Mandibular Right Canine

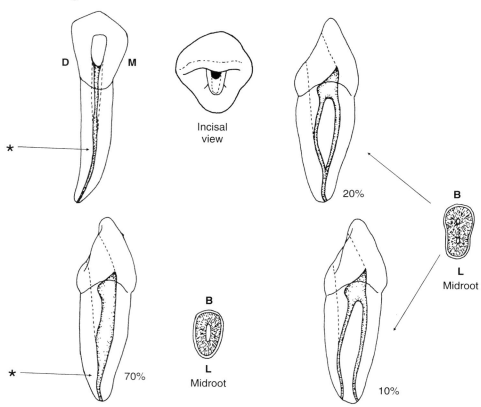

Incisal view

B
L
Midroot

20%

B
L
Midroot

70%

10%

*Most common root curvatures

Mandibular Right First Premolar

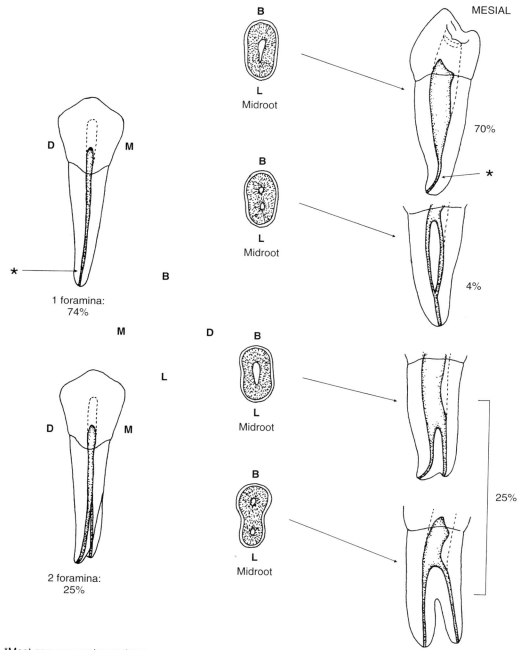

1 foramina:
74%

2 foramina:
25%

B
L
Midroot

B
L
Midroot

B
L
Midroot

B
L
Midroot

MESIAL

70%

4%

25%

*Most common root curvatures

Mandibular Right Second Premolar

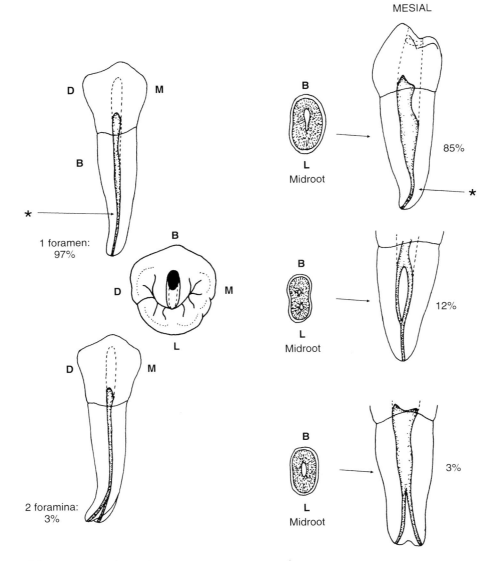

MESIAL

B
L
Midroot

85%

*

B
L
Midroot

12%

B
L
Midroot

3%

D   M

B

*

1 foramen:
97%

B
D   M
L

D   M

2 foramina:
3%

*Most common root curvatures

Mandibular Right First Molar

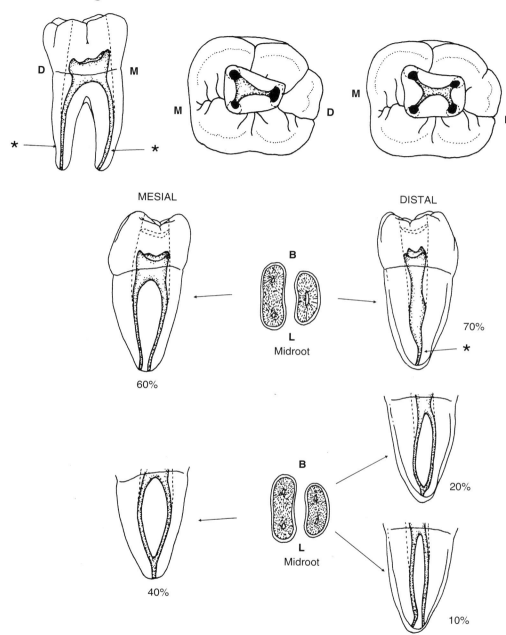

MESIAL

DISTAL

B

L
Midroot

60%

70%

B

L
Midroot

40%

20%

10%

*Most common root curvatures

Mandibular Right Second Molar

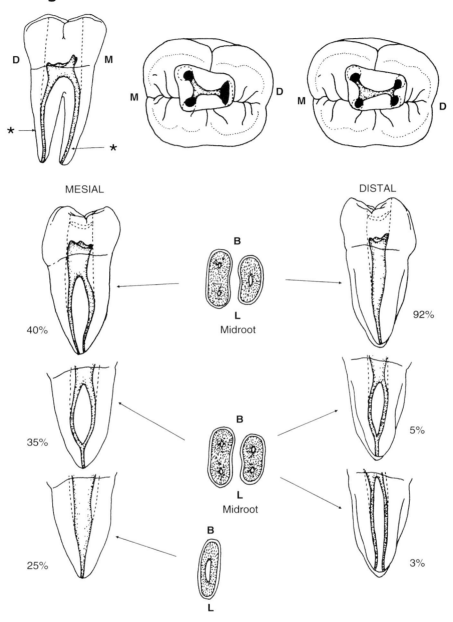

MESIAL

DISTAL

B

L
Midroot

40%

92%

35%

B

L
Midroot

5%

25%

B

L

3%

*Most common root curvatures

Mandibular Right Second Molar

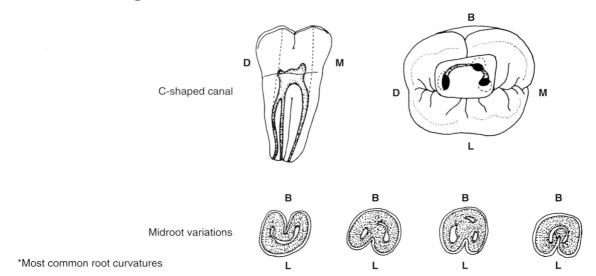

C-shaped canal

Midroot variations

*Most common root curvatures

Some Uncommon Variations

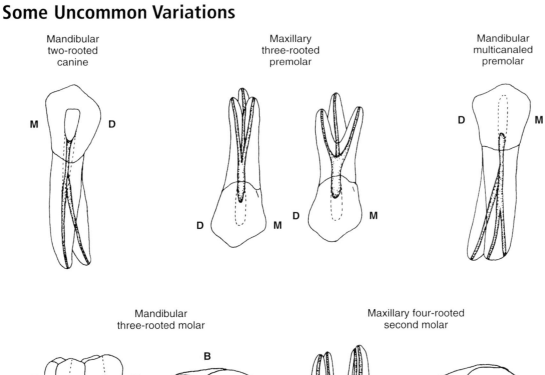

Mandibular
two-rooted
canine

Maxillary
three-rooted
premolar

Mandibular
multicanaled
premolar

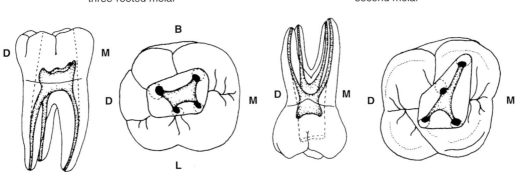

Mandibular
three-rooted molar

Maxillary four-rooted
second molar

Examples of access openings prepared in extracted teeth are given here. It is important to recognize: (1) the location of the access relative to occlusal or lingual landmarks (marginal ridge and cusp tips) and (2) the size and shape of the access relative to the size and shape of the occlusal or lingual surface.

1. Maxillary lateral
2. Mandibular canine
3. Maxillary premolar
4. Four-canal maxillary molar (*arrow* indicates dentin shelf covering mesiolingual orifice)
5. Three-canal mandibular molar
6. Four-canal mandibular molar

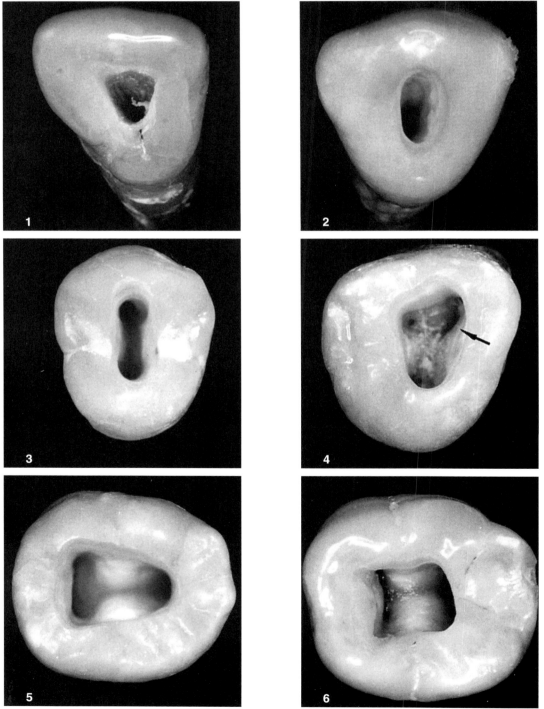

A

Abrasion, 384
Access preparation
    anterior teeth, 195-196, 197f
    burs, 191, 192f-193f
    caries considerations, 187-188
    difficult-to-locate canals, 191
    errors in, 221-222
    misorientation during, 196-198, 198f
    perforation during, 198, 199f, 203,
        311-319
    permanent restoration considera-
        tions, 188
    posterior teeth, 196
    preparations for, 183-187
    straight-line, 183-185, 184f, 195
    techniques for, 191-196
    temporary restoration considera-
        tions, 188-189
    tooth surface conservation, 185-186
Acid etching, 377
Acid-pumice technique, of bleaching,
    419, 419f
Alveolar bone, 22f, 24
Alveolar fractures, 464
Alveolar process, 24
Amalgam, 272-273, 381-382, 409
Amelogenesis imperfecta, 409
Amoxicillin, 541
Anachoresis, 284
Analgesics, 536-537
Anesthesia
    description of, 73
    difficulties, 104-105
    factors that affect, 100-101
    history of, 96f
    incision for drainage, 426
    initial management, 101-102
    mandibular, 103-104
    maxillary, 104
    profound, 301
    referrals for, 73
    selective, 63
    success of, 102-103
    supplemental, 105-112
Anterior teeth
    access preparation of, 195-196, 197f
    retention and core systems for,
        275-276
Antibiotics, 291-292, 539-541
Anxiolytics, 541-542
Apexogenesis, 389
Apical abscess
    acute, 43, 44f, 65t, 66-67, 290, 305f,
        307f
    chronic, 43-44, 65t, 67
Apical canal zipping, 224
Apical clearing, 216, 216f-217f, 253

Apical constriction, 201-203
Apical curvature, 222, 222f
Apical cyst, 41
Apical delta, 7
Apical foramen, 7, 8, 9f, 22f, 173-174,
    176f, 469
Apical fracture, 429
Apical perforation, 184, 203, 320, 322
Apical periodontitis
    acute, 40, 41f, 65t, 66, 289, 301
    chronic, 40-42, 65t, 66, 289
Apical plug, 394
Apical preparation, 211, 213-214
Apical ramifications, 217f
Apical seal, 241-242
Apical stop, 211, 211f
Appointments, 64-66, 94, 553-554
Arachidonic acid, 32
Arterioles, 15, 15f, 18f, 23
Attrition, 384
Avulsion, 461-464
Axons, 18, 19f
Azithromycin, 541

B

Bacteria
    colonization of, 283, 378
    culturing of, 291-292
    ecosystem, 287
    pathoses and, 288-290
    portals of entry, 283-284
    pulpal reaction to, 284
    terminology associated with, 283
    types of, 285t
    virulence factors of, 287-288
Balanced forces method, 230
Bands, 189
Bicuspidization, 438, 440-442, 441f
Bitewing projections, 144, 144f
Biting test, 56f
Bleaching
    complications of, 414-415
    description of, 163
    elderly use of, 558-559
    external techniques, 415-420
    final restoration, 411, 413-414
    internal, 410-414
    laser, 421
    materials for, 410
    mouthguard, 420-421
    thermocatalyic technique, 411
    trauma-related, 414f-416f
    walking bleach technique, 411,
        412f-414f
    when to bleach, 414, 416f-417f
Blood dyscrasias, 409
Blow-out lesion, 474-475, 475f
Body language, 89

Bradykinin, 31-32
Broaches, 156, 158, 212
Burs, 191, 192f-193f, 198, 200f

C

C fibers, 18
Calcific metamorphosis, 36, 36f, 62f,
    69f, 75-76, 76-77f, 349f,
    407-408, 548f
Calcifications, 14f, 14-15, 170, 170f
Calcitonin gene-related peptide, 16, 32
Calcium hydroxide, 233-234, 250-251,
    291, 384, 397, 400f, 414
Canal. See Root canal(s).
Capillary bed, 15, 16f
Capping of pulp, 384-385
Carbamide peroxide bleaching,
    410-411
Carbon dioxide ice testing, 57, 57f
Caries
    access preparation considerations,
        187-188
    depth of penetration assessments,
        61, 63
    microorganisms in, 28
    periapical repair after treatment of,
        385
    pulpal disease and, 284, 383
    removal of, 61, 63
    rubber dam considerations, 127
Cavity preparation, 374-378
Cementodentinal junction, 9, 23, 468
Cementum, 6, 7f, 9, 22-23, 468
Chelators, 219-220
Chemical burns, 415
Chemical irritants, 31, 169-170
Chief complaint, 51
Clamps, 122-124
Clarithromycin, 541
Cleaning and shaping
    accidents during, 319-326
    apical clearing, 216, 216f-217f
    apical preparation, 211, 213-214
    balanced forces method, 230
    débridement, 207-209
    dentin softening, 220-221
    energized vibratory systems, 230-232
    extirpation, 212
    instrumentation, 163, 225-229, 232
    intracanal medicaments, 232-234
    irrigants, 218-220
    ledge formation during, 184,
        222f-223f, 222-223, 319-320, 321f
    lubricants, 221
    master apical file determination, 210
    objectives of, 207
    preparation errors, 221-225
    preparations

Cleaning and shaping—*continued*
  flaring, 212-214
    standardized, 212, 213f
    step-down, 212-216, 213f, 215f
  shaping principles, 209-210
Clindamycin, 541
Clinical tests, 55-56
Cold testing, 57-58
Collagen fibers, 5, 14
Condensing osteitis, 42-43, 43f, 61f, 143f
Cone-image shift, 132, 136-141
Coronal fracture, 415
Coronal leakage, 342f
Coronal root perforation, 322-323
Coronal seal, 241, 269-270, 400, 559
Cracked tooth, 80-81, 500, 501t, 502f,
    505-510
Craze lines, 501-502, 503f, 507
Crown
  cementation of, 378
  formation of, 5
  fracture of, 449-456
  indications, 273-274
  lengthening of, 79, 80f, 120,
    493-494, 494f
  longitudinal fractures of, 63
  perforation of, 83
  placement of, 93f
  preparation of, 374-378
  removal of, 351, 353, 354f
  temporary, 121, 189, 279, 378
Crown-down technique, 214
Crown-root fracture, 270f, 454-456
Culture, 291-292
Cusp fracture, 501t, 502f, 502-505,
    504f-505f
Cytokines, 39

D
Dam. *See* Rubber dam.
Débridement, 207-209, 290, 302
Decalcifiers, 220-221
Dendritic cells, 13, 33, 33f
Dens evaginatus, 176, 177f
Dens invaginatus, 174, 176, 177f
Dental follicle, 7
Dental history, 52, 298-299
Dentin
  age-related changes, 22
  cementum junction with. *See* Cemen-
    todentinal junction.
  desiccation of, 382
  drying of, 376
  excess removal of, 196-198
  formation of, 5, 5f, 9, 10f, 21
  histology of, 11
  hypersensitivity of, 20-21, 21f
  injury-induced formation of, 10
  innervation of, 17-18, 20
  irritant effects, 190
  odontoblasts role in formation of,
    4, 10
  permeability of, 374-375
  resorption of, 36, 37f
  secondary formation of, 21
  softening of, 220-221
  stimulation of, for pulp vitality
    testing, 57
  structural changes in, 270
  tertiary, 10, 372, 372f-373f

Dentinal tubules, 467-468
Dentinoenamel junction, 11
Dentinogenesis, 10-11
Dentinogenesis imperfecta, 409
Dentin-pulp complex, 370
Dentition. *See* Tooth.
Dentogingival junction, 22
Desiccants, 221
Desmosomes, 11-12
Diagnosis, 50-53, 63-64, 64f, 65t, 73
Dilaceration, 176, 179
Discolorations
  aging and, 408, 558-559
  bleaching for. *See* Bleaching.
  causes of, 406-409
  coronal restorations, 409-410
  endemic fluorosis and, 408
  extrinsic, 418-420
  in elderly patients, 558-559
  intrapulpal hemorrhage, 407
  intrinsic, 416-418
  obturation materials, 409
  tetracycline-induced, 408, 416-417
  tooth formation defects as cause of,
    408-409
Disinfection, 125, 163
Doctor
  listening by, 88-89
  patient interactions with, 89-98
  questions frequently asked, 90-97
Drainage
  incision for, 114, 425-426
  infection treatment by, 291
Drains, 304f
Drills, 157-158

E
Ectomesenchymal cells, 4
Elderly
  bleaching, 558-559
  diagnostic approach, 550-551
  differential diagnosis, 552
  endodontic surgery in, 557-558
  healing, 549
  periradicular response, 549
  pulpal response changes, 546-549
  radiographic imaging, 551-552
  restoration considerations in, 556,
    559
  retreatment in, 556
  root canal treatment in, 554-556
  systemic problems in, 549-550
  trauma in, 559-560
  treatment planning in, 552-554
Electronic apex locators, 201-203
Emergencies. *See also specific emergency
    or condition.*
  challenges associated with, 297-298
  definition of, 297
  description of, 296-297
  diagnostic approach, 298-299
  interappointment, 297, 305-307
  postobturation, 297, 307-308
  pretreatment, 297, 300-305
  referral for, 83-84
  treatment planning, 300
Enamel
  formation of, 5, 9
  fracture of, 449
  hypocalcification of, 408

Enamel—*continued*
  hypoplasia of, 418
  spurs, 480
Endemic fluorosis, 408
Endodontics. *See also* Root canal treat-
    ment.
  definition of, 1
  implants, 496-497
  longevity of treated teeth, 269
  pain secondary to, 534-535
  periodontium health and, 470
  pulpal effects, 471
  surgery, 94, 95f
  undergraduate curriculum, 1-2
Endodontist, 85-86
Enostosis, 143f
Enzymes, 288
Epithelial cell rests of Malassez, 6, 23,
    24f
Erosion, 384
Examination
  extraoral, 54
  for emergencies, 299
  intraoral, 54-55
  open apex, 391-393
  pain assessments, 53
  periapical tests, 56
  periodontal, 59, 299
  present illness, 52-53, 447
  pulp vitality tests, 57-59
  radiographic, 59-61, 75
  soft tissue, 54-55
  teeth, 55, 55f
Explorer. *See* Mirror and explorer.
Extirpation, 212
Extracellular vesicles, 288

F
Fatty acids, 288
Fibrinopeptides, 38
Fibroblasts, 12-13
File(s)
  characteristics of, 154f, 155
  cleaning and shaping use of, 226,
    226f
  core material use of, 247
  gutta-percha removal using, 357, 360
  intracanal use of, 158-159
  K-type, 154f, 155
  nickel-titanium, 228
  separation of, 324f
Flaps, 430-434
Flare-ups, 305-307
Focal sclerosing osteomyelitis. *See* Con-
    densing osteitis.
Follicle, 7
Fractures
  alveolar, 464
  categories of, 500-501, 501t
  crown, 449-456
  enamel, 449
  root, 244, 456-458
Frictional heat, 375-376, 382
Furcation perforation, 314-315, 317f

G
Gates-Glidden drills, 157-158, 192f,
    194f, 215
Geriatrics. *See* Elderly.
Gingivectomy, 120

Glass ionomer cements, 381
Gram stain, 292
Ground substance, 14
Gutta-percha, obturation using
  carrier systems, 262
  lateral condensation, 252-257
  removal of, 274-275, 275f, 357, 360,
    360f-361f
  solvent-softened custom cones,
    257-259
  techniques for, 251-252
  vertical condensation, 259-262

H
Hageman factor, 38
Headaches, 528-529
Healing, 44-45, 435-436, 549, 558
Health history, 51-52, 73
Hertwig's epithelium, 5-6, 6f
Hyaline layer of Hopewell-Smith, 6-7
Hydrodynamic theory, of dentin
    hypersensitivity, 20-21
Hydrogen peroxide bleaching, 410
Hyperalgesia, 101, 105, 535b
Hyperplastic pulpitis, 35-36

I
Immune system
  activation of, 371
  cells of, 13
  responses to pulpal injury, 32-33
Immunoglobulins, 32, 32f, 39
Implants, endodontic, 496-497
Infections
  control measures for, 290
  drainage of, 291
  site of, 348
  treatment of, 290-292
Inflammation
  causes of, 91, 91f
  cells involved in, 31
  changes caused by, 36
  neurogenic, 17
  process of, 16-17, 28f, 31-32
  signs and symptoms of, 91, 92f
Informed consent, 89-90, 90b, 90f
Infraorbital block, 104
Injections, 101-102
Instruments
  aspiration of, 324-325
  cleaning and shaping use of, 163,
    225-227
  diagnostic, 161
  disinfection of, 163
  endodontic-specific types of,
    161-162
  engine-driven, 157-158
  extraction of, 362, 365f-366f
  fabrication of, 153
  failure of, 340
  hand-operated, 153f-154f, 153-154
  ingestion of, 324-325
  intracanal use of, 158-159, 208
  nickel-titanium, 156-157, 159, 160f,
    227-229
  nomenclature for, 152
  physical properties of, 154-155
  rotary, 157-158
  separated, 323f-324f, 323-324, 340,
    349f, 360, 362

Instruments—*continued*
  sizing of, 155
  sonic, 231-232
  standardization of, 155-156
  sterilization of, 162-163
  ultrasonic, 230-231
  variations in, 156-157
Intentional replantation, 486-488, 487f
Intracanal medications, 232-234,
    291, 409
Intraosseous anesthesia, 105-107
Intrapulpal hemorrhage, 407
Intrapulpal injection, 111-112, 112f
Irreversible pulpitis, 34, 61, 65t, 66,
    112-113
Irrigants, 218-220, 303, 325-326, 326f
Irritants
  chemical, 28-31, 169-170, 190
  obturation failure caused by, 241
Isolation methods. *See* Rubber dam.

K
Kininogens, 31
Kinins, 31

L
Laser bleaching, 421
Lateral canals, 244, 468, 469f
Lateral channels, 6-7, 8f
Lateral condensation, 160-161,
    252-256, 514
Lateral perforation, 322, 329f
Ledge formation, 184, 222f-223f,
    222-223, 319-320, 321f, 427f
Liners, 382
Lingual groove, 176, 178f
Lipopolysaccharides, 287
Listening, 88-89
Local anesthesia
  blood flow reductions associated
    with, 371
  description of, 73
  difficulties, 104-105
  factors that affect, 100-101
  mandibular, 103-104
  maxillary, 104
  pain management, 538-539
  success of, 102-103
  supplemental, 105-112
Lubricants, 221
Luxation injuries, 459-461
Lymphatic system, 17, 18f

M
Mandibular anesthesia, 103-104
Mandibular molars, 197f
Mantle dentin, 5-6
Mast cells, 31, 32f, 38-39
Master apical file determination, 210
Master cone, 253-254
Maxillary anesthesia, 104
Maxillary molars, 197, 198f
McInnes technique, 419
Medical history, 51-52, 73, 298-299
Mental foramen, 45, 45f
Metronidazole, 541
Microleakage, 379-380
Mineral trioxide aggregate, 389,
    401-402, 402f
Mirror and explorer, 56

Mobility tests, 59
Mouthguard bleaching, 420-421
Myofascial pain, 53

N
Neuritis, 529
Neurogenic inflammation, 17
Neuropeptides, 32, 38
Nickel-titanium instruments, 156-157,
    159, 160f, 227-229
Nonsteroidal antiinflammatory drugs,
    537-538

O
Obturation
  accidents during, 326-328, 341
  apical seal, 241
  coronal seal, 241
  discoloration caused by, 409
  emergencies after, 297, 307-308
  evaluation of, 262-263
  failures in, 240-242
  files, 247
  gutta-percha. *See* Gutta-percha.
  instruments for, 160-161, 163, 255f
  lateral seal, 241
  length of, 241-242, 242f-243f
  materials, 245-248
  objectives of, 240
  overextended, 340
  pastes, 248
  sealers. *See* Sealers.
  sectional, 260
  silver points, 247, 247f
  timing of, 244-245
Odontalgia, 534
Odontoblasts
  cell body of, 11-12, 13f
  dentin formation by, 4, 10
  differentiation of, 5
  displacement of, 376, 376f
  injury to, 376
  morphology of, 11
  number of, 11
  secretory production of, 12
  structure of, 11-12
Open apex
  definition of, 389
  diagnosis of, 391-393
  electrical pulp testing for, 393
  illustration of, 390f
  treatment planning, 393-394
Orofacial pain. *See* Pain.
Orthodontic extrusion, 491-493
Orthograde treatment. *See*
    Retreatment.
Overfills, 241-242, 242f, 258f,
    327-328, 341

P
Pain
  anesthesia for. *See* Anesthesia.
  antibiotic prophylaxis, 539-541
  anxiolytics for, 541-542
  causes of, 33-34
  characteristics of, 524, 530t
  continuous, 53
  deep vs. superficial, 524
  dentinal, 20
  diagnostic procedures, 529-531

Pain—*continued*
flare-ups of, 84
headache-related, 528-529
hypersensitivity theories, 20-21
intensity of, 53
management of, 535-539
mechanisms of, 522-524
myofascial, 53
perception of, 298
percussion, 56
periodontal, 525
physiology of, 33-34
posttreatment, 65
post-treatment, 534-535
procedural, 94-96
psychogenic, 528
pulpal, 10, 525
reaction to, 298
referred, 75, 525-527
significance of, 521-522
spontaneous, 53
spreading, 527-528
terminology associated with, 522b
types of, 522b
Palpation, 56, 56f
Passive step-back technique, 214-216
Pastes, 248
Patient, 88-97
Penicillin, 541
Percolation, 241
Percussion, 56
Perforations
during access preparation, 198, 199f,
203, 311-319
furcation, 315-316, 317f
prognosis, 318-319
retreatment considerations, 348
root, 83, 314, 320-323
stripping, 184-185, 224-225, 315,
316f
Periodontal abscess, 300f
Periodontal ligament
anatomy of, 23, 24f
anesthesia injection, 107-110
function of, 23
mobility tests for evaluating, 59
perforations into, 314
vasculature, 23
Periodontitis
acute apical, 40, 41f, 65t, 66, 289
chronic apical, 40-42, 65t, 66, 289
suppurative apical. *See* Apical abscess, chronic.
Periodontium
anatomy of, 22
blood supply to, 7-8
endodontically involved teeth effects,
470-471
examination of, 59, 299
formation of, 7-8
tissues of, 7
vasculature of, 23
Perio-endo lesion, 473, 474f, 481f-482f
Periradicular lesions. *See also specific
lesion.*
bacterial role in, 29-30
cytokines in, 39
description of, 37-38
healing of, 44-45

Periradicular lesions—*continued*
illustration of, 339f
immunoglobulins in, 39
malignant lesions that simulate, 46
mediators of, 38-39
nonendodontic, 45-46
root canal treatment success and, 333
Periradicular surgery
contraindications, 429-430
description of, 114
indications, 426-429
procedure sequence, 430-435
Periradicular tests, 299
Permanent restorations, 188-190
Phenolics, 233
Phospholipase A$_2$, 32
Pins, 277, 382-383, 409
Plexus of Raschkow, 5
Polyamines, 288
Polycarboxylate cement, 381
Polymicrobial infections, 284-287
Polymorphonuclear leukocytes, 28f,
28-29, 31
Porcelain, 79, 128
Post
for anterior teeth, 275-276
for posterior teeth, 276
removal of, 353, 355f-356f, 356-357
selection of, 274
space preparations for, 274-275,
328-330
temporary, 279
Posterior superior alveolar block, 104
Posterior teeth, 276-277
Predentin, 5
Preodontoblasts, 5, 12
Present illness, 52-53, 447
Probing, periodontal, 59, 472-473,
475f-476f, 482f
Profound anesthesia, 301
Prognosis, 69, 332-333
Prostaglandin E$_2$, 39
Psychogenic pain, 528
Pulp
abscess, 378f
age-related changes in, 21-22, 169,
546-548
anatomy of, 12f, 68f, 167-168
apical region, 173-174
bacteria effects, 283-284, 378-379
blood flow assessments, 59
calcifications, 14f, 14-15, 36, 62f, 69f,
170, 170f, 547
capping of, 384-385, 396-398
caries effects, 284, 383
cells of. *See* Odontoblasts.
characteristics of, 370-371
collagen fibers, 14
coronal, 8
electrical testing of, 58-59, 59f
embryology of, 4-5
extirpation of, 212
frictional heat effects, 382
functions of, 4, 10-11, 373, 373f
ground substance, 14
immune responses of, 32-33
inflammation of. *See* Inflammation.
injury, 16, 31-34
innervation of, 17-21, 30

Pulp—*continued*
intrapulpal pressure, 371
irritants of, 28-31, 169-170, 190
lingual groove, 176, 178f
local anesthesia-induced reductions
in blood flow, 371
lymphatic system of, 17, 18f
morphologic changes in, 21
necrosis of, 29, 36-37, 65t, 66,
113-114, 242f, 244-245, 277f,
287, 301-304, 306, 371, 383,
407, 458b, 469-470
neuropeptides, 32, 38
pain of, 525
pathosis of, 374, 375f
periodontal disease effects, 471
protective measures for, 382
radiographic evaluations of, 61
repair potential of, 373
restorative materials effect on,
378-383
sensations transmitted by, 10-11
size of, 4
stimuli transmission, 19-20
stones, 14f, 14-15, 170
tissue pressure, 16
trauma, 30, 448-449
vasculature of, 15f-18f, 15-18, 21,
30, 59
vitality tests of, 57-59, 299, 472, 551
Pulp chamber
anatomy of, 8f, 75, 76f, 172, 179, 179f
unroofing of, 186-187
Pulp horn
anatomy of, 8, 8f, 172, 176
discoloration caused by, 409
exposure of, 187
removal of, 195-196
Pulp space, 9, 9f
Pulp-dentin complex, 370
Pulpectomy, 212
Pulpitis
hyperplastic, 35-36
irreversible, 34, 61, 65t, 66, 112-113,
277, 301, 393
reversible, 34, 35f, 65t, 66
Pulpotomy, 212, 385, 396-398, 451,
452f, 453b

R
Radiographs and radiography
bitewing, 144, 144f
cone-image shift, 132, 136-141
description of, 59-60
diagnostic, 132, 134, 472
difficulties in obtaining, 75
elderly considerations, 551-552
endodontic uses of, 141-144
exploratory use of, 191
exposure considerations, 136
film-cone placement, 144-148
for emergencies, 299
limitations of, 60
obturation evaluations, 262-263
periapical lesions evaluated using,
60-61
rapid processing, 148
recall, 132-133, 135-136
sequence of, 134-136

Radiographs and radiography—*continued*
  success evaluations, 333, 335f
  treatment uses of, 132
  viewers, 148
  working films, 132-135
Radiolucent lesions, 142, 142f,
    475-476, 477f
Radiopaque lesions, 142-143
Reamers, 157-158
Reaming, 216
Recapitulation, 225, 225f
Referrals, 74-86
Referred pain, 75
Resin composites, 273, 381, 410
Restorations. *See also* Permanent restora-
    tions; Temporary restorations.
  access through, 277
  design principles, 272
  direct, 272-273
  hypersensitivity after, 383
  in elderly, 556, 559
  indirect, 273-274
  microleakage of, 379-380
  patient questions regarding, 96
  removal of, 189-190
  structural and biochemical consider-
    ations, 270-271
  timing of, 271-272
Retreatment
  case selection for, 347-351
  clinician considerations, 348, 351
  communication with patient,
    365, 367
  completion of, 362, 365
  considerations for, 346-347
  crown removal for, 351, 353, 354f
  degree of difficulty, 365
  description of, 342
  disease prevention, 351, 352f-353f
  post and core removal for, 353,
    355f-356f, 356-357
  referrals, 367
  root canal obstructions, 357-362
  short- and long-term outcomes, 365
  tooth considerations, 348
Reversible pulpitis, 34, 35f, 65t, 66
Root
  amputation of, 436-439, 438,
    439f, 442
  curvature of, 76, 78f-79f
  formation of, 5-6
  fractures of, 244, 456-458
  hemisection of, 438-439, 440f, 442
  identification of, 168-169
  length of, 9, 76
  perforation of, 83, 314, 320-323, 436
  resorption of, 81, 171, 171f, 202f,
    261f, 414-415, 436, 548f
  sheath proliferation, 5
  submersion of, 494-496, 495f
  vertical fracture of, 244, 328, 480,
    501t, 513-518, 516f-517f
Root canal(s)
  aberrations of, 216-218
  accessory canals, 173, 244, 468, 469f
  anatomy of, 8f, 9, 172-173
  artificial, 320
  bacteria in, 285t, 285-286
  cone-image shift radiography, 138, 140

Root canal(s)—*continued*
  C-shaped, 179, 179f
  identification of, 168-169
  inability to locate, 84, 191
  ledge formation. *See* Ledge
    formation.
  multiple, 76, 77f-78f
  number of, 76, 77f-78f
  obstruction of, 357-362
  overenlargement of, 222, 227f
Root canal(s)—*continued*
  separation of, 198, 200f
  shape of, 172-173, 209-210
  working length of. *See* Working
    length.
Root canal treatment
  costs of, 96
  evaluation of, 334-337
  failure of, 95f, 334, 335f, 337-342,
    437f
  in elderly, 554-556
  pain associated with, 94-96
  previously started, 189
  procedure, 91f-96f
  success of, 333-334
Root planing, 471
Root-end closure
  case selection, 394
  definition of, 389, 398
  failure of, 402-403
  indications and contraindications, 396
  planning of, 394
  success of, 402, 402f
  technique, 399-401, 401f
  with mineral trioxide aggregate,
    401-402, 402f
Root-end resection, 432-433
Rotary instruments
  characteristics of, 157-158
  gutta-percha removal using, 357
  intracanal use of, 159
  nickel-titanium, 228-229
  passive step-back technique and, 230
  stainless steel, 232
Rubber dam
  application of, 124-125
  equipment for, 121-124
  leaking of, 126
  modifications for difficult situations,
    126-128
  placement of, 120-121, 124-125
  positioning use of, 125
  reasons for using, 119-120, 313
  referrals, 129

S
Sealers, 248-251
Selective anesthesia, 63
Separated instruments, 323f-324f,
    323-324, 340, 349f, 360, 362
Shaping. *See* Cleaning and shaping.
Sharpey's fibers, 7
Silver points, 247, 247f, 360, 363f
Sinus tract type probing, 476-480, 479f
Smear layer, 376-377
Sodium hypochlorite, 290-291, 410
Sodium perborate bleaching, 410
Soft tissue examination, 54-55, 447-448
Solvent-softened custom cones, 257-259

Sonic instrumentation, 231-232
Specialist referral, 84-85
Split dam, 313, 313f
Spoon excavator, 161
Step-back technique, 212-216, 213f,
    215f, 225, 230
Sterilization of instruments, 162-163
Steroids, 539
Stoma parulis, 55
Stones, pulpal, 14f, 14-15, 170
Straight-line access, 183-185, 184f
Stripping perforation, 184-185,
    224-225, 315, 316f
Subodontoblastic plexus of Raschkow,
    18, 20f, 20-21
Substance P, 16
Suppurative apical periodontitis. *See*
    Apical abscess, chronic.
Surgery
  amputation, 436-439, 438, 439f, 442
  corrective, 436
  healing after, 435-436
  in elderly, 557-558
  incision for drainage, 425-426
  periradicular. *See* Periradicular
    surgery.
  referrals, 442-443, 443f

T
T cells, 13, 32, 40f
Temporary restorations
  access preparation considerations,
    188-189
  crowns, 279
  description of, 278
  long-term, 280
  objectives of, 278
  placement of, 278, 279f
  removal of, 189-190
  semipermanent, 271-272
Tertiary dentin, 372, 372f-373f
Tetracycline-induced discoloration,
    408, 416-417
Thermal tests, 57-58
Thermocatalyic technique, 411
Tooth
  access considerations, 185-187
  anatomic regions of, 8-9
  avulsed, 461-464
  canals of, 76, 77f-78f
  control, 56
  cracked, 80-81, 500, 501t, 502f,
    505-510
  examination of, 55, 55f
  extraction of, 394
  fractured, 80-81
  isolation of, 79
  location of, 79, 80f
  luxation injuries of, 459-461
  malpositioning of, 79, 80f
  mobility testing of, 59
  palpation of, 56, 56f
  percussion of, 56
  selective anesthesia, 63
  split, 501t, 502f, 510-513, 511f
  structure of, 270, 272
  surface conservation, 185-187
  trauma, 82, 446-464
Transplantation, 488-491, 489f-490f

Trauma
  examination of, 447-449
  history-taking, 446-447
  in elderly, 559-560
  periodontal defect after, 480
  pulpal, 30, 448-449
Treatment and treatment planning
  adjunctive procedures, 68-69
  appointments, 64-66, 94
  complications that affect, 67, 68f-69f
  description of, 63
  diagnosis-specific approach, 64
  emergencies, 300
  form for, 64f
  modifiers of, 67-69
  referral during, 84
  selection of, 67
  signs and symptoms persisting after,
    83-84
Trigeminal nerve, 17, 19-20
Trigeminal neuralgia, 529

U
Ultrasonic condensation, 256
Ultrasonic instrumentation, 230-231
Underfill, 242, 243f, 326-327, 341

V
Varnishes, 382
Vasoactive intestinal peptide, 16
Venules, pulpal, 15, 15f, 17f-18f
Vertical condensation, 161, 259-262,
  514
Vertical root fracture, 244, 328, 480,
  501t, 513-518, 516f-517f
Vibratory systems, 230-232
Vital pulp therapy
  complications of, 396
  definition of, 389-390
  failure of, 398, 402-403
  indications and contraindications, 395
  planning of, 394
  prognosis, 396
  pulpotomy. *See* Pulpotomy.

Vital pulp therapy—*continued*
  success of, 402, 403f
  techniques, 396-398
Vitality testing, of pulp, 57-59

W
Walking bleach technique, 411,
  412f-414f
Working length
  apical constriction, 201-203
  description of, 200, 201
  electronic apex locators, 201-203
  estimated, 201
  in elderly, 555-556
  patient response, 204
  reference point for, 200-201
  variations in, 201, 202f

Z
Zinc oxide-eugenol, 248, 380-381
Zinc phosphate cement, 381